Clinical Diagnostic Technology

Clinical Diagnostic Technology

The Total Testing Process

Volume 2: The Analytical Phase

EDITORS

Kory M. Ward-Cook

Craig A. Lehmann

Larry E. Schoeff

Robert H. Williams

AACC Press

2101 L STREET, NW, SUITE 202
WASHINGTON, DC 20037-1558

Although the validity of all urls within the text was verified prior to publication, the authors and publisher cannot guarantee url validity post publication as Internet content is subject to change.

1 2 3 4 5 6 7 8 9 0 PCP 07 06 05

Printed in the United States of America

Library of Congress Cataloging-in-Publication Data

Clinical diagnostic technology : the total testing process/editors, Kory M. Ward-Cook . . .
[et al.].
p. ; cm.
Includes index.
Contents: v. 1. The preanalytical phase — v. 2. Analytical — v. 3. Postanalytical.
ISBN 1-59425-034-0 (alk. paper)
1. Diagnosis, Laboratory. 2. Medical laboratory technology. I. Ward, Kory M.
[DNLM: 1. Laboratory Techniques and Procedures—standards. 2. Clinical Laboratory Techniques—methods. 3. Technology, Medical—standards. QY 25 C6412 2003]
RB37.C5875 2003
616.07′56—dc21 2003050275

Contents

Foreword from Volume 1

The authors of this volume look at the big picture of clinical laboratory testing and provide a wealth of important information on the testing process. The participants in this process are the patients, the caregivers, the laboratory workers at all ranks, and the support personnel. The chapters here dissect the many processes and steps that must occur to provide the all-important clinical laboratory services. The needs of the patients are always preeminent, and the full-service laboratory can serve all kinds of patients from tiny preemies to patients of all ages, shapes, and sizes. The usual questions apply: Are the tests appropriate for the patient and is the patient in the proper state for the tests?

The caregivers are defined as all those individuals involved in generating a test order and then responding appropriately to the results. They are those persons with varying responsibilities, training, background, and experience. They are clearly key individuals who share in the responsibilities of generating test orders and acting on reports. The next group is the laboratory workers; they closely or remotely affect the actions of the clinical laboratory. Obtaining a valid specimen is discussed in detail here; it is not a simple task. There are many aspects of a valid specimen, involving the patient, caregivers, and laboratory workers.

Another responsibility of the laboratory and its workers is the optimization of all aspects of the testing process. The latter can be divided into two major phenomena: specimen flow and information flow. In the big picture, there is specimen flow going to the testing site by various means including automated and robotized procedures. There is also extensive use of computer technology in all aspects, from generating orders to performing the tests, and finally to reporting and evaluating test results. Information flow usually starts with the caregivers, continues in the laboratory, and then goes back to those caregivers who have patient responsibilities. Acute needs in specimen flow are the identity and validity of the specimen, appropriateness of the testing process, and timeliness of testing. The specimen and information flow must be harmonized for the benefit of the patient. Information flow that is primarily within the testing site includes quality assurance, quality control, dealing with mistakes and blunders, short- and long-term storage of information, and feedback to and from the caregivers. Information flow may come from all those involved in the testing, internal sources such as laboratory guides and manuals, external sources such as the Internet, and other sources such as consultants and libraries.

A major problem facing laboratories is cost control. In the past, laboratories were a source of income for the testing institution. Now, many laboratories are treated as cost centers, an unhappy change. Laboratory workers have looked at many of the cost-containment schemes discussed here. Automation, robotization, simplification steps, and other tools are in use today to control costs. Robots are in patient areas and in testing sites now, and more and more sophisticated robots are being developed. The automated analyzers of the future will attempt to reduce human input to the testing process as much as possible. People are our biggest cost. Hiring less-trained people is not a solution. Robots now can centrifuge specimens, pull off stoppers, prepare aliquot tubes, carry out the analysis, and store left-over specimen in a space that facilitates recovery. Multifunctional sophisticated robotic systems are dramatically costly and are out of reach for many testing facilities. But if the cost-recovery time goes down and the cost of robots continues to decrease, the amount of such testing can only grow. Robots that can collect a blood specimen are on the horizon. Also, automation is appearing for testing the tiny specimens from babies or the super sick without much human intervention. Noninvasive testing is also coming along. Bloodless testing is surely a worthwhile goal, especially for those individuals who require frequent testing, e.g., patients with diabetes mellitus.

The information explosion has been a boon for all participants. Locally created databases of demographics, medical histories, test data, analog information (X-rays, MRI images, and CAT scans) can be stored and retrieved at remote sites by the patient and others. There is a bounty of external information available within many testing sites. The number of Internet pages dedicated to healthcare, broadly defined, is staggering and growing. The quality of the information is generally good, but caveat emptor still applies. The best sources of information are probably the National Institutes of Health and the National Library of Medicine. Portable databases are now available; some are as small as a credit card but still have a large amount of space for storing analog and digital information.

This volume can clearly serve the needs of all the participants in clinical laboratory testing and help us provide the best service for the patients who depend on us.

John A. Lott, PhD
Professor of Pathology
The Ohio State University

Preface from Volume 1

A void exists in the healthcare industry regarding information about laboratory technology and its application to the testing process. *Clinical Diagnostic Technology—The Total Testing Process* is a three-volume series of books that is intended to fill that void and provide its readers with a comprehensive overview of all analytical techniques/instrumentation and their impact on preanalytical and postanalytical operations toward the delivery of healthcare. With leading experts in their specialty areas as contributing authors, this series is truly one of a kind and the first to consider the entire testing process under one publication series. There have been major advances and developments in the handling of specimens prior to testing, in workstation consolidation, and in new methodologies and analytical systems as well as an expansion of point-of-care testing and an explosion of information technology. This three-volume series is designed to provide the laboratory community with the latest review on these topics. The series is also designed to present the challenges and innovations that should be expected as the technology and our healthcare delivery systems evolve.

The series focuses on the Preanalytical (Volume 1), Analytical (Volume 2), and Postanalytical (Volume 3) phases of laboratory testing. Volume 1 provides the reader with an overview of healthcare and its impact on diagnostic services, the evolution of technology and testing services, workflow analysis, critical pathways and specimen processing, preanalytical laboratory information systems, and preanalytical instrumentation—its technology and evaluation. Volume 2 focuses on the use of technology, quality, and basic principles of instrumentation. Techniques and automated systems of all laboratory testing areas will be presented, including total laboratory automation and point of care. This volume will provide URL addresses to vendors' websites, offering a full view of the instruments and descriptions of their operation. Finally, Volume 3 addresses quality assurance and quality control issues, verification and reporting of results, postanalytical laboratory information systems and telemedicine, biosensors, the virtual clinical laboratory and artificial intelligence, and clinical laboratories in the 21st century.

Editors

Kory M. Ward-Cook, PhD, MT (ASCP), CAE
Chief Executive Officer
National Certification Commission for Acupuncture
and Oriental Medicine (NCCAOM)
Alexandria, Virginia

Craig A. Lehmann, PhD, CC (NRCC), FACB
Dean, School of Health Technology and Management
Professor, Clinical Laboratory Sciences
Health Sciences Center
Stony Brook University
State University of New York
Stony Brook, New York

Larry E. Schoeff, MS, MT (ASCP)
Director and Associate Professor, Medical Technology Program
University of Utah, Department of Pathology
and Education Consultant
ARUP Laboratories, Inc.
Salt Lake City, Utah

Robert H. Williams, PhD, DABCC, FACB, MT (ASCP)
Clinical Scientist/Consultant, Laboratory Administration
Quest Diagnostics, Inc.
and Clinical Associate Professor of Pathology
University of South Florida
Tampa, Florida

Contributors

Jay L. Bock, MD, PhD, DABP
Professor and Acting Chair of Pathology
Stony Brook University School of Medicine
Stony Brook, New York

Larry D. Bowers, PhD
Senior Managing Director
U.S. Anti-Doping Agency
Colorado Springs, Colorado

Karen C. Carroll, MD
Associate Professor, Pathology and Medicine
and Director, Division of Medical Microbiology
Department of Pathology
The Johns Hopkins Medical Institutions
Baltimore, Maryland

Donna D. Castellone, MS, MT(ASCP)SH
Technical Specialist
New York Presbyterian Hospital
Weill Cornell Medical Center
New York, New York
and Clinical Assistant Professor
School of Health Technology and Management
Health Sciences Center
Stony Brook University
State University of New York
Stony Brook, New York

Elizabeth Cascone, MS, MT(ASCP)SBB
The American Red Cross
Southern California Region
Los Angeles, California

Daniel W. Chan, PhD, DABCC
Professor, Pathology, Oncology, Urology, and Radiology
The Johns Hopkins University School of Medicine
and Director, Clinical Chemistry Division
The Johns Hopkins Hospital
Baltimore, Maryland

William Clarke, PhD
Assistant Professor, Pathology
The Johns Hopkins University School of Medicine
and Director, Drug Assay Laboratory and POCT
The Johns Hopkins Hospital
Baltimore, Maryland

Ronald J. Elin, MD, PhD, DABCC, FACB
A. J. Miller Professor and Chair
Department of Pathology and Laboratory Medicine
University of Louisville School of Medicine
Louisville, Kentucky

Kathleen Finnegan, MS, MT(ASCP)SH
Clinical Assistant Professor
Chair, Clinical Laboratory Sciences
School of Health Technology and Management
Health Sciences Center
Stony Brook University
State University of New York
Stony Brook, New York

Deborah Firestone, MA, MT(ASCP)SBB
Clinical Assistant Professor
Clinical Laboratory Sciences Department
School of Health Technology and Management
Health Sciences Center
Stony Brook University
State University of New York
Stony Brook, New York

Craig C. Foreback, PhD
Senior Lecturer
Department of Pathology and Laboratory Medicine
CLS Program
University of Wisconsin Medical School
Madsion, Wisconsin

Candace Golightly, MS
Clinical Assistant Professor
Clinical Laboratory Sciences Department
School of Health Technology and Management
Health Sciences Center
Stony Brook University
State University of New York
Stony Brook, New York

Marc Golightly, PhD
Professor-Director, Clinical Immunology
Department of Pathology
School of Medicine
Stony Brook Medical Center
Stony Brook, New York

Jocelyn M. Hicks, PhD, FRCPath
President
JMBH Associates, Health Care Management Consultants
and Professor Emeritus, Pediatrics and Pathology
George Washington School of Medicine
Washington, DC

Mary Hotaling, MS, MT(ASCP)DLM
Clinical Assistant Professor
School of Health Technology and Management
Health Sciences Center
Stony Brook University
State University of New York
Stony Brook, New York

Noriko Kusukawa, PhD
Assistant Vice-President
New Technology
ARUP Laboratories, Inc.
Salt Lake City, Utah

Stanley S. Levinson, PhD, DABCC
Director of Clinical Chemistry, Toxicology and Immunochemistry
Veterans Affairs Medical Center
and Professor of Pathology and Laboratory Medicine
University of Louisville School of Medicine
Louisville, Kentucky

Rodney S. Markin, MD, PhD
Professor and Vice Chairman
Department of Pathology and Microbiology
Associate Dean for Clinical Affairs, College of Medicine
President, University Medical Associates
University of Nebraska Medical Center
Omaha, Nebraska

James J. Miller, PhD, DABCC, FACB
Associate Professor of Pathology and Laboratory Medicine
Director of Clinical Chemistry and Toxicology
University of Louisville Hospital
University of Louisville School of Medicine
Louisville, Kentucky

Amin A. Mohammad, PhD, DABCC
Director, Laboratory Information Service
Associate Professor, Department of Pathology
University of Texas Medical Branch
Galveston, Texas

Mary C. Newcomb, MT(ASCP)C
Project Manager
Department of Pathology and Microbiology
University of Nebraska Medical Center
Omaha, Nebraska

Anthony O. Okorodudu, PhD, DABCC, FACB
Professor of Pathology
Director of Clinical Chemistry
Department of Pathology/Clinical Chemistry
University of Texas Medical Branch
Galveston, Texas

Christine N. Papadea, PhD, FACB, MT(ASCP)SC
Associate Professor
Director, Clinical Chemistry
Division of Laboratory Medicine
Department of Pathology and Laboratory Medicine
Medical University of South Carolina
Charleston, South Carolina

John R. Petersen, PhD, DABCC
Associate Director of Clinical Chemistry
Department of Pathology
University of Texas Medical Branch Hospitals
Galveston, Texas

Christopher P. Price, PhD, DSc, MCB, FRSC, FRCPath, FACB
Vice President, Outcomes Research
Diagnostics Division, Bayer HealthCare
Newbury, United Kingdom
and Visiting Professor in Clinical Biochemistry
University of Oxford
Oxford, United Kingdom

Larry G. Reimer, MD
Professor
Department of Pathology and Medicine
The University of Utah School of Medicine
and Assistant Dean
Curriculum and Graduate Medical Education
The University of Utah School of Medicine
Salt Lake City, Utah

William L. Roberts, MD, PhD
Associate Professor of Pathology
University of Utah School of Medicine
and Medical Director
Automated Core Laboratory
ARUP Laboratories, Inc.
Salt Lake City, Utah

Richard D. Sciacca
President and Founder
IntMR, LLC
Brookfield, Wisconsin

Andrew St John, PhD, MAACB
Consultant
ARC Consulting
Perth, Western Australia

Carl T. Wittwer, MD, PhD
Professor
Department of Pathology
University of Utah
and Medical Director
ARUP Laboratories, Inc.
Salt Lake City, Utah

Chapter 1

Assessment of Processes in the Clinical Laboratory through Computer Simulation

Amin A. Mohammad, Anthony O. Okorodudu, John R. Petersen, and Richard D. Sciacca

Simulation is defined as a means of seeing how a model of a real system will respond to changes in its structure, environment, or underlying assumptions (1). A **system** may be defined as a combination of elements that interact to accomplish a specific objective. Two types of systems are manufacturing systems such as large production facilities, small jobs shops, machining cells, and assembly lines and service systems which include healthcare facilities, amusement parks, restaurants, and banks. The clinical laboratory is an example of a service system that exists within a larger, more complex service system, the hospital. Some of the many elements of a clinical laboratory are clinical samples, e.g., whole blood, serum, plasma, urine, cerebrospinal fluid, other body fluids, and tissues, different analyzers, and human resources, e.g., medical technologists, technicians, phlebotomists, clerks, and sample processors.

Various well-defined and repetitive activities are performed on each clinical sample by a team of personnel that may come from different sections of a laboratory. A single medical technologist or technician may work at two different workstations, depending on the scope of that station. The processes performed by these laboratory personnel are interrelated and must be designed to produce prompt test results for the ultimate purpose of diagnosing and treating diseases. The simple repetitive steps involved often result in complex interactions that are very difficult to analyze via unaided human intuition. Herbert Simon, a famous economist, called this ability of the human mind to grasp real world complexity "the principle of bounded rationality." This principle states that "the capacity of the human mind for formulating and solving complex problems is very small compared with the size of the problem whose solution is required for objectively rational behavior in the real world, or even for a reasonable approximation to such objective rationality."

The sheer number of clinical samples and the various tasks performed on each sample can stagger the mind. However, it is the interaction of these elements that makes this system so difficult to analyze. The complexities in a clinical laboratory are mainly the function of two factors: (1) interdependencies between elements and (2) variability in overall behavior of different elements of the system. The interdependencies can be readily understood by realizing that generally a given sample has more than one test ordered on it and therefore it must be tested on different instruments, usually by different medical personnel. The unavailability of either the medical personnel or the analyzer will cause delays in test results. The variability in this system arises from the sample arrival patterns, analyzer speed, different processes for different sample types, different number of tests ordered on each sample, or different sample priorities such as routine or stat samples.

WHAT IS SIMULATION?

Simulation is a computer model that is specifically designed to imitate and capture the dynamic behavior of a system in order to evaluate the different ways of improving its efficiency. It is capable of providing insights into the complex dynamics of a system that cannot be obtained by using other techniques. Since simulation accounts for interdependencies and variation, it is the best way to analyze a complex system such as a clinical laboratory. No one knows when the first model of a clinical laboratory or even the first simulation model was constructed. However, testing an idea or a concept via live or mathematical models is well known to both modern and ancient science and can be linked back to the development of basic physical concepts developed by Aristotle and Archimedes. Models are used today to understand and evaluate known phenomena and then to perform experiments to predict the behavior of a real system. Some of the better known examples include the prediction of weather, positions of planets with respect to sun during certain time intervals, the variations in the stock market, forecasting election outcomes, and forecasting product sales volumes. Clinical sciences have thrived on animal models, without them the understanding of and finding cures for various diseases would have been impossible. The clinical observation of a disease, the search for a hypothetical etiology, and, finally, confirmation by recreating the diseased state in an animal and studying the effect of various drugs or treatments on diseased animals can be thought of as modeling. The knowledge gained with this animal model is then used to experiment on human beings and finally to develop a cure.

In simulation, the experimentation is done on a computer by constructing an accurate and representative model. Numerous software programs are available commercially, e.g., MedModel (Promodel Corp., Salt Lake City, UT), Arena (Rockwell Software, Sewickley, PA), and Witness (Lanner Group Inc., Houston, TX). Most of these software products automatically collect performance statistics such as turnaround times for different samples and resource and analyzer utilization and then summarize them for further analysis. Some of them also provide realistic graphical animation of different processes, user interactions, and optimization capabilities.

Two main types of simulation techniques are **discrete event** and **continuous event** models. A discrete event is an instantaneous action that occurs at a unique point in time. An example is a sample arriving in the laboratory. It is loaded into the centrifuge rack, the centrifuge rack is then loaded into a centrifuge, and the centrifuge is started—these are some examples of the numerous discrete events that occur regularly in the laboratory. The occurrence of these events causes a change in system states. In the simulation models, the computer maintains a timing device known as a simulation clock which advances with each event taking place at a fixed point in time. If an event represents an initiation of an activity that will conclude in the future, the simulation will add the completion time to a list of future events and advance the clock to the next time at which an event is due. Discrete event simulation employs statistical methods for generating random behavior and estimating model performance. They are sometimes referred to as Monte Carlo methods because of their similarity to the probabilistic outcomes found in games of chance such as gambling.

A continuous event is an action without stopping. It goes on uninterrupted with time. Biochemical reactions, temperature logs, flow of ocean tides, and river water flow are some good examples of continuous events. These events always involve a change in one of their physical or chemical properties over time and therefore are often represented by differential equations. Changing model variables that are tied to the simulation clock at a well-defined rate best simulates continuous events.

WHY USE COMPUTER SIMULATION FOR LABORATORY MANAGEMENT?

A clinical laboratory is a dynamic system where various well-defined and repetitive processes are applied to a staggering number of samples. Operational decisions are required to provide the best turnaround times (TATs) for specimen test results. "Unusual" events such as the arrival of stat samples and the tests ordered on them are significant variables. The appropriate outcome of the correct test result is highly dependent on the ability of different resources to interact with each other and with the available instrumentation. Management of a clinical laboratory is a daunting task, because every section of the laboratory must work in unison to provide fast and high-quality results. Major challenges facing the clinical laboratory are containing cost and increasing productivity while improving customer satisfaction. Physicians, nurses, other healthcare providers, patients, third-party payers, and consumers are all "customers" of a clinical laboratory. Their satisfaction depends in part on expedient TATs for tests. Generally, the faster a laboratory is able to turn a test around, the happier the customer. The test TATs depend on numerous factors such as the arrival times of routine and stat samples, the test ordering pattern on each sample, available skilled human resources, specific analyzers required, the degree of laboratory automation, and other variables. Of the aforementioned variables, sample arrival patterns and test ordering patterns experience the largest degree of variability and change over time. Therefore, continuous process optimization is required to adapt to these changes. Of the remaining variables described, human resources constitute 60% of total laboratory cost, creating a constant need to find the optimum number of medical personnel and the optimum skill mix to meet the laboratory's operational goals and to minimize overall cost.

The type of analyzer and the degree of automation constitute fixed costs. Once an analyzer is purchased, leased, or rented, it is usually not changed for 3–5 years. However, deciding on an appropriate instrument is an uphill task due to the availability of a wide range of analyzers having different specifications, strengths, and weaknesses. In addition, each analyzer usually involves a large capital investment. Furthermore, manufacturers may complicate the decision making by only releasing the information that is friendly toward their own instruments. Almost all clinical laboratorians base their acquisition decisions on experience, intuition, and experimentation. However, with the current demands and emphasis shifting toward "getting it right the first time" and cost saving, the trial-and-error approach of the recent past is expensive, time consuming, and disruptive. There is a current mentality of "zero tolerance" as it relates to finding the correct analyzer or instrument system. On the other hand, computer simulation provides a powerful planning and decision-making tool which is able to capture system interdependencies, account for the variability in the system, model the analyzer or instrument system, show behavior over time, and provide information on multiple performance measures. The simulation forces attention to details in a design and is less costly. A good simulation model will give the laboratory management team greater freedom to try out different ideas, reduce risks, reduce costs, reduce analysis time, all with no disruption to the current system. Numerous researchers both in Europe and in the United States have applied simulation to study various aspects of the clinical laboratory such as staff assignments, evaluating the queue length, and sample priority handling (2–6). It should be mentioned that the exercise of developing a model itself is highly beneficial since it forces one to work through the operational details of the process and sometimes that is enough to understand and solve a problem.

HOW IS SIMULATION DONE?

Simulation by itself is not a solution tool but rather an evaluation tool. It is essentially a computer model of an existing system created for the purpose of conducting experiments. The development of a simulation model follows the standard scientific protocol which involves:

1. Formulating a hypothesis
2. Setting up an experiment
3. Testing the hypothesis through experimentation
4. Drawing conclusions about the validity of the hypothesis

The first step in developing a hypothesis is asking the right questions. The most common questions that are usually asked by laboratory management are:

- Can the existing process deliver the desired TAT all the time?
- How many full-time equivalents (FTEs) employees are needed to ensure the desired TAT regularly?
- Is it more appropriate to perform chemistry and immunoassay testing on different platforms, or on an integrated platform, or on the same platform?
- How many more FTEs personnel are needed to accommodate a certain increase in test volume?
- What is the best instrument combination for meeting the laboratory's specific TAT goals?
- How will process changes impact overall laboratory efficiency?
- How much buffer capacity (i.e., ability to maintain TAT during labor shortage due to sick leave, vacation, etc.) does a laboratory need?
- What is most appropriate for the laboratory: modular or total laboratory automation?
- What real savings can be expected after implementing a process change?
- What is the impact of an imaging technology such as MICRO 21 on hands-on utilization of medical personnel working in a hematology laboratory?
- What impact will front-end automation have on test TATs and labor utilization of medical personnel working in the receiving and processing area of the laboratory?
- Will total laboratory automation without ability for centrifugation and sample aliquotting work?

After formulating the right hypothesis, the next step is gathering operational details. A simulation model will work with inaccurate data but it cannot work with incomplete operational information. This step is extremely important and there are times when this process itself helps identify solutions and develop various "what if" scenarios. After understanding the operational details, the relevant data for each process are collected. The model is constructed and run for a specific period of interest, which may range from a day to weeks or even a year. The model gathers the performance statistics such as TATs, resource utilization, and instrument utilization and summarizes the data at the end of the run. The simulated TATs are then validated and compared with the actual TATs to calculate the standard error in the model. The model is then optimized to minimize the standard error and used to perform simulated or what if analyses. The process of constructing a simulation model can be illustrated by the following two examples.

Simulating the Receiving and Processing Area of a Laboratory

The receiving and processing area of any clinical laboratory may be its Achilles' heel. This area has the highest liability and is usually staffed with lower paid personnel who have a tendency to churn. The processes occurring in this section are diverse and manual. Figures 1A and 1B show the typical operations occurring in the order-entry and processing areas of a representative U.S. clinical laboratory. Any sample tested in a laboratory has to go through these processes and any errors introduced here will adversely affect all subsequent laboratory processes. A simulation model of the receiving and processing area of a laboratory can be constructed to answer the following primary questions:

- Can the existing process deliver the stipulated TAT of 15 minutes for stat samples and 60 minutes for routine samples?
- What will be the impact on TATs of routine and stat samples when two or three processors call in sick or go on vacation?
- What is the minimum personnel needed to provide the stipulated TATs all the time?
- What is the degree of inefficiencies introduced by continuous arrival of stat samples?
- How much more work can the system handle with the same or reduced personnel?
- What is the optimal number of computer terminals, centrifuges, and refrigerators needed to deliver the stipulated TATs?
- What is the impact of centrifuge downtime on test TATs?
- Can labor saving be achieved by process changes such as physician order-entry?
- What is the impact of front-end automation on test TATs and labor utilization?

Most of the events occurring in the receiving and processing area of a clinical laboratory are discrete in nature; therefore, discrete event simulation is the technique of choice. The changes in the state of the physical system are represented by a series of events that occur at discrete points in the simulation. Figure 2 shows the logic diagram of how discrete event simulation works for the receiving and processing area of the laboratory. At the onset, the model creates a simulation database and programs scheduled events such as sample arrivals. The arrival of a sample is an event 1; since the arrival pattern has already been scheduled at the onset of simulation, it is also called a scheduled event. However, the following event 2, capturing a medical personnel and using him or her for a specified time period, is conditional upon the availability of the medical personnel. Hence, event 2 is called the conditional event. If a medical personnel is not available, then the sample is routed to a waiting queue and will stay there until the availability of a resource (personnel).

Assume the time taken by a medical personnel to complete event 2 is described by a normally distributed random variable as having a mean of 120 seconds and a standard deviation of 30 seconds. Therefore, at the start of event 2, a normal random variate is generated using a random number generator based on the mean and standard deviation, e.g., 90 seconds. This allows the model to schedule the completion of event 2 in advance for that time in the future. In this case, that time will be sample arrival time + 90 seconds. The logic

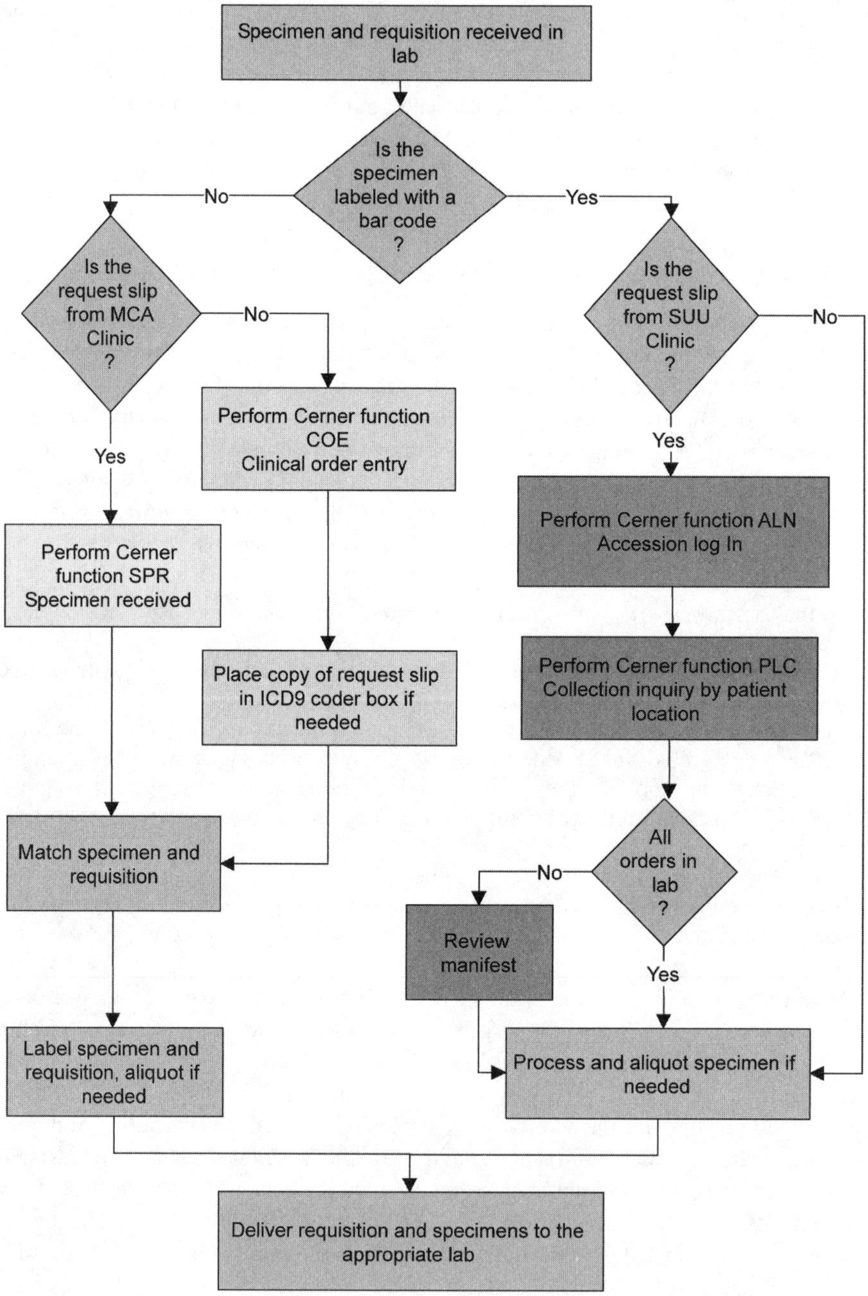

FIGURE 1A. Typical operations occurring in the order-entry area of a representative U.S. clinical laboratory.

associated with event 2 is executed which is use of a medical personnel for 90 seconds. The simulation clock is advanced to the scheduled completion time, i.e., sample arrival time + 90 seconds. Event 2 terminates at this juncture and the medical personnel is set free and made available for the next sample. The model evaluates the set of instructions and decides

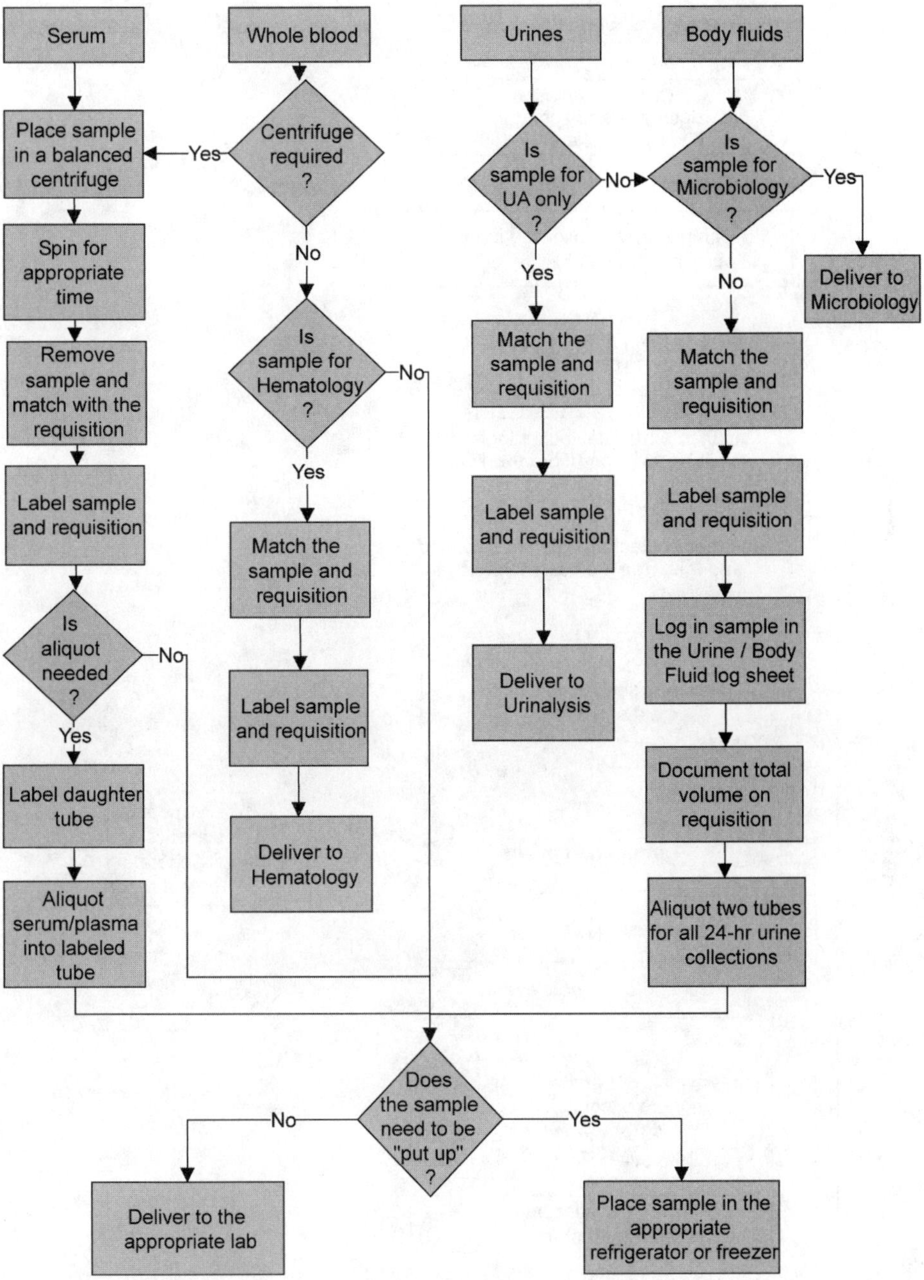

FIGURE 1B. Typical operations occurring in the processing area of a representative U.S. clinical laboratory.

if the process terminates here or moves on to the next step, i.e., event 3. If the sample is a hematology sample and it does not need any further processing, the sample exits the receiving and processing area. The model updates the statistics such as exit time and logs TAT as the difference between the exit and sample arrival times. However, if it is a chemistry sample and it needs further processing, the model moves on and schedules event 3, which may

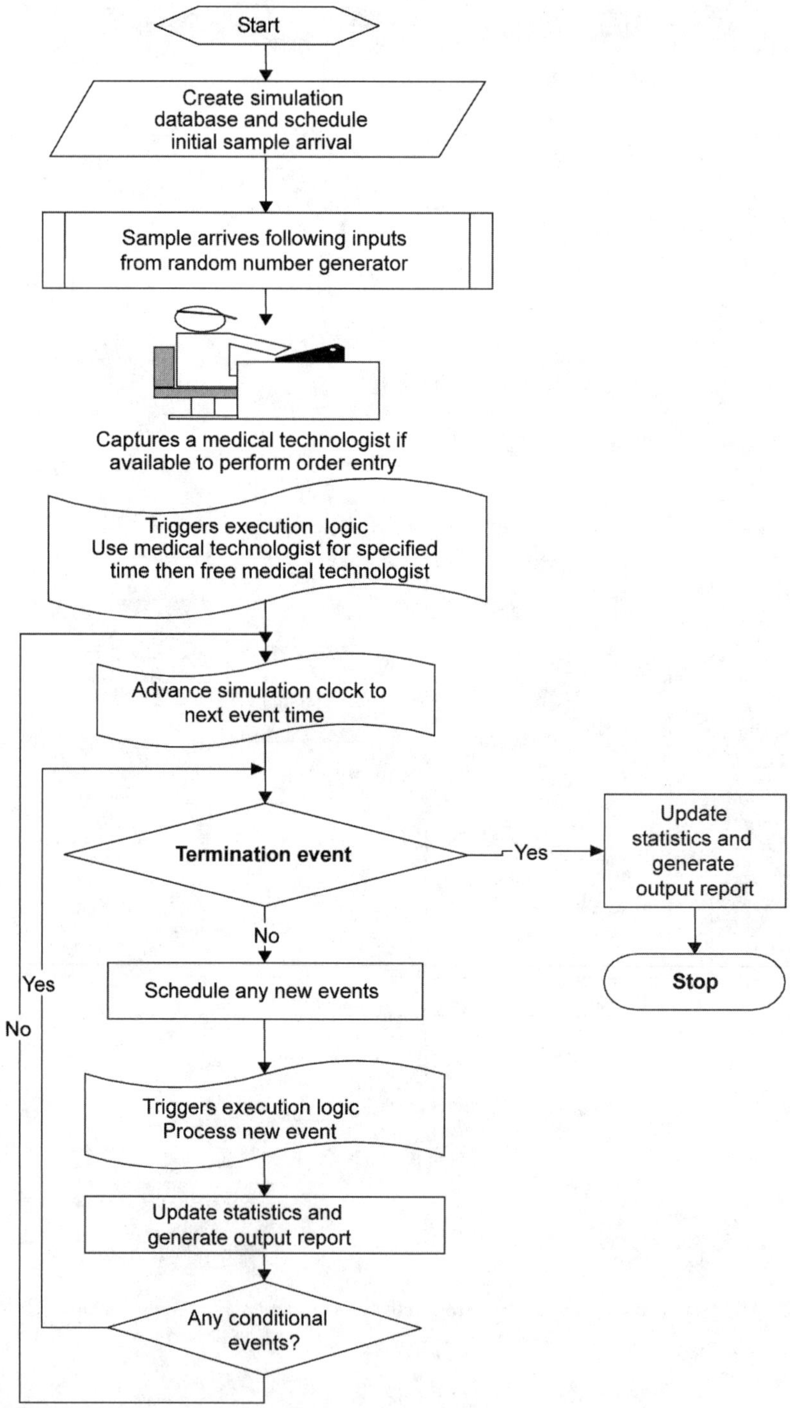

FIGURE 2. Logic diagram of how discrete event simulation works for the receiving and processing area of the laboratory.

be putting the sample into the centrifuge for centrifugation. If there is a wait time associated with event 3, then the model schedules the completion of event 3 by adding the wait time to the existing value on the simulation clock. The simulation clock is again advanced to completion of event 3, any resulting statistics are updated and the decision is made either to advance the model to the next event or terminate the process by exiting the sample.

Thus, the process steps that a sample goes through in a laboratory are broken up into numerous single discrete events. The end of one event is the beginning of the second event and so on and so forth. The model unites these individual events into a continuum by repeating the following sequence:

1. The next scheduled event is
2. Simulation clock variable set to the time equal to the time of the next event
3. Updates statistical inputs wherever required
4. Computes the actions associated with the most current event
5. Schedules the occurrence of next event
6. Moves the simulation clock to the time of occurrence of the next event.

This general logic is applied in simulating the different steps illustrated in Figures 1A and 1B.

In order to construct this model, the following information is needed:

- Arrival pattern of different sample types, i.e., the number of routines, stats, hematology, and coagulation samples arriving per hour
- Test ordering pattern on different sample types. This information provides the number of samples that need aliquotting or need to be tested at more than one station, thus facilitating the simulation of sample delivery to different workstations within a laboratory
- Number of computer terminals available for test accessioning
- Number of available centrifuges
- Shift assignments for different technicians working in receiving and processing area of the laboratory
- Time and motion analysis for various processes occurring in the section. A minimum of 40 readings must be taken for each process occurring in the laboratory. This analysis will also enable one to understand how different personnel handle a process
- The physical layout or floor plan of the existing laboratory

The simulation is typically run for 24 hours and the statistics such as TATs of the different samples, hands-on utilization by medical personnel, and utilization of different computer terminals and centrifuges are recorded and displayed at the end of the run. The number of simulation runs is determined by the confidence level and tolerated error in overall analysis. It can be easily calculated by using:

$$N=[(Z_{\alpha/2}) \times S/e]^2 \tag{1}$$

where α=significance level=1−0.95=0.05 at 95% confidence level
e=tolerated error in overall analysis
S=standard deviation of sample population
Z=derived from standard normal distribution table for 95% confidence level Z=1.96

Typically 10 replication will be able to assert with 95% confidence that the simulated TAT is off by ±10% from the real TAT collected during the data collection phase.

Case Study

The quality assurance report of a clinical laboratory in a major academic medical center revealed a 20% failure in meeting the stat TAT for chemistry samples. Since most of the stat samples come from critical care units such as emergency room, intensive cardiac care unit, and pediatric intensive care unit, it was deemed necessary to evaluate compliance failure and institute a process change. A continuous process improvement committee was formed which examined the different processes occurring in the laboratory over 1 month and came up with the following recommendations:

- Add two processors during the day and evening shifts.
- Assign a dedicated stat station that is staffed all the time and handles only stat samples.
- Add three centrifuges and two computer terminals to speed up test order-entry.
- Acquire a front-end automation system that will automate centrifugation, aliquotting, and sample routing to different areas of the laboratory.
- Develop standard operating procedures for different processes in the laboratory.
- Batch routine samples and handle stat samples as they arrive.

A cost analysis showed that the cost to the institution to implement these changes would be approximately 1 million dollars and there were no guarantees that the changes will improve the TAT. Figure 3 shows the arrival pattern for stat and routine samples. On a typical day, the laboratory processes around 2400 samples. Figure 4 shows the flow diagram of the various processes and the time it takes to finish each one. A simulation model was constructed by taking into consideration the various personnel and their respective shifts, the number of centrifuges, and the number of order-entry stations. Table 1 shows the number of FTEs, centrifuges, and order-entry stations available before process change. Figure 5 shows the layout of the receiving and processing area of the laboratory. The physical layout or floor plan to match the actual laboratory is important, as this will allow estimating the amount of time personnel spend moving from one workstation to another.

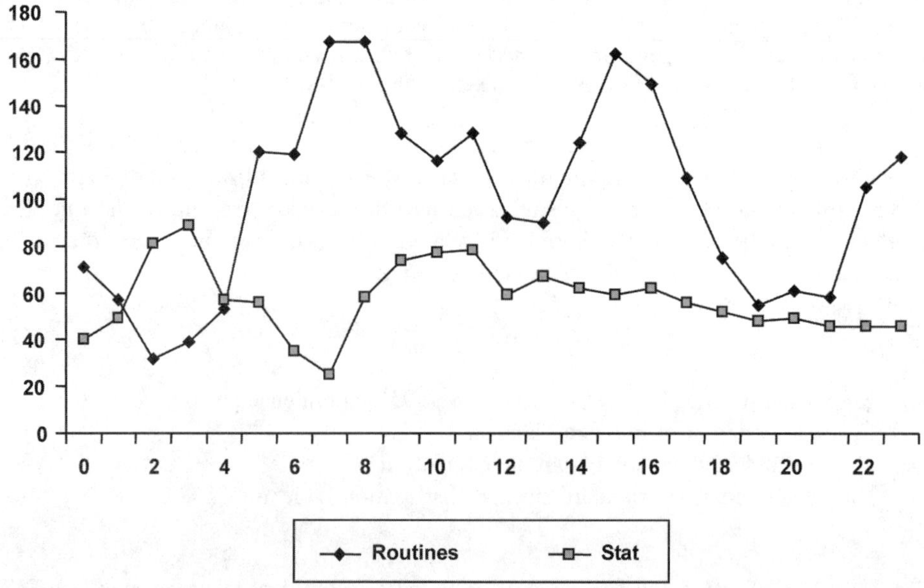

FIGURE 3. Arrival pattern for stat and routine samples.

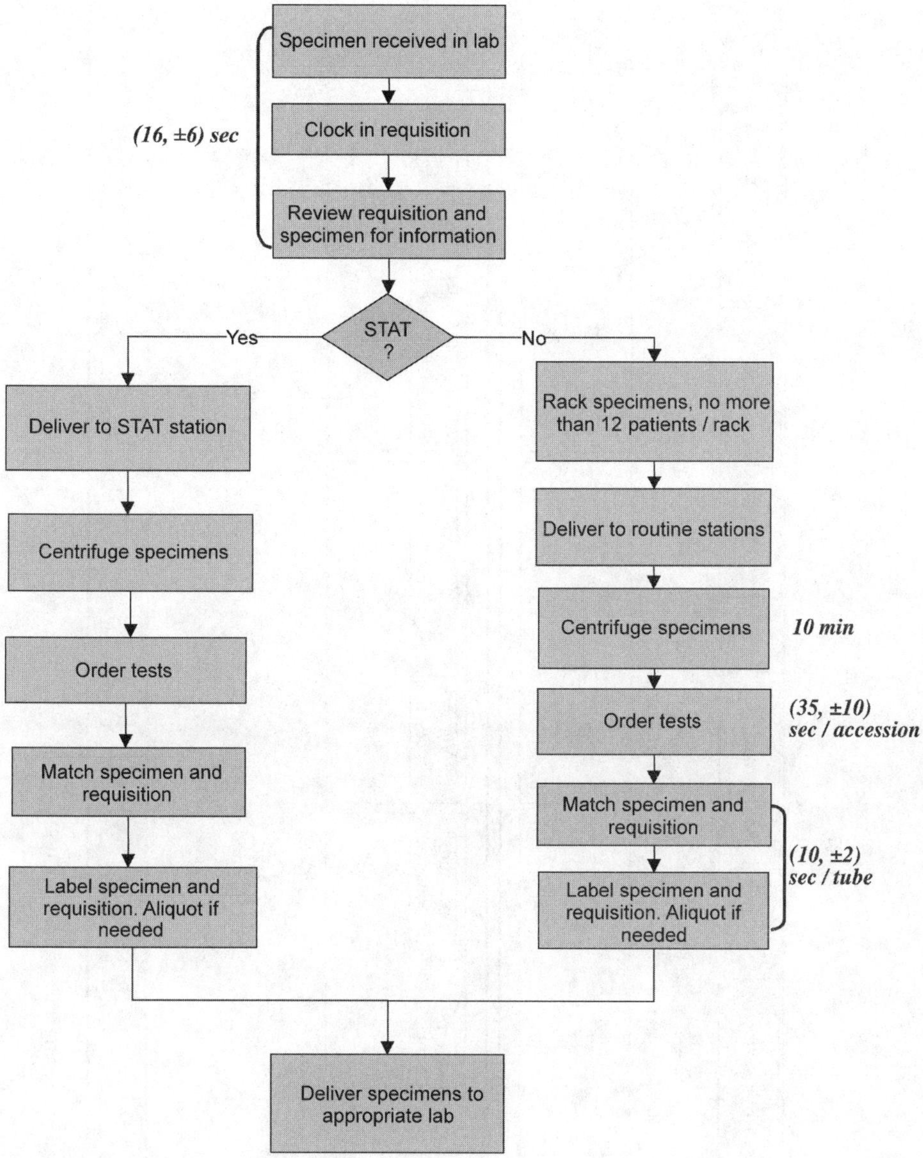

FIGURE 4. Flow diagram of the various processes and the time it takes to finish each one.

TABLE 1. Number of FTE, centrifuges, and order-entry stations before process change

Shifts	FTEs	Centrifuges	Order-entry stations
Day	5	5	5
Evening	6	7	7
Night	5	7	7

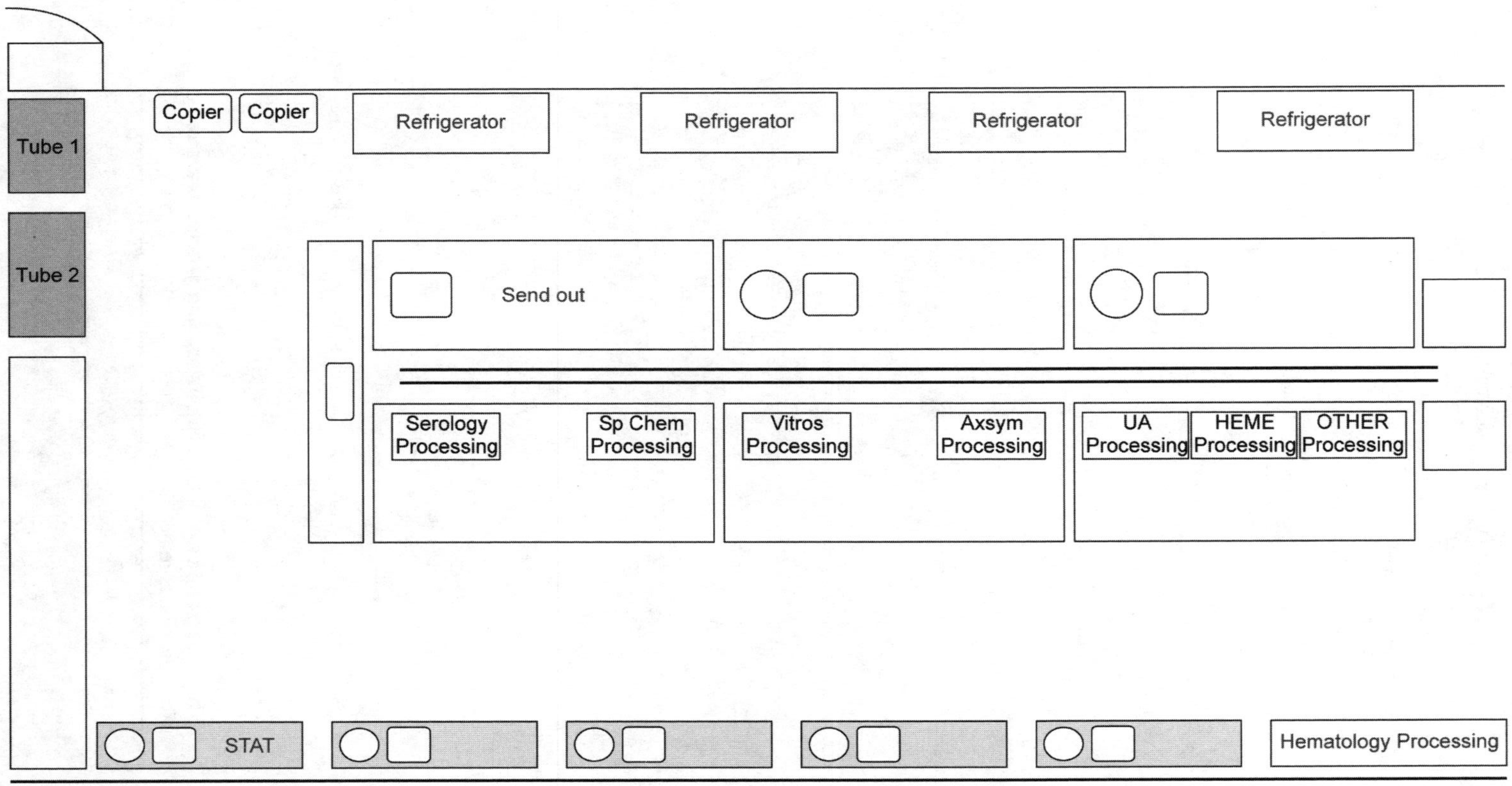

FIGURE 5. Layout of the receiving and processing area of the laboratory.

The model was validated by visual inspections of different processes occurring in the laboratory. Fifteen replications of the model were run and performance statistics such as labor utilization and sample TAT were collected and averaged. Figures 6 and 7 show a comparison between the actual and simulated TAT. According to computer simulations, all of the stat samples should be processed within 30 minutes; however, in reality, only 80% of stat samples are processed within that time frame (Figure 6). A similar discrepancy was noticed for routine samples (Figure 7). Further scrutiny revealed that the laboratory was short two FTEs 60% of the time. This shortage is mainly due to employees calling in sick (call-ins); 95% of call-ins occur during day shift. Reducing the day shift resources by two gave a TAT that compared very well with actual TATs (standard error <8%). The stipulated TAT for stat samples for this laboratory is 30 minutes and, based on computer simulations, it can be achieved 100% of the time if the laboratory is fully staffed. Thus via simulation, the ability of the process to deliver the stipulated TAT was verified.

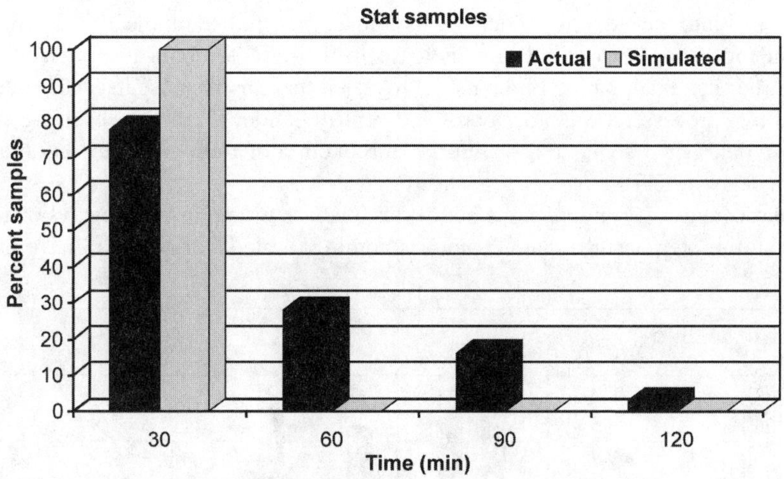

FIGURE 6. Comparison between the actual and simulated TAT of stat samples.

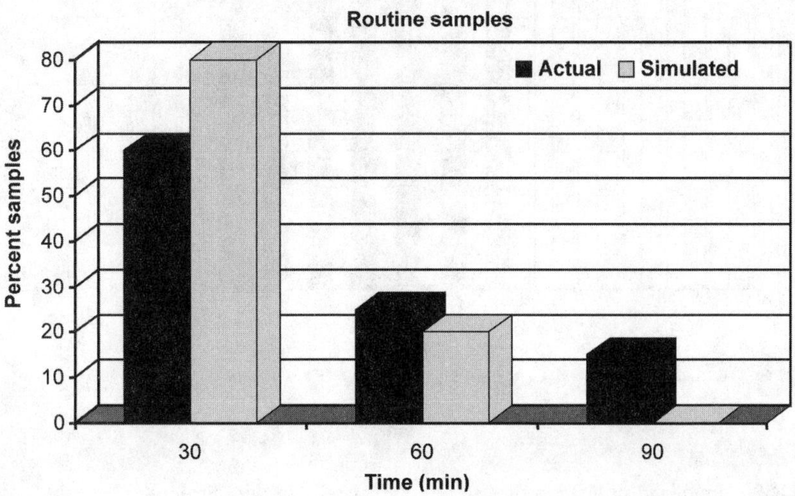

FIGURE 7. Comparison between the actual and simulated TAT of routine samples.

Figure 8 shows the predicted utilization of different personnel working during day, evening, and night shifts. With the exception of two FTEs on the day shift, most of them have less than 70% utilization. It has been the authors' experience that expecting utilization greater than 75% on a regular basis will cause employee burn out and force high turnover. Utilization between 65% and 70% can be considered optimal. From Figure 8 it is also apparent that day and evening shifts have very little buffer capacity in terms of available labor. It was estimated by reducing personnel sequentially per shift and studying its impact on overall TAT of all samples. The study showed no significant deterioration in TAT of stat samples when the personnel in day and evening shifts were reduced by one. However, the utilization of all other FTEs increased by approximately 15%, thus causing their overutilization. A significant increase in TAT for the night shift was observed only when two FTEs were eliminated.

The simulation model of the existing laboratory was then modified to include front-end automation. A simulation model of the FE500, a front-end processor manufactured by Tecan (Tecan AG, Abbott Diagnostics), was constructed and validated. This submodel was then inserted into the existing model and its impact was studied on the TAT. Interestingly, the simulation showed a significant increase in the TAT for both the stat and routine samples. Further examination of the model revealed that this increase in TAT is due to the fact that two processes (i.e., order-entry and centrifugation) that were occurring simultaneously would occur sequentially with the introduction of front-end automation and this caused a delay in TAT.

The recommendation that came out of this analysis was to introduce physician order-entry first; this step ensures that all samples coming to the laboratory will have bar-code

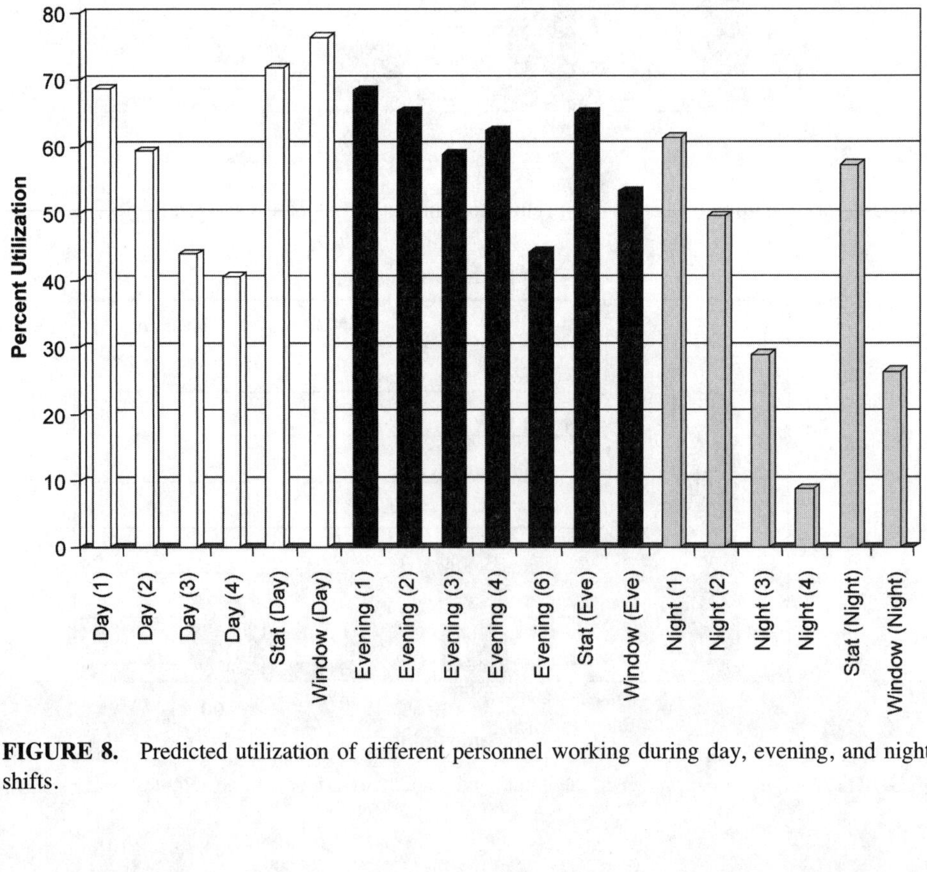

FIGURE 8. Predicted utilization of different personnel working during day, evening, and night shifts.

labels attached on the tubes. Once this is done, then introduce the front-end automation. This stepwise process change, although intuitive, would not have occurred because there were two schools of thought. The first, professing that time gained in automating the aliquotting process will offset the order-entry time and there will be an overall reduction in TAT. The second was that sample order-entry causes the bottleneck and therefore the TAT will increase because of the front-end automation. The savings estimated before simulation were grossly high which caused the estimated return on investment to be off by approximately 2 years.

Another important scenario that was evaluated was assigning one dedicated station to order and process stat samples only. The simulation model showed that this would cause a delay of approximately 50–60 minutes in the TAT of stat samples during peak hours. Therefore, instead of having only one FTE handling the stat samples, all processors were told to process samples in the following order of priority: (1) stat samples, (2) in-hospital routines, (3) in-hospital clinics, and (4) outreach samples. This order ensured the efficient and rapid TAT of stat samples all the time. The addition of more order-entry terminals and centrifuges would not have improved TAT; instead it was determined that the number of routine samples that are batched must be optimized. Simulation optimized this by using the two criteria of time and number of samples. This was achieved by changing the two variables representing time and number of samples in each run until a minimum TAT was obtained for different samples. It was found that batching 24 routine samples in 10 minutes would give minimum TAT and optimum utilization of centrifuges and order-entry stations. The recommendations that resulted from this study are summarized as follows:

- The existing process is capable of providing the stipulated TAT if there are no employee vacancies or call-ins.
- There is no buffer capacity in terms of labor during day and evening shifts. Hence, if more than one person calls in sick during these shifts, it would cause a delay in TAT of approximately 20% of stat samples.
- There are adequate numbers of centrifuges and order-entry terminals.
- The layout of different stations in the laboratory is optimal and only 3% of time is spent on walking from one station to another.
- Implementation of front-end automation without the prior implementation of physician order-entry will cause a delay in TAT of stat samples.
- Implementation of physician order-entry and front-end automation will provide a labor savings of four and three FTEs, respectively.
- Processing hematology samples on the FE500 will not cause any significant delay in TAT of other samples for this laboratory or for the hematology specimens.

Simulating a Clinical Chemistry Analyzer

The evolution of clinical chemistry analyzers began with the introduction of single and multichannel analyzers such as sequential multiple analyzers (SMA) in the 1960s (7, 8). Random-access analyzers such as CX7 by Beckman Coulter and Hitachi 747 by Boehringer Mannheim replaced the SMAs in the early 1980s. The 1990s saw the introduction of random-access immunoassay analyzers such as AxSYM® by Abbott Diagnostics, Immuno 1 by Bayer, and ACS 180 by Ciba Corning. The need for faster analyzers with larger test menus is driven by several factors. One factor is an increasing demand from clinicians and other users of laboratory services for rapid TATs, and another factor is a move to decrease the costs of producing laboratory results and consolidate laboratory testing into fewer workstations. The diagnostic industry responded to this need and currently there are numerous comparable clinical chemistry analyzers that claim to have fast TATs, high

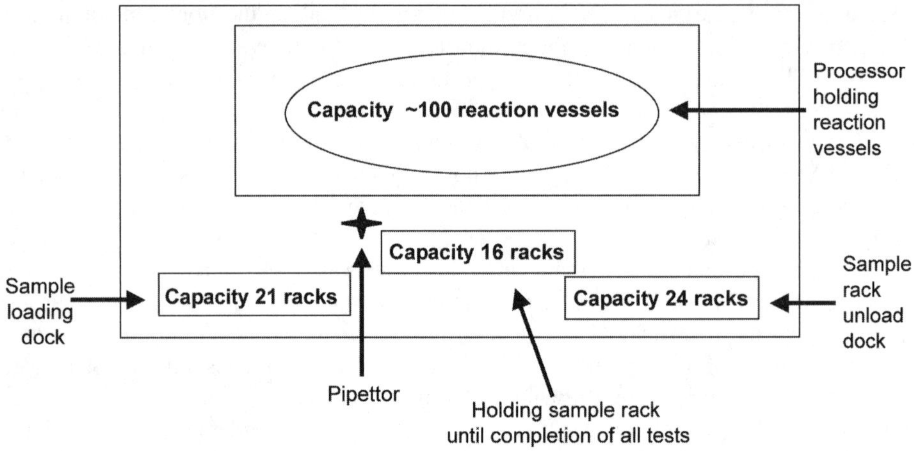

FIGURE 9. Aschematic diagram of a hypothetical immunoassay analyzer.

throughput ranging from 1800 to 2100 tests per hour, and test menus exceeding more than 75 tests per analyzer. In addition to this, every major diagnostic manufacturer has developed hybrid systems that combine the clinical chemistry and immunoassay analyzers on one platform, e.g., the ARCHITECT® series by Abbott Laboratories, the RxL series by Dade Behring, the MODULAR® by Roche Diagnostic, the IMS by Bayer, the VITROS® Fusion by Ortho Clinical Diagnostics/Johnson & Johnson, and the LXI series by Beckman Coulter. With the availability of a wide range of analyzers, selection of the most appropriate analyzer that would meet laboratory needs is no longer a simple exercise of dividing the total number of tests done by the laboratory per day with the analyzer's hourly throughput to determine if it will meet the laboratory TATs. Furthermore, the diagnostic vendors are not very forthcoming with the real throughput of their systems. The real throughput of an analyzer often is dependent on the combination of tests ordered on a sample and can be off by as much as 30% from vendor claims with real samples.

Computer simulation offers an unbiased and a scientific means of evaluating the throughput of an analyzer for a specific laboratory. Depending on the available information, a very accurate simulation model of an analyzer can be constructed using any one of the software packages listed earlier. In fact, the engineering department of most of the diagnostic companies use some sort of simulation during product development and validation, but these models are not released to customers. In the absence of important technical specifications for an analyzer, constructing an exact replica model is an impossibility. However, a relatively accurate model capable of predicting throughput and TATs with 90%–95% confidence can be constructed by using the technical information available in the public domain. In order to understand how such a model can be constructed, it is important to elaborate a little on the different components of a typical clinical analyzer. Figure 9 is a schematic diagram of such a hypothetical immunoassay analyzer. The four main components that must be considered for developing this model are as follows.

Sample Loading Dock Capacity

Every analyzer has an area where an operator loads the samples. The samples are loaded either directly on the loading dock or alternatively they are loaded on a rack which in turn is placed on the loading dock. The number of racks/samples that can be loaded at one given time determines the sample loading capacity, usually ranging from four to 25 racks which translate to 40–125 samples loaded at any given time.

Pipetting Station or Pipettor

The pipettor is a location on the analyzer where an aliquot from the sample tube is drawn and added to the reaction vessel for further processing. Most analyzers have one pipettor and usually the samples are pipetted sequentially. While one sample is getting pipetted, the other samples may remain at the sample loading dock or are placed in the second queue as shown in Figure 9. In the latter case, it is important to know the holding capacity of the queue. The number of aliquots drawn depends on the number of tests ordered on the sample; for a clinical chemistry analyzer it may range from one to 20 aliquots with a mean of seven and for immunoassay it is usually 1.1–1.2 aliquots per sample. The time taken to sample one aliquot is also called sample cycling time and it ranges from 4 to 18 seconds. Samples are brought to the pipettor either by moving the rack holding the sample tube directly below the pipettor or alternatively a robotic arm may pick up the sample tube from the sample rack and hold it below the pipettor syringe. In either case, the time taken to move the sample underneath the pipetting syringe ranges from 1 to 2 seconds and is usually included in the sample cycling time for simulation purposes.

Sample Processor

The sample processor is a temperature-controlled area within an analyzer where addition of reagents, incubation, washings, and photometric readout is carried out. The sample processing area holds a fixed number of reaction vessels and the sample aliquot remains in this area until all of the processes needed to generate a test result are completed. The time spent by the aliquot in the area depends on the test kinetics and can range from 3 to 60 minutes. It is of the utmost importance to capture this time as accurately as possible. Most vendors list this time in their technical briefs, and it is also available in the public domain.

Sample or Sample Rack Unload Dock

After the completion of the sampling process, the sample tubes or sample racks either stay at the sample loading dock or are physically moved to the sample rack unload dock, where they wait until the test is completed. Depending on the test result, the sample tube may be routed back to the pipettor if the sample needs retesting or it may be physically removed by the operator.

Simulation Logic for a Clinical Chemistry Analyzer

Figure 10 depicts the sequence of different steps that needs to be considered in constructing a simulation model of a clinical analyzer. The samples are programmed to arrive as per the sample arrival cycle at a certain location in the model. Upon arrival, the sample is given an identity and is randomly assigned one or more tests based on the test ordering pattern of the institution. This is done by using attributes. The samples are then loaded on the rack. The maximum number of samples that can be loaded on a rack is determined by the holding capacity of the rack. In a typical laboratory, an instrument operator tries to optimize this sample loading either by waiting until the rack is filled completely or by waiting for a certain time after the arrival of the first sample. This is simulated by using the code "LOAD 5 IN N(15,2) seconds." It means that the operator will load five samples if available or will wait for a time period that is randomly selected between 13 and

17 seconds and then load the rack on the analyzer. The rack with the sample is then moved to the pipettor, and, based on the number of test attributes assigned to the sample, the pipettor is used for the assigned sample cycling time per attribute. For example, if a sample has been assigned the attribute for CK-MB and troponin I testing, then the sample may wait at the pipettor for 36 seconds; if it was just CK-MB, it would wait for 18 seconds. Another entity named aliquot is created after the sample cycle time has elapsed and is routed to the processor. The advantages of using the create function is that it attaches all attributes of the mother sample to the daughter aliquot. Once all the samples in a rack are sampled, the rack is held in a queue at the holding sample rack location waiting for the completion of all testing. When the aliquot arrives at the processor, it decreases the capacity of the processor by one and waits there for the time it takes to complete the test. When all the aliquots for a particular sample have waited for the assigned time, they are exited out of the model and this triggers a global variable to change its state either from 1→0 or vice versa. This change in turns tells the software that all tests have been completed on this sample, thereby triggering the log file to capture the TAT for the exiting sample. By using this overall logic, a simulation model of the Centaur® analyzer marketed by Bayer Diagnostics (Tarrytown, NY) was constructed. Some of the model attributes are listed in Table 2. Figure 11 shows the arrival pattern for 1450 samples arriving at a reference laboratory from 1 to 8 pm. By using these inputs, the model predicted a throughput of 225 tests/hour, whereas the throughput claimed by the vendor is 240 tests/hour. Thus, the model is able to predict a test throughput value which is within the 90%–95% confidence interval of the optimum throughput claimed by the vendor. Using this model, it was decided that this laboratory would need two analyzers to get all of its samples tested by 10 pm.

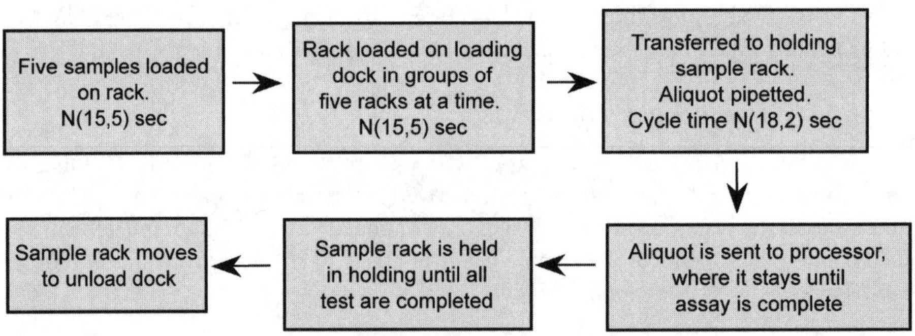

FIGURE 10. Sequence of different steps that needs to be considered in constructing a simulation model of a clinical analyzer.

TABLE 2. Attributes of the Centaur analyzer

Sample cycle time (time taken to sample one aliquot)	18 seconds
Assay time for each assay	16 minutes
Sample loading capacity	21 racks or 105 samples
Samples held in pipetting queue	16 racks or 80 samples
Samples held in unloading dock	24 racks or 120 samples
Processor capacity	100

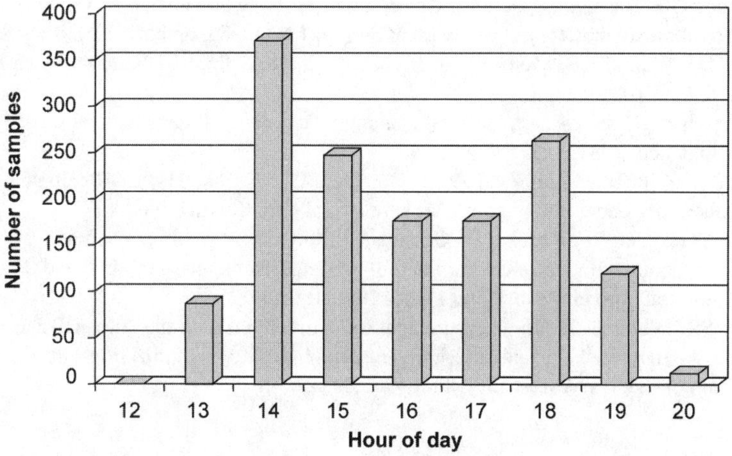

FIGURE 11. Arrival pattern for 1450 samples arriving at a reference laboratory from 1 to 8 pm.

CONCLUSION

Computer simulations have numerous applications in clinical laboratory management. These may include but are not limited to:

- Simulating clinical analyzers to predict optimum throughput
- Evaluating the impact of digital imaging technology on the overall efficiency of a hematology laboratory
- Estimating excess capacity of existing instrumentation
- Optimizing the work flow in the anatomic pathology and histology laboratory
- Scheduling phlebotomy in the outpatient clinic
- Optimizing the work flow in microbiology
- Measuring and optimizing other labor-intensive areas such cytopathology and cytogenetics
- Developing the best courier routes to allow efficient pick-up of samples from outreach clinics.

Simulation by itself is not a solution tool, but rather it is an evaluation tool, and therefore it needs to be performed as a part of a larger process improvement project.

In summary, the various advantages of simulation are:

- It fosters creative problem-solving for the organization.
- It can predict outcomes.
- It can account for system variances.
- It can derive solutions that will minimize the impact of laboratory variances, if not eliminate them entirely.
- It promotes total system exposure to a solution.
- It can reduce costs.
- It forces specific attention to details in a laboratory operational design.

REFERENCES

1. Harrell CR, Bateman RE, Gogg TJ, Mott JRA. System improvement using simulation, 4th ed. Salt Lake City, UT: Promodel Corp., p 1.
2. van Merode GG, Hasman A, Derks J, Schoenmaker B, Goldschmidt HM. Advanced management facilities for clinical laboratories. Comput Methods Programs Biomed 1996;50:195–205.

3. van Merode GG, Hasman A, Derks J, Goldschmidt HMJ, Schoenmaker B, Oosten M. Decision support for clinical laboratory capacity planning. Int J Biomed Comput 1995;38:75–87.
4. Connelly DP, Willard KE. Monte Carlo simulation and the clinical laboratory. Arch Pathol Lab Med 1989;113:750–7.
5. Winkel, P. Operational research and cost containment: a general mathematical model of a workstation. Clin Chem 1984;30:1758–64.
6. Vogt W, Braun SL, Hanssmann F, Liebl F, Berchtold G, Blaschke H, et al. Realistic modeling of clinical laboratory operation by computer simulation. Clin Chem 1994;40:922–8.
7. Mabry CC, Gevedon RE, Roeckel IE, Gochman N. Automated submicrochemistries. A system of rapid sodium, potassium, chloride, carbon dioxide, sugar, urea nitrogen, total and direct reacting bilirubin, and total protein. Am J Clin Pathol 1966;46:265.
8. Gambino SR, Schreiber H. The measurement of CO_2 content with the autoanalyzer. A comparison with 3 standard methods and description of a new method (alkalinization) for preventing loss of CO_2 from open cups. Am J Clin Pathol 1966;45:406–11.

Chapter 2

Quality of the Specimen and the Analytical System

Jay L. Bock

Quality has been defined as "fitness for a purpose," or, more formally, as "the totality of features and characteristics of a product or service that bears on its ability to satisfy given needs" (1). The Institute of Medicine has authored a more medicine-specific definition (2):

> Quality of care is the degree to which health services for individuals and populations increase the likelihood of desired health outcomes and are consistent with current professional knowledge.

For laboratory testing to achieve this type of quality it must first of all be accurate, but it must also possess many other characteristics such as timeliness, affordability, appropriate sample requirements, and effective communication. Analytical quality in the clinical laboratory is essentially a two-pronged task. The laboratory must perform extensive evaluations to ensure that all analytical systems, individual assays, and related products and procedures that it uses have satisfactory performance characteristics. The components of these evaluations will be the subject of the second part of this chapter. The laboratory must also ensure that these performance characteristics are maintained over time. This process is commonly known as "quality control."

The quality of the analytical process begins with the specimen. Every clinical laboratory reports useless and even dangerous results because of problems with specimen collection, identification, transportation, processing, or storage. Considerations for ensuring specimen quality are discussed in the first part of this chapter. The discussion in both parts of this chapter emphasizes general principles rather than detailed protocols. For the latter, references are provided to more detailed publications, including many guidelines published by the Clinical and Laboratory Standards Institute (CLSI, formerly known as the National Committee for Clinical Laboratory Standards or NCCLS).

QUALITY OF THE SPECIMEN

Specimen quality is dependent on many factors. Among the most important are patient preparation, the collection process, delivery of the specimen, and quality assurance in the laboratory.

Patient Preparation

The first specimen quality issue to consider is the condition of the patient. The test result may be adversely affected by conditions such as recent food intake, exercise, posture, time of day, time in menstrual cycle, medications, smoking, and illness unrelated to the condition at hand. Ostensibly the laboratory does not have much control over this important aspect of the testing process, especially when the specimen is collected by non-laboratory personnel. However, it is important that the laboratory document patient preparation requirements in their procedure manuals and make consistent efforts to disseminate this information, through ward manuals, result reports, newsletters, computer screens, educational sessions, etc. Additionally, the laboratory must work with clinical services to foster a culture of proper patient preparation and specimen collection. Not infrequently, the clinical focus is on obtaining a result, even if circumstances indicate that its value may be compromised. Yet a misleading result is much worse than no result at all.

Specimen Collection

The most fundamental requirement for any type of specimen collection, yet one that is not uncommonly abrogated, is proper identification. The laboratory must have clearly defined criteria for specimen identification and for rejection of specimens that are not properly identified. Written procedures and training should emphasize practices to minimize misidentification: for example, tubes should be labeled prior to phlebotomy, not after.

Most clinical laboratory specimens are collected by phlebotomy (venipuncture), which is neither an especially difficult nor a trivial procedure. Its requirements are not too different from those of the analytical procedure itself: documented standard operating procedures, trained personnel, proper supplies and equipment, etc. Phlebotomy has risks of injury to both the patient and phlebotomist, although patients only rarely experience a complication more severe than a hematoma. Improper technique may damage the specimen through several mechanisms including misidentification, contamination from parenteral infusions, contamination from the skin surface (e.g., interference in an alcohol determination due to wiping the skin with alcohol), cross-contamination of materials in the collection tubes, incorrect volume in the collection tube (e.g., erroneous coagulation times due to an improper ratio of plasma to citrate anticoagulant), changes in metabolites due to venous stasis, clotting due to insufficient mixing with anticoagulant, and hemolysis. Yet in most healthcare environments, specimen collection is performed by a wide array of personnel, including dedicated phlebotomists, laboratory technologists, physicians, nurses, medical students, and others. Again it is imperative for the laboratory to be proactive in disseminating the essential information and fostering the attitude that the procedure must be performed correctly **all** of the time.

Quality of a blood specimen for certain tests may be compromised by the specimen containers. Of greatest importance, of course, is that the correct tube be used for the particular test. This is not as trivial as it sounds, because the great variety of collection tubes is often not appreciated. Although the stopper-color coding system is fairly standard, there are many different possibilities for each color. For example, green-stopper tubes may contain the sodium, lithium, or ammonium salt of heparin; gray-stopper tubes may contain oxalate anticoagulant with or without a glycolysis inhibitor; light blue-stopper tubes may contain varying quantities of citrate. Also, undesired ingredients may leach into the specimen. For example, the compound tris(2-butoxyethyl) phosphate, which had been used as a plasticizer in Vacutainer® tube stoppers, was shown to affect measurements of some drugs by diminishing their binding to plasma proteins, thereby causing drug to diffuse into the red-cell compartment (3). Other possibilities are trace metal contamination, binding of trace metabolites to the walls of the tube, or interference from gels or other barrier materials used to separate serum from cells.

The current CLSI standards for venipuncture detail a number of important procedures for ensuring correct identification, safety of the patient and phlebotomist, and integrity of the specimen (4). Requirements for specimen tubes are detailed in another standard (5).

Specimen types other than venous blood present their own challenges for proper collection. In addition to venipuncture, blood specimens may be collected by **arterial puncture** (6), **skin puncture** (7), and, for purposes of neonatal screening, skin puncture onto **filter paper** (8). Arterial puncture is usually performed for purposes of blood gas analysis and therefore requires special attention to maintain anaerobic conditions and to transport the specimen quickly to the laboratory. It also requires procedures to mitigate its additional risks to the patient, mainly the risk that the punctured artery will thrombose (6). Blood obtained by skin puncture contains a variable mixture of venous, arterial, and capillary blood, as well as tissue fluid and intracellular fluid, depending on variables such as site and technique. Poor perfusion, or rapidly changing metabolite levels, can cause measurements in blood obtained by skin puncture to deviate markedly from a simultaneous test on venous blood.

Urine specimens (9) may need to be obtained as a timed (e.g., 24 hour) collection or as a first-morning or "clean-catch" collection, requiring the patient to carefully follow instructions. It can be accidentally contaminated and may be deliberately adulterated, particularly when it is collected for the purpose of drug abuse testing. It deteriorates after approximately 2 hours at room temperature. Timed collections are frequently not properly collected. Measuring urine creatinine is of some use in detecting incomplete collections but is only a very crude measure.

Cerebrospinal fluid and other body fluid specimens must be meticulously collected by skilled operators, usually physicians. Specimen quality can be readily compromised by contamination by blood or by skin flora or by delay in transport to the laboratory; having to re-obtain a specimen in these cases is obviously a very undesirable, and sometimes impossible, option.

Sweat testing (10) is a critical procedure for diagnosis of cystic fibrosis. Deviations from correct procedure, such as allowing sweat to evaporate, contaminating the sweat, or collecting an insufficient quantity, can easily lead to diagnostic error.

Specimens for **detection of microorganisms** include blood for culture (4), blood for parasite examination (11), stool for parasite examination (12), sputum, body fluids, and swabs of wounds and diverse body sites. Stringent requirements for collection and transport must be established to minimize the risk of contamination, yet maximize the opportunity to detect true pathogens. Depending on the collection site and the organisms of interest, specific collection devices, procedures, and transport media are generally necessary.

Specimens for cytologic examination include cervical smears (13), urine and other body fluids (14), and fine-needle aspirations (15). Their main purpose is the detection of cancer via microscopic detection of subtle cellular changes. Hence, the focus is on preserving cellular detail, generally requiring immediate fixation of the specimen.

Specimen Delivery

Specimen quality can potentially be lost during delivery, due to excessive delay, adverse temperature, or mechanical trauma to the specimens. Delivery may be a multistep process, e.g., specimens may be initially delivered to a central receiving area and then transported to specific workstations. Means of transport include human couriers, robotic-style devices, and pneumatic tubes. Preservation of specimen integrity in the process must be ensured, but selection of systems will also depend on cost, convenience, and safety issues.

Specimen Quality Assurance in the Laboratory

Not all deviations in specimen quality can be detected once the specimen reaches the laboratory, but the laboratory must have criteria for unacceptable specimens. Foremost is the requirement for proper specimen identification. The exact requirements for specimen labeling will vary among institutions. Laboratories are frequently faced with the problem of improperly identified specimens for which re-collection is impossible or very inconvenient, yet test results are critical, or so it is claimed. If identification can be established with certainty, these specimens may be accepted, but there should be clear documentation of the circumstances and acceptance of responsibility by the person who made the original error.

Before further processing specimens, the laboratory should establish that they meet basic requirements for the test or tests ordered (e.g., sufficient volume, proper anticoagulant or preservative) and that there is no evidence of undue delay or other mishandling of the specimen. If a specimen is unsatisfactory, a replacement should be promptly requested.

Some problems with the specimen may only become apparent later, in the course of its analysis. For a common example, hemolysis will only be visible after a whole blood specimen is centrifuged. That would invalidate measurements of components that have high concentration in the red cell, such as potassium and lactate dehydrogenase. (A disadvantage of direct analysis of whole blood for these components is that hemolysis is not visible.) In addition, anything causing high optical absorbance by a specimen (e.g., hemolysis, icterus, lipemia) can potentially interfere with spectrophotometric assays. Automated chemistry analyzers should have the ability to check for these types of interferences, and the laboratory procedures should have explicit criteria for specimen rejection.

Specimen quality has to be preserved within the laboratory. Specimens must not be allowed to evaporate or to stand at room temperature for an excessive period prior to analysis. Care must be taken not to interchange or cross-contaminate specimens. Most laboratories will retain specimens in refrigerators or freezers for some period in case repeat or additional testing is needed. The temperature of these should be well controlled and monitored.

QUALITY OF THE ANALYTICAL SYSTEM

The quality of an analytical system can be considered in two aspects. The quality of the **process** describes how well the system fits into laboratory workflow and helps to achieve clinical goals; its evaluation is in large part subjective. The quality of the **result** depends on the accuracy of the test and must be evaluated with the aid of rigorous statistical procedures, although subjective judgments are still involved.

Quality of the Process

Many operational issues affect the quality of an analytical method with respect to the needs of a particular laboratory and clinical setting. The laboratory needs to evaluate these based on manufacturers' claims, published evaluations, site visits to other laboratories, and in-house trial.

Degree of Automation

Greater automation can reduce labor and help ensure uniformity, although it may also introduce the hazard of dependence on a complex system. The most advanced and widely used automation in modern clinical laboratories applies to the actual performance of assays; only recently have systems become generally available that automate specimen processing and delivery to workstations, nearing the goal of "total laboratory automation." All methods designated "automated" are not equivalent, since some may require much more operator involvement than others. The amount of effort needed for calibration, troubleshooting, and maintenance as well as for routine operation is an important consideration.

Consolidation

Workflow, labor costs, maintenance, training, and space utilization are improved if tests can be consolidated on as few workstations as possible. Again the drawbacks of heavy reliance on individual systems must be considered, and some redundancy is usually necessary. Consolidated workstations should allow convenient "random access" to whatever tests are desired on a particular specimen.

Speed

Speed is important for two reasons: results may be needed quickly (and at any time of day) for clinical reasons, and speed may be needed to process a large number of specimens in a reasonable amount of time. The former consideration is especially important in a hospital, whereas the latter may be more important in commercial laboratories. Speed should be measured as both time to result for a single specimen, and number of results that can be generated per hour.

Cost

The total cost of a particular method may be difficult to calculate. It includes costs of equipment, maintenance, overhead, labor, reagents, control specimens, and supplies, all of which depend on a workload that may not be entirely predictable. Vendors offer many different types of payment plans, varying in whether equipment is purchased, leased, or paid for with reagent costs, whether all supplies are included, etc. The laboratory should carefully consider "hidden" costs such as certain supplies, re-runs in case of failures, quality control, and maintenance, preferably shifting these to the supplier insofar as possible. The laboratory may also be able to diminish cost by entering into longer-term agreements with suppliers, but in so doing will sacrifice flexibility.

Reliability

Reliability is a crucial quality issue, relative to both laboratory operations and accurate results, but it is one of the most difficult to assess. Instrument breakdowns or other failures can have effects ranging from mild inconvenience to very stressful disruptions of the entire laboratory operation. Evaluation should begin with the reputation of the supplier/manufacturer:

- Does it have an excellent track record?
- Does it appear that it can meet maintenance and support needs?
- Are communications satisfactory?
- Does it appear to have long-term stability?

Customers should carefully interview other sites and perform as lengthy an in-house evaluation as can be negotiated.

Other Commercial Issues

Most clinical laboratory assays have been well established for many years and use dedicated automation platforms and reagents purchased from commercial vendors. For newer or very esoteric tests, commercial assays may not be available. Reliance on commercial assays has a very large overall benefit, mainly in terms of efficiency, but it can cause some difficulties. The quality of the laboratory is intimately tied to the quality of the vendor. Although most diagnostics vendors are strongly committed to quality, they also have marketing and other concerns that may conflict with quality. For example, they may be hesitant to make improvements or introduce new assays that would only be of interest to a small number of their customers. Patent issues may restrict the use of the best technologies. Laboratory customers can do a great deal to improve quality of the industry by demanding the best and by close communication with vendors to identify and resolve the many problems that will inevitably arise in running state-of-the-art assays.

The nature of laboratory–vendor arrangements can influence quality in many important ways. For example, using fewer vendors, and entering into longer-term agreements, may limit expense but also decrease flexibility and possibly force use of inferior methods in some cases.

Laboratories also, of course, use many assays that are designed in-house, often referred to as "homebrew" assays. For many of the more esoteric tests there may be no alternative. Homebrew tests allow the laboratory greater flexibility but also place much greater demands for method documentation. Laboratories may also need to make modifications to commercial assays and must proceed with great caution and impeccable documentation when doing so.

Quality of the Result

The quality of an analytical result is its closeness to the correct result. This definition raises two questions:

- How can one ever know the correct result?
- If one could know the correct result, how much deviation from it is acceptable?

Neither question is completely answerable. For some tests the idea of an absolutely correct result is at least approachable. For well-defined, simple chemical substances in plasma, such as sodium, glucose, or cholesterol, **primary** methods, formerly sometimes referred to as **definitive** methods, can be designed, usually based on the principles of isotope dilution. The idea behind these is that the compound to be measured, modified only by labeling it with a stable isotope, serves as an internal standard with virtually identical chemical properties. It is then possible to purify the sample exhaustively, removing possible interferences, without worrying about recovery since the ratio of internal standard to analyte remains constant. The final measurement, performed with a mass spectrometer, is a ratio of labeled substance (standard) to unlabeled substance (analyte), which can be reduced to the original concentration of analyte in the sample based on a parallel measurement on an accurate standard. For many clinical laboratory assays, a fundamentally accurate underpinning of this sort is not possible. Protein analytes, for example, are complex molecules which may have polymorphic primary structure, multiple subunits, glycosylation, phosphorylation, peptide nicks, and other types of heterogeneity. These variations may affect the biological activity of the protein, and it is in general not even possible to define what would constitute an absolutely accurate measurement. For some analytes, physiological concentration may be below the detection threshold of the most accurate techniques. And some tests are of a functional nature, e.g., erythrocyte sedimentation rate or clotting times, making problematic the concept of a fundamentally accurate standard.

The question of how much deviation from a hypothetical true result can be accepted has been debated for many years. Some workers have used a statistical approach to this question. The earliest publication frequently cited is by Tonks (16), who suggested that allowable error, measured as twice the standard deviation, should be no more than one-fourth the magnitude of the reference range. Cotlove et al. (17) suggested that the day-to-day analytical variance of a biochemical test should not exceed 25% of the average within-person biological variance of that test in healthy subjects. Harris (18) expanded on this concept, specifying limits of acceptable imprecision and bias for eight common chemistry tests. Glick (19) proposed that for tests used to monitor values in the neighborhood of a normal range or therapeutic range, the upper limit of random error should equal 20% of the difference between the limits of the range. These proposals are all based on professional judgment rather than any rigorous statistical derivation (20).

A second approach is to base analytical goals on the state-of-the-art, as evidenced, for example, on interlaboratory proficiency surveys. A third approach is to attempt to determine actual customer needs or desires, e.g., by surveying physicians (21). Clearly this approach is subjective, but it has the merit of relating test accuracy to goals for clinical care. The various approaches to determining requirements for test accuracy each have advantages and drawbacks (20, 22). If test specifications are made too rigorous, then expense and other resources are wasted in meeting them; on the other hand, test methods that are too inaccurate will not be able to meet clinical needs. Indeed, certain applications of lab tests may never even be discovered if widely used methods have insufficient accuracy.

In some cases, analytical goals have been set for a test by an expert committee examining that particular test. A notable example is the first report of the Adult Treatment Panel of the National Cholesterol Education Panel, which decreed that in order for physicians across the country to be able to relate patients' cardiac risk to serum cholesterol measurements, the imprecision and bias of those tests both need to be less than 3% (23). Regulatory or accrediting agencies may also set standards for test accuracy that clinical laboratories must meet (presumably these are chosen based on the sort of criteria already discussed, but a specific justification is usually not given). In the United States, the Clinical Laboratory Improvements Amendments of 1988 set established specific accuracy targets for proficiency testing for many common analytes. Some examples of these are shown in Table 1 (24).

Error in laboratory results is generally considered to have two components: random and systematic. **Random error,** or imprecision, is easier to determine since it does not require an absolute standard of truth. **Systematic error,** or bias, often cannot be directly determined, but it can be approximated by studies of sensitivity, linearity, recovery, interference, and agreement with a comparative method. Protocols for determining these different aspects of result quality are summarized in the following sections.

Precision

The International Union of Pure and Applied Chemistry (IUPAC) has defined precision as (25):

> Closeness of agreement between independent test results obtained under prescribed conditions.

TABLE 1. Examples of accuracy targets for proficiency testing specified by CLIA '88

Analyte	Criteria for acceptable performance—target plus or minus
Sodium	4 mmol/L
Potassium	0.5 mmol/L
Chloride	5%
Alkaline phosphatase	30%
Calcium	1 mg/dL
Magnesium	25%
Uric acid	17%
pCO_2	5 mm Hg or 8%, whichever is greater
Cholesterol, total	10%
Cholesterol, high-density lipoprotein	30%
Digoxin	20% or 0.2 ng/mL, whichever is greater
Hemoglobin	7%
Hematocrit (excluding spun hematocrit)	6%
Leukocyte count	15%
ABO group	[100% accuracy]
Antibody identification	[80% accuracy]
Antinuclear antibody	2 dilutions

It is a measure of reproducibility, or random error. Assessments of precision are almost always related to the **Gaussian distribution** (Figure 1), which is the mathematical representation of the familiar bell-shaped curve. The Gaussian distribution (commonly known in statistics as the **normal** distribution, although this is misleading in a clinical context) arises from an important mathematical result called the central limit theorem. This theorem essentially states that if many random variables, whatever their individual distributions, are summed together to give a new random variable, the distribution of that new variable will follow the Gaussian distribution. If a histogram is plotted of results of a laboratory measurement repeated many times, its shape will usually be Gaussian. Intuitively, this is because variability in the measurement results from many small, independent, random sources of error. If instead there was a single, dominant, and possibly nonrandom source of variability (say, the temperature in the room or the technologist performing the test), then the actual distribution could be much more irregular.

The Gaussian is a symmetric function described by only two parameters: the mean, μ, which locates the center of the curve (central tendency), and the standard deviation, σ, which describes the width of the distribution (dispersion) (*see* Figure 1). The parameter σ is what is usually given as a descriptor of a method's precision. It is often convenient to convert it to a dimensionless number, known as the coefficient of variation, or CV:

$$CV = \frac{\sigma}{\mu} \times 100\% \quad (1)$$

An exact determination of μ and σ is impossible, because it would require an infinite number of measurements. In practice, what is determined from a finite number of measurements are the **sample mean**, m, and the **sample standard deviation**, s. They are

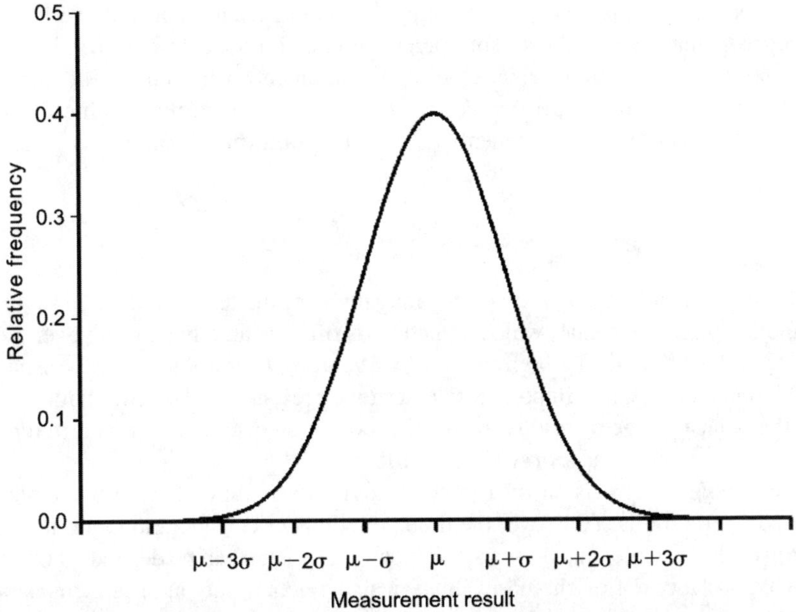

FIGURE 1. Graph of the Gaussian distribution function, also known as the normal distribution, or bell-shaped curve. The graph describes the relative frequency of a measurement as a function of the value of that measurement. The function is derived from two parameters: μ, which is the mean, and σ, which is the standard deviation. The exact mathematical formula is: $f(x) = 1/\sqrt{2\pi}\sigma\, e^{-(x-\mu)^2/2\sigma^2}$, where e is the base of the natural logarithms. Important properties of the function are:

- It is symmetric about the value $x = \mu$, where the function is at its maximum.
- It has a finite value for any positive or negative value of x. However, its value rapidly becomes exceedingly small for $x > \mu + 3\sigma$ or $x < \mu - 3\sigma$.
- The curve is normalized so that the total area under it is exactly 1; 68.27% of the area lies within the limits $\mu \pm \sigma$, meaning the percentage of measurements that will fall in this range; 95.45% of the area is within $\mu \pm 2\sigma$, and 99.73% is within $\mu \pm 3\sigma$.

given by the formulas:

$$m = \Sigma x_i / N \tag{2}$$

$$s = \sqrt{\frac{\Sigma (x_i - m)^2}{N - 1}} \tag{3}$$

where N is the number of observations. The larger the value of N, the closer the sample statistics m and s are to the population statistics μ and σ. Confidence intervals can be calculated using formulas available in statistics textbooks. Generally about 20 measurement points will give good results in practice.

The main difficulty with precision determinations is that, as indicated in the definition above, precision relates to repeated measurement **under prescribed conditions**. When the conditions of measurement are allowed to vary, the precision can vary, e.g., if repeated measurements are all done within a very short time, or throughout the day, or over several weeks; using one bottle of reagent, or one lot of reagent, or multiple lots, etc. To some degree it may be possible to split precision into components, e.g., within-run, within-day, and day-to-day. A convenient fact is that imprecision from different sources adds as the root-mean square, i.e., if imprecision has contributions from a within-day component, s_{wd}, and a day-to-day component, s_{dd}, then the **total imprecision** s_T is given by:

$$s_T = \sqrt{s_{wd}^2 + s_{dd}^2} \tag{4}$$

Precision depends importantly on the magnitude of the test result, i.e., σ is, in general, a function of μ (their ratio, which is the CV, is often relatively constant over the range of clinical values but will be high at very low values). Therefore in the assessment of a clinical laboratory test, it is important to determine precision at the low, middle, and high end of the clinical range of results. A specification of precision at several different measurement levels is known as a **precision profile**.

Determining the precision of a method obviously requires having a sample whose analyte concentration is stable over the time period under consideration. For analytes that are intrinsically unstable, this presents a difficulty. Precision can be dependent on the sample matrix, so laboratories should evaluate it using actual patient specimens as well as artificial quality control materials.

The actual reproducibility of a method is often affected by certain types of nonrandom error. For example, test results may tend to drift in a steady direction over time. Results may be subject to carry-over (cross-contamination of one specimen by another) or other phenomena that relate to the exact manner in which specimens are processed. Methods are also variably subject to outlier results, i.e., results that, because of some sporadic human or instrumental malfunction, are many standard deviations from the mean and therefore wildly improbable based on the Gaussian distribution. All of these types of error can be more difficult to quantify than random imprecision, but a method's vulnerability to them is an essential aspect of its quality.

The CLSI protocol EP5-A gives detailed protocols for determining the precision of laboratory methods, including a procedure for verifying whether in-house data for a method are consistent with a manufacturer's claims (26).

Sensitivity, Limit of Detection, and Limit of Quantification

The **sensitivity** of an assay is often defined as the lowest quantity of substance that the assay can detect. In nomenclature of IUPAC, however, this latter quantity is referred to as the **limit of detection**. The sensitivity of a method is instead defined as "a measure of the magnitude of the response caused by a certain amount of analyte" (27–29). Of more practical importance is the **limit of quantification**, which is "the lowest amount or concentration of analyte in a sample which can be quantitatively determined with an acceptable level of precision and accuracy." Thus, the limit of quantification is intimately tied to the precision of the assay and can be determined, based on user needs, from the precision profile. This assay property is crucial for those assays such as thyrotropin where quantification at very low levels provides important diagnostic information.

Calibration, Linearity, Reportable Range, and Recovery

All assays produce a measurable signal that is related to a substance concentration (or other reported result) through a process of **calibration**. Calibration requires one or more materials (calibrators) that behave similarly to the specimens to be tested and for which the true result is known. (As already discussed, the availability of such materials can sometimes be problematic.) In general it is desirable to use several calibrators, with values that span the range of clinical interest. In the most favorable case, the assay response is **linear** over this range, meaning that the assay response is exactly proportional to analyte concentration. If linearity is assured, then linear regression techniques can be applied to optimize the calibration curve, and it may be possible to use as few as two calibrators. In the more general case, the response signal is not linear, and the calibration curve is constructed using point-to-point methods or regression to a more complex function. Even in this latter case, however, the assay should achieve **linearity** in the sense that measured concentration should be proportional to true concentration over the **reportable range** of the assay. All clinical laboratory assays must possess linearity in this sense, and the laboratory must take care to determine the reportable range and adhere to it.

Linearity is commonly assessed by obtaining or preparing two samples, one with a high concentration and one with a low concentration of analyte. Several precise mixtures of these are then prepared, and all of the samples are analyzed two to four times. Even if the concentrations of the original samples are not known with absolute accuracy, the concentrations of the mixtures can be expressed as functions of those. Unfortunately, it is not entirely clear how to best assess or describe deviation from linearity in the measured results. Simple visual inspection of a plot is a reasonable approach, but it is subjective and does not quantify any deviation from linearity. Objective statistical methods to document linearity or quantify deviation from linearity have been described, but they present certain difficulties and have not been widely adopted (30–32). The reportable range is assigned based on the concentration range over which the assay is demonstrably linear. The reportable range can often be extended on the high end by dilution of the specimen, but a standard operating procedure for specimen dilution (specifying the diluent to be used, the pipets to be used, etc.) should be established and validated, rather than leaving the means for dilution up to the discretion of the operator.

For an acceptably linear and calibrated assay it should be possible to demonstrate **recovery**, meaning that if a known quantity of material is added to a specimen, that exact amount should be measured by the assay. Recovery is measured as a percentage, with the ideal being 100%. Again, for some of the more difficult analytes, it may not be possible to obtain a definitively known amount of material. Even for simpler analytes, which can readily be obtained in pure form, a recovery experiment may be problematic, because the material may not readily dissolve or may not attach to transport proteins in the same manner as native material, or the addition may require some dilution of the sample matrix. A recovery experiment is best conducted by starting with a material that is known to have a zero concentration of analyte. This is possible for many analytes, e.g., drugs, but it may be difficult or impossible for some endogenous metabolites. Alternatively one can begin with an arbitrary material and measure the concentration both before and after the addition, but the need to take the difference between two measurements adds error.

Interferences

Interferences are one of the most troublesome aspects of assay quality, in part because not all interferences can be anticipated. An interference can be said to occur when any specimen component other than the analyte itself influences the concentration measurement. An interference may be caused by a single, identifiable substance or may relate to a bulk property of the material such as viscosity or turbidity. In the latter case, the interference is frequently described with the somewhat ambiguous term "matrix effect."

An interference study is an important part of the method validation. Potential interferents to be examined include ones with general importance (e.g., hemolysis, icterus, lipemia, high or low protein) and those with specific importance to the assay (e.g., chemicals closely related to the analyte). These are generally tested by spiking the relevant substance into test materials. Two limitations of this type of interference testing are noted:

- The effect of a compound added in vitro may differ from the effect when the compound is naturally occurring. For example, if a patient is taking a drug, his or her blood will typically contain not only that drug but also one or more metabolites, some of which may not be well characterized.
- A compound may have both positive and negative interfering effects, which could offset at the concentration being tested but not at other concentrations.

An additional opportunity to detect interferences arises from a properly performed method comparison study (*see* next section).

Method Comparison

The final step in establishing the accuracy of an analytical system is demonstrating that it gives equivalent results to a trusted analytical system. This presents a number of difficulties. First, what trusted method can be used for the comparison? Ideally this would be a definitive method, or at least a reference method. Unfortunately, as already discussed, these may not be available at all or may only be available at prohibitive cost. In practice, one frequently has to compare the new method to an existing routine method that has been used for an extended period of time with apparently satisfactory results. The next hurdle is to set up an experimental protocol for comparing the methods that does not introduce its own sources of bias. For example, if the comparative assay is always run at a later time than the candidate assay, there may be a tendency for the comparative results to be higher, due to sample evaporation, or lower, due to analyte deterioration. Third, and a source of some controversy and confusion, is the performance of a valid and informative statistical analysis of the data (33).

As usual, the first step in data analysis should be careful visual inspection of the data. The CLSI guideline on intermethod comparisons (34) recommends examining two types of plot: a **scatterplot**, which is a graph of the candidate method results on the y-axis versus the reference method results on the x-axis; and a **bias plot**, which is a graph of the intermethod difference on the y-axis versus the reference method result on the x-axis.

Presentation of comparative data in a scatterplot is traditionally accompanied by some type of linear regression analysis. This is sometimes referred to as a "correlation" analysis, but that term is inappropriate, because the goal is not to detect whether the methods correlate (they must, unless one or both are totally invalid!), but rather to quantify how well they agree. Mathematically, however, correlation analysis is essentially identical to the simplest type of linear regression analysis, which estimates the "best" linear fit to the comparative data. That line should ideally be the line of identity, with a slope of 1 and an intercept of zero. The actual slope and intercept for the comparative data can be calculated by linear regression, providing an estimate of proportional and fixed bias, respectively, of the candidate assay relative to the reference assay. The statistical software used should provide confidence intervals for both of these parameters, since, as usual, the sample data are only an approximation to the population data.

Different regression techniques use different definitions of the "best" linear fit and hence will give different estimates of these parameters (though the differences are slight if agreement between the methods is good). The simplest standard regression technique minimizes the sum of the squared distances from each data point to the fitted line, measured vertically. This approach essentially assumes that the results of the reference method are perfectly accurate. If one instead measures the distances horizontally (or interchanges the x- and y-variables), a slightly different line is obtained in general. A more complicated method, commonly known as "Deming's method" although described earlier by other workers, accounts for imprecision in both variables by employing a parameter, λ, which represents the ratio of the variance of the candidate method to the reference method (35). When $\lambda=1$ this method minimizes the distances measured perpendicular to the fitted line. A third popular approach is that of Passing and Bablok: being a non-parametric method, it offers the theoretical advantage of not making any assumptions about the data, but its calculations are the most laborious (36). With any of these methods, estimates of slope and intercept can be adversely affected when the data are **heteroscedastic** (precision varies with analyte level), when outliers are present, or when the range of values tested is not well distributed; special procedures may be used to discard outliers and correct for heteroscedasticity. Linear regression will also be misleading, of course, when the true relationship between methods is some function other than a straight line.

Besides determining best fit it is important to quantify how far individual data points may deviate from that curve. A commonly reported statistic, although really not suitable for this purpose, is the **correlation coefficient**, r. This number reaches its maximum value of 1 when the data points fall exactly on a straight line with positive slope. It is zero when the data points exhibit completely random scatter, and it is negative when the regression line has negative slope. It is generally just slightly less than 1 for real-world method comparison studies. Although a value of r close to 1 indicates minimal scatter about the regression line, the number is highly dependent on the range of values tested, since choosing a narrow range effectively magnifies the relative amount of scatter. A more useful parameter is the **standard error of the estimate**, S_{xy}, which is a number in the units of measurement related to how much difference one may expect between the measured y-value and the y-value estimated from the measured x-value. [It should be calculated using standard regression formulas, **not** the Deming method (34).] Another way to examine scatter is through a residual plot or bias plot, e.g., as described by Bland and Altman (37). Data points with an unusual amount of intermethod disagreement (i.e., outliers) should be carefully examined. It is best to have sufficient volume of all specimens to do repeat analyses in these cases, in order to eliminate the possibility of a blunder. If a major discrepancy is reproducible, then it generally indicates some type of interference in one method or the other. Further analysis of the specimen may be able to identify the cause of the interference. Important information may also be obtained by investigating the patient who was the source of the specimen; however, this is only possible if the specimens were not collected anonymously, which may raise issues of confidentiality.

CONCLUSION

Ensuring the quality of laboratory testing requires fastidious attention to all aspects of the testing process: test ordering, specimen procurement, delivery to the laboratory, analysis, and result reporting. This can only take place in a milieu that emphasizes the constant need for improvement.

REFERENCES

1. ANSI/ASQC. Quality systems terminology. Milwaukee, WI: ASQC, 1978.
2. Lohr KN. Medicare: a strategy for quality assurance. Washington, DC: National Academy Press, 1990.
3. Borga O, Piafsky KM, Nilsen OG. Plasma protein binding of basic drugs. I. Selective displacement from alpha 1-acid glycoprotein by tris(2-butoxyethyl) phosphate. Clin Pharmacol Ther 1977;22:539–44.
4. National Committee for Clinical Laboratory Standards. Procedures for the collection of diagnostic blood specimens by venipuncture; approved standard, 5th ed. NCCLS Document H3-A5. Wayne, PA: NCCLS, 2003.
5. National Committee for Clinical Laboratory Standards. Tubes and additives for venous blood specimen collection; approved standard, 5th ed. NCCLS Document H1-A5. Wayne, PA: NCCLS, 2003.
6. National Committee for Clinical Laboratory Standards. Procedures for the collection of arterial blood specimens; approved standard. NCCLS Document H11-A3. Wayne, PA: NCCLS, 1999.
7. National Committee for Clinical Laboratory Standards. Procedures and devices for the collection of diagnostic blood specimens by skin puncture; approved standard, 4th ed. NCCLS Document H4-A4. Wayne, PA: NCCLS, 1999.
8. National Committee for Clinical Laboratory Standards. Blood collection on filter paper for newborn screening programs; approved standard, 4th ed. NCCLS Document LA4-A4. Wayne, PA: NCCLS, 2003.
9. National Committee for Clinical Laboratory Standards. Urinalysis and collection, transportation, and preservation of urine specimens; approved guideline, 2nd ed. NCCLS Document GP16-A2. Wayne, PA: NCCLS, 2001.
10. National Committee for Clinical Laboratory Standards. Sweat testing: sample collection and quantitative analysis; approved guideline, 2nd ed. NCCLS Document C34-A2. Wayne, PA: NCCLS, 2000.
11. National Committee for Clinical Laboratory Standards. Laboratory diagnosis of blood-borne parasitic diseases; approved guideline. NCCLS Document M15-A. Wayne, PA: NCCLS, 2000.
12. National Committee for Clinical Laboratory Standards. Procedures for the recovery and identification of parasites from the intestinal tract; approved guideline. NCCLS Document M28-A. Wayne, PA: NCCLS, 1997.
13. National Committee for Clinical Laboratory Standards. Papanicolaou technique; approved guideline, 2nd ed. NCCLS Document GP15-A2. Wayne, PA: NCCLS, 2001.
14. National Committee for Clinical Laboratory Standards. Nongynecologic cytologic specimens: collection and cytopreparatory techniques; approved guideline. NCCLS Document GP23-A. Wayne, PA: NCCLS, 1999.
15. National Committee for Clinical Laboratory Standards. Fine needle aspiration biopsy (FNAB) techniques; approved guideline, 2nd ed. NCCLS Document GP20-A2. Wayne, PA: NCCLS, 1996.
16. Tonks DB. A study of the accuracy and precision of clinical chemistry determinations in 170 Canadian laboratories. Clin Chem 1963;9:217–33.
17. Cotlove E, Harris EK, Williams GZ. Biological and analytic components of variation in long-term studies of serum constituents in normal subjects. III. Physiological and medical implications. Clin Chem 1970;16:1028–32.
18. Harris EK. Proposed goals for analytical precision and accuracy in single-point diagnostic testing. Theoretical basis and comparison with data from College of American Pathologists proficiency surveys. Arch Pathol Lab Med 1988;112:416–20.
19. Glick JH Jr. Expression of random analytical error as a percentage of the range of clinical interest. Clin Chem 1976;22:475–83.
20. Doumas BT. The evolution and limitations of accuracy and precision standards. Clin Chim Acta 1997;260:145–62.

21. Barnett RN. Medical significance of laboratory results. Am J Clin Pathol 1968;50:671–6.
22. Kaplan LA. Determination and application of desirable analytical performance goals: the ISO/TC 212 approach. Scand J Clin Lab Invest 1999;59:479–82.
23. Report of the National Cholesterol Education Program Expert Panel on Detection, Evaluation, and Treatment of High Blood Cholesterol in Adults. The Expert Panel. Arch Intern Med 1988;148:36–69.
24. Clinical Laboratory Improvement Amendments of 1988. Code of Federal Regulations, revised as of October 1, 2000. Federal Register 2000.
25. Thompson M, Wood R. Harmonised guidelines for internal quality control in analytical chemistry laboratories. Pure Appl Chem 1995;67:649–66.
26. National Committee for Clinical Laboratory Standards. Evaluation of precision performance of clinical chemistry devices; approved guideline. NCCLS Document EP5-A. Wayne, PA: NCCLS, 1999.
27. IUPAC. Harmonised guidelines for the in-house validation of methods of analysis (technical report). Research Triangle Park, NC: IUPAC, 2002. (Available at *http://www.iupac.org/divisions/V/501/draftoct19.pdf*, accessed 5/02).
28. Pardue HL. The inseparable triad: analytical sensitivity, measurement uncertainty, and quantitative resolution. Clin Chem 1997;43:1831–7.
29. Ekins R, Edwards P. On the meaning of "sensitivity." Clin Chem 1997;43:1824–31.
30. National Committee for Clinical Laboratory Standards. Evaluation of the linearity of quantitative measurement procedures; approved guideline. NCCLS Document EP6-A. Wayne, PA: NCCLS, 2003.
31. Kroll MH, Emancipator K. A theoretical evaluation of linearity. Clin Chem 1993;39:405–13.
32. Burnett RW. Quantitative evaluation of linearity. Clin Chem 1980;26:644–6.
33. Strike PW. Statistical methods in laboratory medicine. Oxford: Butterworth-Heinemann, 1991. Chapter 9, Method comparison studies, pp 307–30.
34. National Committee for Clinical Laboratory Standards. Method comparison and bias estimation using patient samples; approved guideline, 2nd ed. NCCLS Document EP9-A2. Wayne, PA: NCCLS, 1995.
35. Cornbleet PJ, Gochman N. Incorrect least-squares regression coefficients in method-comparison analysis. Clin Chem 1979;25:432–8.
36. Passing H, Bablok W. A new biometrical procedure for testing the equality of measurements from two different analytical methods. J Clin Chem Clin Biochem 1983;21:709–20.
37. Bland JM, Altman DG. Statistical methods for assessing agreement between two methods of clinical measurement. Lancet 1986;1:307–10.

Chapter 3

Interferences in Laboratory Tests

James J. Miller, Stanley S. Levinson, and Ronald J. Elin

The clinical laboratory must produce accurate results for quality patient care. Unfortunately, some endogenous and many exogenous components of patients' samples compromise accuracy by interfering with the analysis. Interference can be defined as "the effect of a substance present in the sample that alters the correct value of the result for an analyte" (1). The major endogenous sources of interference include hemoglobin, lipemia, and bilirubin. The major exogenous sources of interference are drugs and additives from collection containers. One of the earliest (1973) compilations (2) of factors affecting laboratory tests included not only analytical interferences but preanalytical variables and physiological effects as well. Later, the review by Kroll and Elin (1) in 1994 provided an excellent update on interferences in clinical laboratory analyses. Glick et al. (3) published the second edition of their well-known *Interferographs* in 1991. This book graphically presents interferences by hemoglobin, bilirubin, and lipemia for most routine clinical chemistry analytes on many of the automated instruments in common use at that time. Two of the books in the "Effects" series by Donald Young are especially important resources for information on interferences: *The Effects of Preanalytical Variables on Clinical Laboratory Tests* (4), in its second edition, and *Effects of Drugs on Clinical Laboratory Tests* (5), now in its fifth edition. Finally, the CLSI (NCCLS) guideline EP7-A (6) is an indispensable resource for properly performing and interpreting tests of interference.

Although the magnitude of the problem of interference on clinical laboratory analyses is difficult to determine, some estimates are available. Glick et al. (7) evaluated the major endogenous interferents in 2599 serum samples. Hemolysis greater than 1+ (about 50 mg/dL hemoglobin) was present in 244 (9.4%) of samples; icterus greater than 1+ (about 1.9 mg/dL bilirubin) was present in 525 (20.2%) of samples; and, lipemia greater than 1+ (about 430 mg/dL triglycerides) was present in 69 (2.6%) of samples. Thus, there were 838 specimens (32%) that had at least 1+ for hemolysis, icterus, or lipemia (turbidity). The frequency of interference in clinical chemistry tests by drugs was reported in a study of 100 outpatients (8). The percentage of tests affected by interference increased from 7% in patients taking one drug to 100% in patients taking five drugs. While there has been some improvement in the specificity of laboratory tests since this study was published in 1971, there also has been a great increase in the number of drugs available. As an indication of the increase in the magnitude and recognition of the problem of drug interferences in laboratory tests, the first edition of Young's "drug file" in 1972 (9) had 263 pages but subsequent editions have grown steadily to the two-volume fifth edition published in 2000 (5) with approximately 2000 pages, which includes more than 10,000 more entries than did the fourth edition in 1995.

In this chapter, the sources and mechanisms of interference are reviewed and guidance is provided for evaluating and recognizing interference. While most cases of interference reported in the literature affect general chemistry tests and immunoassays, to illustrate the fact that no laboratory section is immune, examples of interferences in other areas of laboratory medicine are given. Also provided are recommended techniques for the evaluation of interference during method evaluation and the detection and reporting of interference during routine use of assays. Illustrative examples are given but there is no attempt to be encyclopedic since, as already noted, excellent reviews and compilations of specific interferences are available.

The chapter concludes with some recommendations for laboratorians and reagent manufacturers. It is unrealistic to anticipate that the problem of interference will improve significantly in the foreseeable future. However, substantial improvement in the quality of laboratory test results can be made if laboratorians know how to recognize and investigate interferences. The goal of this chapter is to provide this knowledge.

GENERAL CONCEPTS

Interference causes inaccuracy or bias in clinical laboratory results. This bias may be positive if the interferent increases the measured result or negative if the interferent decreases the measured result. In addition, cases have been reported in which positive interference is caused by some concentrations and negative interference is caused by other concentrations (10, 11), which may occur if the interferent affects the assay by two or more mechanisms (*see* section on Analyte-Dependent Interference later). Similarly, a particular interferent may cause positive interference in one method for a particular analyte and negative interference in another method for the same analyte. For instance, bilirubin causes negative interference in a phenol-aminophenazone peroxidase method for creatinine (12) but positive interference in a 3,5-dinitrobenzoate method (13). For particular samples, interferences may be even more complex, with more than one interferent present at the same time. For example, hemoglobin causes negative interference and bilirubin causes positive interference in one enzymatic method for creatinine (14). These effects may cancel each other if both interfering substances are present.

Clinically Significant Interference

Whether or not the bias due to interference is clinically significant depends on the use of the test results and on the error allowable. Many publications and package inserts indicate the interferent concentration that causes 10% error, implying that only error greater than 10% is clinically significant. Realizing that some assays cannot tolerate 10% error and other assays can tolerate more than 10% error, other authors have used the Clinical Laboratory Improvement Amendments of 1988 (CLIA '88) criteria for acceptable performance in proficiency testing (PT); however, these criteria are for total error (TE), which includes imprecision, method-specific bias, and sample-specific bias or interference (6). It is beyond the scope of this chapter to discuss the concepts of setting analytical quality goals. It is important to remember that bias due to interference needs to be evaluated in terms of its effect on TE. If the assay already has some analytical bias, less additional bias from interference in the same direction can be tolerated. Similarly, if the assay has greater than desirable imprecision, less bias can be tolerated.

Analysis of biological variation is an objective and practical method to help determine quality goals for imprecision, bias, and TE. The book *Biological Variation: From Principles to Practice* (15) lists the coefficients of variation for intraindividual and interindividual biological variation in Appendix 1 and quality goals derived from them in Appendix 2. The interindividual biological variation (reference interval) of analytes may be as low as 1% for sodium and 40% or more for enzymes, hormones, and tumor markers. Intraindividual biological variation is usually lower. The lower the biological variability, the less analytical error can be tolerated if the assay is to be able to differentiate this variability from pathological changes. Many commonly measured analytes have bias goals of less than 10%, in particular, the bias goal for sodium is 0.3% and that for calcium is 0.8%.

Analyte-Dependent Interference

Interfering substances may cause interference by a variety of mechanisms, sometimes more than one at the same time. One way to classify these effects is based on whether the degree of interference is dependent or independent of analyte concentration. Analyte-dependent interference means that the degree of interference caused by a certain concentration of interferent varies with the concentration of the analyte. If the interferent simply absorbs light of the same wavelength as the product of the analytical reaction or reacts in the assay similar to the reaction of the analyte, the interference is likely to be analyte-independent. On the other hand, if the interferent and the analyte interact in some way, e.g., if they react with each other, the interference is likely to be analyte-dependent. It is possible for both types of interference to occur simultaneously.

Analyte-dependent interference can be detected by analyzing two or more concentrations of interferent each at two or more concentrations of analyte. This concept was first described by Kroll et al. (16). They exemplify each type of interference by the analysis of hemoglobin interference in a creatinine assay (analyte-independent), a total bilirubin assay (analyte-dependent), and a direct bilirubin assay (combined analyte-independent and analyte-dependent). For each analyte, they prepared four serum pools with concentrations of analyte spaced across the analytical range. They then added four concentrations of hemoglobin to aliquots of each pool. This provided 16 samples with varying analyte and interferent concentrations. The apparent analyte concentrations were measured and the results were analyzed by multiple linear regression analysis using the model equation:

$$F = c_0 + c_1[A] + c_2[I] + c_3[A][I] \tag{1}$$

where F is the measured result, [A] is the analyte concentration, [I] is the interferent concentration, [A][I] is their product, and c_0, c_1, c_2, and c_3 are the respective coefficients. The coefficients derived from the regression analysis are shown in Table 1. The signs of the coefficients indicate the direction of interference, positive or negative. The values in parentheses are the probabilities (p) that the coefficients are not significantly different from zero. The coefficient c_0 represents the blank (no analyte and no interferent) and should be close to zero. The coefficient c_1 represents the recovery of analyte in the absence of interferent and should always be near 1 and, obviously, always significantly different from zero. The coefficient c_2 represents the analyte-independent interference and the coefficient c_3 represents the analyte-dependent interference. For hemoglobin interference in the creatinine assay, c_2 is significant and negative (negative analyte-independent interference); in the total bilirubin assay, c_3 is significant and negative (negative analyte-dependent interference); and, for direct bilirubin, c_2 is significant and positive and c_3 is

TABLE 1. Value of coefficients for F = $c_0 + c_1[A] + c_2[I] + c_3[A][I]$

	Analyte		
	Creatinine	Total bilirubin	Direct bilirubin
c_0	0.43 (>0.39)	–0.59 (>0.35)	–0.16 (>0.65)
c_1	0.99 (<0.001)	0.99 (<0.001)	0.98 (<0.001)
c_2	–0.35 (<0.01)	–0.24 (>0.01)	0.24 (<0.001)
c_3	–0.00074 (>0.35)	–0.016 (<0.001)	–0.013 (<0.001)

The probabilities that the coefficients are not significantly different from zero (null hypothesis) are shown in parentheses. [Reprinted with permission from Kroll et al. (16)]

significant and negative (positive analyte-independent interference combined with negative analyte-dependent interference).

Three-dimensional response surfaces (Figure 1) can be constructed in order to better visualize the effect of the interference. The analyte-independent interference in the creatinine assay (Figure 1, top) is characterized by a flat response surface and a constant degree of interference by hemoglobin across the range of creatinine concentrations. Analyte-dependent interference is illustrated in Figure 1, center. Here, hemoglobin has little or no interference in the total bilirubin assay at low bilirubin concentration, but as the concentration of bilirubin increases, the negative interference of hemoglobin increases. Combined interference is shown in Figure 1, bottom. At low direct bilirubin concentrations, the graph shows that hemoglobin causes positive interference; however, at higher direct bilirubin concentrations, the negative analyte-dependent interference predominates and the interference by hemoglobin is negative.

It is important to determine the type of interference. When there is analyte-dependent interference, an interference study performed at only one concentration of analyte will underestimate or overestimate the degree of interference. Furthermore, when there is mixed positive and negative analyte-dependent interference, as in the case of hemoglobin interference in the direct bilirubin assay, the study may miss the presence of interference entirely. Note that at 18 mg/L of direct bilirubin, hemoglobin causes no interference.

The response surfaces shown in Figure 1 allow one to visualize the effects of the interferent, the analyte, and their interaction on assay results; however, this type of graph is not very useful to the bench tech who must decide whether or not to report a result. Kazmierczak et al. (17) described another type of graph that allows one to determine if the interference is excessive, provided the interference equation is known and the interferent concentration can be measured. The interference coefficients in Table 1 can be used to calculate combinations of measured results and interferent concentrations that would represent clinically significant bias. Figure 2 illustrates this for the described creatinine and total bilirubin assays. The calculations necessary to construct Figure 2 are given in Appendix A. As mentioned previously in the section on Clinically Significant Interference, different limits for allowable interference have been used. As seen for creatinine (Figure 2A), more than one decision point can be included on the same graph. Here both the CLIA '88 criteria for acceptable performance for total error (3.0 mg/L or 15%; lower right corner) and the more stringent maximum bias goal (15) based on biological variability (<0.68 mg/L or 3.4%) are plotted. To use the graph, the technologist would measure the analyte and interferent concentrations and find the point on the graph corresponding to these results. If the point is in

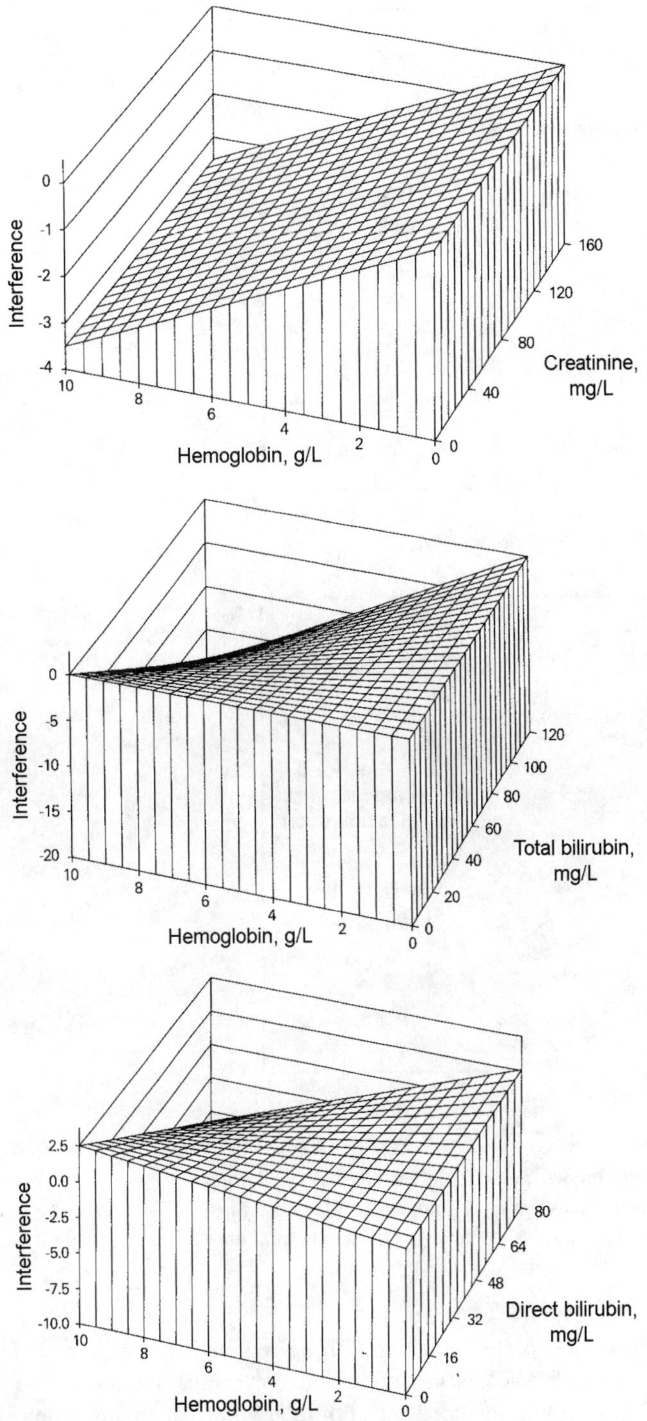

FIGURE 1. Response surfaces for the interference by hemoglobin.
Top: Analyte-independent: Creatinine; interference $= -0.35 \times$ [hemoglobin].
Center: Analyte-dependent: Total bilirubin; interference $= 0.016 \times$ [total bilirubin] $\times$ [hemoglobin].
Bottom: Combined: Direct bilirubin; interference $= 0.24 \times$ [hemoglobin] $- 0.013 \times$ [direct bilirubin] $\times$ [hemoglobin]. [Reprinted with permission from Kroll et al. (16)]

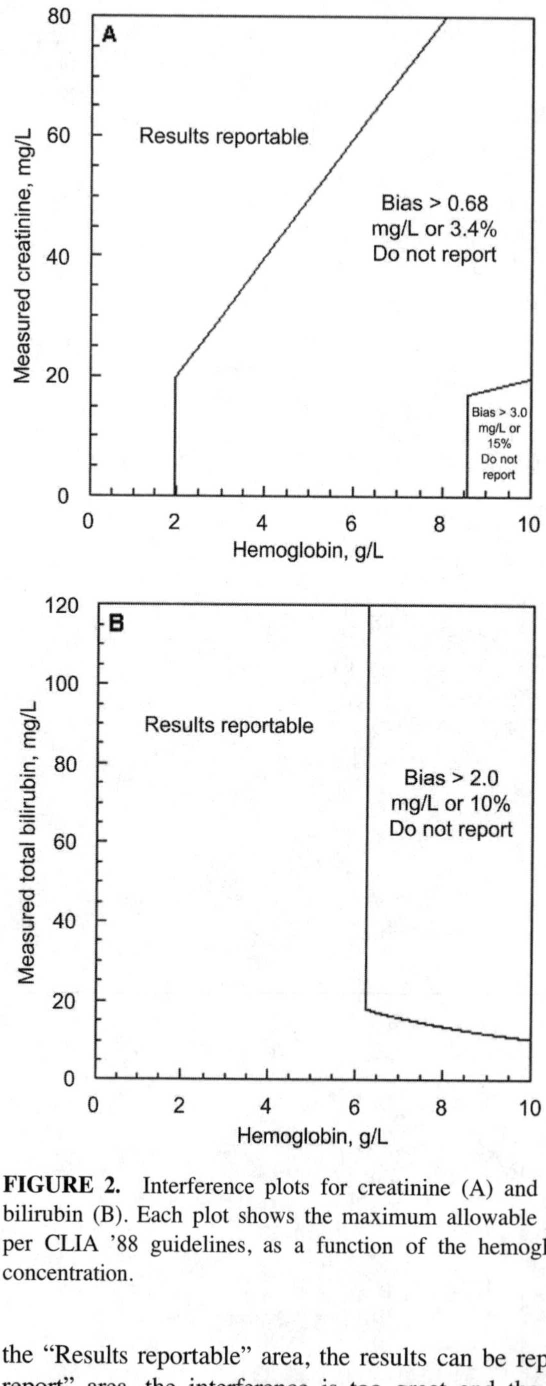

FIGURE 2. Interference plots for creatinine (A) and total bilirubin (B). Each plot shows the maximum allowable bias, per CLIA '88 guidelines, as a function of the hemoglobin concentration.

the "Results reportable" area, the results can be reported. If the point is in the "Do not report" area, the interference is too great and the results should not be reported (*see* Reporting Results with Interference later). For total bilirubin, only the limits based on biological variability (2.0 mg/dL or 10%) are plotted since no values in the range of the graph exceeded the CLIA '88 criteria for acceptable performance. For direct bilirubin, no results in the plotted range exceeded either the CLIA '88 criteria for acceptable performance or the limit based on biological variability. It is important to note that the results with excess bias do not necessarily indicate that the measured result is too high. In fact, in these cases the measured results are too low due to the negative interference.

ENDOGENOUS INTERFERENTS

The three major sources of endogenous interferents in patients' samples are hemolysis, lipemia (turbidity), and bilirubin. In addition, proteins, especially paraproteins and other antibodies with more specific effects, are a significant source of endogenous interference. An indispensable resource for these and many other endogenous interferents is *Effects of Preanalytical Variables on Clinical Laboratory Tests* (4). A summary of the major sources of endogenous interferents is found in Table 2.

Hemolysis and Hemoglobin

Hemolysis releases the contents of erythrocytes into the serum or plasma, including hemoglobin and several commonly measured components present in high concentration in erythrocytes. For example, in the cytoplasm of erythrocytes the concentration of lactate dehydrogenase is about 160-fold greater, potassium 22-fold greater, and magnesium 3-fold greater than the normal concentrations in serum or plasma (18, 19). Thus, hemolysis sufficient to produce 1 g/L of hemoglobin in the serum will increase the concentrations of lactate dehydrogenase by 670 U/L, potassium by 3 mmol/L, and magnesium by 0.12 mg/dL (18–20). Other erythrocyte constituents may interfere as well. For example, hemolysis may affect the determination of creatine kinase (CK) activity through the release of adenylate kinase (AK), which catalyzes the removal of the ADP substrate of CK assays (21). Most current CK assays include diadenosine pentaphosphate to inhibit AK activity (21).

Hemolysis may occur in vivo or in vitro. If hemolysis occurs in vivo, increases in these components are not considered interferences, but their elevation may help to diagnose the condition (22). Hemoglobin released from erythrocytes due to in vivo hemolysis is diluted into the total intravascular blood volume and much of it becomes bound to haptoglobin with the hemoglobin–haptoglobin complex being removed from the circulation. However, hemolysis in vivo may still increase the hemoglobin concentration enough to cause interference after blood is collected. Most hemolysis occurs in vitro due to mechanical destruction during specimen collection, transport, processing, or storage (if serum or plasma remains in contact with the cells after centrifugation). Hemolysis can also be caused by freezing, hyperosmotic shock, detergents, exhaustion of glucose in the sample, and increased erythrocyte fragility due to inherited diseases (23). Serum begins to appear hemolyzed at a hemoglobin concentration of about 0.1–0.2 g/L (24); however, bilirubin or lipemia may mask even greater concentrations of hemoglobin (25).

TABLE 2. Summary of endogenous interferences

Interferent	Mechanism	Direction of interference
Hemoglobin	Spectral	Usually positive
	Reactivity	Usually negative
Lipemia	Light scatter	Positive or negative
	Volume displacement	Negative
	Lipophilic sequestering	Negative
Bilirubin	Spectral	Usually positive
	Reactivity	Usually negative

Hemoglobin itself may interfere due to its spectral properties or due to the chemical reactivity of its iron atoms. Although the spectral absorbance peak of hemoglobin is about 420 nm, it absorbs significantly between 340 and 440 nm. This absorption is probably the cause of interference in most assays in which the interference is positive, such as in the bromcresol green procedure for albumin (26). Negative interference by hemoglobin is likely due to its reaction, or that of its iron, with reagent components or the analyte, e.g., in the Malloy-Evelyn (27) and Jendrassik-Grof (28) methods for bilirubin.

As already indicated, the difference between hemolysis and hemoglobin interference is due to the release of other intracellular contents of erythrocytes into the serum. In addition, erythrocyte membrane fragments in hemolyzed samples may interfere with some assays; for example, hemolysis, but not hemoglobin, was reported to cause false elevations of troponin I on the Behring Opus-1 (29). Positive interference of hemolysis was also reported in the Ortho Clinical Diagnostics Troponin I and the Roche Troponin T assays (30), which was most significant at the lower clinical cutoffs used for risk stratification of patients with acute coronary syndromes.

Hemoglobin-based oxygen carriers (HBOC) are acellular, hemoglobin derivatives, stabilized by cross-linking, that are given intravenously in place of blood transfusions. Technically, these are exogenous interferents such as drugs, but they are covered here because samples appear hemolyzed. Since these blood substitutes are acellular, they are not removed by centrifugation and serum or plasma collected from patients who have received them will appear markedly hemolyzed. In general, HBOC interference mimics the effect of hemoglobin following hemolysis, but without the release of other erythrocyte constituents. Interference of HBOC has been reported for alkaline phosphatase, alanine and aspartate aminotransferases, bilirubin (17, 31), creatinine (32), cholesterol (17), immunoassays for hepatitis B surface antibody, hepatitis B surface antigen, prealbumin and haptoglobin (33), and whole blood hemoglobin (34). Because of the major impact of these products, a number of techniques have been investigated to reduce or eliminate HBOC from serum samples. These include ultrafiltration (35) and polyanionic ligands with binding affinity for HBOC (36).

Lipemia and Turbidity

Lipemia is the result of increased serum concentrations of lipoproteins, which cause interference by three mechanisms:

- Light scattering due to their large size
- Volume exclusion effect also due to their large size and hydrophobic nature
- Dissolution of hydrophobic analytes, reagents, or reaction products into the lipid interior due to their lipophilic nature (37)

The terms lipemia and turbidity are frequently used interchangeably, but they may not be equivalent. The lipoproteins that are the primary cause of turbidity are the triglyceride-rich very low density lipoprotein (VLDL) and chylomicron fractions. Sometimes the triglyceride concentration is used as a surrogate marker of lipemia. However, Glick et al. (7) found a lack of correlation between triglyceride measurements and visual estimation of lipemia, a subjective measure of turbidity. Other possible causes of turbidity in serum include erythrocyte debris, platelets, white blood cells, fibrin clots, or contaminating particulate matter. Regardless of the cause of turbidity, it results in light scattering. In the absence of a sample blank, light scattering from the sample decreases the spectral operating (linear) range and causes positive interference. Light scattering also may have marked effects on methods based on light scattering, e.g., nephelometry and turbidimetry.

The large lipid particles cause a volume displacement effect such that a measured volume of sample is significantly greater than the aqueous volume in the sample. This volume displacement effect may cause negative interference in some methods for analytes such as electrolytes that are present primarily in the aqueous phase of the serum. Although this effect can be detected in chloride and potassium results, it is most obvious for sodium because of its low biological variability. This has lead to the concept of pseudohyponatremia (38). Sodium methods are not affected by lipemia if the analysis is made in the aqueous fraction by ion-selective electrode (ISE) methods and there is no sample dilution (so-called direct ISE methods). ISE methods that include a dilution of the sample (indirect ISE methods) and other methods that include sample dilution (e.g., flame photometry) will be affected negatively by lipemia (38).

Besides light scattering and volume displacement, lipemia may interfere with assays by partitioning of nonpolar analytes, reagents, or reaction products into lipoprotein particles. Examples of nonpolar analytes subject to partitioning errors include steroid hormones and hydrophobic drugs such as Dilantin® and phenobarbital (37).

Two methods have been used to treat lipemic specimens in order to obtain clear samples for analysis. The most commonly used method is ultracentrifugation using small, air-driven centrifuges such as the Beckman Airfuge (39, 40). The other method utilizes a lipemia-clearing reagent, LipoClear, from StatSpin, Inc. (41, 42).

Bilirubin

The third major endogenous interferent is bilirubin. Interference by bilirubin arises from its strong absorbance between 400 and 500 nm and from its chemical reactivity. Generally, spectral interference causes increased results and chemical reactivity causes decreased results. In some cases, both effects occur simultaneously (43, 44). The interference by bilirubin in assays where hydrogen peroxide is an intermediate have been studied extensively (43–46), e.g., in various methods for cholesterol, glucose, triglycerides, and uric acid. This interference is negative due to reaction of bilirubin directly with hydrogen peroxide or with other reaction intermediates (44). Some methods such as the Kodak Ektachem avoid the problem by using a chromogen that reacts with hydrogen peroxide but not with bilirubin (44). It should be noted that positive interference by bilirubin in methods using wavelengths where bilirubin does not absorb also have been reported. For example, bilirubin recently was reported to cause positive interference in an enzymatic method for acetaminophen using a wavelength of 600 nm (47), although the mechanism of interference was not determined.

Most reported studies of bilirubin interference did not test both conjugated and unconjugated bilirubin and it is generally assumed that they are equivalent. However, one study reported negative interference by conjugated, but not unconjugated, bilirubin in an assay for inorganic phosphorus (48).

Bilirubin interference can be reduced or eliminated by the addition of ferrocyanide to the reagents (44, 49), pretreatment of serum samples with peroxidase and hydrogen peroxide (50), or pretreatment with bilirubin oxidase (51).

Proteins

Markedly elevated paraprotein concentrations as found in multiple myeloma or other hematological diseases may interfere with some assays. The mechanisms of paraprotein interference include chemical interference, volume displacement, and increases in sample viscosity. Sonnenblick et al. (52) reported on three patients where paraproteins interfered with phosphate determination by the ferrous sulfate/ammonium molybdate method, presumably by an undetermined chemical mechanism. Although most patients with paraproteins did not have spuriously elevated phosphate measurements, Larner (53) states that paraproteinemia is the most common cause of pseudohyperphosphatemia. Another positive interference by paraproteins was reported for the o-phthalaldehyde method for urea (54). Again, not all sera from patients with paraproteins exhibited this effect, which was believed to be due to precipitation in the acid conditions of the reaction. As with lipemia (*see* Lipemia and Turbidity), the very high protein concentrations present in paraproteinemia may cause false decreases in sodium measurements (pseudohyponatremia) due to volume displacement (38). As with lipemia, only methods that require the serum to be diluted are affected, while direct ion-specific electrode methods are not. Recently, Steinberger et al. (55) reported that intravenous immunoglobulin therapy may increase the serum protein concentration sufficiently to cause pseudohyponatremia.

Paraproteins and hyperproteinemia in general may cause interference by increasing the viscosity of the samples. The Johnson and Johnson VITROS® analyzer uses dry slide technology, i.e., the reagent slides are dry and all of the liquid in the reaction mixture is derived from the sample. The sample must spread across the slide and dissolve the reagents. One might expect that the rate of spreading and, thus, the reaction kinetics would vary with sample viscosity. While many effects of protein concentration on VITROS methods have been reported (4, 56, 57), only a few are listed in the limitations section of the current VITROS product labeling (cholesterol, C-reactive protein, and salicylate show negative interference from increased protein, while glucose, lactic dehydrogenase, and phenytoin show positive interference). The shorter list from the VITROS product labeling may be a reflection of methodological changes. For example, the older ultraviolet aspartate aminotransferase procedure had positive interference from elevated protein, but the newer visible procedure does not.

Besides the relatively nonspecific effects of paraproteins, antibodies may bind various analytes in serum specifically (58). For large analytes, usually proteins, the large analyte–antibody complex is often referred to as a "macro-analyte." Examples have been reported for most commonly measured enzymes, e.g., macro-amylase (59), macro-creatine kinase (CK) (60), macro-alkaline phosphatase, and macro-lactic dehydrogenase (61, 62), and for several peptide hormones, e.g., macro-prolactin (63), macro-parathormone (64), and macro-insulin (65, 66). There have also been reports of endogenous antibodies to thyroglobulin (67–69) and TnI, causing positive (70) or negative (71) interference. Sturk and Sanders (72) and Mifflin et al. (73) reviewed macro-enzymes and Cattaneo et al. reviewed macro-prolactinemia (74). These immune complexes may interfere is several ways. The most common effect for the macro-enzymes is prolonged clearance leading to elevated concentrations in the blood.

The finding of elevated amylase due to macro-amylase has been long known (59). Misdiagnoses as a result of macro-amylase complexes in persons with abdominal pain unrelated to pancreatitis can occur. Macro-amylase can also be perplexing in patients who exhibit this state along with coexisting pancreatitis. In such cases, it is important to determine if macro-amylase is present. There are two clues that should lead one to suspect that an elevated amylase is the due to macro-amylase. First, it is very unlikely that anyone with an elevated amylase but a normal lipase is affected by acute pancreatitis. Second, in acute pancreatitis, the level of amylase and lipase rise and fall over a period of days, while with macro-amylasemia the level remains constant for months or years. Patients with elevated amylase levels falling into the above two categories should be screened further by measuring urinary amylase. In acute pancreatitis, the urinary amylase level is elevated, while with macro-amylasemia, although the serum amylase is elevated, the urinary amylase level is low. This finding of low urinary amylase in the presence of elevated levels of serum amylase confirms the presence of macro-amylasemia. If desired, final confirmation can be made by electrophoresis, where macro-amylases appear as a smeared band which changes its migration pattern after treatment with antibodies to human immunoglobulins (73).

Recently, Sanchez-Munoz et al. (75) reported on a case of hypertransaminasemia due to a macro-aspartate aminotransferase. On the other hand, Hirano et al. (62) reported on a patient with very low lactate dehydrogenase caused by an antibody that blocked the active site of the enzyme. Years ago, when CK isoenzymes were commonly assayed by electrophoresis, macro-CK, although usually migrating between CK-MM and CK-MB, could cause confusion by co-migrating with CK-MB (76, 77). Macro-CK causes variable effects on immunological tests for CK-MB (78). In the immunoinhibition assay, the serum is reacted with an exogenous antibody against the M subunit prior to the assay which blocks the active site of the enzyme. The antibody inactivates M, but not B subunits. Normally, of the typical isoenzymes, only MM is found in the serum of adults, while MB is elevated after an myocardial infraction (MI). Therefore, in the usual case, after an MI, the only activity measured is the B activity of MB. This activity is multiplied times two, because it represents only 1/2 of the MB activity. The difficulty occurs in unusual cases where macro-CK or BB is present. In these cases, a positive result is elicited in the absence of MB, false positive for MI. Furthermore, the calculated values may be very high because the "atypical" activity is multiplied by 2. Although less common, interfering antibodies have been reported for small molecules as well. For example, Cissewski et al. (79) reported a paraprotein that caused spurious elevations of both thyroxine and triiodothyronine.

Matrix Effects

Most of the interferences already described result from relatively specific causes. For matrix effects, it is somewhat more difficult to specify the cause. The matrix of a sample (patient, control, or standard) refers to the milieu or environment of the analyte and includes characteristics such as pH, ionic strength, and protein and lipid concentrations. A matrix effect is an interference caused by a difference in the reactivity of the analyte due to a difference in its environment in the sample. Some of the effects already described under Proteins may be considered matrix effects. The difficulty in matching the artificial matrix of standards, controls, and proficiency samples and the matrix of patient samples often causes marked biases between different assays. In addition, changes in specimens during processing or storage may cause them to respond differently in an assay even when the analyte is stable.

Control material is usually processed (e.g., lyophilized), preserved (e.g., sodium azide, antibiotics), and stabilized (e.g., dithiothreitol, acetylcysteine) differently than serum specimens, which frequently introduces matrix effects. In addition, the serum base and added analytes of control material are often from nonhuman sources (e.g., bovine, equine), which may introduce additional components of matrix effect (80). Many proficiency testing samples are subject to the same types of matrix effects since these samples are usually identical to control material. Differences in matrix components between patient samples are usually less marked, but occasionally can cause significant inaccuracies.

There are several situations in which matrix effects can be particularly important. When the analyte must be extracted either to remove cross-reactive compounds or to increase sensitivity, it is likely that the extracted sample may have a different matrix than the calibrators unless the calibrators are also extracted. When a result is greater than the analytical range of the assay and the sample must be diluted, use of an appropriate diluent matrix is critical for obtaining accurate results. It is important to demonstrate that a series of dilutions with the chosen diluent generates a linear response as the matrix changes. Matrix interference is common when an assay is performed on body fluids other than the fluid for which the assay was designed.

INTERFERENCE IN IMMUNOASSAYS

Immunoassays include one or more antibodies in the reagent. Both endogenous and exogenous substances may interfere. Some interferences in immunoassays are essentially the same mechanistically as interferences for general chemistry assays; some are uniquely pertinent to immunoassays. Categories of interference in immunoassays include:

- Cross-reactivity and heterogeneous antigens
- The hook effect
- Interfering antibodies
- Signal interference and
- Matrix effects

A number of references review these interferences in detail (81–89).

There are four major design classifications of immunoassays (90, 91):

- Label free assays: agglutination, precipitation (turbidimetry and nephelometry), and immunosensors
- Reagent-excess assays: one-site assays (immunostaining, Western blots); two-site "sandwich" immunometric assays (immunoenzymometric assays, immunofluorometric assays, etc.)
- Reagent-limited assays: labeled antigen or antibody assays [RIA, enzyme immunoassays (EIA)] and separation-free homogeneous assays: fluorescence polarization immunoassay (FPIA); cloned enzyme donor immunoassay (CEDIA)
- Ambient analyte assays: microarrays, microchip assays

Although most categories of immunoassay interference may affect any of the immunoassay designs, some types of interference predominate in certain design types. These will be noted in the material to follow. Most of the examples given in this section will involve the reagent-limited assays, reagent-excess assay, and turbidimetry/nephelometry, since these are the most commonly used assays. A summary of interferences in immunoassays is shown in Table 3.

TABLE 3. Summary of interferences in immunoassays

	Interference type				
Immunoassay type	Cross-reactivity	Hook effect	Antibody	Signal	Matrix effect
Competitive	Usually +	Minimal	Minimal	+ or –	+ or –
Nephelometric/ turbidimetric	+ or –	–	Usually +	Usually +	+ or –
Immunometric	Minimal (+ or –)	– (if 1-step)	Usually +	+ or –	+ or –

Cross-Reactivity and Heterogeneous Antigens

Cross-reactivity between the analyte and other components of the sample is one of the most common types of interference in immunoassays. Cross-reactivity represents nonspecificity and is essentially the same as nonspecificity in general chemistry assays except that only noncovalent binding of the analyte to the antibody is involved instead of a chemical reaction. Cross-reactivity usually causes positive interference, but negative interference is possible (92, 93). Cross-reactivity can affect any type of immunoassay, but it is most problematic in reagent-limited, competitive binding assays. Cross-reactivity occurs because a component of the assay other than the analyte has structural similarity to the analyte and therefore binds to the antibody. Cross-reactants may be other members of the same class as the analyte, e.g., luteinizing hormone cross-reactivity in older human chorionic gonadotropin (hCG) assays; metabolites or precursors of the analyte, e.g., conjugated cortisol metabolites in urinary cortisol assays; or coadministered drugs of similar structure, e.g., tricyclic antidepressants. Usually the similarity in structure is obvious, but sometimes the similarity is difficult to appreciate without the aid of three-dimensional molecular models. For example, cyproheptadine, an antihistamine with only partial structural similarity to tricyclic antidepressants, was reported to cause a false-positive serum tricyclic antidepressants screen (94). The binding of the cross-reactant is usually of lower affinity than that of the analyte itself and usually must be present at somewhat higher concentration than the analyte to interfere. This is not always the case. For example, one immunoassay for cortisol had much higher affinity for hydrocortisone (>700% cross-reactivity) and fludrocortisone (320% cross-reactivity) than for cortisol (95).

In the past, most quantitative immunoassays for analytes of any size were performed by competitive immunoassays, usually RIA. In these assays, the analyte competes with a labeled derivative of the analyte (tracer) for binding to a single antibody (polyclonal or monoclonal) relatively specific for the analyte (although some methods use a second antibody to separate bound and unbound tracer). With the development of two-site "sandwich" assays, most analytes big enough to simultaneously bind two antibodies are assayed by this technique. The binding sites of antibodies can accommodate molecules of about 700 Daltons. Analytes of this size or smaller continue to be measured by competitive assays. Two-site assays are much less prone to cross-reactive interference because both reagent antibodies must bind the analyte simultaneously, making a "sandwich," in order to generate a signal. This makes two-site assays much less prone to cross-reactive interference. It is possible and more likely, for a cross-reactant to bind one or the other, but not both of the reagent antibodies, which would keep the "sandwiches" from forming and would be expected to cause negative interference. However, since this type of assay is run under reagent excess conditions, even if a cross-reactant ties up some antibodies, there is usually sufficient excess antibody to quantitatively measure the analyte unless the cross-reactant concentration is very high.

It should be noted that cross-reactivity is not always undesirable. The most obvious example is related to screens for drugs of abuse, in which each assay is designed to detect a class of drugs, e.g., barbiturates or opiates, and a relatively balanced degree of immunoreactivity among various members of the class is desirable. Many of the drugs monitored therapeutically by immunoassays have pharmacologically active metabolites. For example, carbamazepine 10,11-epoxide, the major metabolite of carbamazepine is 100% pharmacologically active (96). In addition, the relative concentrations of the parent drug and the metabolite vary greatly among individuals. Although it has not been documented, a carbamazepine assay with 100% cross-reactivity with the epoxide should correlate better with clinical efficacy than an assay with low cross-reactivity with the metabolite.

There are many reports of cross-reactive interference in digoxin assays (97–99). There are several reasons for this, but the most interesting is the presence of endogenous steroid derivatives, synthesized by the adrenal cortex (100), with structural similarity to digoxin (101), which are elevated in the serum of some patients. These compounds, called digoxin-like immunoreactive factors (DLIF) or substances (DLIS), can be quite problematic for digoxin assays. Most current digoxin assays were developed with special attention to minimizing cross-reactivity with DLIF (102–104).

For many protein analytes, there may be variable proportions of several forms present in samples, referred to as heterogeneous antigens. In some cases, it is desirable to detect these various forms and in other cases it is best not to detect them. Cardiac troponin (Tn) is present in a large number of forms in serum. There is a small amount of uncomplexed TnI and TnT molecules present with the majority being complexed with each other and with TnC (IT, IC, TC, and ITC complexes). In addition, the subunits may be intact or partially cleaved by proteases and have disulfide bonds reduced or oxidized. All of these variations can affect the immunoreactivity and it is recommended that all forms be detected equally. As another example, hCG may exist in serum as intact hCG, free beta-subunits, and as beta-subunit fragments. In normal pregnancy, mainly the intact protein is secreted by the placenta, but in malignant trophoblastic disease, fragments and the free beta-subunit may be secreted in the absence of the intact molecule. In fact, a molar ratio of beta-hCG to intact hCG greater than 5 is considered indicative of malignant disease. The problem here is not that the subunits interfere with the assay but that a malignant tumor may be overlooked if the assay does not detect them. As a result, most commercial testing methods measure both intact hCG and free beta-subunits.

Cross-reactivity may be reduced or eliminated by various means, the most obvious of which is to develop more specific antibodies. Small molecules must be chemically attached to larger carrier proteins in order to make them immunogenic. Within the constraints of chemically reactive groups within the structure of the analyte, the specificity of the antibodies generated can be modulated by the type and position of the attachment to the protein (105). Monoclonal antibodies are often thought to be more specific than polyclonal antibodies, but this is a misconception. Monoclonal antibodies have specificity for one particular site (epitope). Cross-reactivity may still occur at that site. Polyclonal antisera have antibodies that bind multiple sites on the molecule, providing increased likelihood for cross-reactive interference. The great advantage of monoclonal antibodies is that many clones with different properties are typically available and these can be screened for desirable properties including high analytical sensitivity and specificity (106, 107).

Another way to reduce or eliminate cross-reactivity is to separate the cross-reactant from the analyte. Of course, separation is a way to eliminate any interferent from the analyte. Any separation technique, e.g., extraction, chromatography, or precipitation, may be useful. It is important to confirm that the recovery of the analyte is quantitative. To some extent cross-reactivity can be reduced by adjustments of the reaction time and temperature. Vining et al. (108) showed that increasing the incubation time of steroid assays decreases the cross-reactivity of structurally similar compounds. This is a general phenomenon and cross-reactivity decreases to a minimum at equilibrium. Unfortunately, it may take 24 hours or more to reach equilibrium in some immunoassays. The use of short incubation times to improve the turnaround time may compromise specificity. Finally, the use of two-site immunometric assays can greatly decrease cross-reactivity, but this is only feasible for molecules large enough to simultaneously bind two antibodies.

The Hook Effect

The hook effect may occur in turbidimetric and nephelometric assays and in two-site immunometric assays performed in one step (109–111). The hook effect represents the condition of antigen excess, whereby very high concentrations of the analyte saturate all available antigen binding sites on the reagent antibodies without forming complexes. Thus, above a certain concentration of analyte, progressively lower results are produced (Figure 3).

The hook effect has been reported for hCG (109, 112), CA 19-9 (113), CA 125 (114–116), quantitative immunoglobulin assays (111), prostate-specific antigen (117), myoglobin (118), and many other analytes. In turbidimetric and nephelometric assays, which rely on the light-scattering effect of large immune complexes between antigen and antibody, high concentrations of the analyte saturate all available antigen-binding sites on the antibody without forming immune complexes (Figure 4A). Modern nephelometers and dedicated turbidimeters have built-in checks for antigen excess. Turbidimetric assays performed on routine chemistry analyzers may not be able to perform an antigen excess check. Similarly, in immunometric (sandwich) assays performed in one step, i.e., the antigen (sample), capture antibody, and detection antibody are incubated together, high concentrations of the antigen can saturate all binding sites so that no "sandwich" bridges are formed (Figure 4B). The hook effect can be eliminated from immunometric assays by employing a two-step procedure in which there is a wash step between the incubation of the sample and the capture antibody and the addition of the detection antibody (Figure 4B).

Interfering Antibodies

Endogenous and exogenous antibodies can interfere with immunoassays. Because of their reagent-excess conditions, two-site immunometric assays are prone to interference from endogenous antibodies that can bind reagent antibodies (81, 83, 85, 87, 119–123). This is illustrated in Figure 5.

There are two general types of endogenous antibodies that interfere with immunometric assays, anti-animal antibodies and heterophile antibodies. Both types interfere with

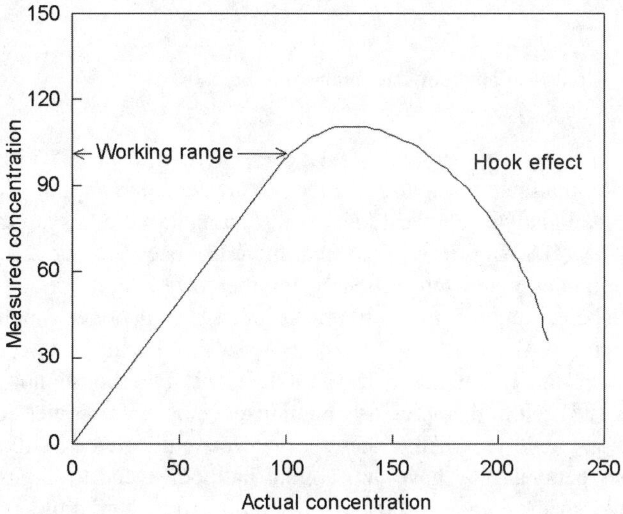

FIGURE 3. Illustration of the hook effect.

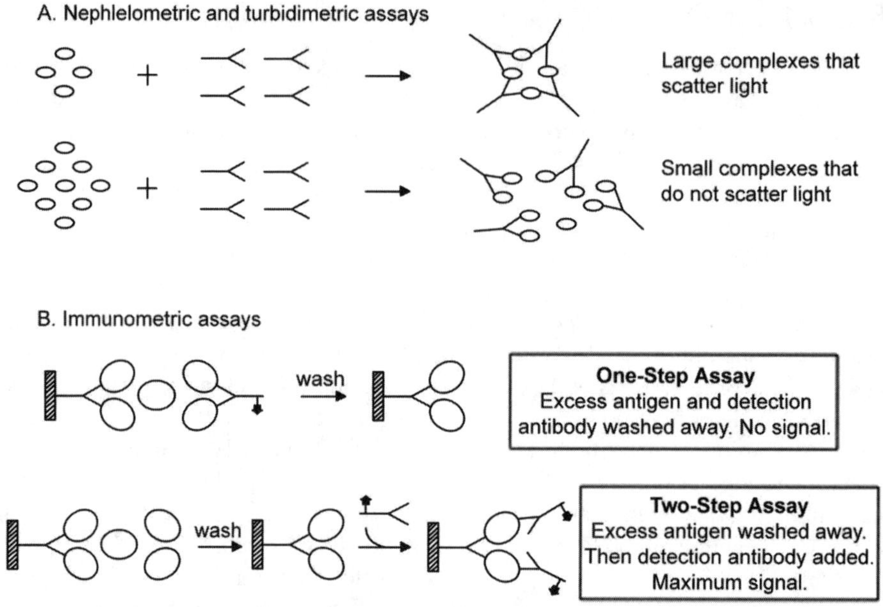

FIGURE 4. Mechanism of the hook effect.

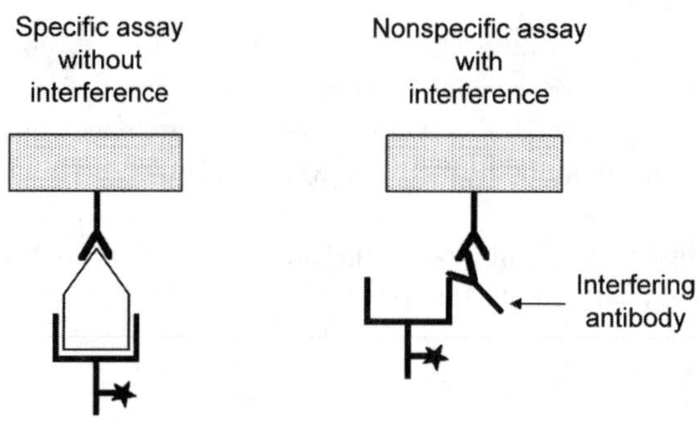

FIGURE 5. Illustration of antibody interference in immunometric assays.

two-site assays by binding the capture antibody to the detection antibody in the absence of the specific antigen analyte. The best known anti-animal antibodies are the **human anti-mouse antibodies (HAMA)**. In recent years, there has been an increasing use of mouse monoclonal antibodies given intravenously for therapeutic purposes or for location of tumors using labeled monoclonal antibodies, and some patients generate an immune response producing HAMA (124, 125). The HAMA formed may cause false-positive or falsely increased results in immunometric assays that use two mouse monoclonal antibodies as reagents (85). New therapies use humanized mouse antibodies to minimize this immune response. However, whether these humanized antibodies are still immunogenic is unknown. Other persons may have anti-animal antibodies due to exposure to antigens from a particular species, e.g., vaccines from rabbit or chicken, anti-snake venom from horse, or calcitonin from salmon or from occupational or casual contact with pets and other animals (85). Because of homology between antibodies from different species, these may exhibit sufficient cross-reactivity to interfere with assays using mouse, sheep, or goat capture and detection antibodies.

It is difficult to predict if a particular serum will cause false elevations in a particular assay for several reasons. Although HAMA usually interfere with assays that use mouse monoclonal antibodies, occasionally they do not. If the concentration of HAMA is low, some assays have sufficient blocking agent to inhibit the interference. Finally, anti-animal antibodies may cross-react with antibodies from other species (126).

Heterophile antibodies are poorly defined antibodies generated against no easily identifiable antigen (86, 127). In some cases, these may be natural antibodies that bind other endogenous antibodies as part of the regulation of the normal immune response (128). In other cases, they may be autoantibodies that have broad specificity against a variety of antigens including immunoglobulins. Antibodies with broad specificities are called polyspecific antibodies. Rheumatoid factor, frequently present in patients with rheumatoid arthritis, may cause false increases by binding to the Fc region of reagent antibodies. The terms anti-animal antibodies and heterophile antibodies are frequently used loosely and interchangeably since both antibodies interfere by the same mechanism. But there are important differences between these antibodies. Their sources are different and heterophile antibodies usually have weaker binding and less specificity than anti-animal antibodies (129).

Regardless of these subtle differences, there are many reports of anti-animal and heterophile antibody interferences in immunometric assays (119, 120). A short list of examples includes falsely elevated values for thyrotropin (123, 130, 131), CA 125 (132), FSH (133), C-reactive protein (134), TnI (135), and hCG (123, 136–138). The false positivity in hCG assays has lead to inappropriate chemotherapy and surgery in a number of women (136, 138–140). Most reports of antibody interference in immunometric assays have been false increases. As with cross-reactivity in immunometric assays and for the same reason, negative interference is less common, but it has been reported (85, 141).

Polyspecific antibodies also may interfere by binding to components of the reagent system other than the capture and detection antibodies. Thus, Ritter et al. (142) reported on antibodies that bound fluorescein-thyroxine conjugate, causing a false decrease in an FPIA for T4. This same group reported on an antibody to thyroxine-glucose-6-phosphate dehydrogenase conjugate that caused a false decrease in the EMIT T-uptake assay (143).

Endogenous antibodies may also interfere with immunoassays by binding to the analyte. Antibody complexes with large analytes are usually called macro-enzymes or macrohormones, such as macro-amylase or macro-prolactin. These have already been described. For small molecules, most reports have concerned antibodies against thyroxine, triiodothyronine (79, 144 –146), and digoxin (147, 148), but there is also a report of an antitestosterone antibody, which caused positive interference (149).

The reagents for all immunometric assays, and probably most other immunoassays as well, include blocking agents to minimize the possibility of heterophile and anti-animal antibody interference. However, this type of interference is still possible and does occur in all immunometric assays (unless samples are pretreated to remove all antibodies before the assay is performed). Some assays may be more prone to interference than others because insufficient blocking agent was included. It is very difficult to determine how much blocking agent is required and no type or amount of blocking agent can block all interfering antibodies. When interference by endogenous antibodies is suspected, it is useful to have one or more techniques available to help in the investigation.

A variety of physical and chemical techniques can be used to treat a serum sample to remove interfering antibodies, including ultrafiltration (147); protein A (150) or protein G (144) treatment, which removes immunoglobulin G; precipitation of protein with trichloroacetic acid (147) or ethanol (151); precipitation of immune complexes and antibodies with polyethylene glycol 6000 (130 g/L) (144); and denaturation of antibodies with sulfhydryl agents and detergents (152). These methods are time consuming and not suitable for routine use, but they may be helpful for investigating suspicious samples. When using any of these techniques, it is important to run controls, presumed not to contain interfering antibodies, to ensure that the treatments do not also remove or damage the analyte.

The main technique for investigating potential heterophile antibody interference is the use of blocking agents, which have been reviewed (85). Blocking agents in this context are nonimmune serum, partially purified immunoglobulin fractions, and various commercially available preparations specifically designed to block interfering antibodies. These last two blocking agents are theoretically stronger treatments, but unprocessed, whole, nonimmune serum has the advantage that it contains a diverse mixture of proteins that may adsorb out many types of interfering antibodies. Historically, nonimmune globulin from the species used to produce the test antibodies was used. For assays that use a capture antibody and a detection antibody from different species, addition of nonimmune globulin from each species is recommended (119, 132). If two mouse monoclonal antibodies are used, it has been suggested that bovine immunoglobulin be added in addition to mouse immunoglobulin, since the bovine immunoglobulin seems to supplement the ability of mouse serum to block interfering antibodies (86).

The commercially available, specifically designed preparations include the following: Immunoglobulin Inhibiting Reagent (IIR; Bioreclamation) (153), Heterophile Blocking Reagent (HBR; Scantibodies), Heterophile Blocking Tube (HBT; Scantibodies), Heteroblock (Omega Biologicals), and polymerized nonimmune (irrelevant) monoclonal antibodies (MAK-33) (154, 156). The Heterophile Blocking Tubes contain predispensed, lyophilized binders suitable for treating individual 0.5-mL sample aliquots without dilution (156, 157). These blocking agents work well against most heterophile antibodies and anti-animal antibodies, but none is perfect (153, 154, 158). The authors recommend that at least one or two of these be available in laboratories for investigating antibody interferences. The convenient, single sample packaging of some commercial blocking agents makes them easier to use than animal serum.

Exogenous antibodies may interfere with immunoassays as well. Digibind® is the antigen-binding fragment (Fab) derived from specific anti-digoxin antibodies given as an antidote for digoxin intoxication. The ability of Digibind to interfere in digoxin immunoassays has been well documented (159–162). As Digibind binds digoxin, large amounts are drawn out of tissues into the blood, greatly increasing the total circulating digoxin concentration. In most digoxin assays, the digoxin dissociates from the Digibind causing very high measured digoxin. Digibind may also compete with the reagent antibodies for binding the tracer, which may cause falsely low results. Therefore, the effect of Digibind on digoxin assays is unpredictable (163, 164). It has been proposed that it would be helpful to measure the free, unbound digoxin concentration during Digibind therapy (165), which may be achieved by ultrafiltration of the serum or with selected immunoassays for digoxin (166).

Signal Interference

Immunoassays require an indicator mechanism to detect the antigen–antibody complex (e.g., radioactive tracer, enzyme reaction, light scatter). Some samples may contain endogenous or exogenous compounds that artifactually increase or decrease the magnitude of the indicator response without affecting antigen–antibody binding. This is called signal interference. Because there are many types of indicator mechanisms used in immunoassays, there are many types of signal interference. A few examples are illustrated here.

Spectral interferences by bilirubin, hemoglobin, and turbidity described previously can interfere in immunoassays as well. For example, the fluorescence of bilirubin was reported to interfere with an FPIA method for monoethylglycinexylidide (167), giving a high blank error by the instrument rather than an erroneous result. Eosin, which is fluorescent and sometimes applied to burns, can be absorbed in sufficient amounts to cause negative interference with an FPIA method for vancomycin (168). A final example of spectral interference is the report that an aspirin metabolite in urine, salicyluric acid, could interact with NADH in such a way as to diminish its absorbance at 340 nm and cause false-negative drug screens by EMIT assays (169, 170). Usually, these spectral interferences do not affect two-step assays where a wash step would remove the interfering substance.

For EIA, elevated activity of the detection enzyme in the sample may cause false increases in the measured result (171, 172). For example, Butch et al. (173) reported that high-molecular-mass forms of alkaline phosphatase found in some serum samples could cause false elevations in the Stratus creatine kinase MB assay, which uses an alkaline phosphatase label. Similarly, purified alkaline phosphatase added to serum caused false increases in the Stratus TnI assay (174). Many immunoassays take advantage of the high affinity binding of biotin to streptavidin. With very high serum concentrations of biotin obtainable during high-dose biotin therapy, this biotin–streptavidin interaction can be dissociated, causing false-negative results (175). As new mechanisms of nonisotopic detection in immunoassays are developed, expect new examples of signal interference in the future.

Matrix Effects

Matrix effects in immunoassays are essentially the same as matrix effects in other assays (previously discussed). However, antigen–antibody binding reactions are often quite sensitive to variations in the matrix and differences in the matrix may also alter the efficiency of separation of bound and unbound fractions and the extent of nonspecific binding of the tracer.

EXOGENOUS INTERFERENTS

There are thousands of exogenous substances that have the potential to interfere with laboratory tests. This is exemplified by the encyclopedic drug files that list interferences by medications (5, 176–178). Hemoglobin base oxygen carriers, although exogenous, were covered under Hemolysis because of the similarity. Besides drugs, materials given to patients for diagnostic purposes and specimen additives such as anticoagulants and preservatives may interfere with some assays. There are also characteristics of nonspecimens, i.e., calibrators, controls, and proficiency testing samples that may make them behave differently than human specimens in some assays. Differences in these test materials can be considered interferences as well. Rather than list examples of exogenous interferences, some key issues pertinent to these three categories of exogenous interferences follow.

Drugs and Diagnostic Materials

Many medications interfere with laboratory tests. Most drugs are small organic molecules (<1 kDa) with a variety of polar and nonpolar functional groups. Metabolites of drugs may interfere with the same analyses as the parent drugs do, and they may interfere with the measurement of the parent drug. The most common metabolic transformations are oxidations; reductions; ester and amide hydrolysis; conjugation with glucuronide, glycine, or sulfate; and acetylation, which take place in the liver (179). Liver disease may alter the metabolic rate and circulating proportions of parent drug and metabolite. Most nonpolar drugs are metabolized to more polar forms, so they can be excreted in the urine (179). In patients with renal insufficiency, metabolites may accumulate in the blood. Many of the metabolites have the potential to be more reactive than the parent drugs. Hydroxylation, aldehyde formation, and the addition of acetyl groups often make drugs more reactive in assays. Phenytoin and its primary metabolite, 5-(p-hydroxyphenyl)-5-phenylhydantoin, can cause false-positive barbiturates screens (180). The hydroxylated and demethylated metabolites of cyclosporin G have highly variable cross-reactivity (5%–100%), depending on the assay (11). Furosemide itself does not interfere with the Jaffe method for creatinine, but one of its metabolites causes a negative interference (181). The interferences by the metabolites of drugs may be difficult to detect because of the unpredictability of the metabolite concentration.

Exogenous substances that may interfere with laboratory tests are sometimes given to patients for diagnostic purposes. For example, the results of laboratory tests performed after fluorescein angiography may be erroneous because of interference by intravenous fluorescein (182). Interference may also be caused by radiopaque materials administered for radiologic studies (183).

Additives

A variety of materials are added to the blood collection tubes for anticoagulation, to inhibit glycolysis, or to seal the stopper. All of the common anticoagulants [heparin, ethylenediaminetetraacetic acid (EDTA), citrate, and oxalate] have been reported to interfere with assays for many analytes (4). The antiglycolytic additives fluoride and iodoacetate may interfere with methodologies for a variety of analytes (4). Fluoride and iodoacetate inhibit glycolytic enzymes (184) and the latter inhibits CK activity (185). Finally, the silicone-coated stoppers used in some evacuated collection tubes may contaminate specimens with silicone and interfere with the measurement of ionized magnesium with an ion-selective electrode (186, 187).

Test Materials

Calibration, control, and proficiency testing materials are often made from a defibrinated plasma base with added substances that may interfere with analyses. Some components of the plasma base may be removed and other components, often of nonhuman origin, added to obtain the desired concentrations of various analytes. After the manufacturing process, these materials may contain very high concentrations of bilirubin, glucose, and multiple drugs. The final composition of these materials is frequently very different from the composition of typical human samples. Differences in assay response between these materials and human samples may go unnoticed because the differences are constant throughout the lot. This situation is more problematic with proficiency survey material because analytical results are compared with those of other laboratories. Interfering components of the proficiency testing material are likely to give different responses in different methods for the same analyte (188–190). For example, the therapeutic drug monitoring proficiency survey material of the College of American Pathologists contains many drugs, including lithium. One ion-selective electrode method for lithium gave consistently higher results than methods using other electrodes (191). Further investigation demonstrated a relationship between the measured lithium concentration and the quinidine concentration (191). Thus, in this case, the presence of many drugs in the survey material revealed that quinidine caused interference with one of the ion-selective electrode methods for lithium. Lastly, ascorbic acid causes a negative interference with the glucose oxidase method, but not the hexokinase method, for glucose (192, 193). Therefore, glucose oxidase methods show a negative bias compared with hexokinase methods when proficiency survey materials contain ascorbic acid. These examples demonstrate that proficiency testing results are a useful resource for the identification of interferences among methods for a given analyte.

INTERFERENCES IN NONCHEMISTRY TESTS

Interference may also occur for laboratory tests performed in hematology, microbiology, immunology, molecular diagnostics, and transfusion medicine, but to a lesser extent than clinical chemistry. In hematology, interference may produce spurious counts for cells or platelets. A well-known example of interference is spurious thrombocytopenia that occurs in samples from 0.1% to 2.0% of patients due to in vitro platelet clumping in the presence of anticoagulants (194). In addition to the thrombocytopenia, an elevated mean platelet volume and elevated platelet distribution width characterize this anomaly. Most anticoagulants may produce this anomaly: EDTA to the greatest extent and acid–citrate–dextrose (ACD) to the least extent (195). The anticoagulant-induced pseudothrombocytopenia is caused by antibodies that bind to platelets in vitro in the presence of anticoagulants, leading to platelet clumping. Studies suggest that expression of the GpIIb/IIIa complex may be altered by the anticoagulant, particularly EDTA, in certain patients (195). Other examples of interferents affecting the automated cell count are spuriously low eosinophil counts in HIV-infected patients due to degranulation of the cells (196) and a traumatic femoral venipuncture resulting in contamination of the blood sample with subcutaneous adipose tissue which causes a spurious increase in the white blood cell count (197). Furthermore, malaria-infected red blood cells and amphotericin B lipid complex have been reported to spuriously increase the platelet count (198, 199). If the cell or platelet count from an automated instrument is flagged or inconsistent with the patient's status, a review of the peripheral smear is indicated.

Transfusion medicine, microbiology, immunology, and molecular diagnostics frequently utilize test systems that involve antigen–antibody reactions or molecular probes for defined sequences. In general, these test systems are somewhat less subject to exogenous or endogenous interferents. Since the antibody composition for the patient is unique and, for the most part, unknown to the testing laboratory, cross-reactivity by an unknown antibody may affect a laboratory test result. For example, it has been reported that Lyme antibodies may interfere with tests for antinuclear antibodies (200). In transfusion medicine, frequently the serum sample is treated to remove certain constituents, usually antibodies during the process of antibody identification. The treatment may have unknown effects that alter the final result. As an example, rabbit erythrocyte stroma is frequently used to absorb cold autoantibodies from serum. A recent report identified that this reagent also absorbed anti-Vel antibodies that were then missed by the laboratory (201). Thus, reagents used to treat serum may also affect uncommon alloantibodies. As microbiology moves more toward molecular diagnostics for organ identification, the risk of interference with biochemical tests will be replaced by more accurate molecular tests. As an example, a study that compared molecular with phenotypic methods for identification of mycobacteria found that molecular tests were not only more rapid but also more accurate than traditional typing (202). With the move to more molecular testing, the risk for interferents should be reduced.

EVALUATION OF INTERFERENCE DURING METHOD VALIDATION

Detection of interference can be very difficult. The best opportunity to detect and characterize interferences is during the evaluation of an assay. Before putting an assay into routine use, laboratories are required to validate the procedure, i.e., confirm that the manufacturer's claims in the package insert are achievable in their laboratory. The validation process includes estimations of precision, accuracy, method comparison, linearity (and sometimes recovery), and interference studies. Besides the interference studies per se, tests of linearity and recovery and the method comparison can also provide information about potential interfering substances and their characteristics. These will be discussed in this section. The strategy is to identify known or likely interfering substances and to identify samples that appear to have or are likely to have interfering substances present and then to characterize these substances and samples. This process of experimental discovery will help tremendously after the assay is put into routine use, at which time recognition of inaccurate results due to interferences is quite difficult. However, the first step is the collection and review of as much information about the assay as possible.

Information Sources

While gathering information about the new assay, information should also be obtained about the comparison method (the old assay). Even if information about the old assay was collected previously, new information may have become available. If there is no old assay, i.e., this test is being added to the laboratory's repertoire, the results will still need to be compared to results from a referral laboratory and information about that assay will be necessary. There are a number of resources available. The Internet and resources like PubMed and the availability of many electronic journal articles make a thorough literature search extremely easy today. One would like to find out not only as much as possible about the specific assay under study, but also what is known about other methods that use the same analytical principle. Review the current edition of Young's drug (5) and preanalytical variables (4) files for information about the new and old assays. Both of these resources should be available in all laboratories. The preanalytical variables file lists interferences from hemolysis, bilirubin, lipemia, and various additives such as EDTA. *Interferographs* (3) also gives graphical representations of interferences by hemolysis, bilirubin, and lipemia in methods on a variety of automated instruments. Carefully review the "Limitations of the Procedure" section of the package inserts, which lists not only known interferences, but also substances that have been tested and found not to interfere. Again, remember to collect information about the old method. From time to time, both during method evaluation and during routine use of the assay, it may be helpful to compare results with results by another method. Develop a collegial and cooperative relationship with neighboring laboratories, including a referral laboratory, and find out what method they use and what substances interfere with their method. Finally, every laboratory should have the latest edition of the NCCLS Evaluation Protocols, which give detailed procedures for each experiment in a method validation. The interference protocol EP-7A (6) also gives a good deal of general information about interferences.

Interference Study

The **first step** is to decide what to test. Most laboratories test for interference from hemoglobin, bilirubin, and lipemia, but there may be a variety of other substances that should be tested. A literature search and review of other informational resources may have identified known or potential interfering substances. There may be suspect substances identified during the method comparison study (see below). It may be helpful to test drugs or endogenous substances with structures similar to the analyte. Lastly, consider the mechanism of the assay. For example, if it includes biotin–streptavidin in the reagent, biotin may interfere, and if the assay is an EIA using alkaline phosphatase, elevated alkaline phosphatase in patients' sera may interfere.

The **second step** is to produce or obtain preparations of the potential interfering substances. Preparation of a hemolysate is simple and the concentration of the stock hemolysate is usually high enough to measure on hematology analyzers. Conjugated bilirubin is available from chemical supply companies, but few of them have unconjugated bilirubin. Since conjugated bilirubin is more soluble and, therefore easier to work with, most laboratories use this form for interference studies, but differences in interference properties between conjugated and unconjugated bilirubin have been reported (48). Both forms of bilirubin must be protected from light. Testing for interference by lipemia typically has used Intralipid, a suspension of triglycerides for nutritional support, which is available in most hospital pharmacies. However, the CLSI (NCCLS) interference guidelines, EP7-A (6), no longer recommends the use of Intralipid to test for interference by lipemia due to reported differences between interference assessed with Intralipid or with lipoproteins (203, 204). They recommend using natural triglyceride-rich lipoproteins (VLDL and chylomicrons), which can be collected by ultracentrifugation. Detailed instructions on the preparation, handling, and use of hemolysates, bilirubin, and Intralipid or lipoproteins for interference testing are available (3, 6). Drugs and other compounds can usually be obtained from the pharmacy or chemical companies.

The **third step** is to prepare samples with the interfering substances added and analyze them. In order to detect analyte-dependent interference, the authors recommend preparing at least two pools from patient samples. The analyte concentrations of these pools should be near medical decision concentrations, but one concentration should be relatively low and one should be relatively high. Also stock preparations of the substances to be tested should be spiked into each pool at two concentrations (or more), one relatively low and one high concentration. Thus, there are two concentrations of interferent in the low analyte pool and two concentrations of interferent in the high analyte pool. If no interference is detected, the four samples give greater confidence in the results. If interference is detected and the amount of bias caused by a given concentration of interferent is essentially the same at the two analyte concentrations, then the interference is independent of analyte concentration. One can extrapolate these data to determine the bias across the range of interferent concentrations and to determine what concentrations will cause clinically significant bias. If a given concentration of interferent causes a different amount of bias at the two analyte concentrations, the interference is analyte-dependent. In this case, additional samples with a range of analyte and interferent concentration would be needed to fully characterize the interference (205, 206). For example, Table 4 shows the results of this four-sample interference experiment for hemoglobin interference in a hypothetical urea nitrogen assay and the creatinine and total bilirubin assays previously described in Analyte-Dependent Interference. There is no interference by hemoglobin in the urea nitrogen assay. In the creatinine assay, the negative bias is dependent on the hemoglobin concentration but not the creatinine concentration, so the interference is analyte-independent. For the total bilirubin assay, the negative bias varies with hemoglobin concentration and bilirubin concentration, so the interference is analyte-dependent. In this case, further studies with additional concentrations of bilirubin and hemoglobin should be performed. Manufacturers may assist with these more complex interference studies. Figure 6 is a flow chart for interference studies.

Method Comparison

In method comparison studies, samples are assayed by the new method and a comparison method, usually the old method or a reference method, and a regression analysis is performed. The main reason for this study is to document the relationship between the new method and the comparison method, but information about interferences can also be obtained. It is recommended that at least 40 samples with a wide range of concentrations be compared (CLSI/NCCLS). The authors recommend including other samples known or suspected of containing interfering substances. Samples giving atypical comparisons, i.e., outliers, are likely to contain an interferent. To increase the chances of finding these samples, one could include samples with hemolysis, elevated bilirubin, and turbidity; different types of samples (serum, plasma, etc.); samples from patients taking medications that may interfere; samples from patients with a variety of acute and chronic diseases, especially liver and kidney disease; and from patients with potentially interfering antibodies such as rheumatoid factor, antinuclear antibodies, and HAMA. If potential interfering substances are identified, additional samples may be collected to confirm the observation or, if possible, the specific interferent may be studied in the interference testing. While analyzing

TABLE 4. Results from a four-sample interference study

Analyte	Analyte concentration	Hb concentration, g/L	Result	Bias	Conclusion
Urea N, mg/L	100	2	100	0	No interference
	500	2	500	0	
	100	10	100	0	
	500	10	500	0	
Creat, mg/L	10	2	9.3	−0.7	Analyte-independent interference
	100	2	99.3	−0.7	
	10	10	6.5	−3.5	
	100	10	96.5	−3.5	
T Bil, mg/L	10	2	9.7	−0.3	Analyte-dependent interference
	100	2	96.9	−3.1	
	10	10	8.4	−1.6	
	100	10	84.3	−15.7	

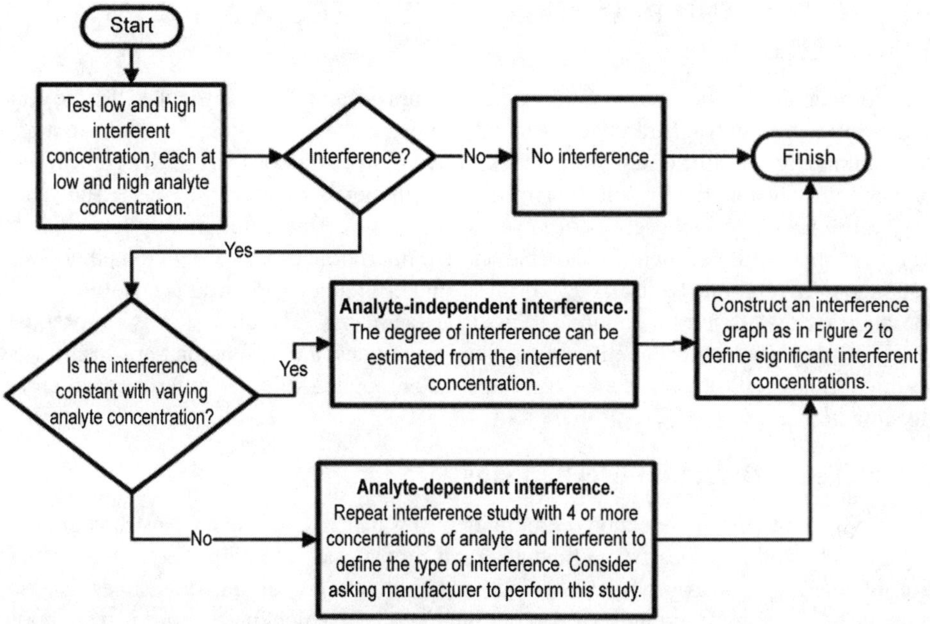

FIGURE 6. Flow chart for interference studies.

these data, keep in mind that the interference may be in the comparison method rather than in the new method and that interference affecting both assays equally will not be detected by the comparison study. Finally, attempts to separate the analyte from the interfering substance or to separate heterogeneous forms of the analyte, along with suitable controls, by various extraction, chromatographic, or electrophoretic techniques may be pursued. The separated fractions can be reanalyzed by both methods to see if the bias was eliminated. If a suitable separation technique is identified, it can be used for troubleshooting suspicious samples after the assay is put into routine use.

Linearity and Recovery

In linearity studies, often referred to as tests of parallelism in the case of immunoassays, it is wise to test dilutions of a few patient samples in addition to high standards or controls. Samples suspected of containing an interfering substance in the method comparison study (and nonsuspicious samples, as controls) can be checked for linearity upon dilution. Often samples with interferents present will display nonlinearity upon dilution or nonparallelism (with the standard curve), because the effect of the interferent is diminished by dilution or reacts by a different mechanism. Nonlinearity confirms that an interfering substance is present, but linearity does not guarantee the absence of interference because the effect of some interfering substance is linear.

In recovery studies, a known amount of pure analyte, if available, or a small volume of a calibrator, control, or patient sample with a high analyte concentration is spiked into samples and analyzed for the expected increase in concentration. Samples identified in the method comparison study as possibly containing an interferent can serve as the sample receiving the added analyte. Recovery significantly different from 100% (different enough to cause clinically significant bias) suggests the presence of an interfering substance in the samples to which the analyte is spiked.

DETECTING AND REPORTING INTERFERENCE DURING ROUTINE USE

Detection of interference during routine use of an assay can be very difficult. The true concentration of the analyte is rarely known and, therefore, there is no basis on which to judge the accuracy of a result. Usually the only clue is a result that does not fit the clinical picture or a grossly abnormal result. It is important to remember that an interfering substance may cause results to be falsely normal whether the true result is abnormally low or high. The best opportunity to identify and characterize interferences is during the method validation studies (previously discussed). If these studies are thorough, troubleshooting possible aberrant results during routine use will be facilitated. The first step is to establish detection mechanisms for identifying patients, specimens, and results that are suspicious. In the second step, several techniques can then be applied to see if interference can be documented.

Interference Detection Mechanisms

A thorough interference detection program identifies patients, specimens, instrument readings, results, and inquiries from clinicians requiring special attention. The initial evaluation of interferences may have identified certain clinical conditions, e.g., liver disease, renal insufficiency, autoimmune disease, or pregnancy, in which interference is more common. In addition, the evaluation may have identified one or more drugs that can interfere with the analysis. In many cases, this information will not be available. In the hospital setting, a fully integrated hospital and laboratory information system (LIS) may be able to flag orders for the test on patients with these conditions or receiving these drugs. If this information is available, results from patients in these categories or taking these drugs may be scrutinized more thoroughly.

If hemolysis, elevated bilirubin, or lipemia interfere, it is important to visually inspect the samples. If the interference is only significant above a certain concentration, some objective measurement of the interfering substance is recommended because subjective visual estimates are not accurate (7). It is useful to have an instrument that can measure serum indices, but specific measurements of hemoglobin, bilirubin, and triglyceride can be used as well. Serum indices are quantitative estimates of hemoglobin, bilirubin, and turbidity (lipemia) that have been incorporated into several general chemistry analyzers (207, 208). These indices are helpful for the detection of these endogenous interferences and several authors have proposed using the indices along with interferographs or mathematical equations to correct results for interference (209–211).

Most instruments will print various error codes such as for a high blank, etc., whether or not a quantitative result is produced as well. These should always be checked carefully and may indicate a sample with an interfering substance is present. In assays that have a high frequency of anomalous results, extreme measures to test for interferences may be necessary, such as testing sample blanks or nonspecific binding on all samples or analyzing two dilutions on all samples.

Results can be screened for possible interference in three ways. The delta check is a comparison of the patient's current result with the previous result. If an interfering substance is varying in concentration, this might be detected with a delta check. The second way to screen results for possible interference is by checking the results of two or more physiologically related assays run simultaneously. For example, although the combination of elevated free thyroxine and elevated thyroid-stimulating hormone can occur in secondary hyperthyroidism, it is rare. When this combination of results does occur, it may be due to interference in one or both of these assays. The last way is to have the LIS screen all results for outliers, e.g., the most extreme 1% or 2% of results. Investigation of highly unusual results may identify an interferent.

The final component of a thorough interference screening program is clinician inquiry. Many times clinicians provide valuable information by calling the laboratory with concerns about results that are unexpected or inconsistent with the patient's clinical picture.

Techniques to Document Interference

Three major techniques can be used to investigate and document whether an interfering substance is present in a sample:

- Test the sample by another method.
- Perform linearity studies on it.
- Treat the sample to see if an interfering substance can be removed, destroyed, or inhibited.

Laboratories rarely have two methods for the same analyte readily available. That is why it is very helpful to have a relationship with neighboring laboratories, including the primary referral laboratory, to help each other out from time to time by analyzing suspicious samples. Obviously the other laboratory must use a different method and preferably a method that uses a different methodological principle. For example, an interferent with the alkaline picrate method for the determination of creatinine is unlikely to interfere with an enzymatic creatinine method.

The easiest test for potential interference is to check for nonlinearity upon dilution. The authors recommend preparing and analyzing three or more dilutions, the results of which can be plotted against the expected results. If the dilutions are nonlinear, this is strong evidence for the presence of an interfering substance. However, the effect of some interferents is linear upon dilution, so the finding of linearity does not rule out the presence of an interferent.

Finally, the sample can be treated to attempt to remove, destroy, or inhibit the interfering substance. Possible treatments include extraction, chromatography, ultrafiltration, and addition of a heterophile-blocking preparation. Addition of a heterophile-blocking preparation is quite easy and quick. The other techniques are time consuming. All of these procedures need to be checked with control samples. In addition, the identity of the interfering substance is usually not known at this point so one cannot predict what treatment, if any, will work. Several treatments may need to be tried.

Reporting Results with Interference

Technologists frequently annotate results from specimens with visually apparent endogenous interferents, such as hemoglobin, increased bilirubin, and turbidity. However, this practice may be insufficient. A simple notation such as "hemolyzed" is insufficient because the physician has no way of knowing whether the hemolysis has any effect on the result or in what direction. In addition, hemolysis may adversely affect only one or a few tests on a multianalyte panel. A more complete statement is preferred, e.g., "Specimen moderately hemolyzed. This is likely to cause the potassium and lactic dehydrogenase results to be falsely increased and the bilirubin result to be falsely decreased. No change is expected for the other results." Individual results that would have extreme bias may be suppressed and this action should be included in the notation as well.

The laboratory should have policies for rejecting specimens with visually apparent interferents and criteria for the specimen recollection. This is especially true for hemolysis, which is usually caused by poor specimen collection or handling, whereas elevated bilirubin or lipemia is likely to be present in a recollected sample as well. Colored charts are available to assess visually the amount of hemolysis, degree of bilirubin elevation, and lipemia/turbidity. Some samples are difficult or impossible to recollect. The ordering physician should be consulted before rejecting samples. In addition, sometimes even an inaccurate result may be helpful to the physician, as when the interpretation of the result would be the same with or without the interference. For example, if the creatinine is elevated and bilirubin is present in sufficient concentrations to cause a negative interference, it would be clear that creatinine is elevated. In addition, as already mentioned, not all tests on a panel may be affected.

Some authors have suggested correcting results for interference (within limits) for hemoglobin if its concentration can be measured (210, 211). This approach could be done for other interferents that can be measured, e.g., bilirubin or I-index, triglycerides or L-index, glucose. The creatinine result in the previous example could be even more informative to the physician if one could estimate the true value of creatinine given the bilirubin concentration. If a lab decides that correcting results for interference is feasible, the actual result should be reported along with the corrected result in the annotation, e.g., "Specimen moderately hemolyzed (200 mg/dL hemoglobin). Based on our interference studies, the true potassium concentration is approximately 4.5 mmol/L and the true lactic dehydrogenase activity is approximately 200 U/L. No change is expected for the other results."

It may be possible to report results on samples that have had an interferent removed. For example, if lipemia interferes, it is generally considered acceptable to report results from the clear infranate of a lipemic sample after ultracentrifugation. A more controversial situation is a result of an immunometric assay that decreases after treatment with a heterophile antibody blocking agent. For example, if troponin is spuriously elevated and treatment of the sample with a blocking agent reduces the result to normal, the normal result probably could be reported, but the original result and the action taken should be included in the report. However, if the elevated result is reduced, but still elevated, one cannot be sure that all of the interferent was removed. Again, this can be included in the report.

SUMMARY AND RECOMMENDATIONS

There are many endogenous and exogenous sources of interferences in laboratory tests. It is easy to recognize the visually apparent endogenous sources, hemolysis, elevated bilirubin, and lipemia, but endogenous compounds like glucose, creatinine, and endogenous antibodies cannot be detected by eye. Similarly, most exogenous interfering substances, primarily medications and sample additives, cannot be detected visually. In this chapter, some general concepts regarding interferences were reviewed and specific examples of endogenous and exogenous interferences were given, including several unique aspects of interferences in immunoassays. Recommendations have been provided on the evaluation of interferences during method validation studies and on the detection and investigation of interference during the routine use of an assay. With this in mind, the authors now make some recommendations to laboratory personnel and to manufacturers of laboratory assays and instruments.

Recommendations to Laboratory Personnel

Recognition of samples and results that may be affected by an interfering substance and investigation of those samples is usually handled by laboratory personnel. Sometimes the unexpected results are brought to the attention of the laboratory by physicians, but it is still laboratory personnel that must investigate and resolve the issue. A thorough evaluation of interferences, including a thorough review of the literature, should be a major component of the validation of methods. Knowledge gained at that time will be invaluable for investigating spurious results after the assay is in routine use. A complete summary of this information should be included in the procedure so all technologists can make use of the information. A good working relationship with the physicians the laboratory serves is helpful. Under those circumstances, physicians are more likely to mention unexpected results and provide the clinical information that may provide clues to the cause of interference.

Laboratories should establish a multipronged interference screening program. This program might include special attention to specimens and results from particular categories of patients or patients on certain medications. Such a program would require an integrated information system with access to diagnoses, pharmacy orders, and laboratory orders and could be programmed to flag those combinations that are frequently problematic. For example, the current "drug file" (5) is available in electronic form and the LIS could be programmed to compare pharmacy orders with the file for possible interferences. Specimens should be checked visually or with serum indices for hemolysis, elevated bilirubin, and turbidity and the results on samples with these endogenous interferents annotated appropriately or suppressed. Instrument printouts should be checked carefully for error codes. The use of one or more result screening methods, e.g., delta checks, discordant result checks, and extreme result checks, is recommended. Finally, laboratory personnel should keep up with the literature and carefully read manufacturers' customer bulletins since new interferences may be reported.

When the interference screening program identifies suspicious samples, the laboratory should utilize the various methods of documenting interference, such as testing linearity upon dilution, testing by another method, and various treatments to remove interference. Testing by another method typically requires sending the specimen to another laboratory. It is important to be sure the other laboratory is using a different method, preferably with a different method principle. For endogenous antibody interference, it is most desirable to check a two-site assay by a competitive inhibition assay, if possible. Heterophile interference usually will be reduced in a two-site method from a different manufacturer (86). On the other hand, suspected interference by HAMA may be similar for all assays using mouse antibodies for both capture and detection. Thus, in this case, it would be desirable to check the analysis with an assay using at least one antibody from another species. Neighboring laboratories can help each other out by providing this service at no charge. If there is a clinically meaningful difference between the two methods, interference is likely.

It is advisable to have available various sample treatment procedures, such as one or more endogenous antibody-blocking agents and a small ultracentrifuge, such as an airfuge, to clear lipemic specimens. If drug interference is suspected, discuss this possibility with the patient's physician. It may be possible to discontinue the medication or relate the interference to the dosing schedule. In addition, the pharmacy can be consulted to identify other patients taking the drug and to obtain a sample of the drug for interference testing. If a new interfering substance is identified, notify the manufacturer and return to the interference testing procedure to further investigate. If the interference appears to be analyte-dependent, ask the manufacturer to investigate more thoroughly. Contact the reagent or instrument manufacturer to obtain the most recent information from other users about interference with the assay. Finally, it is important to send samples to the manufacturer for confirmation of results and other studies. Working with manufacturers allows them to be aware of the problem, notify other users, and, hopefully, to correct the problem.

Recommendations to Manufacturers

During assay development, manufacturers of analytical methods and instruments should do their best to design an assay that is free from interference. However, it is probably impossible to eliminate interferences totally and a rigorous evaluation of interference and communication of this knowledge to customers is essential. The authors recommend that manufacturers test potential interfering substances with the described four-sample procedure and follow this up with more thorough studies on substances that display analyte-dependent interference. Also, instrument manufacturers should include in the instrument design methods for detecting interference such as serum indices and antigen excess testing.

Manufacturers are required by the Food and Drug Administration to include detailed information on interference in their package inserts. The information should include the basic design of the interference study and the concentrations of interferents and analytes evaluated. For analyte-dependent interference, the model used and multiple regression parameters should be included. It would also be helpful to include graphs such as those in Figures 1 and 2. Manufacturers could provide software programs and expert systems to help their customers analyze interference, both during method evaluation and during routine use. The mathematics and graphics involved with analyte-dependent interference especially may be beyond the capabilities of many laboratories. For example, a program to calculate the estimated true result given the measured result, the interferent concentration, and the laboratories maximum allowable bias limit would be very useful to the bench technologist. Such a program could be linked to an expert system that would generate an appropriate interpretive comment for annotating results. It may be feasible for manufacturers to include these aids in the package insert, on separate compact disks, or by download from the company's web site.

Manufacturers should be prepared to provide advice and support for the resolution of customers' interference problems, especially as users raise suspicions. This would include sharing any similar reports of interference from other laboratories and providing confirmation testing on particular samples and additional studies as necessary to characterize fully the interferences and, if possible, to work out the mechanism. In general, the cost of interference testing can be a financial strain on laboratories, but of minor consequence to manufacturers. Manufacturers should assist their customers with this cost, perhaps by providing extra reagents. The results of these investigations, whether or not interference is documented, should be made available to the customer. It is not practical to update package inserts frequently; however, these notifications and reports can be sent by email and made available on the company's web site.

APPENDIX

A. Calculations Necessary to Construct the Graphs of Figure 2

In general, using the interference model and coefficients (Table 1), an equation relating the measured analyte concentration to the interferent concentration is needed for each performance criterion (Figure 2).

The overall equation for the measured result in the model used for analyte-dependent interference is $F = c_0 + c_1[A] + c_2[I] + c_3[A][I]$, where F is the measured analyte concentration, [A] is the true analyte concentration, [I] is the interferent concentration, [A][I] is their product, and c_0, c_1, c_2, and c_3 are the respective coefficients. The terms $c_0 + c_1[A]$ simply represent the response of the analyte in the assay and are unrelated to the bias due to interference. The terms $c_2[I] + c_3[A][I]$ represent the bias. Set this part of the response equal to the allowable bias criteria or CLIA '88 total error criteria of the assay.

Creatinine: $c_2 = -0.35$, c_3 is not significant, bias limits ±0.68 mg/L or ±3.4%.

Bias = c_2[I] = –0.35[I]

–0.35[I] = ±0.68

[I] = ±0.68 Only –0.68 makes physical sense because [I] must be positive.

[I] = 1.97 This defines the vertical line near 2 g/L hemoglobin in Figure 2A.

For percent bias, divide the bias by [A] and express 3.4% as a fraction (0.034).

–0.35[I]/[A] = ±0.034	Derive the equation relating F to [I].
F = [A] + (–0.35[I])	Solve for [A] and insert it in the prior equation.
[A] = F + 0.35[I]	
–0.35[I]/(F + 0.35[I]) = ±0.034	As above, only –0.034 makes physical sense.
–0.35[I] = –0.034 × (F + 0.35[I])	
–0.35[I] = –0.034F – 0.0119[I]	
0.034F = 0.35[I] – 0.0119[I] = 0.338[I]	
F = 9.94[I]	This defines the angled line above 2 g/L hemoglobin in Figure 2A.

These steps can be repeated for the CLIA '88 total error criteria (3.0 mg/L or 15%) to solve for [I] = 8.57 and F = 1.98[I].

Total Bilirubin: $c_3 = -0.016$, c_2 is not significant, bias limits ±2.0 mg/L or ±10%.

Bias = c_3[A][I] = –0.016[A][I] = ±2.0

[A] = ±2.0/(–0.016[I])	Only a negative 2.0 makes physical sense.
[A] = (125/[I])	
F = [A] + Bias = [A] + (–0.016[A][I])	
F = (125/[I]) – {0.016 × (125/[I]) × [I]}	The [I]s cancel in the second term.
F = (125/[I]) – 2	This defines the curved line at the bottom of Figure 2B.

For percent bias, divide the bias by [A] and express 10% as a fraction (0.1).

Bias/[A] = (–0.016[A][I])/[A] = ±0.1	The [A]s cancel.
–0.016[I] = ±0.1	Only a negative 0.1 makes physical sense.
[I] = 6.25	This defines the vertical line at 6.25 g/dL hemoglobin on Figure 2B.

For each set of criteria, the equations define two lines that intersect to form four quadrants. Values for F and [I] can be entered into the bias equations to determine which quadrant has excess bias.

REFERENCES

1. Kroll MH, Elin RJ. Interference with clinical laboratory analyses. Clin Chem 1994;40: 1996–2005.
2. Schwartz MK. Interferences in diagnostic biochemical procedures. Adv Clin Chem 1973; 16:1–45.

3. Glick MR, Ryder KW, Glick SJ. Interferographs: user's guide to interferences in clinical chemistry instruments, 2nd ed. Indianapolis: Science Enterprises, Inc., 1991.
4. Young DS. Effects of preanalytical variables on clinical laboratory tests, 2nd ed. Washington, DC: AACC Press, 1997.
5. Young DS. Effects of drugs on clinical laboratory tests, 5th ed. Washington, DC: AACC Press, 2000
6. Powers DM, Boyd JC, Glick MR, Miller WG. Interference testing in clinical chemistry; approved guideline. NCCLS Document EP7-A. Wayne, PA: NCCLS, 2002.
7. Glick MR, Ryder KW, Glick SJ, Woods JR. Unreliable visual estimation of the incidence and amount of turbidity, hemolysis, and icterus in serum from hospitalized patients. Clin Chem 1989;35:837–9.
8. Munzenberger P, Emmanuel S. The incidence of drug-diagnostic test interferences in outpatients. Am J Hosp Pharm 1971;28:786–91.
9. Young DS, Thomas DW, Friedman RB, Pestaner LC. Effect of drugs on clinical laboratory tests. Clin Chem 1972;18:1041–303.
10. Datta P, Dasgupta A. Bidirectional (positive/negative) interference in a digoxin immunoassay: importance of antibody specificity. Ther Drug Monit 1998;20:352–7.
11. Yatscoff RW, Langman LJ, LeGatt DF. Cross-reactivities of cyclosporin G (NVa^2 cyclosporin) and metabolites in cyclosporin A immunoassays. Clin Chem 1993;39:1089–92.
12. Eng CD, Delgado R, Kroll MH. Complex analyte-dependent and analyte-independent interferences with conjugated bilirubin in the enzymatic phenol-aminophenazone peroxidase (PAP) method for creatinine determination. Eur J Clin Chem Clin Biochem 1993;31:839–50.
13. Kroll MH, Olson D, Rawe M, King C, Hagengruber C, Elin RJ. Comparison of creatinine as determined with the Ames Seralyzer and by three Jaffe-based methods. Clin Chem 1985;31:1900–4.
14. Schlebusch H, Gruenn U, Schneider Ch. Simultaneous interference of bilirubin and hemoglobin in creatinine determinations. Clin Chem 1993;39:1144.
15. Fraser CG. Biological variation: from principles to practice. Washington, DC: AACC Press, 2001.
16. Kroll MH, Ruddel M, Blank DW, Elin RJ. A model for assessing interference. Clin Chem 1987;33:1121–3.
17. Kazmierczak SC, Catrou PG, Boudreau D. Simplified interpretative format for assessing test interference: studies with hemoglobin-based oxygen carrier solutions. Clin Chem 1998;44:2347–52.
18. Meites S, Hogg CK. Direct spectrophotometry of total serum bilirubin in the newborn. Clin Chem 1960;6:421–8.
19. Elin RJ, Hosseini JM. Magnesium content of mononuclear blood cells. Clin Chem 1985;31:377–80.
20. Brydon WG, Roberts LB. The effect of haemolysis on the determination of plasma constituents. Clin Chim Acta 1972;41:435–8.
21. Greenson JK, Farber SJ, Dubin SB. The effect of hemolysis on creatine kinase determination. Arch Pathol Lab Med 1989;113:184–5.
22. Blank DW, Kroll MH, Ruddel ME, Elin RJ. Hemoglobin interference from in vivo hemolysis. Clin Chem 1985;31:1566–9.
23. Guder WG. Haemolysis as an influence and interference factor in clinical chemistry. J Clin Chem Clin Biochem 1986;24:125–6.
24. Behrendt H. Chemistry of erythrocytes. Springfield, IL: Charles C. Thomas, 1957.
25. Caraway WT. Chemical and diagnostic specificity of laboratory tests. Am J Clin Pathol 1962;37:445–64.
26. Flood J, Liedtke R, Mattenheimer H, Rothouse L, Trundle D, Vroon D, et al. A multicenter evaluation of the Boehringer Mannheim/Hitachi 717 system. Clin Biochem 1990;23:477–88.
27. Shull BC, Lees H, Li PK. Mechanism of interference by hemoglobin in the determination of total bilirubin. I. Method of Malloy-Evelyn. Clin Chem 1980;26:22–5.

28. Shull BC, Lees H, Li PK. Mechanism of interference by hemoglobin in the determination of total bilirubin. II. Method of Jendrassik-Grof. Clin Chem 1980;26:26–9.
29. Wenk RE. Mechanism of interference by hemolysis in immunoassays and requirements for sample quality. Clin Chem 1998;44:2554.
30. Hammett-Stabler CA, Snyder JA, Chapman JF, Rogers MW, King MS, Phillips JC. Hemolysis interferes with troponin I and troponin T immunoassays. Clin Chem 2003;49:A89.
31. Christenson RH, Gregory LC, Duh SH, Mackenzie C, Trump BF. Hemoglobin based blood substitutes: Interference with routine chemical tests. Clin Chem 1993;39:1129.
32. Ali AC, Mihas CC, Campbell JA. Interferences of o-raffinose cross-linked hemoglobin in three methods for serum creatinine. Clin Chem 1997;43:1738–43.
33. Glick MR, Pieper JM, Ryder KW, Danielson CA. Interference by stabilized human hemoglobins on immunochemistry and special chemistry tests. Clin Chem 1996;42:S312.
34. Leissing N, Mattia-Goldberg C, Balma D. Modification of hematology methods to overcome interferences from diaspirin cross-linked hemoglobin (DCLHb). Clin Chem 1993;39:1142.
35. Leissing N, Mattia-Goldberg C, Oskroba D. Modification of clinical chemistry methods to overcome interferences from diaspirin crosslinked hemoglobin (DCLHb). Clin Chem 1993;39:1144.
36. Albertson D, Nelson D, Pereira D, Hai TT, Goldberg C. Evaluation of two solid phase adsorbents for the selective removal of diaspirin crosslinked hemoglobin (DCLHb) from clinical samples. Clin Chem 1996;42:S193–4.
37. Creer MH, Ladenson J. Analytical error due to lipemia. Lab Med 1983;14:351–5.
38. Aw TC, Kiechle FL. Pseudohyponatremia. Am J Emerg Med 1985;3:236–9.
39. Miyada D, Tipper P, Jantsch D, Simpkins H, Steele W, Flores O. The effect of hyperlipidemia on Technicon SMAC measurements. Clin Biochem 1982;15:185–8.
40. Heller C, Hinzmann R, Hofmann M, Kaufhold S, Henkel E, Oellerich M. Lipid interference in the determination of the concentration of haemoglobin in plasma using the ACA SX analyzer. Eur J Clin Chem Clin Biochem 1996;34:811–6.
41. Rogers LC, Smith FA. Evaluation of Lipoclear, a non-ionic polymer system, for the removal of interfering lipemia. Clin Chem 1989;35:1103.
42. Hung TL, Shiesh SC. The effectiveness of LipoClear in eliminating lipemic interference in biochemical analyzers. J Biomed Lab Sci 1996;8:33–7.
43. Witte DL, Brown LF, Feld RD. Effects of bilirubin on detection of hydrogen peroxide by use of peroxidase. Clin Chem 1978;24:1778–82.
44. Spain MA, Wu AH. Bilirubin interference with determination of uric acid, cholesterol, and triglycerides in commercial peroxidase-coupled assays, and the effect of ferrocyanide. Clin Chem 1986;32:518–21.
45. Guy JM, Legg EF. Bilirubin interference in determinations of creatinine with the Hitachi 737 analyzer. Clin Chem 1990;36:1851–2.
46. Weber JA, van Zanten AP. Interferences in current methods for measurements of creatinine. Clin Chem 1991;37:695–700.
47. Bertholf RL, Johannsen LM, Bazooband A, Mansouri V. False-positive acetaminophen results in a hyperbilirubinemic patient. Clin Chem 2003;49:695–8.
48. Alvarez F, Whalen K, Scott MG. Conjugated, but not unconjugated, bilirubin negatively interferes in Hitachi 747 assay of inorganic phosphorus. Clin Chem 1993;39:1–6.
49. O'Leary N, Pembroke A, Duggan PF. A simplified procedure for eliminating the negative interference of bilirubin in the Jaffe reaction for creatinine. Clin Chem 1992;38:1749–51.
50. Rajs G, Mayer M. Oxidation markedly reduces bilirubin interference in the Jaffe creatinine assay. Clin Chem 1992;38:2411–3.
51. Wu TW, Kwan WK, Fung KP, Savage T. Enzymatic diminution of interference due to bilirubins on the Jaffe reaction of creatinine in a Cobas FARA II analyzer. Clin Chem 1995; 41:S162–3.
52. Sonnenblick M, Eylath U, Brisk R, Eldad C, Hershko C. Paraprotein interference with colorimetry of phosphate in serum of some patients with multiple myeloma. Clin Chem 1986;32:1537–9.
53. Larner AJ. Pseudohyperphosphatemia. Clin Biochem 1995;28:391–3.

54. Pierce GF, Garrett NC, Koenig J, Lichti DA, Chan KM. Interference by monoclonal proteins in the o-phthalaldehyde method for blood urea nitrogen. Clin Chim Acta 1986;154:233–6.
55. Steinberger BA, Ford SM, Coleman TA. Intravenous immunoglobulin therapy results in post-infusional hyperproteinemia, increased serum viscosity, and pseudohyponatremia. Am J Hematol 2003;73:97–100.
56. Kulpmann WR, Maibaum P, Sonntag O. Analyses with the KODAK-Ektachem. Accuracy control using reference method values and the influence of protein concentration. Part I. Electrolytes. J Clin Chem Clin Biochem 1990;28:825–33.
57. Kulpmann WR, Maibaum P, Sonntag O, Schumann G, Siekmann L. Analyses with the KODAK-Ektachem. Accuracy control using reference method values and the influence of protein concentration. Part II. Substrates. J Clin Chem Clin Biochem 1990;28:835–43.
58. Pudek MR, Nanji AA. Antibody interference with biochemical tests and its clinical significance. Clin Biochem 1983;16:275–80.
59. Andrews PA, Thomas PA. Macro-amylasaemia as a cause of persistently raised serum amylase. Br J Surg 1988;75:1035.
60. Bohner J, Stein W, Steinhart R, Wurzburg U, Eggstein M. Macro creatine kinases: results of isoenzyme electrophoresis and differentiation of the immunoglobulin-bound type by radioassay. Clin Chem 1982;28:t-23.
61. Fujita K, Takeya C, Saito T, Sakurabayashi I. Macro lactate dehydrogenase: an LDH-immunoglobulin M complex that inhibits lactate dehydrogenase activity in a patient's serum. Clin Chim Acta 1984;140:183–95.
62. Hirano T, Matsuzaki H, Miura M, Kojima E, Tamura N, Sekine T. An immunoglobulin G inhibiting lactate dehydrogenase activity. Clin Chim Acta 1986;159:17–25.
63. Bonhoff A, Vuille JC, Gomez F, Gellersen B. Identification of macroprolactin in a patient with asymptomatic hyperprolactinemia as a stable PRL-IgG complex. Exp Clin Endocrinol Diabetes 1995;103:252–5.
64. Cavaco B, Leite V, Loureiro MM, Ferreira MF, Pereira MC, Santos MA, et al. Spontaneously occurring anti-PTH autoantibodies must be considered in the differential diagnosis of patients with elevated serum PTH levels. J Endocrinol Invest 1999;22:829–34.
65. Arnqvist H, Olsson PO, von Schenck H. Free and total insulin as determined after precipitation with polyethylene glycol: analytical characteristics and effects of sample handling and storage. Clin Chem 1987;33:93–6.
66. Sapin R. The interference of insulin antibodies in insulin immunometric assays. Clin Chem Lab Med 2002;40:705–8.
67. Ligabue A, Poggioli MC, Zacchini A. Interference of specific autoantibodies in the assessment of serum thyroglobulin. J Nucl Biol Med 1993;37:273–9.
68. Erali M, Bigelow RB, Meikle AW. ELISA for thyroglobulin in serum: recovery studies to evaluate autoantibody interference and reliability of thyroglobulin values. Clin Chem 1996;42:766–70.
69. Dai J, Dent W, Atkinson JW, Cox JG, Dembinski TC. Comparison of three immunoassay kits for serum thyroglobulin in patients with thyroid cancer. Clin Biochem 1996;29:461–5.
70. Plebani M, Mion M, Altinier S, Girotto MA, Baldo G, Zaninotto M. False-positive troponin I attributed to a macrocomplex. Clin Chem 2002;48:677–9.
71. Bohner J, von Pape KW, Hannes W, Stegmann T. False-negative immunoassay results for cardiac troponin I probably due to circulating troponin I autoantibodies. Clin Chem 1996;42:2046.
72. Sturk A, Sanders GT. Macro enzymes: prevalence, composition, detection and clinical relevance. J Clin Chem Clin Biochem 1990;28:65–81.
73. Mifflin TE, Bruns DE, Wrotnoski U, MacMillan RH, Stallings RG, Felder RA, et al. University of Virginia case conference. Macroamylase, macro creatine kinase, and other macroenzymes. Clin Chem 1985;31:1743–8.
74. Cattaneo F, Kappeler D, Muller B. Macroprolactinaemia, the major unknown in the differential diagnosis of hyperprolactinaemia. Swiss Med Wkly 2001;131:122–6.

75. Sanchez-Munoz D, Romero-Gomez M, Moro A. Macro-AST as cause of unknown hypertransaminasaemia. Eur J Gastroenterol Hepatol 2003;15:103–4.
76. Jay DW. Macro-creatine kinase co-migrating with CK-MB on electrophoresis. Clin Chem 1988;34:1920.
77. Medeiros LJ, Greco FA, Walsh D, Gerson B. Macro creatine kinase type 1 with electrophoretic mobility identical to that of the MB isoenzyme. Clin Chem 1985;31:1393–6.
78. Jacobs E, Anzalone T, Sarkozi L. Immunoprecipitation method for CK-MB analysis reevaluated: influence of CK-BB and macro-CK on blank activities. Clin Chem 1988;34:585–8.
79. Cissewski K, Faix JD, Reinwein D, Moses AC. Factitious hyperthyroxinemia due to a monoclonal IgA in a case of multiple myeloma. Clin Chem 1993;39:1739–42.
80. Rej R. Accurate enzyme activity measurements. Arch Pathol Lab Med 1993;117:352–64.
81. Weber TH, Kapyaho KI, Tanner P. Endogenous interference in immunoassays in clinical chemistry. A review. Scand J Clin Lab Invest 1990;201(Suppl):77–82.
82. Miller JJ, Levinson SS. Interferences in immunoassays. In: Diamandis EP, Christopoulos TK, eds. Immunoassay. San Diego: Academic Press, 1996:165–90.
83. Ward G, McKinnon L, Badrick T, Hickman PE. Heterophilic antibodies remain a problem for the immunoassay laboratory. Am J Clin Pathol 1997;108:417–21.
84. Selby C. Interference in immunoassay. Ann Clin Biochem 1999;36:704–21.
85. Kricka LJ. Human anti-animal antibody interferences in immunological assays. Clin Chem 1999;45:942–56.
86. Levinson SS, Miller JJ. Towards a better understanding of heterophile (and the like) antibody interference with modern immunoassays. Clin Chim Acta 2002;325(1-2):1–15.
87. Bjerner J, Nustad K, Norum LF, Olsen KH, Bormer OP. Immunometric assay interference: incidence and prevention. Clin Chem 2002;48:613–21.
88. Marks V. False-positive immunoassay results: a multicenter survey of erroneous immunoassay results from assays of 74 analytes in 10 donors from 66 laboratories in seven countries. Clin Chem 2002;48:2008–16.
89. Emerson JF, Ngo G, Emerson SS. Screening for interference in immunoassays. Clin Chem 2003;49:1163–9.
90. Gosling JP. A decade of development in immunoassay methodology. Clin Chem 1990;36:1–27.
91. Gosling JP. Immunoassay: a practical approach. Oxford, U.K.: Oxford University Press, 2000.
92. Jortani SA, Miller JJ, Helm RA, Johnson NA, Valdes R Jr. Suppression of immunoassay results by cross-reactivity. J Clin Ligand Assay 1997;20:177–9.
93. Steimer W, Muller C, Eber B, Emmanuilidis K. Intoxication due to negative canrenone interference in digoxin drug monitoring. Lancet 1999;354:1176–7.
94. Wians FH Jr, Norton JT, Wirebaugh SR. False-positive serum tricyclic antidepressant screen with cyproheptadine. Clin Chem 1993;39:1355–6.
95. Berthod C, Rey F. Enormous cross-reactivity of hydrocortisone hemisuccinate in the "RIA-NEN" RIA kit for cortisol determination. Clin Chem 1988;34:1358.
96. Shen S, Elin RJ, Soldin SJ. Characterization of cross reactivity by carbamazepine 10,11-epoxide with carbamazepine assays. Clin Biochem 2001;34:157–8.
97. Szefler SJ, Koup JR, Giacoia GP. Paradoxical behavior of serum digoxin concentrations in an anuric neonate. J Pediatr 1977;91:487–9.
98. Graves SW, Brown B, Valdes R Jr. An endogenous digoxin-like substance in patients with renal impairment. Ann Intern Med 1983;99:604–8.
99. Valdes R Jr, Graves SW, Brown BA, Landt M. Endogenous substance in newborn infants causing false positive digoxin measurements. J Pediatr 1983;102:947–50.
100. Shaikh IM, Lau BW, Siegfried BA, Valdes R Jr. Isolation of digoxin-like immunoreactive factors from mammalian adrenal cortex. J Biol Chem 1991;266:13672–8.
101. Qazzaz HM, Jortani SA, Poole JM, Valdes R Jr. Evidence for presence of a reduced form of digoxin-like immunoreactive factor (dihydro-DLIF) in mammalian tissues. Clin Chem 1996;42:1092–9.

102. Jiang F, Wilhite TR, Smith CH, Landt M. A new digoxin immunoassay substantially free of interference by digoxin immunoreactive factor. Ther Drug Monit 1995;17:184–8.
103. Miller JJ, Straub RW Jr, Valdes R Jr. Analytical performance of a monoclonal digoxin assay with increased specificity on the ACS:180. Ther Drug Monit 1996;18:65–72.
104. Datta P, Dasgupta A. Interference from digitoxin-like immunoreactive factors reduced in a new monoclonal chemiluminescent digitoxin assay. Ther Drug Monit 1998;20:663–8.
105. Pratt JJ. Steroid immunoassay in clinical chemistry. Clin Chem 1978;24:1869–90.
106. Ghosh SK. Production of monoclonal antibodies to estriol and their application in the development of a sensitive nonisotopic immunoassay. Steroids 1988;52:1–14.
107. Parvaz P, Mathian B, Patricot MC, Garcia I, Revol A, Mappus E, et al. Production of monoclonal antibodies to dehydroepiandrosterone-sulphate after immunization of mouse with dehydroepiandrosterone-bovine serum albumin conjugate. J Steroid Biochem 1989;32:553–8.
108. Vining RF, Compton P, McGinley R. Steroid radioimmunoassay—effect of shortened incubation time on specificity. Clin Chem 1981;27:910–3.
109. Wheeler CA, Davis S, Degefu S, Thorneycroft IH, O'Quinn AG. Ovarian choriocarcinoma: a difficult diagnosis of an unusual tumor and a review of the hook effect. Obstet Gynecol 1990;75:1–9.
110. Fernando SA, Wilson GS. Studies of the 'hook' effect in the one-step sandwich immunoassay. J Immunol Methods 1992;151:47–66.
111. Butch AW. Dilution protocols for detection of hook effects/prozone phenomenon. Clin Chem 2000;46:1719–21.
112. Khosravi MJ, Diamandis EP. Immunofluorometry of choriogonadotropin by time-resolved fluorescence spectroscopy, with a new europium chelate as label. Clin Chem 1987;33:1994–9.
113. Wu JT, Christensen SE. Effect of different test designs of immunoassays on "hook effect" of CA 19-9 measurement. J Clin Lab Anal 1991;5:228–32.
114. Pesce MA. "High-dose hook effect" with the Centocor CA 125 assay. Clin Chem 1993;39:1347.
115. Barbati A, Di Renzo GC, Cosmi EV. Hook effect in immunoradiometric assay of CA 125 in peritoneal fluid: evidence of high CA 125 concentrations by a comparative immunoblotting analysis. Clin Chem 1993;39:1548–9.
116. Barbati A, Cosmi EV, Spaziani R, Ventura R, Montanino G. Serum and peritoneal fluid CA-125 levels in patients with endometriosis. Fertil Steril 1994;61:438–42.
117. Furuya Y, Cho S, Ohta S, Sato N, Kotake T, Masai M. High dose hook effect in serum total and free prostate specific antigen in a patient with metastatic prostate cancer. J Urol 2001;166:213.
118. Kikuchi H, Ohta A, Takahashi Y, Shibata A, Ohtake T, Watanabe K. High-dose hook effect in an immunochromatography-optical quantitative reader method for myoglobin. Clin Chem 2003;49:1709–10.
119. Boscato LM, Stuart MC. Incidence and specificity of interference in two-site immunoassays. Clin Chem 1986;32:1491–5.
120. Boscato LM, Stuart MC. Heterophilic antibodies: a problem for all immunoassays. Clin Chem 1988;34:27–33.
121. Kricka LJ. Interferences in immunoassay—still a threat. Clin Chem 2000;46:t-8.
122. Klee GG. Human anti-mouse antibodies. Arch Pathol Lab Med 2000;124:921–3.
123. Ismail AA, Walker PL, Barth JH, Lewandowski KC, Jones R, Burr WA. Wrong biochemistry results: two case reports and observational study in 5310 patients on potentially misleading thyroid-stimulating hormone and gonadotropin immunoassay results. Clin Chem 2002;48:2023–9.
124. Frodin JE, Harmenberg U, Biberfeld P, Christensson B, Lefvert AK, Rieger A, et al. Clinical effects of monoclonal antibodies (MAb 17-1A) in patients with metastatic colorectal carcinomas. Hybridoma 1988;7:309–21.
125. Kimball JA, Norman DJ, Shield CF, Schroeder TJ, Lisi P, Garovoy M, et al. The OKT3 Antibody Response Study: a multicentre study of human anti-mouse antibody (HAMA) production following OKT3 use in solid organ transplantation. Transpl Immunol 1995;3:212–21.

126. Thompson RJ, Jackson AP, Langlois N. Circulating antibodies to mouse monoclonal immunoglobulins in normal subjects—incidence, species specificity, and effects on a two-site assay for creatine kinase-MB isoenzyme. Clin Chem 1986;32:476–81.
127. Kaplan IV, Levinson SS. When is a heterophile antibody not a heterophile antibody? When it is an antibody against a specific immunogen. Clin Chem 1999;45:616–8.
128. Hurez V, Kaveri SV, Kazatchkine MD. Expression and control of the natural autoreactive IgG repertoire in normal human serum. Eur J Immunol 1993;23:783–9.
129. Hennig C, Rink L, Fagin U, Jabs WJ, Kirchner H. The influence of naturally occurring heterophilic anti-immunoglobulin antibodies on direct measurement of serum proteins using sandwich ELISAs. J Immunol Methods 2000;235:71–80.
130. Zweig MH, Csako G, Benson CC, Weintraub BD, Kahn BB. Interference by anti-immunoglobulin G antibodies in immunoradiometric assays of thyrotropin involving mouse monoclonal antibodies. Clin Chem 1987;33:840–4.
131. Landau-Levine M, Way BA, Clutter WE, Scott MG, Gronowski AM. Antibody interference with the Abbott AxSym immunoassay for thyroid-stimulating hormone. Clin Chim Acta 1999;281:177–80.
132. Boerman OC, Segers MF, Poels LG, Kenemans P, Thomas CM. Heterophilic antibodies in human sera causing falsely increased results in the CA 125 immunofluorometric assay. Clin Chem 1990;36:888–91.
133. de Koning CH, Popp-Snijders C, Martens F, Lambalk CB. Falsely elevated follicle-stimulating hormone levels in women with regular menstrual cycles due to interference in immunoradiometric assay. J Assist Reprod Genet 2000;17:457–9.
134. Benoist JF, Orbach D, Biou D. False increase in C-reactive protein attributable to heterophilic antibodies in two renal transplant patients treated with rabbit antilymphocyte globulin. Clin Chem 1998;44:1980–5.
135. Fitzmaurice TF, Brown C, Rifai N, Wu AH, Yeo KT. False increase of cardiac troponin I with heterophilic antibodies. Clin Chem 1998;44:2212–4.
136. Cole LA, Rinne KM, Shahabi S, Omrani A. False-positive hCG assay results leading to unnecessary surgery and chemotherapy and needless occurrences of diabetes and coma. Clin Chem 1999;45:313–4.
137. Butler SA, Cole LA. Use of heterophilic antibody blocking agent (HBT) in reducing false-positive hCG results. Clin Chem 2001;47:1332–3.
138. Rotmensch S, Cole LA. False diagnosis and needless therapy of presumed malignant disease in women with false-positive human chorionic gonadotropin concentrations. Lancet 2000;355:712–5.
139. Hussa RO, Rinke ML, Schweitzer PG. Discordant human chorionic gonadotropin results: causes and solutions. Obstetr Gynecol 1985;65:211–9.
140. Cole LA. Phantom hCG and phantom choriocarcinoma. Gynecol Oncol 1998;71:325–9.
141. Butler J. Negative interference in immunoassays. Clin Chem 1995;41:481–2.
142. Ritter D, Stott R, Grant N, Nahm MH. Endogenous antibodies that interfere with thyroxine fluorescence polarization assay but not with radioimmunoassay or EMIT. Clin Chem 1993;39:508–11.
143. Ritter D, Brown W, Nahm MH, Ladenson JH, Scott MG. Endogenous serum antibodies that interfere with a common thyroid hormone uptake assay: characterization and prevalence. Clin Chem 1994;40:1940–3.
144. Despres N, Grant AM. Antibody interference in thyroid assays: a potential for clinical misinformation. Clin Chem 1998;44:440–54.
145. John R, Othman S, Parkes AB, Lazarus JH, Hall R. Interference in thyroid-function tests in postpartum thyroiditis. Clin Chem 1991;37:1397–400.
146. Norden AG, Jackson RA, Norden LE, Griffin AJ, Barnes MA, Little JA. Misleading results from immunoassays of serum free thyroxine in the presence of rheumatoid factor. Clin Chem 1997;43:957–62.

147. Liendo C, Ghali JK, Graves SW. A new interference in some digoxin assays: anti-murine heterophilic antibodies. Clin Pharmacol Ther 1996;60:593–8.
148. Ingels M, Rangan C, Morfin JP, Williams SR, Clark RF. Falsely elevated digoxin level of 45.9 ng/mL due to interference from human antimouse antibody. J Toxicol Clin Toxicol 2000;38:343–5.
149. Torjesen PA, Bjoro T. Antibodies against [125I] testosterone in patient's serum: a problem for the laboratory and the patient. Clin Chem 1996;42:2047–8.
150. Hunter WM, Budd PS. Circulating antibodies to ovine and bovine immunoglobulin in healthy subjects: a hazard for immunoassays. Lancet 1980;2:1136.
151. Levine S, Noth R, Loo A, Chopra IJ, Klee GG. Anomalous serum thyroxin measurements with the Abbott TDx procedure. Clin Chem 1990;36:1838–40.
152. Muller W, Mierau R, Wohltmann D. Interference of IgM rheumatoid factor with nephelometric C-reactive protein determinations. J Immunol Methods 1985;80:77–90.
153. Nicholson S, Fox M, Epenetos A, Rustin G. Immunoglobulin inhibiting reagent: evaluation of a new method for eliminating spurious elevations in CA125 caused by HAMA. Int J Biol Markers 1996;11:46–9.
154. Reinsberg J. Different efficacy of various blocking reagents to eliminate interferences by human antimouse antibodies with a two-site immunoassay. Clin Biochem 1996;29:145–8.
155. Reinsberg J, Schmolling J, Ackermann D. A simple and sensitive assay for determination of human anti-idiotypic anti-B72.3 antibodies, which is not affected by the presence of tumour-associated glycoprotein 72. Eur J Clin Chem Clin Biochem 1996;34:237–44.
156. Preissner CM, O'Kane DJ, Singh RJ, Morris JC, Grebe SK. Phantoms in the assay tube: heterophile antibody interferences in serum thyroglobulin assays. J Clin Endocrinol Metab 2003;88:3069–74.
157. Tommasi M, Brocchi A, Cappellini A, Raspanti S, Mannelli M. False serum calcitonin high levels using a non-competitive two-site IRMA. J Endocrinol Invest 2001;24:356–60.
158. Sosolik RC, Hitchcock CL, Becker WJ. Heterophilic antibodies produce spuriously elevated concentrations of the MB isoenzyme of creatine kinase in a selected patient population. Am J Clin Pathol 1997;107:506–10.
159. Rainey PM. Effects of digoxin immune Fab (ovine) on digoxin immunoassays. Am J Clin Pathol 1989;92:779–86.
160. Banner W Jr, Bach P, Burk B, Freestone S, Gooch WM III. Influence of assay methods on serum concentrations of digoxin during FAB fragment treatment. J Toxicol Clin Toxicol 1992;30:259–67.
161. Ujhelyi MR, Robert S, Cummings DM, Colucci RD, Green PJ, Sailstad J, et al. Influence of digoxin immune Fab therapy and renal dysfunction on the disposition of total and free digoxin. Ann Intern Med 1993;119:273–7.
162. Dodds HM, Norris RL, Johnson AG, Pond SM. Evaluation and comparison of the TDxII, Stratus, and OPUS digoxin assays. Ther Drug Monit 1995;17:68–74.
163. Rainey PM. Digoxin immune Fab (Digibind) markedly affects the results of immunoassays for digoxin. Clin Chem 1989;35:1165.
164. Lehrer M, Catinella M. Observations of a renal patient treated with Digibind; comparison of digoxin levels by Abbott TDx and Opus. Clin Chem 1993;39:1240.
165. Ujhelyi MR, Robert S. Pharmacokinetic aspects of digoxin-specific Fab therapy in the management of digitalis toxicity. Clin Pharmacokinet 1995;28:483–93.
166. Hursting MJ, Raisys VA, Opheim KE, Bell JL, Trobaugh GB, Smith TW. Determination of free digoxin concentrations in serum for monitoring Fab treatment of digoxin overdose. Clin Chem 1987;33:1652–5.
167. Schutz E, Shipkova M, Niedmann PD, Wieland E, Armstrong VW, Oellerich M. Determination of monoethylglycinexylidide by fluorescence polarization immunoassay in highly icteric serum samples: modified precipitation procedure and HPLC compared. Clin Chem 1998;44:1269–74.

168. Leal T, Dupret P, Hassoun A, Wallemacq PE. Topical application of eosin to burns produces interference in measurement of serum vancomycin by fluorescence polarization immunoassay. Clin Chem 1997;43:1238–40.
169. Wagener RE, Linder MW, Valdes R Jr. Decreased signal in Emit assays of drugs of abuse in urine after ingestion of aspirin: potential for false-negative results. Clin Chem 1994;40:608–12.
170. Linder MW, Valdes R Jr. Mechanism and elimination of aspirin-induced interference in Emit II d.a.u. assays. Clin Chem 1994;40:1512–6.
171. Pesce AJ, Michael JG. Artifacts and limitations of enzyme immunoassay. J Immunol Methods 1992;150:111–9.
172. Maxey KM, Maddipati KR, Birkmeier J. Interference in enzyme immunoassays. J Clin Immunoassay 1992;15:116–20.
173. Butch AW, Goodnow TT, Brown WS, McClellan A, Kessler G, Scott MG. Stratus automated creatine kinase-MB assay evaluated: identification and elimination of falsely increased results associated with a high-molecular-mass form of alkaline phosphatase. Clin Chem 1989;35:2048–53.
174. Dasgupta A, Chow L, Wells A, Datta P. Effect of elevated concentration of alkaline phosphatase on cardiac troponin I assays. J Clin Lab Anal 2001;15:175–7.
175. Henry JG, Sobki S, Arafat N. Interference by biotin therapy on measurement of TSH and FT4 by enzyme immunoassay on Boehringer Mannheim ES700 analyser. Ann Clin Biochem 1996;33:162–3.
176. Salway JG. Drug-test interactions handbook. London: Chapman and Hall Medical, 1990.
177. Tryding N, Roos KA. Drug interferences and drug effects in clinical chemistry, 5th ed. Stockholm: Apoteksbolaget, 1989.
178. Siest G, Galteau MM. Drug effects on laboratory test results: analytical interferences and pharmacological effects. Littleton, MA: PSG Publishing, 1988.
179. Benet LZ, Sheiner LB. Pharmacokinetics: The dynamics of drug absorption, distribution and elimination. In: Gilman AG, Goodman LS, Rall TW, Murad F, eds. Goodman's and Gilman's The Pharmacological Basis of Therapeutics. New York: Macmillan, 1985:13–22.
180. Siff KS, Finkler AE. False-positive barbiturate test in urine owing to phenytoin and 5-(p-hydroxyphenyl)-5-phenylhydantoin. Clin Chem 1988;34:1359–60.
181. Murphy JL, Hurt TL, Griswold WR, Peterson BM, Rodarte A, Krous HF, et al. Interference with creatinine concentration measurement by high dose furosemide infusion. Crit Care Med 1989;17:889–90.
182. Bloom JN, Herman DC, Elin RJ, Sliva CA, Ruddel ME, Nussenblatt RB, et al. Intravenous fluorescein interference with clinical laboratory tests. Am J Ophthalmol 1989;108:375–9.
183. Blitzer MG, Wilkie PL, Shapira E. Interference of radiopaque diagnostic contrast material (diatrizoate meglumine) in assays of urinary amino acids. Clin Chem 1986;32:559.
184. Marbach EP, McLean M, Scharn M, Jones T. Sodium iodoacetate as an antiglycolytic agent in blood samples. Clin Chem 1975;21:1810–2.
185. Price NC. The reaction of rabbit muscle creatine kinase with some derivatives of iodoacetamide. Biochem J 1979;177:603–12.
186. Sachs C, Marsoner HJ, Ritter C, Kindermas C, Ghahramani M. Ionized magnesium measurement in serum. Clin Chem 1993;39:1176.
187. Marsoner HJ, Spichiger UE, Ritter C, Sachs C, Ghahramani M, Offenbacher H, et al. Measurement of ionized magnesium with neutral carrier based ISE's. Progress and results with the AVL 988-4 magnesium analyzer. Scand J Clin Lab Invest Suppl 1994;217:45–51.
188. Middle JG, Libeer JC, Malakhov V, Penttila I. Characterisation and evaluation of external quality assessment scheme serum. Discussion paper from the European External Quality Assessment (EQA) Organisers Working Group C. Clin Chem Lab Med 1998;36:119–30.
189. Ross JW, Miller WG, Myers GL, Praestgaard J. The accuracy of laboratory measurements in clinical chemistry: a study of 11 routine chemistry analytes in the College of American

Pathologists Chemistry Survey with fresh frozen serum, definitive methods, and reference methods. Arch Pathol Lab Med 1998;122:587–608.
190. Steele BW, Wang E, Palomaki G, Klee GG, Elin RJ, Witte DL. Sources of variability: a College of American Pathologists Therapeutic Drug Monitoring study. Arch Pathol Lab Med 2001;125:183–90.
191. Witte DL. Matrix effects in therapeutic drug monitoring surveys. Proposed protocol to identify error components and quality improvement opportunities. Arch Pathol Lab Med 1993; 117:373–80.
192. Lott JA, Turner K. Evaluation of Trinder's glucose oxidase method for measuring glucose in serum and urine. Clin Chem 1975;21:1754–60.
193. Siest G, Appel W, Blijenberg GB, Capolaghi B, Galteau MM, Heusghem C, et al. Drug interference in clinical chemistry: studies on ascorbic acid. J Clin Chem Clin Biochem 1978;16: 103–10.
194. Bartels PC, Schoorl M, Lombarts AJ. Screening for EDTA-dependent deviations in platelet counts and abnormalities in platelet distribution histograms in pseudothrombocytopenia. Scand J Clin Lab Invest 1997;57:629–36.
195. Schrezenmeier H, Muller H, Gunsilius E, Heimpel H, Seifried E. Anticoagulant-induced pseudothrombocytopenia and pseudoleucocytosis. Thromb Haemost 1995;73:506–13.
196. Thomson S, Sheridan B. Erroneous automated eosinophil counts in HIV-infected individuals. Br J Biomed Sci 1995;52:165–6.
197. Whiteway AJ, Bain BJ. Artefactual elevation of an automated white cell count following femoral vein puncture. Clin Lab Haematol 1999;21:65–8.
198. Beyan C, Cetin T, Kaptan K, Ural AU, Yalcin A. Does amphotericin B lipid complex (Abelcet) affect haematological parameters erroneously? Haematologia 2001;31:245–9.
199. Crabbe G, Van Poucke M, Cantinieaux B. Artefactually-normal automated platelet counts due to malaria-infected RBC. Clin Lab Haematol 2002;24:179–82.
200. Lovece S, Stern R, Kagen LJ. Effects of rheumatoid factor, antinuclear antibodies and plasma reagin on the serologic assay for Lyme disease. J Rheumatol 1991;18:1813–8.
201. Mechanic SA, Maurer JL, Igoe MJ, Kavitsky DM, Nance ST. Anti-Vel reactivity diminished by adsorption with rabbit RBC stroma. Transfusion 2002;42:1180–3.
202. Springer B, Stockman L, Teschner K, Roberts GD, Bottger EC. Two-laboratory collaborative study on identification of mycobacteria: molecular versus phenotypic methods. J Clin Microbiol 1996;34:296–303.
203. Nanji AA, Poon R, Hinberg I. Lipaemic interference: effects of lipaemic serum and intralipid. J Clin Pathol 1988;41:1026–7.
204. Cobbaert C, Tricarico A. Different effect of Intralipid and triacylglycerol rich lipoproteins on the Kodak Ektachem serum cholesterol determination. Eur J Clin Chem Clin Biochem 1993;31:107–9.
205. Kroll MH. Analyte-dependent interference and multi-interference. Dtsch Ges Klin Chem Mitt 1991;22:13–20.
206. Kroll MH, Chesler R. Rationale for using multiple regression analysis with complex interferences. Eur J Clin Chem Clin Biochem 1992;30:415–24.
207. Glick MR, Ryder KW, Vroon D, Masters BE, Sonntag O. Practical uses of serum indices to reduce errors from lipemia, icterus, and hemolysis. Clin Chem 1990;36:1008.
208. Pearson JR, Wells R, Wells A. Serum index identifies lipemic samples causing interference with bilirubin assay on Hitachi 717. Clin Chem 1991;37:2014–5.
209. Randall AG, Garcia-Webb P, Beilby JP. Interference by haemolysis, icterus and lipaemia in assays on the Beckman Synchron CX5 and methods for correction. Ann Clin Biochem 1990;27:345–52.
210. Jay DW, Provasek D. Characterization and mathematical correction of hemolysis interference in selected Hitachi 717 assays. Clin Chem 1993;39:1804–10.
211. von Eyben FE, Petersen PH, Lindegaard ME, Blaabjerg O, Norgaard PB, Arends J. Correcting for contamination from hemolysis in measurements of lactate dehydrogenase isoenzyme 1 in serum from patients with testicular germ cell. Clin Chem 1993;39:2199.

Chapter 4

Basic Principles of Instrumentation: Spectrophotometry, Fluorometry, Turbidimetry, and Nephelometry

Mary Hotaling

Photometry literally means light measurement and in the clinical laboratory it is used as a generic term describing analytical methods measuring light intensity. Currently in the clinical laboratory, the clear majority of analytical instruments are based on photometric measurement, making photometry the most utilized analytical method encountered by the clinical laboratory scientist. Photometric instrumentation takes advantage of physical phenomena resulting from light energy interacting with matter. The main photometric-based clinical laboratory methods involve measurement of molecular light absorption, emission, reflectance, and scatter to determine sample analyte concentration.

Molecular absorption methods include photometry and spectrophotometry. Molecular emission methods include fluorometry and chemiluminescence. Fluorometry, discussed in detail later in this chapter, is based on light emitted by sample fluorophores after excitation by light energy. Sample fluorophore concentration is proportional to the intensity of light emitted. Chemiluminescence involves chemical reactants that produce light and is covered more extensively in Chapter 7. Light reflectance methods include reflectometry, which is the basis for a number of point-of-care testing devices used in alternate site testing. These instruments are covered in Chapter 17. Particle concentration in solution may be measured by the light-scattering methods of turbidimetry and nephelometry. Particles in solution scatter light and the sample concentration is proportional to the intensity of light scattered. Additional particle counting clinical applications will be discussed in Chapter 14. Regardless of the precise type of light interaction with molecules and the particular measuring method, these photometric methods involve comparing an "unknown" sample concentration with one or more "known" standard or reference concentration(s). To understand how photometric measurements are made and how they are useful for determination of analyte concentration, a discussion of the nature, behavior, and subsequent interaction of light with matter is essential.

PROPERTIES OF LIGHT AND INTERACTION WITH MATTER

Light is a form of electromagnetic radiation energy consisting of visible and near-visible wavelengths. This radiant energy has both wave-like and particle-like properties such that light is most simply described as photons of energy traveling in waves. **Photons** are light particles or packets produced by vibrating electrical charges from the electrons of atoms and by the vibrations of atoms within molecules.

Light Wavelength, Amplitude, and Frequency

Light is generally described in terms of color that the eye observes. However, light is more precisely characterized using the terms wavelength, amplitude (intensity), and frequency. Using these terms, a single light wave consists of wavelength and amplitude (Figure 1A), where **wavelength** is the distance from a point on a wave to the same point on the next cycle of the wave. The wavelength corresponds to the color of light and is expressed in units of nanometers (nm), i.e., 10^{-9} meters, and is sometimes represented by the symbol lambda (λ). **Amplitude** is the peak height of a light wave and refers to light intensity. Photodetectors used in various photometric methods measure light intensity as opposed to wavelength and frequency. As light intensity increases, the electrical output from the photodetector increases proportionately. **Frequency** refers to the number of cycles of a wave generated in 1 second (c/s) and may be expressed in units of Hertz (Hz).

Interrelationships Among Energy, Wavelength, and Frequency

As stated earlier, light has wave and particle (photon) properties that are interrelated. The physicist, Max Planck, expressed the relationship between energy and frequency by stating that the energy of a photon (E) is directly proportional to the frequency (ν):

$$E \propto \nu \quad (1)$$

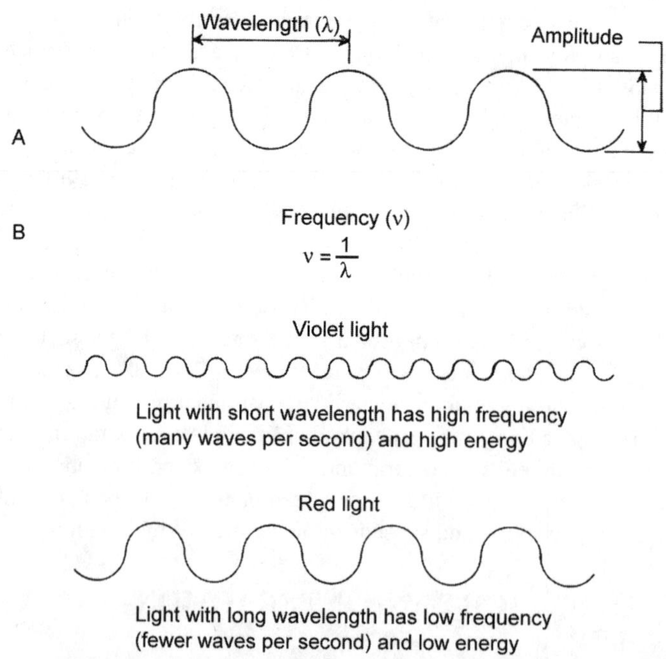

FIGURE 1. Characteristics of light waves: A shows wavelength and amplitude and B shows frequency.

TABLE 1. Interrelationships among wavelength, frequency, and energy

Energy and frequency	Energy and wavelength	Frequency and wavelength
$E = h\nu$	$E = \frac{hc}{\lambda}$	$\nu = \frac{c}{\lambda}$
where E = energy (photons) h = Planck's constant ν = frequency	where E = energy (photons) h = Planck's constant c = speed of light λ = wavelength	where ν = frequency c = speed of light λ = wavelength

The resulting proportionality constant is called Planck's constant (h). Derived equations that further define the interrelationships among light energy, frequency, and wavelength are given in Table 1. As can be seen in these equations, frequency (ν) is inversely proportional to the wavelength (λ). Consequently, as light frequency changes, so does its wavelength and energy content, such that shorter wavelengths contain more energy than longer wavelengths. This relationship is represented in Figure 1B.

Electromagnetic Spectrum

The electromagnetic spectrum is divided into regions based on how the waves are produced or detected. Figure 2 illustrates the relationships of wavelength (λ), frequency (ν), and energy (E) within the electromagnetic spectrum. As can be seen, the electromagnetic spectrum includes short-wavelength, high-energy gamma and x-rays, through the long-wavelength, low-energy radiowaves. Most often, visible light (380–750 nm) and ultraviolet (UV) light (220–380 nm) and occasionally short infrared (750–2000 nm) wavelengths are used in the modern analytical instruments in the clinical laboratory.

Interaction of Light with Matter

Light interacts with matter resulting in various phenomena including light absorption, reflection, refraction, emission, and scattering. These processes are currently employed as analytical techniques in one manner or another in many clinical instruments.

Absorption

Light absorption occurs as molecules or molecular compounds in solution interact with specific visible and UV wavelengths of light based upon the molecule's electron structure. Absorption of light energy is enough to excite certain orbiting electrons to a higher energy level (excited state). As the excited electrons fall back to the unexcited (ground) state, excess energy may be released as heat and/or light. Measurement of the interaction of visible and UV light with matter is broadly called **absorption spectrophotometry** and is used to determine the concentration of a target substance. Light absorption is the basis for **atomic absorption**, and **molecular absorption spectrophotometry** methods in the clinical laboratory. In molecular absorption spectrophotometry methods, the sample concentration is determined by measuring the amount of light the solution absorbs or transmits. These measurements are then compared to the absorbance or transmittance of known concentration standard solutions.

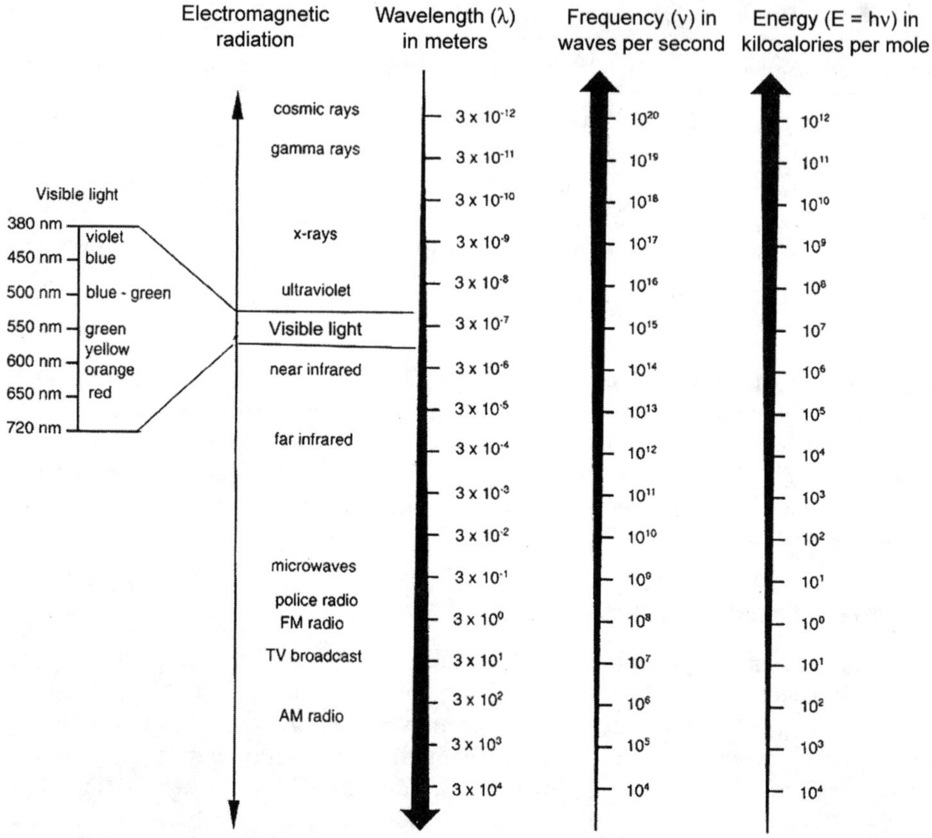

FIGURE 2. Electromagnetic spectrum.

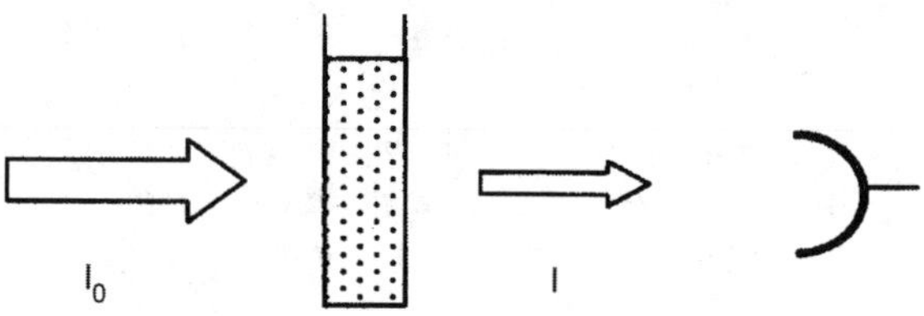

$$\%T = \frac{I}{I_0} \times 100$$

FIGURE 3. Percent transmittance (%T) defined; I = incident light, I_0 = transmitted light.

Transmittance

The concept of light transmittance is important because only the light transmitted through a solution to a photodetector is actually measured in absorbance spectrophotometry methods. As Figure 3 illustrates, when monochromatic light of intensity I_0 strikes a solution, some of the light is absorbed by the molecules, while the remainder is mostly transmitted through the solution (I). Transmittance is generally expressed as percent transmittance

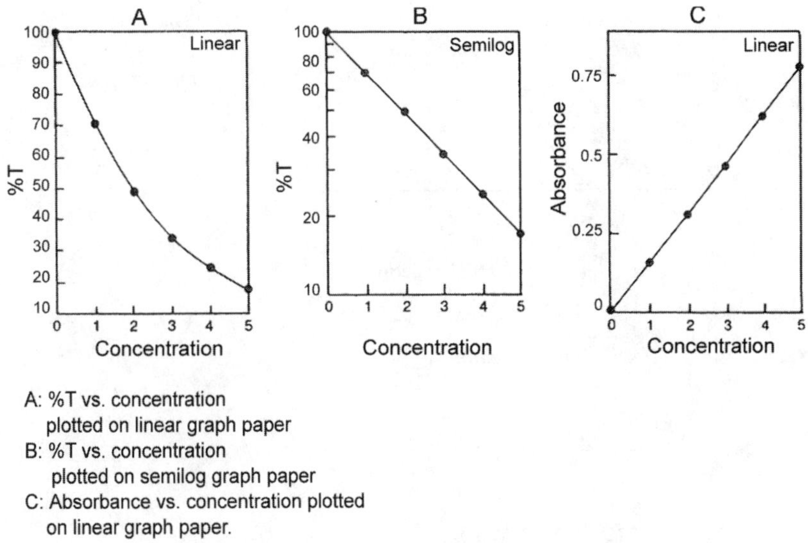

FIGURE 4. %T versus concentration and absorbance versus concentration.

(%T), and this is the ratio of the amount of light transmitted through the sample compared to the amount of light striking the sample. The values of %T and concentration have an inverse log relationship such that as the concentration of the solution increases, the %T decreases nonlinearly as depicted graphically in Figure 4. When %T versus concentration is plotted on linear graph paper, it is nonlinear (Figure 4A); when plotted on semilog graph paper, the line is straight with a negative slope (Figure 4B). For convenience, and to avoid the use of logs, %T is related to the light absorbed by a solution by the equation:

$$A = \log (100/\%T) = 2 - \log\%T \tag{2}$$

where A = absorbance. Absorbance is directly related to concentration and gives a straight line when represented graphically (Figure 4C).

Reflection and Refraction

Beside light transmittance and absorbance, phenomena of reflection and refraction may occur when light interacts with matter as illustrated in Figure 5. **Reflection** occurs when light is deflected by the surface of a substance. The reflected light ray is in the same plane as the incident ray and is perpendicular to the reflecting plane. Probably the most intuitive illustration of reflectance is referred to as specular reflectance. Specular reflectance occurs when light is reflected from a smooth mirror-like surface, as opposed to diffuse reflectance that occurs when light is reflected from an irregular surface.

Specular reflectance is exploited as an analytical technique used to measure sample concentration in **reflection photometry (reflectometry)** instruments. Reflectometry instruments (reflectometers) measure the amount of light reflected by a colored reaction product present on a reflective test surface composed of plastic or paper. An example of a reflectometer is depicted in Figure 6. The term reflection density is used to describe the quantity of light absorbed by the colored reaction product on the test surface and is inversely related to the light intensity reflected by the sample. The greater the sample

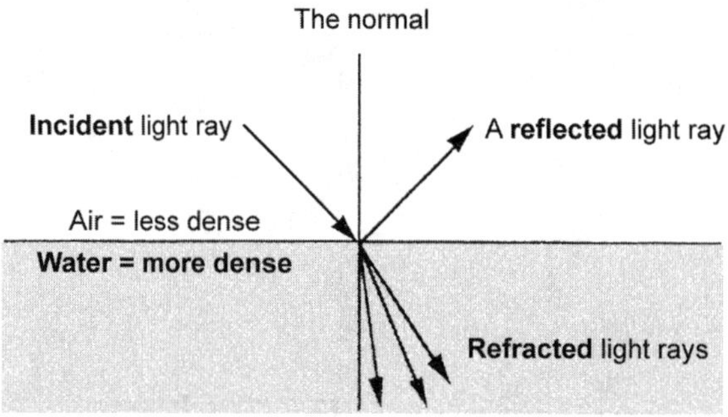

FIGURE 5. Light reflection and refraction.

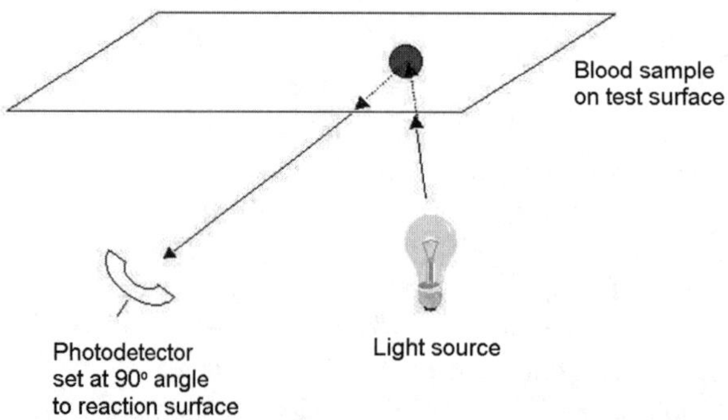

FIGURE 6. Reflectometer.

concentration, the more intense the color and the lower the reflection density. A white surface (maximum reflection) serves as the zero concentration standard and a black surface (zero reflection) serves as the high concentration standard. The relationship between concentration and reflectance is inverse and nonlinear and requires the use of a mathematical algorithm to linearize the data to determine sample concentration.

Refraction

Refraction is the change of direction of a light ray as it passes from one medium into a second medium as seen in Figure 5. Refraction is the phenomenon that is employed by a prism to disperse white light into its constituent wavelengths or colors as depicted in Figure 7. Because the velocity of light is a function of its wavelength, each wavelength in turn is refracted (bent) to a different degree (or angle), thereby dispersing white light into its constituent colors, producing the visible spectrum of violet, blue, green, yellow, orange, and red. A nonlinear spectrum results from refraction by a prism because the longer wavelengths (red) are not refracted as much as the shorter wavelengths (violet).

Refractometry is an analytical method routinely used to estimate urine specific gravity and to rapidly assess serum total protein concentration using a refractometer instrument. The refractive index of urine is linearly related to the specific gravity up to 1.035 g/mL.

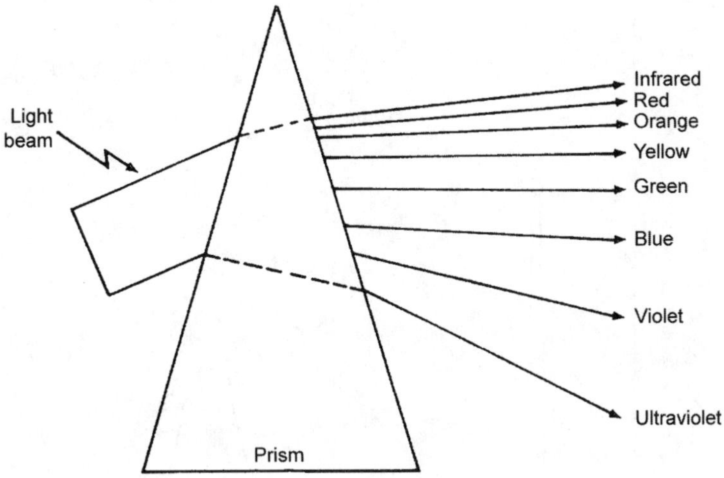

FIGURE 7. Refraction of white light by a prism.

SPECTROPHOTOMETRY AND PHOTOMETRY: PRINCIPLES OF LIGHT MEASUREMENT

Absorbance is the amount of monochromatic light of specific wavelength absorbed by a solution. The use of monochromatic light ensures accurate measurement of light absorption to determine analyte concentration. Absorbance has no units and can be expressed in terms of %T, where the relationship is: $A = 2 - \log\%T$ as given in Equation 2. Absorbance is directly proportional to concentration of the absorbing species when the appropriate wavelength of light is used and if Beer's law is followed. It is important to remember that absorbance is not a directly measurable quantity, and it can only be obtained mathematically by calculation from %T data.

Absorbance Spectra

A spectral absorbance curve is a graph of light absorbance data for a substance plotted at various wavelengths. Figure 8 represents an idealized spectral absorbance curve for a substance. The spectral absorbance curve is unique to each substance and reveals the substance's absorbance minima and maxima. This information is vital when choosing the optimum wavelength for clinical assay methods. In addition to identifying absorbance maxima, selection of the optimum assay wavelength depends upon other factors including the slope of the absorption maxima peak and the absorption spectra of potential interfering substances. For instance, if the shape of the absorbance peak is too sharp (*see* λ_1 in Figure 8), small errors in wavelength isolation may cause large errors in absorbance measurement and therefore inaccurate sample analyte concentration. In Figure 8, λ_2 is not an absorbance maximum, and therefore λ_3 would be the optimal assay wavelength for this substance. Ideally, selection of an assay wavelength in close proximity to or within the absorbance spectra of a likely interfering chromogen should be avoided.

Absorbance Laws

Beer's Law

Beer's law states that monochromatic light absorbance varies directly with the concentration of the solution. For example, if a 0.5% solution yields a 0.20 absorbance reading, a

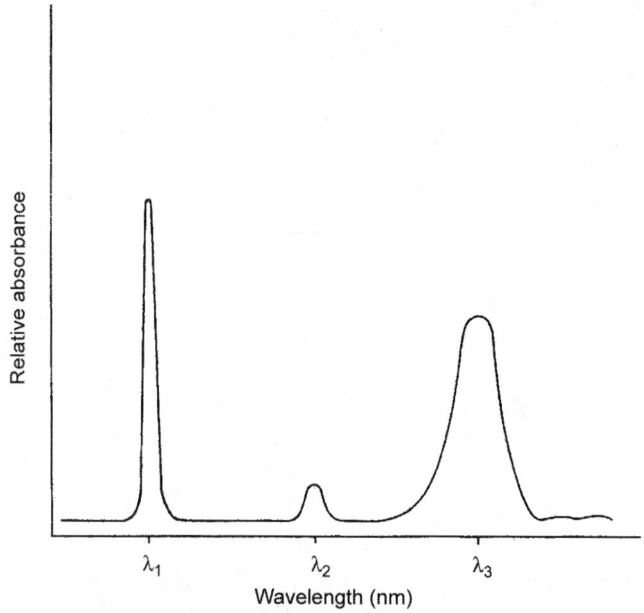

FIGURE 8. Spectral absorption curve.

1.0% solution of the same substance should yield a 0.40 absorbance reading. Solutions of known concentration (standards) of a substance that obeys Beer's law can be used to construct a standard curve by plotting each standard solution absorbance reading versus the concentration. The standard curve may then be used to determine the concentration of an unknown solution of the same substance based on its absorbance.

Bouguer–Lambert Law

Bouguer–Lambert law states that the absorbance of a solution depends upon the number of light-absorbing molecules in the light path. If the light path increases, the number of molecules in the light path increases and as a result, the absorbance increases proportionally. For example, when the absorbance of a solution in a 1-cm light path is 0.05, and then the same solution is measured using a 2-cm light path, the absorbance reading is expected to be 0.10 since the light path is twice as long.

Beer-Lambert Law

The combined Beer-Lambert law states:

$$A = abc \tag{3}$$

where A = absorbance
a = molar absorptivity; a constant for a compound at a given wavelength in a 1-cm light path
b = light path (cm)
c = concentration of the absorbing compound

When molar absorptivity (a) and light path (b) are kept constant, this formula can be used to calculate an unknown concentration from the absorbance measurement:

$$Au/Cu = As/Cs \tag{4}$$

where Au = absorbance of unknown
Cu = concentration of unknown
As = absorbance of standard (known)
Cs = concentration of standard (known)

Equation 4 may be rearranged to solve for the unknown concentration:

$$Cu = Au/As \times Cs \tag{5}$$

This equation is applicable only if Beer's law is obeyed and stray light is minimized. When a single standard solution is used to obtain the unknown concentration, an upper limit of linearity must be known and cannot be exceeded. If the unknown concentration is above the assay linear limit, a dilution must be made and the sample reassayed. Alternately, when a standard curve is constructed to determine the unknown concentration, assay linearity can only be assumed up to the concentration of the highest standard. If an unknown sample concentration exceeds the highest standard concentration, a sample dilution must be made and the sample reassayed.

SPECTROPHOTOMETRY INSTRUMENTATION: PHOTOMETERS AND SPECTROPHOTOMETERS

Photometers are a general class of photosensitive devices that measure light intensity. A colorimeter measures the transmittance or absorption of **colored** light by a solution. In this instrument, simple glass filters produce colored light, i.e., light of more than one wavelength. The spectrophotometer measures the transmittance or absorption of monochromatic light by a solution.

Spectrophotometer

The major spectrophotometer components are illustrated in Figure 9 and include the light source, monochromator (wavelength selector), sample cell, photodetector, and readout device. The source light is passed through a monochromator to select the desired light wavelength. The selected monochromatic light passes through a sample cell where a portion of the light is absorbed by the solution, depending on its nature and concentration. Light that is not absorbed by the solution is transmitted to a photodetector. The

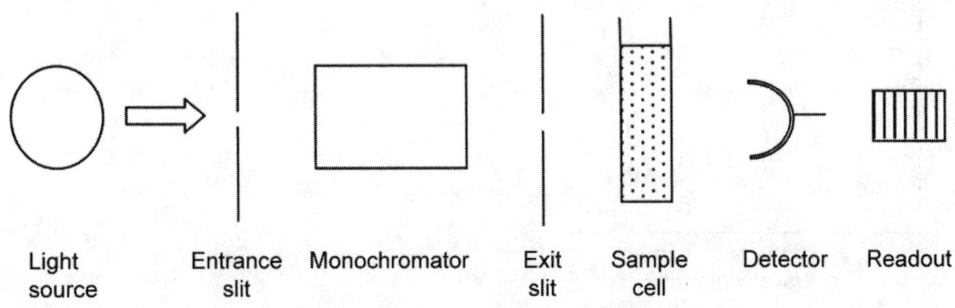

FIGURE 9. Major components of a single-beam spectrophotometer.

photodetector converts light energy to electrical energy and the amplifier (if needed) increases the electrical signal that is registered on a meter or recorder.

Components of Photometers

Light Source. It is important to recognize that the light produced by any particular light source is not constant over a continuous range of wavelengths and that different types of lamps vary in the spectra they produce. A source light that is often used is the tungsten-halogen or quartz-halogen lamp as these provide good output in a continuous spectrum through the near UV (~340–380 nm), visible, and near infrared regions. The quartz-halogen lamp produces better light in the near-UV region than the tungsten-halogen light source (1). If strict UV wavelengths are needed, then a hydrogen or deuterium lamp is preferred. Some dedicated, special purpose photometric-based instruments sometimes use light-emitting diodes (LEDs) as a light source. These very low energy light sources are used in some point-of-care testing instruments and in some automated microbiology systems to detect bacterial growth and metabolism. In contrast, lasers produce an intense and pure monochromatic light with minimum scatter; however, different types of lasers are needed to produce different light wavelengths.

Monochromator. The monochromator system isolates the light of the desired wavelength(s) from a polychromatic light source by excluding unwanted wavelengths using one or more filters, a prism, or a diffraction grating. With conventional light sources such as lamps, a single light wavelength cannot be achieved; instead a range of wavelengths called either bandpass or **bandwidth** is produced. Specifically, the bandpass (bandwidth) is defined as the range of wavelengths between the points at which transmittance is one-half the peak transmittance as illustrated in Figure 10. The bandpass of the spectrophotometer describes the purity of light passing through the sample and is dependent upon the efficiency of the monochromator system to isolate wavelength bands. As an example, Figure 10 depicts the bandpass curve produced by a 10-nm bandpass spectrophotometer. When 550 nm is selected as the desired wavelength, in reality, a 10-nm range of wavelengths from 545 to 555 nm is produced. The various monochromators produce different typical bandpass ranges, e.g., glass filters = >30 nm, interference filters = 10–20 nm, prisms and diffraction gratings = <5 nm (2).

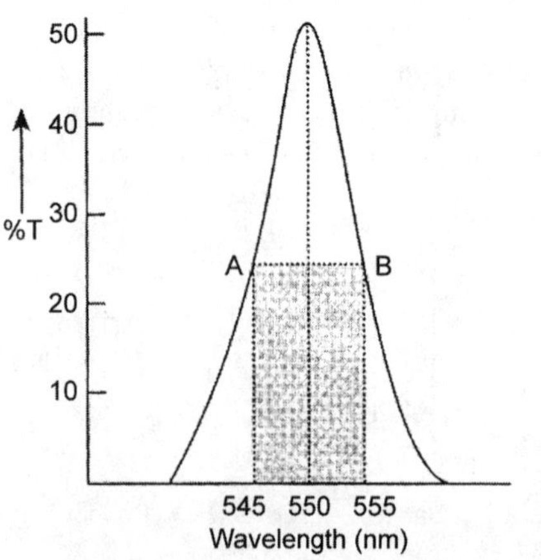

FIGURE 10. Bandpass of a spectrophotometer.

Filter Monochromators

Glass filters are the simplest monochromators and have characteristically wide bandpass as this light includes more than one color. The glass filters function by absorbing the unwanted wavelengths and transmitting the desired wavelengths of light. Although glass filters are the least efficient monochromators, they are generally sufficiently accurate and economical for routine testing in dedicated photometers, such as hemoglobin concentration determinations performed in automated hematology cell counter analyzers.

Interference filters provide a narrow bandpass and are composed of layers of semitransparent film on both sides of a thin transparent layer. When light strikes the semitransparent film, some is reflected from the front surface, and some penetrates and is reflected by the film surface on the other side of the transparent layer. If the two reflected rays are in phase, the intensity is doubled. If the rays are out of phase, they destroy each other. Interference filters transmit multiples (harmonics) of the desired wavelength, e.g., a 620-nm filter transmits some 310- and 1240-nm light unless another filter eliminates these.

Prisms and Diffractions Grating Monochromators

The most widely used true monochromators consist of several major parts depicted in Figure 11 and include an entrance slit, a prism or diffraction grating to disperse light into its various wavelengths, and an exit slit to select the wavelength(s) allowed to pass into the sample cell. The entrance slit is designed to limit the amount of source light allowed to strike the prism or grating. This minimizes reflected light that can contribute significantly to stray light of the instrument.

As can be seen in Figure 7, as white light strikes a prism, it is dispersed into its constituent wavelengths (colors) forming a nonlinear spectrum, as the shorter wavelengths are refracted (bent) more than the longer wavelengths. Prisms are not generally used any longer in good quality spectrophotometers as economical, high-quality diffraction gratings are readily available and these produce linear, high-quality spectra from a polychromatic light source. The diffraction grating consists of engraved reflective parallel grooves of up to 1000–2000 lines/mm. The more etched lines the better the resolution. When white light strikes the grating, each of the grooves creates a tiny linear spectrum. The spectrum falls onto the monochromator wall where a very narrow exit slit permits only a small portion of

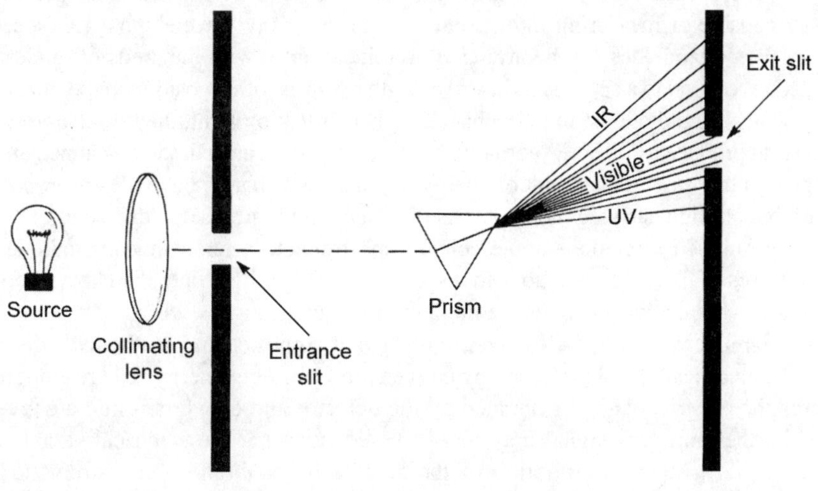

FIGURE 11. Principle monochromator elements.

the spectrum to emerge from the monochromator pass-through and to strike the sample cell. The exit slit size directly influences the magnitude of the instrument bandwidth.

Sample Cells. Sample cells hold the sample reaction and must be clean and free of fingerprints, scratches, and clouding. Most sample cells have the standard 1-cm light path, while a longer light path is useful for more accurate readings of dilute samples. Square-shaped sample cells present a flat surface to the incident light and are less susceptible to light reflectance errors than round-shaped sample cells. Quartz glass or special-type optical glass samples cells must be used for methods involving UV light wavelengths since the lime in ordinary glass absorbs these wavelengths. Steps need to be taken to prevent room light from entering the sample cell chamber such as placing a light shield over the sample cell compartment to avoid stray light errors. Light transmitted through the sample solution strikes the photodetector.

Photodetectors. Photodetectors detect light energy and proportionately convert it to electrical energy using photosensitive or photoemissive materials that release electrons upon exposure to light. Two main types are used: photomultiplier tubes and photodiodes.

Photomultiplier Tube Photodetectors. The photomultiplier tube (PMT) is an electron tube that internally amplifies the initial light signal to improve detection sensitivity. A photomultiplier tube consists of a cathode that emits electrons, up to 16 photosensitive electrodes (dynodes) that multiply the initial energy, and an anode that collects the amplified electrons. When light strikes the cathode, emitted "primary" electrons are attracted to the first dynode. This causes the emission of 3–6 more "secondary" electrons that strike the second dynode, and the cascading electron effect continues through the entire series of dynodes until the electrons reach the anode. This chain reaction results in an amplified electric current, up to a million times the initial energy. The resultant electric current is measured and is directly proportional to the light intensity striking the photomultiplier tube.

Photodiodes (Light-Sensing Diodes) Photodetectors. Semiconductor photodetectors such as photodiodes have begun to replace conventional photomultiplier tubes in modern clinical laboratory instruments. Some photodiode designs use silicon chips that convert light energy to an electrical signal for measurement. Photodiodes are popular photodetectors, as these are capable of measuring light simultaneously at many wavelengths with speed and accuracy (3). Photodiodes can be arranged in a linear array with hundreds of diodes, each calibrated to respond to a specific light wavelength by virtue of its position in the linear array. Electronically, each diode is initially charged; when struck by light, they discharge (release electrons) to produce a current. Alternatively, after discharge, each diode is scanned and then recharged; in this case, the amount of energy required to recharge the diodes is proportional to the amount of light striking the diode. As illustrated in Figure 12, the diffraction grating is typically positioned **after** the sample cell for spectrophotometers using photodiode array photodetectors. This design functions to disperse transmitted light onto the photodiode array detector so that many wavelengths are monitored simultaneously.

The **signal processing unit or readout device** amplifies and mathematically manipulates the electrical signal produced by conversion from light energy. The readout device measures the electrical signal generated by the detector and converts it into a convenient format. Furthermore, the signal may be processed such that the electrical signal can be directly related to the concentration of the analyte by calibrating an instrument in the proper units, e.g., concentration, transmittance, absorbance, fluorescence.

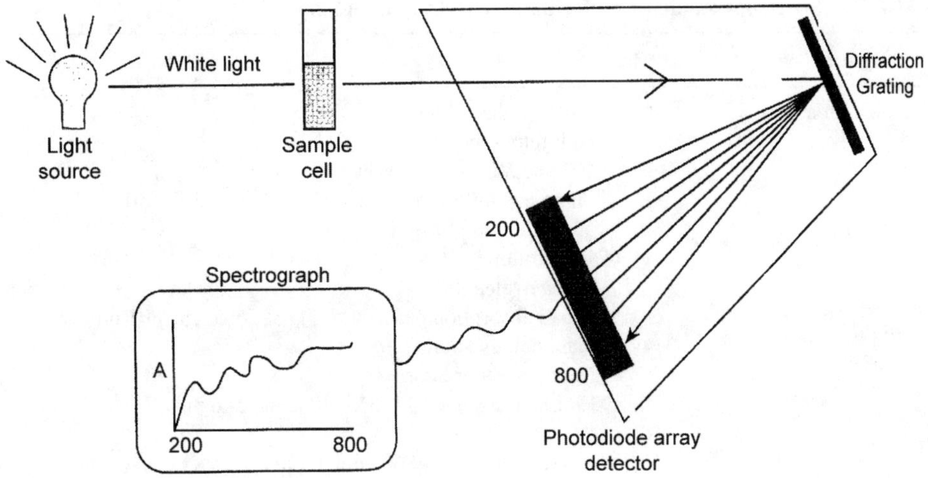

FIGURE 12. Photodiode array spectrophotometer.

Limitations/Sources of Error

Spectrophotometer analytical problems may be due to stray light, nonlinearity of the instrument response, wide bandwidth, and wavelength inaccuracy. When these inaccuracies are minor, they usually do not cause large errors in measurement since known concentration standard solutions are used to verify linearity. However, spectrophotometer performance checks are needed to ensure reliability of routine testing.

Quality Assurance

Instrument spectrophotometric performance checks and calibration are essential analytical quality assurance program components. These performance checks are required periodically and as needed when a major photometric component is replaced or serviced and include wavelength accuracy, stray light, photometric linearity, and accuracy (4, 5). A summary of spectrophotometer performance check methods is provided in Table 2.

Wavelength Accuracy. Wavelength accuracy verifies that the wavelength selected is actually the wavelength of light striking the sample. For instance, when the wavelength selector is set at 520 nm the monochromator may actually produce light at a different, unexpected wavelength. Wavelength inaccuracy can occur when the light source is replaced, as this may change the precise angle at which light strikes the diffraction grating and thus the spectrum produced. Wavelength accuracy checks are important because if wavelength selection accuracy changes, then sample absorbance changes according to its characteristic spectral curve. Deviations from the expected light wavelength often cause falsely decreased absorbance measurements as the superfluous inaccurate wavelengths are transmitted through the sample, rather than absorbed by the molecules in the solution.

There are three methods to perform wavelength accuracy; these include using **rare-earth glass filters**, substituting the source lamp with a mercury or deuterium lamp, and using chromogenic standard solutions. Using the rare-earth didymium or holmium oxide glass filters is among the most common and convenient methods. Didymium filters are

TABLE 2. Spectrophotometer performance checks and methods

Performance check	Method
Wavelength accuracy	▪ Rare-earth glass filters a. Holmium oxide UV and VIS wavelengths Sharp absorption peaks at 241, 279, 287, 333, 361, 418, 453, 536, and 636 nm b. Didymium VIS wavelengths Broad absorption peaks at 537, 586, 685, and 801 nm ▪ Radiant energy sources a. Mercury vapor lamp Emission lines at 313, 365, 405, and 546 nm b. Deuterium lamp Emission lines at 486 and 656 nm ▪ Chemical solutions a. Holmium nitrate (50 g/L) Sharp absorption peaks at 362, 418, 453, 474, 538, and 643 nm b. Commercial green food coloring (French's). Dilute 0.5 mL to 2.0 L Absorption peaks at 257, 410, and 630 nm
Stray light	▪ Glass cut-off filters Absorb all light at a given wavelength
Photometric linearity	▪ Neutral density glass filter sets Different absorbance values for use at several different wavelengths compared to given certified values, e.g., National Institute of Standards and Technology (NIST) ▪ Chemical solutions Chemicals such as those used to verify wavelength accuracy diluted to several different concentrations
Photometric accuracy	As above for photometric linearity as manufacturer usually provides each standard set (glass filters or chemicals) as a series of known absorbance values

useful to calibrate wide bandpass instruments over the visible spectrum since didymium has characteristic broad absorbance peaks within this region. Holmium oxide filters are used for narrow bandpass instruments for visible and UV wavelengths since holmium oxide has characteristic sharp absorption peaks within these regions. Several standard **chemical solutions** may be prepared or purchased that also have characteristic absorbance peaks. For example, holmium nitrate solution has characteristic sharp absorption peaks over the visible spectrum. Although various standard solutions and standard filters of didymium and holmium oxide can be reliable and convenient to use, the most accurate wavelength calibration method is accomplished by substituting the source lamp with a **mercury or deuterium lamp**. Although this is the most accurate method, it is not routinely performed. Stray light is another parameter to be evaluated when verifying spectrophotometer performance.

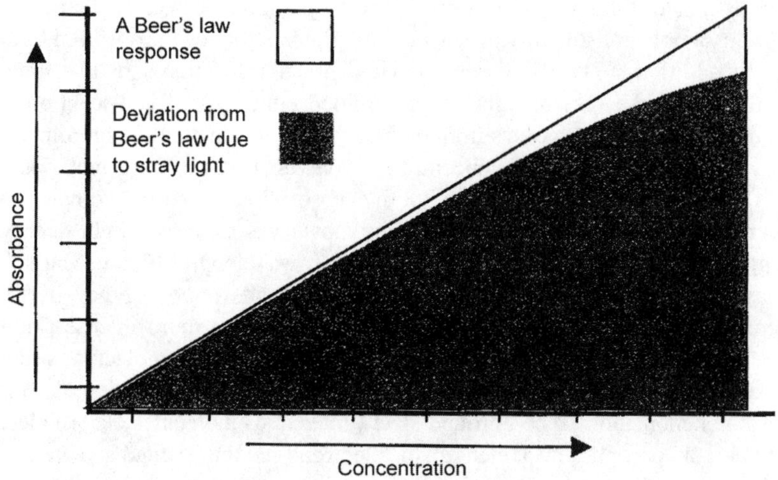

FIGURE 13. Effect of stray light on absorbance measurements.

Stray Light. Stray light is defined as light reaching the photodetector at a wavelength other than that selected and all light that did not pass through the sample. Excessive stray light may be caused by leakage of extraneous light, light scattering by dust or scratches on optical surfaces, and light from the next higher or lower wavelength from that selected. Stray light is measured with blocking filters that absorb all light at a given wavelength, thus any light reaching the detector is stray light. Excessive stray light causes falsely decreased absorbance and decreased high-end assay linearity as illustrated in Figure 13. Excessive stray light shows a greater effect at high solution concentration because at this level, stray light makes up a larger proportion of %T as compared to the %T of lower solution concentration.

Photometric Linearity and Accuracy. Photometric linearity means that for a change in concentration a photometer yields a proportional change in absorbance. The photometric linearity of an instrument ensures a true Beer's law relationship between absorbance and sample concentration. Methods of checking photometric linearity include neutral density filters and chemical solutions known to follow Beer's law. Photometric accuracy checks should be performed after wavelength calibration, stray light, and photometric linearity checks are verified to be within expected ranges.

Photometric accuracy verifies that the absorbance displayed by the instrument is the true absorbance of the solution. A measure of photometric accuracy gives an overall indication of spectrophotometer performance including wavelength calibration (accuracy), linearity, and freedom from stray light. Loss of photometric accuracy is generally caused by large bandwidth and excessive stray light. Neutral density glass filters or the same chemical standards used to verify wavelength accuracy are measured at several different wavelengths to verify photometric accuracy.

FLUOROMETRY

The advantages of fluorescence as an analytical method lie in its superior sensitivity and specificity over routine absorption spectrophotometry. The increased sensitivity is a result of the fact that the emitted fluorescent light comes directly from the sample. The specificity is greater than that of absorption spectrophotometry because there is no interference from sample constituents or reagent components that can absorb light but do not fluoresce. In addition, no two substances have identical absorption and emission spectra.

Fluorometry makes use of light energy emitted either by a fluorescent analyte or a fluorescent label used in numerous immunoassay detection methods. Fluorometry is particularly suited to measuring low concentration analytes because these methods are typically 10–100-fold more sensitive than routine absorption spectrophotometry methods. Fluorescence is a property that allows certain substances to absorb light energy at one wavelength and then emit a portion of it at a longer wavelength. Fluorescent substances tend to have conjugated (overlapping) double or triple bonds and/or rigid cyclic structures. Some molecules have high fluorescence efficiency and give more intense fluorescence than those of lower fluorescence efficiency due to their particular molecular structure.

To better appreciate the fluorescence process, it is helpful to review the molecular basis for the phenomenon. When ground state (unexcited) molecules absorb electromagnetic radiation of appropriate wavelength, the electrons become excited and are driven into vacant higher energy orbitals. Excited molecules are unstable and tend to dissipate excess energy rapidly and return to ground state. Many excited molecules release this excess energy to the surrounding environment as heat. In addition to heat, particular molecules release a portion of this excess energy by light emission at a longer (lower energy) wavelength. The difference in energy between the excitation light and emission light is called the **Stokes shift**. This shift to a longer emission wavelength is due to the loss of energy from the unstable excited molecule before light emission occurs due to molecular collision with solvent, other molecules, and intramolecular vibration and rotation.

Fluorescence, Phosphorescence, and Chemiluminescence

Fluorescence and phosphorescence are two types of light emission that may occur when certain molecules absorb light energy and become excited. Fluorescence emission is characterized by a rapid decay time ($\sim 10^{-8}$ second) (6), and those molecules capable of fluorescence are called fluorophores. Phosphorescence is essentially the same process as fluorescence except that light emission has a longer decay time ($\sim 10^{-4}$ to greater than 1 second) (7). Molecules can also absorb **chemical** energy and become excited to higher energy levels. After becoming excited, these molecules behave as if they were excited by the light absorption. When chemically excited molecules emit light, the process is called **chemiluminescence** (8). Chemiluminescence is an even more sensitive analytical method than fluorescence and will be discussed further in Chapter 7. To better understand the subtle differences between fluorescent and phosphorescent light emission requires a discussion of **electrons and electronic states** of an excited molecule.

Most ground state molecules contain an even number of electrons as the electrons fill the orbitals in pairs with their spins in opposite directions. When the spin of the excited electron pair is in opposite directions, this is called the singlet state (S) (*see* the energy level diagram in Figure 14). The terms S_0 is the ground state and S_1 and S_2 are the first and second singlet excitation levels, respectively. When the spin of excited electrons is in an unpaired condition, this is referred to as a triplet (T). Like the singlet, the triplet may have first and second excitation states T_1 and T_2, respectively.

As mentioned earlier, a molecule excited to a higher energy level dissipates its excess energy and returns to ground state rapidly. Initially, excess energy transfers efficiently to other molecules by molecular collisions, and further dissipates through intramolecular vibration or rotation to achieve the lowest vibrational level. For example, possible

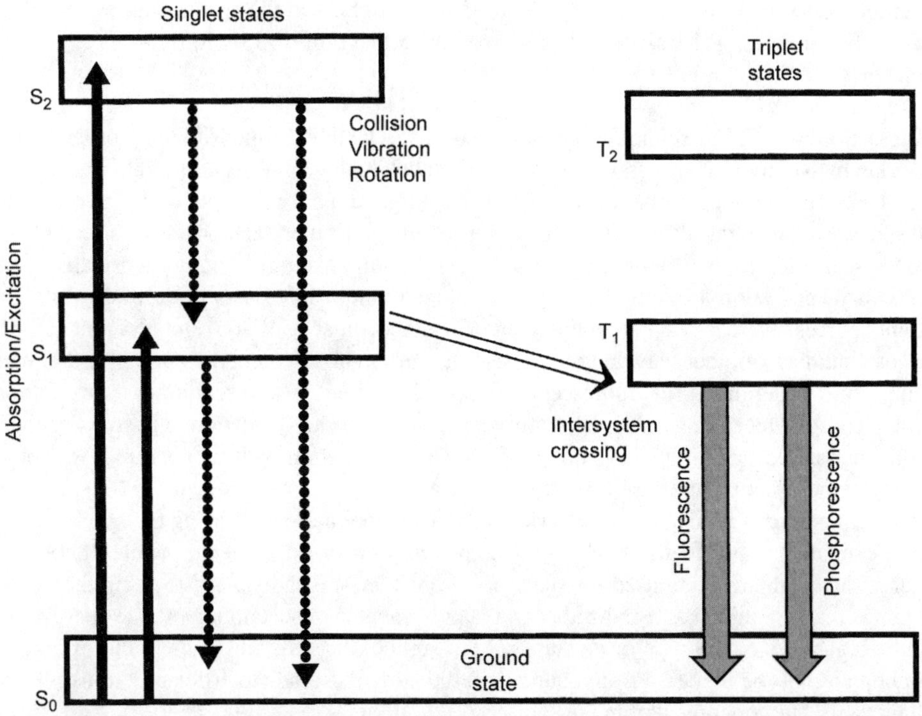

FIGURE 14. Energy level diagram. Singlet states are represented by S_0, S_1, and S_2. Triplet states are T_1 and T_2.

transitions that can occur include S_2 to S_1, S_1 to S_0, or S_1 to T_1, and T_1 to S_0 energy states. Light emission processes of fluorescence and phosphorescence occur last. Light emission from a singlet excited state molecule is called fluorescence. Specifically, an S_1 to S_0 transition results in fluorescence. Phosphorescent light emission occurs from a molecule in a triplet state and is represented by a T_1 to S_0 transition. In either case, after light emission, the molecule returns to the ground state. Phosphorescence is not generally used in current clinical applications and will not be discussed further.

Fluorometer Instrumentation

Fluorescence is a technique used to measure clinical analyte concentration for a variety of analytes often using immunoassay-based methods. These include hormones, therapeutic drugs, and other special clinical chemistry analytes. The fluorescence intensity produced by the sample or immunoassay fluorescent label is directly proportional to the excitation light intensity and the fluorophore concentration. Fluorescence intensity is known to obey Beer's law at relatively low fluorophore concentration.

Fluorometer Components

Fluorescence intensity is measured using either a fluorometer or spectrofluorometer instrument that contains the following basic components that are essentially the same equipment found in a basic absorbance spectrophotometer, but with some important differences: excitation light source, monochromators, sample cell, and detector. The key difference between the fluorometer and spectrofluorometer is that a fluorometer uses filter monochromators to isolate excitation and emission light, and the spectrofluorometer uses a diffraction grating like the spectrophotometer. A diagram of a basic right-angle fluorometer is shown in Figure 15.

Light Source. The excitation light source needs to be a high-intensity lamp or laser producing high output in the ultraviolet and short-wavelength visible spectra. Both of these criteria are crucial owing to the fact that fluorescent light emission intensity is proportional to the intensity of light absorbed by the fluorophore molecules, and that emission light is always of a longer wavelength (lower energy) than the excitation light energy absorbed. Mercury and xenon arc lamps and quartz-halogen lamps and lasers are useful excitation light sources. Mercury lamps produce major line spectra at 254, 365, and 366 nm, as well as at a number of other wavelengths. These discrete light wavelengths may limit the mercury lamp's usefulness for fluorescent compounds and labels that require other excitation wavelengths. Depending on the laboratory's needs, a superior excitation light source choice is the xenon arc lamp or quartz-halogen lamp. These excitation light sources are less intense than mercury lamps and lasers but they emit a continuous spectrum in the 200–800-nm range, allowing analysis of a wide variety of fluorophore molecules using the specific optimal excitation wavelength(s). Mercury lamps are used in fluorometers, while xenon and quartz-halogen lamps are used for spectrofluorometers. A disadvantage to using the xenon lamp is that it requires a specialized power supply capable of sustaining a stable energy output. Regardless of the type of excitation light source selected, all optics in the excitation light path must be prepared from quartz or fused silica materials to efficiently transmit UV light to the fluorophores within the sample.

Monochromators. Fluorometers require two monochromators; the primary monochromator selects the excitation light wavelength(s) absorbed by the sample, while the secondary monochromator selects the specific emission light wavelength(s) emerging from the excited sample such that only emission light strikes the photodetector. As an additional preventative measure, the secondary or emission light monochromator is routinely positioned at a 90° angle to the excitation light source to further minimize the potential interference

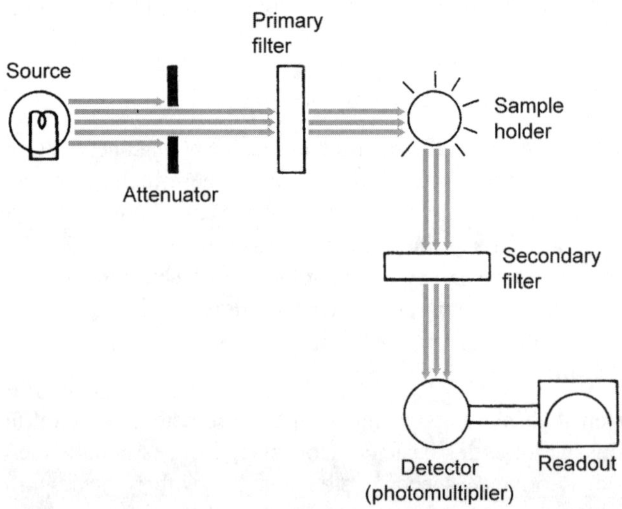

FIGURE 15. Basic right-angle fluorometer.

that occurs if excitation light reaches the photodetector. A basic fluorometer uses filters for wavelength isolation, while a spectrofluorometer uses diffraction gratings for wavelength isolation.

Sample Cells. Rectangular cells are preferred over round cuvets to minimize excitation light scatter interference. The sample cells must be composed of UV-light-transmitting materials to permit the UV excitation light to pass into the sample in the cuvet. Materials that transmit UV light well include quartz or fused silica materials. Ordinary glass does not permit efficient UV light transmission. If UV light is not transmitted to the sample, poor or no fluorescence results.

The sample cell is often placed at the 90° angle intersection point between the excitation light path and emission light path. Alternatively, the sample can be placed at other angles in relation to the excitation light and detector to accommodate different system configurations such as that used to measure front-surface fluorescence of a turbid solution or solid-support matrix. The solid-support matrix mechanically holds the fluorophore molecules for optical measurement. For example, the MEIA technology employed by the Abbott AxSYM immunoassay analyzer (9) uses an inert glass fiber matrix as a mechanical support for the bound immune complex sandwich (antibody–antigen–antibody). The alkaline phosphatase immune complex label catalyzes the hydrolysis of the fluorogenic substrate 4-MUP (4-methylumbelliferyl phosphate) to the fluorescent product 4-MU (4-methylumbelliferone). Front-surface fluorometry methods offer excellent linearity over a wide range of analyte concentrations.

Detectors. Sensitive photodetectors are generally required because sample fluorescent light emission is characteristically weak; therefore, a photomultiplier tube or similarly sensitive photodetector is often used to amplify and measure the emission light. The photodetector is positioned at a 90° angle to the excitation light source. This orientation of the photodetector and excitation light source is essential to minimize potential stray light interference from the excitation light source.

Results

Fluorescence intensity is directly proportional to the sample fluorophore or fluorescent label concentration at low levels (6). When known concentrations of an analyte (calibrators) are measured, a calibration curve is mathematically derived that best characterizes the analyte concentration–response relationship. Unknown patient sample analyte concentration is calculated using this calibration curve.

Limitations/Sources of Error

The most widely recognized interference in fluorescence techniques is quenching. **Quenching** is an overall reduction in fluorescent light emission intensity and may be due to intermolecular collisions that transfer energy to other fluorophore molecules, to nonfluorophore molecules (quenchers), or to the solvent itself. Quenching is often caused by "inner filter effect," pH and temperature variations, and high fluorophore concentration. Besides quenching, another well-recognized source of error in fluorescence techniques is light scatter.

Inner Filter Effect. A form of quenching that does not involve direct energy transfer is the inner filter effect whereby emission light never reaches the detector because it is absorbed by nonfluorescent molecules. Another mechanism involves the formation of a chemical complex (charge transfer complex) involving electron transfer between the excited fluorophore and the quencher. Excessive molecular quenching can be caused by factors that increase the number of molecular collisions in the test solution, including high temperature and high fluorophore concentration.

pH and Temperature Variations. Most fluorophores have an optimal pH range for maximal fluorescence intensity. Fluorescence intensity by fluorophores containing ionizable groups can be affected by the pH of the solvent as a result of changing the ratio of the charged and uncharged species. Temperature also affects fluorescence and generally the lower the temperature, the less efficient the quenching process, especially for those mechanisms involving intermolecular collisions described earlier. For some fluorophores, a change in fluorescence intensity can be as much as 50% with a relatively small change (10–15°) in temperature (7). Another important variable affecting fluorescence is fluorophore concentration.

High Fluorophore Concentration. High fluorophore concentration can result in "self-quenching" and "self-absorption." In **self-quenching**, excitation light absorbance by fluorophores is high and most light is absorbed before it reaches molecules near the center of the sample cell so that these do not become excited. This process causes the fluorescence signal to be significantly diminished given that most of the light reaching the detector normally arises from the inner volume of the sample cell as illustrated in Figure 16. Self-absorption occurs as excited fluorophores in the center of the sample cell have the emission light absorbed by other molecules and as a result it does not reach the photodetector. This process occurs when the Stokes shift is small, i.e., when the excitation and emission spectra overlap or are close together. High fluorophore concentration problems can be corrected by using dilute solutions, shortening the pathlength of the sample cell, or using front surface fluorescence techniques as discussed earlier.

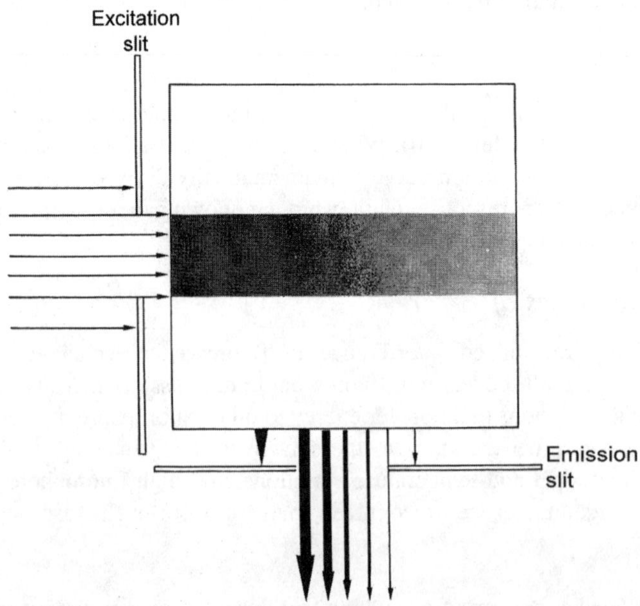

FIGURE 16. Effects of optical configuration and concentration on fluorescence detection.

Light Scatter. Excitation light scatter toward the photodetector reduces assay sensitivity and contributes to background signal "noise" and can occur even when the detector is positioned at a right angle to the excitation light path. Light scatter is a significant problem in the presence of sample turbidity or when the sample cell is round. It also presents a problem especially when the fluorophore Stokes shift is small. This problem can be minimized by proper excitation and emission wavelength selection so that overlap is reduced as much as possible.

TURBIDIMETRY AND NEPHELOMETRY

Light scatter, transmission, absorption, and reflection are physical effects of light colliding with molecules in solution. Turbidimetry and nephelometry are analytical methods used to measure light scatter by particles suspended in solution. Specifically, **turbidimetry** measures the reduction in source light **transmitted** through a colloidal solution and is used to assay smaller particles at higher concentrations. This attenuation of light transmission through the solution of particles is due to light scattering, reflectance and absorption. **Nephelometry** is based upon detection of that portion of light **scattered** or reflected by the particles in a solution toward a detector at an angle not in the direct path of the transmitted light (10). Nephelometry is the method of choice for assaying larger particles at lower concentrations.

There are numerous clinical turbidimetry and nephelometry applications throughout the clinical laboratory. For example, various automated microbiology analyzers employ turbidimetric measurements to detect bacterial growth in broth culture media and assess minimal microbial inhibition for antibiotic sensitivity from such cultures. Turbidimetry is used in automated coagulation analyzers to detect fibrin clot formation for routine assays including prothrombin time (PT), activated partial prothrombin time (aPTT), and fibrinogen quantitation. In addition, the clinical chemistry as well as immunology laboratory routinely quantifies specific proteins such as immunoglobulins in blood and body fluids. Hematology and flow cytometry laboratories use cell counters and flow cytometers that analyze cells based upon light-scattering as well as other characteristics. Currently, some of the most frequently encountered light scattering clinical applications involve quantitation of immunocomplex (antigen–antibody complex) formation in various immunoassays. To better understand the principles of turbidimetric and nephelometric assays, it is useful to begin with a discussion of both immunocomplex formation and light scattering.

Principles of Light-Scattering Methods: Nephelometry and Turbidimetry

Immunocomplex (Antigen–Antibody Complex) Formation

A basic principle of antigen–antibody reactions is that, when an antigen (Ag) reacts with its specific antibody (Ab), an Ag–Ab immunocomplex forms. As can be seen in Figure 17, antigen–antibody immunocomplex formation follows three discernible developmental stages: antibody excess, antigen–antibody equivalence, and finally antigen excess. Within the zone of antibody excess, increasing the antigen concentration results in ever-increasing immunocomplex formation until the zone of equivalence is reached. At this stage, there is maximal immunoprecipitation whereby formerly soluble immunocomplexes become insoluble complexes that precipitate out of solution. Beyond the zone of equivalence, as more and more antigen is added to the system, immunocomplex precipitation declines steadily owing to antigen excess. Similarly to other types of particles in

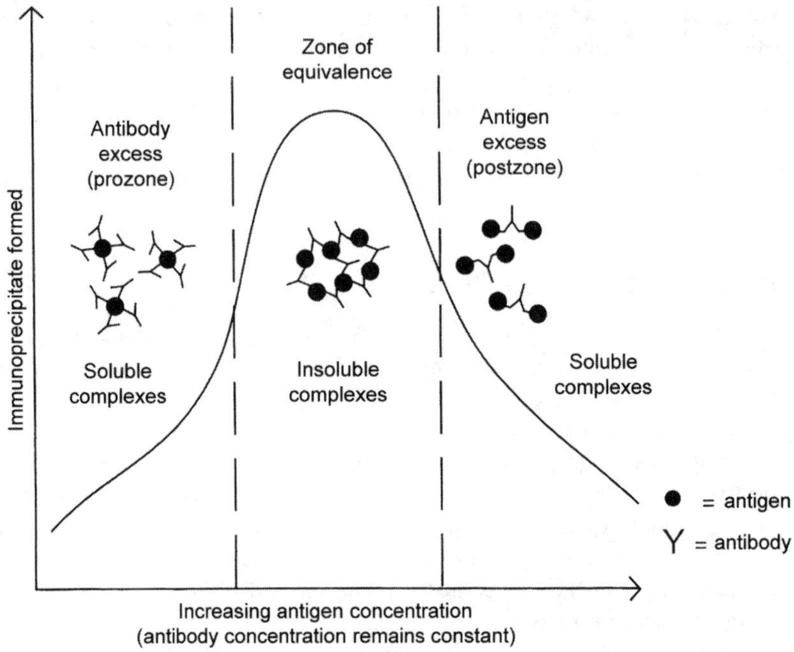

FIGURE 17. Antigen–antibody immunoprecipitation curve with schematic diagrams of immune complexes through the stages of immunoprecipitation reaction.

solution, light of an appropriate wavelength striking an immunocomplex can be transmitted, absorbed, reflected, or scattered. Turbidimetric and nephelometric immunoassays detect the presence of these particles in solution by their ability to transmit and scatter light, respectively.

Light-Scattering Properties of Particles in Solution

Rayleigh first described the light-scattering properties of particles in solution over a century ago. Light scattered by a homogeneous population of particles depends upon the relationship between the incident light wavelength (λ) and particle size (d). Figure 18 illustrates the three types of light scatter: Rayleigh, Mie, and Rayleigh-Debye. Rayleigh scatter describes the phenomenon whereby incident light is scattered nearly symmetrically about a small particle, resulting in a scattered light intensity minima at a 90° angle to the incident light. Rayleigh type of scatter occurs when the incident light wavelength is significantly greater than the particle diameter ($d < 0.1\lambda$). Rayleigh scatter best predicts the light scatter properties of dilute solutions of small particles such as immunoglobulins. Mie type of light scatter occurs when the incident light wavelength is significantly smaller than the particle diameter ($d > 10\lambda$). These very large particles cause most of the incident light to appear to be scattered in the forward direction because of destructive out-of-phase backward-direction scatter. Mie scatter may be used to quantitate very large particles such as red blood cells and bacteria. Rayleigh-Debye type of light scatter occurs when the incident light wavelength is approximately equal in size to the particle diameter ($d \approx \lambda$). In this case, light scatter is preferentially in a forward direction as opposed to a backward direction (11). Rayleigh-Debye light scatter is often used to quantitate high molecular weight plasma proteins, e.g., some IgM class immunoglobulins and immunocomplex (antigen–antibody) formation reactions.

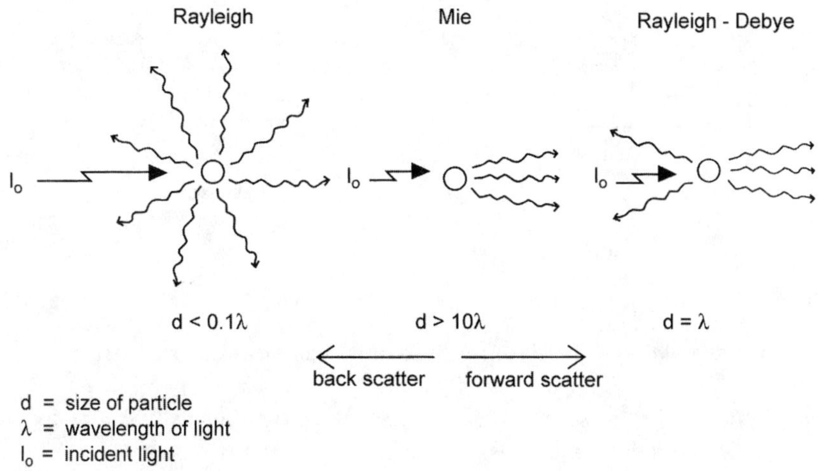

FIGURE 18. Light-scattering properties of particles in solution: Rayleigh, Mie, and Rayleigh-Debye types.

Immunocomplex-forming reactions essentially produce Rayleigh-Debye light scatter since they are often heterogeneous, containing free antigen, and antibody, along with their resultant soluble and insoluble immunocomplexes as the reaction proceeds through the three stages described earlier. Immunocomplex monitoring systems generally use a source light wavelength in the 320–650-nm range to observe light scatter caused by particles with diameters ranging from 250 to 1500 nm. Rayleigh-Debye light scatter is effectively monitored using a nephelometer to sensitively detect forward light scatter at a 15–90° angle of observation.

Light Scatter Instrumentation: Turbidimeter and Nephelometer

The basic components of the instrumentation used to measure turbidimetric and nephelometric properties of particles in solution are illustrated in Figure 19. These instruments are similar and include a light source, sample cell, and a photodetector.

Turbidimeter

Turbidimetry is in many aspects analogous to absorption spectrophotometry. For example, sample solution turbidity is determined by measuring light transmission to a photodetector placed at 180° from the incident light beam as seen in Figure 19. Given that the spatial arrangement of the light source, sample holder, and photodetector is the same for absorption spectrophotometry and turbidimetry analysis, turbidimetric assays are routinely performed along with color development assays using a standard automated spectrophotometer-based analyzer.

Nephelometer

In contrast to turbidimetric assays, a dedicated nephelometer instrument is required for nephelometric assays. A nephelometer uses a high-intensity light source focused onto the sample cell and the sample particles scatter some of the incident light in the forward direction owing to Rayleigh-Debye or Mie type of scatter. The scattered light is collected and focused onto a sensitive photodetector that can be located at a selected fixed angle,

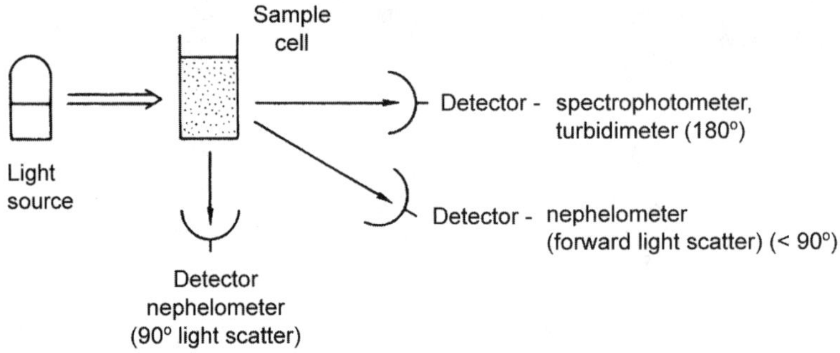

FIGURE 19. Nephelometer, turbidimeter, and spectrophotometer instrument design.

usually 30°, 70°, or 90°, as seen in Figure 19. Scattered light intensity is directly proportional to the concentration of particles in the sample solution.

Instrument Components: Nephelometer and Turbidimeter

Light Source and Wavelength Selection. High-intensity light sources such as lasers, tungsten-halogen, or xenon lamps are frequently used for nephelometry. Lasers are especially well suited for this purpose as they provide stable, highly collimated intense beams of monochromatic light. These features of laser light sources provide substantial improvements in sensitivity (ability to detect weak light scattering) over conventional high-intensity lamps. Although it is recognized that scattered light intensity increases as shorter wavelengths of incident light are used, this range is best avoided when assaying serum samples. The source light wavelength selected is generally different than that of what the particles would normally absorb. The wavelength selected is typically in the 320–380-nm or 500–650-nm ranges to avoid absorption by protein at <300 nm and by some serum chromogens, especially porphyrins at 400–425 nm (12). Wavelength selection for conventional light sources may be accomplished using interference filters. Laser light sources provide monochromatic light and do not require a mechanism for wavelength selection.

Collimating Optics. Conventional tungsten-halogen or xenon lamps require collimating optics to further intensify and narrow the source light beam to minimize stray light. Laser light sources are already highly collimated and hence require no additional collimating or light collection optics.

Sample Cell. The sample cell may be composed of glass or plastic, depending on the selected source light wavelength. When the source light is within the UV light range, the sample cells need to be composed of quartz or other UV light transmissible materials since UV light is not transmitted well through ordinary glass and some plastics.

Photodetector. Both photomultiplier tubes and photodiodes are used and placed at an angle to the incident light, i.e., 180° for a turbidimeter and 30°, 70°, or 90° fixed angle for the nephelometer. The precise angle is chosen to maximize the sensitivity of the measurement and is dependent upon the light-scattering properties of the particles in solution (13).

Nephelometry Reaction Methods. Immunocomplex formation may be monitored by either rate (kinetic) or endpoint (equilibrium) methods. These reaction-monitoring methods differ as to whether readings are taken at the end of the reaction (endpoint) or during active immunocomplex formation (rate).

Rate (Kinetic)

Immunocomplex (antigen–antibody complex) reactions begin with an initial lag phase followed by a rapid, linear increase in light scatter as larger particles (immunocomplexes) form over time. The rate of immunocomplex formation slows to a plateau when flocculation and precipitation appear. After the plateau is reached, antigen becomes in excess and light scatter begins to diminish. Rate (kinetic) analysis of light scattering is illustrated in Figure 20. Rate (kinetic) methods take light scatter measurements within the first few minutes after antigen and antibody are combined. During this period, the largest **rate of change** of scattered light intensity occurs. Kinetic methods offer several distinct advantages over endpoint methods. Generally, rate methods are faster and can be assayed in a fixed time during the most rapid rate of change of light scattering. These methods do not require a separate sample blank measurement since rate of change is monitored, as opposed to absolute light scatter in the endpoint analysis method.

Endpoint (Equilibrium)

Endpoint (Equilibrium) reaction methods measure light scattering when the immunocomplex reaction reaches equilibrium. Figure 21 depicts an example of the endpoint reaction analysis method. A single light scatter measurement is taken during this steady-state time period when rate of change is small (*see* R in Figure 21). Endpoint methods require an incubation period before this single measurement is made. In addition, a serum blank measurement (B) may be needed to correct for high background light scattering owing to sample turbidity caused by lipids and other macromolecules. Making a large serum dilution or sample pretreatment to remove the interfering substances can minimize this potential problem.

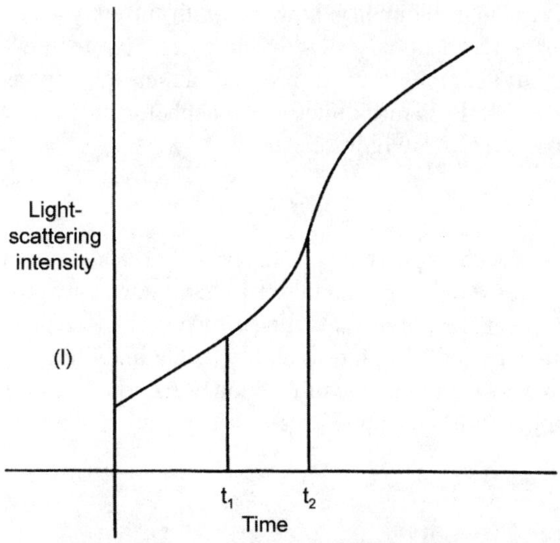

FIGURE 20. Rate (kinetic) nephelometry reaction measures light-scattering signal at two or more time intervals: t_1 = time period one, t_2 = time period two, and I = light-scattering intensity.

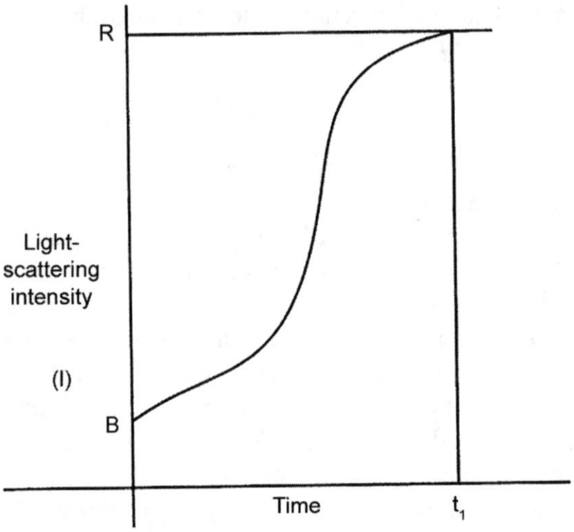

FIGURE 21. Endpoint (equilibrium) nephelometry reaction measures light-scattering signal at t_1 (time 1) during steady-state (R); B = sample blank measurement and I = light-scattering intensity.

Limitations/Sources of Error

Turbidimetry and nephelometry have numerous similarities to absorption spectrophotometry and can suffer from many of the same sources of interference and errors. In addition, nephelometry has some unique features and some specific limitations and errors will be discussed.

Sensitivity of Turbidimetry versus Nephelometry

In theory, nephelometry is more sensitive than turbidimetry; however, with currently available instruments and methods, the nephelometer is only slightly more sensitive for low-level immunocomplex (antigen–antibody complex) reactions and about equally as sensitive for specific protein quantitation (14). Both turbidimetric and nephelometric assay sensitivity depends primarily on the absence of stray light scatter.

Polymer Enhancement

The use of nonionic hydrophilic polymers such as polyethylene glycol (PEG) and dextran in nephelometric reactions has greatly improved the speed and sensitivity of the assay procedures. In immunocomplex reactions, the PEG polymers compete for water molecules, thus decreasing their availability and thereby reducing the solubility of the immunocomplex in the solution. The net effect is an increase in the rate of reaction. Reaction times for endpoint assays have dropped from hours to minutes and kinetic assay peak rates have increased as much as 10-fold (15).

Sources of Error

High Background Scatter. Nephelometric assay sensitivity is largely controlled by the amount of background scatter from sample and reagents. Relatively high background scatter should be avoided. Sample background scatter is related to sample macromolecules,

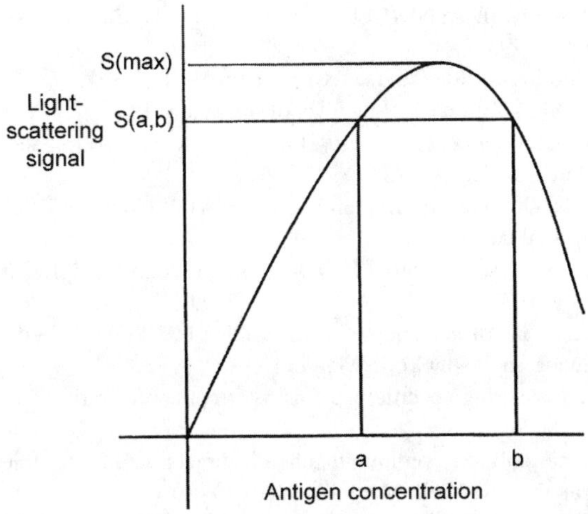

FIGURE 22. Antigen excess curve. Effects of increasing antigen concentrations beyond S(max) representing maximum light scattering. Different antigen concentrations (a) and (b) each give equivalent light-scattering signal responses, shown as S(a,b).

especially lipids. If endpoint reactions are used, correct with sample dilution or by using a sample blank measurement. If rate reactions are used, the instrument electronically corrects for the sample background scatter. Furthermore, reagents can contain dust particles and filtering of reagents may avoid this problem.

Antigen Excess. Antigen excess is a potential problem that is observed more frequently in endpoint reactions than in rate reactions. As discussed earlier, the immunocomplex reaction begins with antibody excess and proceeds into equilibrium where peak light scattering occurs. After equilibrium, the reaction enters into antigen excess phase and light scattering diminishes. As can be seen in Figure 22, if light-scattering measurements are made during the antigen excess phase represented by point S(b), peak light scattering is missed and this can result in falsely decreased light scatter to be measured. Most commercially available nephelometers now have an integrated means to detect antigen excess (16).

REFERENCES

1. Schoeff LE. Molecular absorption spectroscopy. In: Schoeff LE, Williams RH, eds. Principles of laboratory instruments. St. Louis: Mosby, 1993.
2. Ward KM, Harris E. Spectrophotometry. In: Ward KM, Lehmann CA, Leiken AM, eds. Clinical laboratory instrumentation and automation: principles, applications, and selection. Philadelphia: WB Saunders, 1994.
3. De Cresce RP, Lifshitz MS. Chemistry instrumentation: new technology for the 1980s and beyond. Lab Med 1986;17:267–70.
4. Karselis TC. The pocket guide to clinical laboratory instrumentation. Philadelphia: FA Davis, 1994:67–71.
5. Alexander LR, Barnhart ER. Photometric quality assurance instrument check procedures. Atlanta, U.S. Department of Health and Human Services, Centers for Disease Control, Bureau of Laboratories, 1980.
6. Tiffany TO. Fluorometry, nephelometry, and turbidimetry. In: Burtis CA, Ashwood ER, eds. Tietz textbook of clinical chemistry, 3rd ed. Philadelphia: WB Saunders, 1999.

7. Bowie LJ. Molecular emission spectroscopy. In: Schoeff LE, Williams RH, eds. Principles of laboratory instruments. St. Louis: Mosby, 1993.
8. Kricka LJ. Chemiluminescent and bioluminescent techniques. Clin Chem 1991;37:1472–81.
9. Abbott AxSYM System Operations Manual. Volume 1, Principles of operation, 1996.
10. Kusnetz J, Mansberg HP. Optical considerations: nephelometry. In: Ritchie RF, ed. Automated immunoanalysis, Part 1. New York: Marcel Dekker, 1978.
11. Pesce AJ, Frings CS, Gauldie J. Spectral techniques. In: Kaplan LA, Pesce AJ, Kazmierczak SC, eds. Clinical chemistry: theory, analysis and correlation, 4th ed. St. Louis: Mosby, 2003.
12. Schoeff LE. Nephelometry and turbidimetry. In: Schoeff LE, Williams RH, eds. Principles of laboratory instruments. St. Louis: Mosby, 1993.
13. Gauldie J. Principles and clinical applications of nephelometry. In: Kaplan LA, Pesce AJ, eds. Non-isotopic alternatives to radioimmunoassay. New York: Marcel Dekker, 1981.
14. Sternberg JC. A rate nephelometer for measuring specific proteins by immunoprecipitin reactions. Clin Chem 1977;23:1456–64.
15. Hellsing K. Enhancing effects of nonionic polymers on immunochemical reactions. In: Ritchie RF, ed. Automated immunoanalysis. Part 1. New York: Marcel Dekker, 1978.
16. Hills LP, Tiffany TO. Comparison of turbidimetric and light scattering measurements of immunoglobulins by use of a centrifugal analyzer with absorbance and fluorescence light scattering optics. Clin Chem 1980;26:1459–66.

Chapter 5

Chromatography and Mass Spectrometry in the Clinical Laboratory

Larry D. Bowers

The development of chromatographic separation and detection technologies and the advances in the understanding of biological systems have been closely linked. The ability to separate individual compounds of interest from complex biological matrices such as blood and urine has contributed to the basic understanding of biochemistry and pharmacology. Separation of the chiral components of drugs, for example, has resulted in a better understanding of drug metabolism and activity. Rapid separation and sensitive detection of compounds such as cholesterol and steroids have lead to the development of chromatographic reference methods for the clinical laboratory. Quantification, in addition to reliable information regarding identification, has resulted in the application of chromatographic techniques to workplace and emergency care drug testing. The ability to separate, identify, and quantify individual components in complex mixtures has contributed to the revolution in proteomics and metabonomics. Thus, chromatographic separations have played, and will continue to play, a key role in clinical laboratory science.

THE CHROMATOGRAPHIC PROCESS

The International Union of Pure and Applied Chemistry (IUPAC) defines chromatography as "a physical method of separation in which the components to be separated are distributed between two phases, one of which is the **stationary phase** while the other, the **mobile phase**, moves in a definite direction" (1–5). The stationary phase can be a solid, a gel, or a liquid. If the stationary phase is a liquid, it can be coated, chemically bonded, or immobilized (e.g., polymerized or cross-linked) onto a solid support to keep it from moving. The solid support may or may not be involved in the separation process. The mobile phase can be a gas, a liquid, or a supercritical fluid. This discussion is restricted to a system in which the mobile phase is percolated continuously through the chromatographic bed during the separation process, although there are several other techniques for separating components by chromatography. The components of the sample are separated from each other into zones or bands along the chromatographic bed.

When the stationary phase/solid support bed is in the form of a tube, the component bands are eluted from the tube and transported to a detector by the mobile phase. The plot of detector response as a function of time (or volume) is called a chromatogram (Figure 1). The detector signal observed when only mobile phase is eluting from the column is called the baseline. When a component is eluted from the column and observed by the detector, the signal generally takes the form of a bell-shaped curve and is called a chromatographic peak.

Chromatographic phase systems can be classified in several ways. A separation technique in which the stationary phase/solid support bed is contained within a tube is commonly called **column chromatography**. High-performance liquid chromatography (HPLC) is an example of column chromatography. When the bed of stationary phase/solid support is present in a flat sheet, the technique is commonly called planar or **open-bed chromatography**. Thin-layer chromatography (TLC) is an example of open-bed chromatography. A second means of classification is the physical state of the mobile phase,

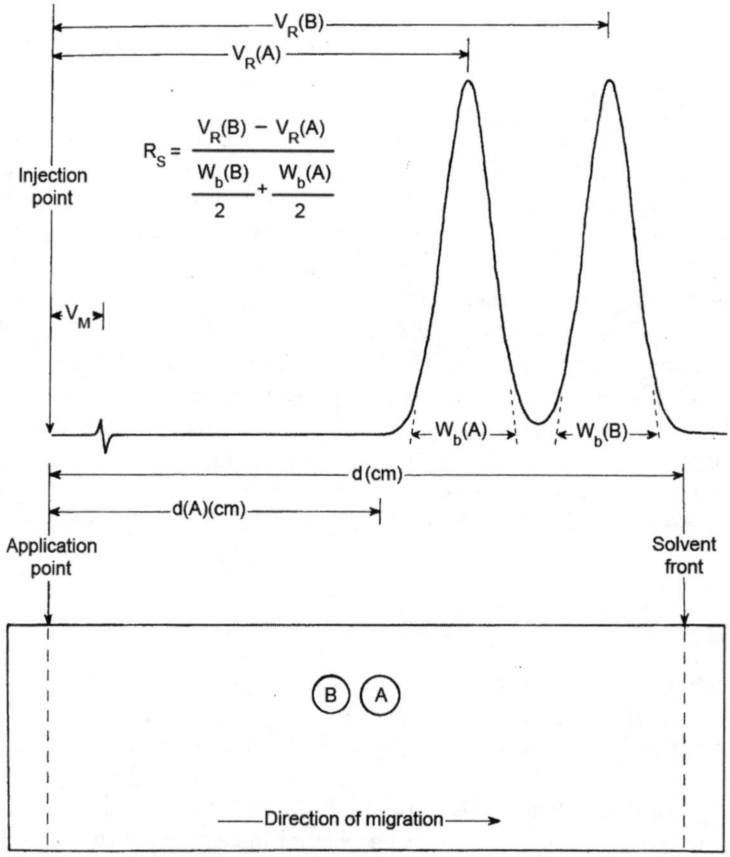

FIGURE 1. Schematic diagram of a separation using elution column chromatography and planar chromatography. Note that for elution techniques, more retained compounds elute at a longer time while for planar techniques, retained compounds fall further behind the solvent front. (*Reprinted from Tietz textbook of clinical chemistry, 3rd ed., Burtis CA, Ashwood ER, eds., p. 167, Copyright 1999, with permission from Elsevier*)

which gives rise to gas chromatography (GC), liquid chromatography (LC), and supercritical fluid chromatography (SFC). In some cases, the physical state of both phases is used, for example, by convention in gas–liquid chromatography (GLC), the mobile phase is a gas and the stationary phase is a liquid.

A third way of classifying chromatographic phase systems is the mechanism of the separation. **Adsorption chromatography** is based on the selective interactions of molecules to be separated with the active groups on the surface of a solid stationary phase. The difference in solubility of various components between the mobile and stationary phases forms the basis of **partition chromatography**. Since there is a much wider selection of pairs of mobile phases and stationary phase liquids, the basis of most separations is partitioning. Reversed-phase (RP) HPLC is one frequently used form of partition chromatography. A difference in the molecular size and shape can be used to separate molecules by steric exclusion or gel permeation chromatography.

Ion-exchange chromatography makes use of interactions between positively or negatively charged sites on the analyte with an oppositely charged group on the stationary phase. Separation of negatively or positively charged analyte molecules is called anion-exchange chromatography or cation-exchange chromatography, respectively. Specialty columns, e.g., SAX, WAX, SCX, and WCX are used with this type of chromatography. **Affinity chromatography** makes use of biological selectivity, such as the interaction of an antigen or hapten with an antibody, to cause a differential separation. Many other selective analyte–ligand interactions also have been used to separate molecules of biological interest. Separation of **chiral** compounds also can be achieved readily (6). The critical step in the development of a successful chromatographic analysis is to recognize a molecular difference between the compounds that need to be separated and to select a chromatographic phase system that exploits those differences.

Chromatographic phase systems also are used for sample clean-up. Small beds of stationary phase/solid support have been developed for use in **solid-phase extraction** (SPE). SPE columns are frequently contained in 1- or 3-mL polypropylene syringe formats and used for rapid removal of matrix interferences and concentration of the compounds of interest. The SPE process for liquid samples consists of three steps: application of the sample; a wash with one or more solvent systems that elute interferences but do not displace the compound(s) of interest; and elution of the analytes. Sample components of interest can be concentrated prior to injection into the chromatographic system when a large volume of sample is placed on the SPE column and the components of interest eluted in a much smaller volume. Usually the solid support used in SPE columns is about 50 μm in diameter to allow a slight vacuum to draw fluid through the bed. More recently, membranes containing totally porous microparticulate (5 μm) support particles have been used. The structure of the membrane allows sufficiently high permeability for a small pressure or vacuum to pull solvent through the particle bed. This approach results in membranes that have the ability to bind large amounts of sample component and can be eluted with small volumes of solvent. Another extraction system, **solid-phase microextraction** (SPME), uses stationary phase immobilized in a fused silica needle and allows transfer of the sample components into either a gas or liquid mobile phase without solvent elution. Furthermore, immunoaffinity-based solid-phase clean-up can be extremely useful in extracting compounds from complex biological samples (7). A recent review addresses modern extraction techniques including restricted access media and molecularly imprinted polymers (8).

Equilibrium Aspects of Chromatography

Chromatographic separation occurs as a result of a near-equilibrium distribution of the analyte molecules between the stationary and mobile phases. The distribution constant, K_c, can be represented as:

$$K_c = \frac{C_{i(S)}}{C_{i(M)}} = \frac{W_{i(S)}/V_S}{W_{i(M)}/V_M} = \frac{W_{i(S)}}{W_{i(M)}}\frac{V_M}{V_S} = k \bullet \beta \quad (1)$$

where $C_{i(S)}$ and $C_{i(M)}$ are the concentration of compound i in the stationary and mobile phases, respectively, $W_{i(S)}$ and $W_{i(M)}$ are the mass of compound i in the stationary and mobile phases, respectively, and V_S and V_M are the volume of stationary and mobile phase, respectively. The ratio of the mass of compound i in the stationary and mobile phases is the **retention factor**[1], **k**, and the ratio of the volume of the mobile and stationary phases is called the **phase ratio**, β. Since the distribution constant is fixed under a particular set of conditions, decreasing the amount of stationary phase relative to mobile phase decreases the retention factor. The development and use of open-tubular capillary GC columns with a very thin annulus of stationary phase coated or immobilized on the inner surface of the tube results in a system with a large phase ratio. This development has made possible the GC analysis of many nonvolatile compounds such as steroids and drugs. From a practical standpoint, once a column chromatographic system is purchased, the β is constant, and thus altering any parameter that changes K_c results in a change in k.

If the compound of interest does not interact with the stationary phase, both K_c and k will be zero. The development of sample introduction and detection systems in the chromatographic system that are physically separated from the column means that the molecules have to be transported from the site where the sample was introduced into the mobile phase and to the site where they are detected. Thus, a compound that does not interact with the stationary phase appears at the detector in a volume of mobile phase given by:

$$V_M = V_{col} + V_{ext} \quad (2)$$

where V_M is the observed hold-up volume which is made up of the mobile phase volume in the column (V_{col}) and in any tubing or other area outside of the chromatographic column (V_{ext}) that is swept by the mobile phase. In practice, every effort should be made to minimize V_{ext}. If V_{ext} is small relative to V_{col}, it can be ignored in a practical discussion of chromatographic theory, even though the chromatographic process is initiated only when an analyte comes in contact with the phase system. Extracolumn volumes do have a role in determining the appearance of the chromatographic peaks, even though they are not involved in the chromatographic process.

For a compound that does interact with the stationary phase, its rate of movement through the chromatographic bed is retarded relative to the rate of mobile phase movement and thus it will be retained. The adjusted retention volume, V'_R, which reflects the retention relative to the mobile phase, is the difference between the total retention volume, V_R,

[1] The retention factor previously was known as the capacity factor, designated by the symbol k', but the use of this term is now discouraged.

and the hold-up volume, V_M. The k also can be thought of as the relative amount of time the compound spends in the stationary phase relative to the mobile phase, and thus $k = V'_R/V_M$. As a result,

$$V_R = V'_R + V_M = V_M\,(k+1) \tag{3}$$

Although retention has been presented in terms of volumes, it can also be discussed in terms of retention time, t_R, since $t_R = V_R/F_c$ where F_c is the volumetric flow rate in the As a practical matter, the highest point on the chromatographic peak is taken as a measure of the retention time or volume (*see* Figure 1). While this is a good approximation for a symmetrical peak, it is not theoretically correct for peaks that are asymmetrical.

In column chromatography, the compound of interest is carried along by the mobile phase and is eluted from the bed and detected. The sample is introduced into the mobile phase stream as a pulse, either by injection or sample valve. In contrast, the compounds in open-bed chromatography usually are visualized in some way while they are still associated with the separation medium. In this case, instead of an elution volume, the retention behavior of a compound is described as the retardation factor, R_F, defined as the distance to the center of the sample component spot [d(A)] relative to the distance traveled by the mobile phase front (d; Figure 1). By definition, R_F is always less than one and is related to k by:

$$R_F = \frac{1}{(1+k)} \tag{4}$$

Thus, the retention behavior of a compound can be compared for open-bed and column systems having the same mobile and stationary phases. Planar chromatography techniques continue to develop with improved phases for higher separation ability and electro-osmostic or forced fluid flow to achieve constant flow velocity (9).

The principal reason for using a chromatographic analysis system is the separation of two or more compounds or the separation of a compound of interest from the complex biological matrix. The separation factor, α, is the ratio of the adjusted retention volumes, V'_R, of two adjacent peaks. By definition, α is always greater than one[2]:

$$\alpha = \frac{V'_{R2}}{V'_{R1}} = \frac{t'_{R2}}{t'_{R1}} = \frac{k_2}{k_1} \tag{5}$$

The separation factor indicates the ability of the chromatographic system to retain selectively one compound of interest relative to another and is the major parameter to consider in developing an efficient analytical scheme based on chromatography.

Dynamic Aspects of Chromatography

If equilibrium were the only process at work in chromatography, all molecules of the compound of interest would emerge from the column at the same instant. For various reasons related to the flow of the mobile phase and molecular diffusion, this is not the case and the molecules emerge from the column as a Gaussian-shaped peak. In an open-bed system, the fact that the final spot diameter is larger than the application spot is the result of similar

[2] The term "selectivity" was used in the past for the separation factor, but its use is now discouraged.

processes. For a Gaussian peak, the standard deviation is a measure of the peak width, and so a measure of chromatographic peak width expressed as the plate number, N, for the peak corresponding to compound A is defined as:

$$N = \left[\frac{V_R(A)}{s(A)}\right]^2 \tag{6}$$

where s is the standard deviation of the peak. Since it is difficult in practice to measure the standard deviation of a peak, several approaches to measuring the width of the peak have been reported, based on the relationships shown in Figure 2. Because almost no chromatographic peak is really symmetrical near the baseline, the recommended method is to measure the peak width at a height half-way to maximum height, thus N is given by:

$$N = 5.54\left[\frac{V_R(A)}{w_h(A)}\right]^2 \tag{7}$$

where $w_h(A)$ is the width of the peak half way between the baseline and the peak maximum and the 5.54 factor comes from the relationship between $w_h(A)$ and s(A). The units of retention and peak width must be the same when computing N, since the number of plates has no units. The plate number is reflective of column performance; a column with

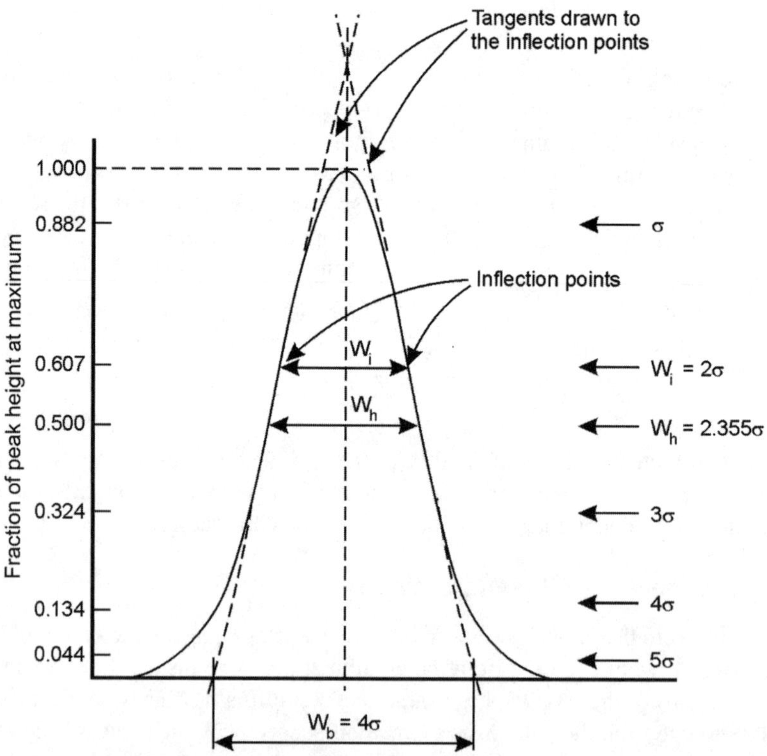

FIGURE 2. Relationship between various measures of peak width and the standard deviation of a Gaussian peak. (*From Ettre LS. Nomenclature for chromatography. Pure Appl Chem 1993; 65:819–72. © 1993 IUPAC*)

a larger number of theoretical plates is more efficient. Narrower, sharper peaks have a number of advantages, such as better detection limits and the ability to separate more peaks per unit time. Note also that since N should be constant for a particular system, the width of a peak increases with increased retention.

Another equation used to calculate N is based on three parameters easily measured by digital integrators:

$$N = 2\pi \left(\frac{t_R h'}{A} \right)^2 \tag{8}$$

where t_R is the elution time (sec), h' is the peak height (volts), and A is the peak area (volt-sec). This equation is used frequently by computer-based integration systems to measure N.

To this point, it has been implied that the column is the only source of chromatographic band broadening. The total peak width observed is the product of a number of processes:

$$W^2_{total} = W^2_{column} + W^2_{injector} + W^2_{tubing/connectors} + W^2_{detector} \tag{9}$$

where w_{column} is the effect due to the column, $w_{injector}$ is the broadening due to the sample introduction system, $w_{tubing/connectors}$ is the contribution from the tubing and connections linking the column to the sample introduction and detection systems, and $w_{detector}$ is due to broadening that occurs in the detector. The most common source arising from the column is the presence of more than one interaction between the analyte and the stationary phase. An example would be the interaction of an organic base with the negatively charged silanol groups on the surface of silica gel during a separation whose primary mechanism is partitioning into nonpolar octadecyl hydrocarbons bonded to the silica gel surface. Another possible cause of peak tailing is a nonlinear relationship between k and concentration of the analyte.

The sample introduction process contributes both to peak broadening and to peak tailing. For example, injection of large sample volumes in GC or HPLC results in broadened peaks. In GC, the injection process itself results in a tailed peak due to the gas dynamics in sweeping out the injector volume. The contribution from tubing can be minimized by using tubing of the smallest practical internal diameter and minimizing the length of the tubing. It is also important to use good technique in making connections between tubing and columns or other devices, as a poorly made connection can lead to dramatic peak broadening and tailing. The contributions from the detector arise from the volume and the flow dynamics of the detection cell and also from the electronic processing of the signal. If all broadening factors are less than about one-third of that due to the column, they can be ignored.

Another term of theoretical significance is the height equivalent to a theoretical plate, HETP or H. As the name suggests, this is the length of column that corresponds to one theoretical plate: The value of H is calculated from the length of the column, L, and N:

$$H = \frac{L}{N} \tag{10}$$

As will be seen in subsequent sections, the proper selection of flow rate, mobile phase composition, column diameter, and support particle size minimizes H, resulting in an optimum value for N.

Peak tailing can be a problem as mentioned earlier; asymmetric peaks frequently are encountered in routine chromatography. Peaks that have a longer trailing trace are referred to as "tailed," while those that have an elongated leading portion are referred to as "fronted." There are two primary analytical outcomes of an asymmetric peak. First, N, as measured at half-height, is an overestimate of the real efficiency of the system. There have been various attempts to calculate a corrected N, such as the Dorsey–Foley equation (10):

$$N_{corrected} = \left(\frac{t_R}{w_{0.1}}\right)^2 \left(\frac{41.7}{(B/A)+1.25}\right) \quad (11)$$

where $w_{0.1}$ is the width of the peak one-tenth of the way from the baseline to the peak apex (*see* Figure 2), and A and B are the distances from a line dropped vertically from the apex to the front and back, respectively, of the peak envelope one-tenth of the way from the baseline to the peak apex. The more tailed the peak (B>A), the smaller the value of N. In the case of a fronted peak, the quantity (A/B) is substituted for (B/A). The **asymmetry factor**, A_s, has been described to quantify the asymmetry of a peak; A_s is the ratio (B/A) just described. Symmetrical peaks should have an A_s between 0.95 and 1.10.

The second analytical outcome is that when a tailed peak elutes just before another peak, a larger portion of the first peak is found under the second. As a result, quantification of the peaks, particularly using peak area, is less accurate. This topic is covered in more detail under *Considerations for Quantitative Analysis.*

Peak Resolution

Since the purpose of a chromatographic analysis is to separate one compound from another, it is important to have a way of describing the quality of a separation. Peak resolution, R_s, is the difference of the volumes (or times) of the peak maxima relative to the width of the chromatographic peak:

$$R_s = \frac{V_R(B) - V_R(A)}{\frac{w_b(B)}{2} + \frac{w_b(A)}{2}} = \frac{V_R(B) - V_R(A)}{w_b(B)} \quad (12)$$

where $w_b(B)$ is the width at baseline of the second peak, assuming that the two peak widths are equal. Note that in order for the signal to reach baseline between the two peaks, an R_s of 1.5 is required. The R_s is increased either by increasing the distance between the peak maxima or by decreasing the peak width. Substituting previously defined terms:

$$R_s = \frac{\sqrt{N}}{4}\left(\frac{k}{k+1}\right)\left(\frac{\alpha-1}{\alpha}\right) \quad (13)$$

From this equation, it can be seen that there are three ways to improve the resolution of a particular chromatographic separation. Increasing N improves the narrowness of the peaks. While N is an important contributor to resolution, an increase in N is usually used to fine-tune a separation. This is because an increase in N by a factor of 10, which is not easy to achieve, results in an increase of resolution only by a factor of 1.4. The distance between the peak maxima is increased either by increasing the separation factor or by increasing the retention factor. The optimal value for k is between 2 and 10. For some difficult separations, k may have to be adjusted to between 1 and 20. When k = 10, for example, its contribution to R_s is at 91% of its maximum value. Increasing k from 10 to 15 would only add 2.7% to R_s but would increase the time of analysis by 45%. Increasing α, however, is a powerful way to increase resolution, since an increase in α from 1.01 to 1.05 increases R_s by 480%. The key to developing an effective, valid chromatographic method is an understanding of how to adjust experimental parameters to optimize α, k, and N.

General Elution Problem

Chromatographic theory deals with retention behavior in systems in which the equilibrium conditions are consistent across the length of the column. In GC, this requires that the temperature be constant, which is referred to as an **isothermal** condition. In LC, the composition of the mobile phase (and temperature) must be held constant, which is referred to as an **isocratic** (same strength) condition. For some analytical problems, the range of k values for the compounds of interest is such that it is impossible to find a single set of isothermal or isocratic conditions under which all compounds of interest elute under optimal conditions and in a reasonable amount of time. For example, to perform a drug screen for sedative-hypnotic drugs, it would be impossible to find a single isothermal GC condition that would allow this separation to occur. This is known as the **general elution problem**. As will be discussed in a coming section, the solution to this problem is to alter the elution conditions during the separation. Two commonly used techniques are **temperature programming** in GC and **solvent strength programming** (gradient elution) in HPLC. Since one analytical strength of chromatography is separating a large number of compounds, temperature programming and, to a lesser extent, gradient elution are used frequently used in bioanalytical separations. Changing elution conditions changes both the elution time and the peak shape. Altering the elution conditions during the run also means that the system must be reequilibrated to the initial conditions before the next sample can be analyzed, which decreases sample throughput.

CHROMATOGRAPHIC METHOD DEVELOPMENT

Fitness for Purpose

Chromatographic applications have a number of beneficial uses in the clinical laboratory. In general, chromatography can be implemented for improved assay specificity for the compound of interest, qualitative identification of compounds, and quantification of compounds. Since chromatographic assays would fall in the Clinical Laboratory Improvement Act category of "complex assays" and in most cases would have been developed within the laboratory for its own use, it is important that the assay be fit for purpose (11). In order to establish the suitability of a method for measurement of a particular analyte, it is necessary to validate the method. For a unique method developed "in-house," validation approaches have been described in detail elsewhere (12). The initial step is to define method applicability including the analyte(s) being measured, its concentration range, the sample matrix (e.g., urine), and the purpose of the measurement. Based on this definition of method applicability, a set of method specifications can be developed to ensure that the method is suitable for achieving the analytical objectives. During method development, the following parameters should be characterized:

- Trueness (bias)
- Precision
- Selectivity (or specificity)

- Sensitivity (calibration)
- Range
- Limit of quantification
- Limit of detection
- Robustness and ruggedness

Accuracy reflects the closeness of an analytical result to the "true" value and is composed of both systematic (trueness) and random errors (precision) associated with a method. **Precision** may be measured as repeatability, intermediate precision, or reproducibility. Analytical **selectivity** of a method is its ability to measure the analyte accurately in the presence of the sample matrix. Analytical **sensitivity** is the slope of the response–concentration curve. **Range** specifies the lowest and highest concentrations for which the method can be used. The **limit of detection** represents the smallest concentrations that can be reliably distinguished from the background signal. The **limit of quantification** is the lowest concentration that can be determined with acceptable accuracy and precision. **Robustness** is the ability of the method to provide the same results in the face of small changes in method conditions. **Ruggedness** can be determined by deliberately altering analytical conditions such as analyst, instrument, column, and reagents. (See references 11 and 13 for a more detailed discussion.) A measure of system suitability should be made for each analytical run—including chromatographic measures of merit such as N, peak asymmetry, and peak resolution of a known pair of components; retention time consistency with reference materials; and, where applicable, quantitative results within acceptable limits.

Considerations for Quantitative Analysis

Although the primary purpose of a chromatographic method is to separate the analyte from other compounds and matrix components, on-line detection systems and computer-based data reduction make quantitative analyses feasible. The concentration of the compound of interest at any time is given by the equation for a Gaussian peak:

$$C_t = \frac{C_s V_s}{V_R}\sqrt{\frac{N}{2\pi}}\exp\left[-\frac{N(t-t_R)^2}{2t_R^2}\right] \quad (14)$$

where C_t is the concentration at time t, C_s is the concentration in the sample, and V_s is the volume of sample introduced into the chromatographic system. At the peak apex ($t = t_R$), the concentration is given by:

$$C_{t_R} = \frac{C_s V_s}{V_R}\sqrt{\frac{N}{2\pi}} \quad (15)$$

This equation provides guidance on maximizing the peak height. Increasing the concentration of the analyte in the injection solution and increasing the volume of solution injected increases the signal. As mentioned earlier, increasing the volume of sample will, at some point, result in broadened peaks, lowered effective N, and decreased peak height. Decreasing k or V_M reduces the retention volume (*see* Equation 3), although the effect of k on resolution also must be considered. A reduction in V_M is accomplished most effectively by decreasing the column diameter, particularly in HPLC systems. Increasing N results in narrower, taller peaks with greater height relative to area.

Two types of detectors are used with chromatographic systems: mass-flow dependent and concentration dependent. For a concentration-dependent detector, the measured peak height is given by $h' = S_h C_{tR}$ where h' is the height of the peak and S_h is the response factor for the detector. Integrating the peak for a concentration-dependent detector, the $A = S_A(W_i/F_c)$ where A is the peak area and S_A is the response factor. Thus, if there is an increase in flow rate during the elution of the peak envelope, the area is decreased while the peak height is not. For a mass-flow sensitive detector, the observed peak height is given by $h' = S_h C_{tR} F_c$, while the peak area is given by $A = S_A W_i$. In this case, an increase in flow rate increases the peak height but has no affect on the peak area. Peak area was used in the early development of GC because the flame ionization detector is a mass-flow dependent detector and control of the flow rate was not as precise as that obtained with modern flow controllers. As a result, more precise quantitative results were obtained with peak area measurements.

Modern digital integrators have eliminated the need for other forms of chromatographic peak recording (14). The difficulty for the computer in accurately determining the peak characteristics, particularly for trace analysis, is to recognize the start and end of the peak on a baseline that may be drifting and have noise superimposed on it. All digital integrators use some form of noise filtering to reduce the effect of noise on peak start/stop points and peak area and peak height measurements. In general, the computer uses an algorithm based on signal change relative to a threshold value or rate of signal change (first derivative of the signal) to recognize the beginning and end of a peak. A combination of the first and second derivatives of the signal is used to recognize the peak apex, the peak inflection points, and even unresolved peaks. Various proprietary algorithms are used to determine whether to broaden the peak start/stop points to improve peak height and area allocation, whether to use valley points or peak skim approaches to allocate peak area, or whether to report peaks that do not have sufficient peak height or area to exceed a threshold value.

Snyder et al. (15) and Meyer (16) dealt with the issue of errors in peak area for incompletely resolved peaks. Figure 3 illustrates two points for a pair of peaks with an area ratio of 8:1 (15). The black dot near the apex of each peak is the actual position (time and height) of the "theoretical" peak apex, whereas the line tracing would be the observed chromatogram. Note that at a R_s of 0.8 for Gaussian-shaped peaks, the peak height measurements are accurate to about 1% for both peaks. The measurement of the height of the second peak becomes less accurate with increased peak tailing (17). Peak overlap and peak tailing degrade accurate measurement of peak area much more rapidly. In general, computer-based integrators partition area by dropping a vertical line to baseline from the minimum valley point between the two peaks. This results in misallocation of some area of each peak. Even at an R_s of 1.25, when the asymmetry factor is 2, the area of the smaller, later eluting peak is overestimated by more than 30% while the area of the larger, earlier eluting peak is underestimated by about 5% (16). Thus, while digital integrators have broad capabilities to compensate for drifting baselines, asymmetric peaks, and incompletely resolved peaks, the analyst must recognize the integrator actions, evaluate their appropriateness, and reintegrate chromatograms when necessary.

The choice between peak height and peak area for quantification should be based on aspects of the analysis system other than flow control or data reduction. As previously mentioned, peak height measurements yield better accuracy when peak resolution is less than optimal, whether this is due to closely spaced analytes or the unexpected appearance of sample-specific matrix interference. Peak height measurements also perform better in trace analysis situations where determination of the peak start and stop points is difficult due to baseline noise. Peak area measurements provide better results when

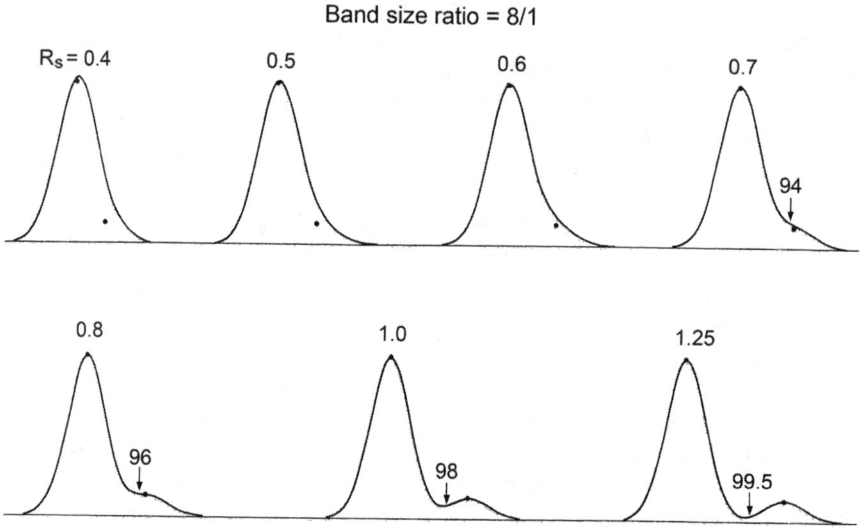

FIGURE 3. Appearance of chromatographic peaks in an eight-to-one concentration ratio at various values of resolution (R_s). The dots on the curves represent the true peak height and retention time for the two peaks. (*From Snyder LR. A rapid approach to selecting the best experimental conditions for high speed liquid chromatography. Part I. Estimating initial sample resolution required by a given problem. J Chromatogr Sci 1972;10:202. Reproduced from the Journal of Chromatographic Science by permission of Preston Publications, A Division of Preston Industries, Inc.*)

the concentration–response relationship is not linear; when well-resolved, tailed peaks are encountered; or when maximum precision is required for large peaks.

The final consideration in a quantitative chromatographic analysis system is the method of calibration. **External standard calibration** utilizes a series of solutions of known concentration analyzed, usually at the same time as the unknown sample. The concentration of the unknown is then determined by interpolation from the peak height or area versus concentration curve. A major source of error using external standard calibration is the reproducibility of injection volume and technique. **Internal standard calibration** requires that a specific amount of a reference compound, the internal standard, be added to the standard and unknown solutions. The peak height ratio or peak area ratio of the analyte to the internal standard is plotted as a function of analyte concentration, and the unknown concentration is determined by interpolation from this curve. The advantage of internal standard calibration is that if the internal standard is added prior to any sample preparation steps, and if the internal standard has chemical behavior similar to the analyte, then both losses in sample preparation and any variation in injection can be eliminated. The ideal internal standard in GC–MS or HPLC–MS analysis is a compound in which ^{2}H or ^{13}C has been substituted for ^{1}H or ^{12}C in the analyte. In this case, the chemical behavior of the internal standard is identical to the analyte, yet the detector is able to distinguish the analyte and internal standard on the basis of mass. The suitability of an internal standard must be determined by the purpose of the analysis. The final calibration method, **standard addition**, is rarely used in the clinical laboratory setting because it requires analysis of each sample twice. A known amount of the compound is added to the sample itself, and the sample is analyzed before and after addition. The difference between the peak heights or areas is then due to the amount of added material, and the initial concentration can be calculated.

An area that has received increased attention in recent years is measurement **uncertainty** (18). According to the ISO/IEC 17025:1999 General Requirements for the

Competence of Calibration and Testing Laboratories (19), every certificate of analysis or laboratory report should be accompanied by an estimate of the uncertainty. Uncertainty is a measure of the range of values possible based on the measurement result. Uncertainty in quantitative measurements should include reproducibility, bias, calibration uncertainties, and other parameters that significantly affect the result. One approach to the estimation of method uncertainty is the development of an uncertainty budget (18) where the contribution of each step in the analysis, as determined by statistical or other information, is summed as their variance into a combined standard uncertainty, u_c. A recent example of this approach was published for a chromatographic method for quantifying biogenic amines (20). Other approaches to determining uncertainty also have been proposed (21). Once u_c is determined, an expanded uncertainty, U, is often computed using a coverage factor, k, based on statistical probabilities. Thus, a report could state that the true value, Y, is included within the range $y \pm ku_c$ ($y \pm U$) with 95% confidence (where $k \approx 2$ at 95% confidence level). Caution must be exercised in applying this process to clinical situations!

Considerations for Qualitative Analysis

One application of chromatography is the identification of an unknown compound. An example would be the detection of an unknown drug using a GC screening procedure for sedative-hypnotic drugs. The identification is generally based on the agreement between the retention time of a peak in the chromatogram of a sample and that of either a standard or a retention time from a library. Although a match of retention times can be consistent with the presence of a particular compound, **it does not prove identity**—another compound also could have the same retention behavior under the particular chromatographic conditions used.

Several approaches can be taken to decrease the uncertainty in identification. The compound could be analyzed using another type of column. For example, in GC it is possible to insert two capillary columns with different stationary phases into the same injection port. Simultaneous analysis of the sample on two columns occurs, and if the retention behavior on both columns is consistent with a single compound, there is increased confidence that the identity is correct.

A second approach is to use either a selective detector or to compare the response of the compound on two detectors in parallel. For example, the two columns from the previous example could be connected simultaneously to flame-ionization and thermionic-specific detectors. The ratio of the responses is an indication of the chemical makeup of the compound, and a match of retention time and detector response ratio between the unknown and a standard provides additional certainty to the identification. In HPLC, the use of a parameter such as peak purity based on diode-array spectra also could be used. The use of a detector that provides structural information, such as a mass spectrometer, contributes to reliable identification.

Absolute retention time data cannot be used for compound identification due to the dependence of retention behavior on mobile phase flow rate, column length, stationary phase, and temperature. As a result, the relative retention time is used more frequently. The relative retention time usually is calculated as the ratio of the retention time of the unknown peak to the retention time of a reference compound. In its simplest form, the reference compound is a compound added to each sample as an internal standard. The **Kováts GC retention index (I) system** compares retention behavior of compounds across various columns. A homologous series of hydrocarbons is used as a reference framework. By using hydrocarbons, the retention behavior is, by definition, independent of the polarity of the phase. When the compounds are analyzed at a constant temperature, I is calculated from the relationship:

$$I = 100z + 100\,\frac{\log t'_R(x) - \log t'_R(z)}{\log t'_R(z+1) - \log t'_R(z)} \qquad (16)$$

where z is the number of carbons of the standard eluting just before the unknown component, x. A hydrocarbon with 15 carbons has, by definition, an I of 1500. A compound with a log t_R' value midway between C-15 and C-16 has an I of 1550. Compendia of retention index data have been developed for drugs, environmental toxins, and many other compounds. Use of such lists helps in obtaining a preliminary identification of the compound. Unfortunately, there are two limitations to this retention index approach: most separations are not done under isothermal conditions; and hydrocarbons do not produce a response on selective detectors such as the thermionic-specific detector. As a result, other compounds, such as alkyl nitriles, have been proposed as the reference set for comparing retention behavior when using thermionic-specific detectors (TSD).

To address the issue of temperature-programmed analysis, a similar value, called the **linear retention index (I^T)**, can be calculated for linear temperature-programmed GC analyses:

$$I^T = 100z + 100\,\frac{\Theta(x) - \Theta(z)}{\Theta(z+1) - \Theta(z)} \qquad (17)$$

where Θ is the elution temperature of the unknown (x) or the hydrocarbon. The elution temperature is a function of the initial temperature, the rate of temperature increase, the phase ratio and column length, and the inverse of the flow rate. As a result, care must be taken when comparing results from two laboratories. In general, the values obtained for I^T and I on the same column will not be the same.

While the concept of uncertainty in quantitative measurements is widely used, the concepts regarding the expression of the uncertainty in qualitative measurements are not as well developed (22, 23). The certainty in identification of a drug, for example, will be related to its concentration in the biological matrix. At some concentration, the method will fail to identify the compound reliably. Similarly, while the precision of identification cannot be expressed as a standard deviation, it may be possible to express the fraction of attempts in which a true or false positive result is obtained. The lack of statistical foundation for assessing the uncertainty of qualitative methods and the amount of work required to acquire valid estimates of uncertainty may limit progress toward uncertainty expressions in qualitative methods.

Optimization of a Separation

Any separation involves the interplay between resolution, speed, and capacity; it is possible to obtain a reasonable compromise between two of the three parameters, but not all three.

The parameters effecting peak resolution (R_s) were presented in Equation 13. In order to have a robust quantitative analytical system, it is recommended that the R_s between the peak of interest and any other matrix component or other interference be at least 1.5. In order to maximize R_s, the k value should be between 2 and 10; the α should be maximized by selection of appropriate chromatographic conditions (mode, column, etc.); and the N should be as large as practical.

To minimize the time required for a separation:

$$t_R = N\frac{H}{u}(k+1) \tag{18}$$

where u is the mobile phase linear velocity calculated as the column length divided by the hold-up time ($u = L/t_M$). For the present discussion, the retention time will be that of the peak of interest. Unlike the situation with peak resolution, where increased k increases R_s, speed of analysis considerations require minimizing k. While Equation 18 suggests that decreasing N is good, it is actually minimization of the column length (*see* Equation 10) that reduces analysis time. A decrease in H is good for minimizing time, as is an increase in mobile phase linear velocity. Understanding the relationship between H and u, which allows selection of optimal conditions, is critical to minimizing analysis time. Remember that for an isothermal or isocratic separation, analysis time is determined by the last peak to elute from the column.

The capacity of a column is the amount of compound that can be placed on the column before significant peak distortion occurs. The capacity of a column depends on its characteristics. For example, the capacity of a 0.25-mm diameter capillary GC column with a 0.25-μm film thickness is approximately 40–80 ng of compound. Due to the low capacity of capillary GC columns, special injection techniques have been developed to inject a fraction of the sample onto the column. The capacity of the column increases with increasing column diameter, thicker stationary phase films, and increased solubility of the compound in the stationary phase. Note that the characteristics that increase capacity are the opposite of those that increase chromatographic resolution and speed of analysis. The capacity of an HPLC column for small molecules, due to the large surface area of totally porous, microparticulate support particles, is on the order of 200 mg. Thus, for analytical-scale HPLC separations, sample capacity does not pose a problem.

GAS CHROMATOGRAPHY

Optimizing Resolution

The primary parameters used to optimize a separation by GC and their effect on separation are:

Polarity of the stationary phase	α
Derivatization of analyte	k, α
Phase ratio	k, sample capacity, N
Column diameter and length	N, pressure drop, sample capacity
Carrier gas type and velocity	N, pressure drop, k
Temperature	k, effective N, pressure drop

In GC, the initial decision in developing a separation is selection of a stationary phase. Since the mobile phase in GC does not play an active role in determining k or a, the selection of the stationary phase is critical. Most phases are based on silicon polymers because the stationary phase must be a liquid at separation temperatures of up to 350 °C. The development of polysiloxane and polysilarylene stationary phase backbones has improved stationary phase stability significantly and decreased column bleed. Incorporation of nonpolar side chains (such as methyl and phenyl), and polar groups (such as glycols) provides for a wide range of interaction, and selectivities. Kováts indices also can be used to assist in column selection. Table 1 provides a list of the most popular GC stationary phases.

TABLE 1. Typical gas chromatographic stationary phases

Stationary phase	Composition	Polarity	Applications	Comments
OV-1 (DB-1, DB-1ms, HP-1, HP-1ms, HP-101, Ultra-1, SPB-1, CP-Sil 5 CB Low Bleed/MS, Rtx-1, BP-1, 007-1(MS), SP-2100, SE-30, CP-Sil 5 CB MS, ZB-1, AT-1, MDN-1)	Dimethylpolysiloxane	Nonpolar	Volatile amines, anabolic steroids, anticonvulsants, bacterial identification, drug screens, fatty acid methyl esters (FAMEs)	Highest temperature operating range
OV-101 (DB-5, DB-5ms, HP-5, HP-5ms, Ultra-2, SPB-5, CP-Sil 8 CB, Rtx-5, BP-5, OV-5, 007-2(MPS-5), SE-52, SE-54, XTI-5, PTE-5, HP-5MS, ZB-5, AT-5, MDN-5)	(5%-Phenyl)-methylpolysiloxane	Nonpolar	TMS-derivatives of amphetamine and metabolites, bacterial identification, TMS-derivative of cocaine and metabolites, drug screens, FAMEs, derivatives of THC, narcotics, tricyclic antidepressants	Polysilarylene phases, where the phenyl group bridges the polymer backbone between silyl groups, greatly increasing the temperature stability and decreasing column bleed. The polysilarylene phases have a slightly different separation factor than their siloxane counterparts. These columns are frequently labeled as "MS" or "low bleed" columns.
DB-35, HP-35, Rtx-35, SPB-35, AT-35, Sup-Herb, HP-35, BPX-35	(35%-Phenyl)-methylpolysiloxane	Intermediate	Barbiturates	

OV-17 (DB-17, DB-17ms, HP-50+, Rtx-50, CP-Sil 24 CB, 007-17(MPS-50), HP-17, SP-2250, SPB-50, ZB-50, AT-50)	(50%-Phenyl)-methylpolysiloxane	Intermediate	Underivatized steroids, drug screens	As the polarity of the stationary phase increases, its sensitivity to O_2 and H_2O degradation increases. As a result, the upper temperature limit of the column decreases.
OV-225 (DB-225, SP-2330, CP-Sil 43 CB, Rtx-225, BP-225, AT-225)	25%-Trifluoropropyl–25%-phenyl–50%-methylsiloxane	Intermediate	cis- and trans-FAMEs	
Polyethyleneglycol (DB-Wax, HP-20M, SUPELCOWAX 10, CP-WAX 52CB, SUPEROX II, CB-WAX, Stabilwax, BP-20, Carbowax, HP-Innowax, Rtx-WAX, ZB-WAX)	Polyethylene glycol	Polar	Volatile alcohols, aldehydes, ketones, phenols, FAMEs	Custom polar phases for blood alcohol analysis have been made, including DB-ALC1, DB-ALC-2, HP-ALC, Rtx-BAC1, Rtx-BAC2
Chiral columns (CycloSil-B, LIPODEX C, Rt-β DEXm, β-DEX 110, β-DEX 120)	Hepatkis (2,3-di-O-methyl-6-O-*tert*-butyl dimethylsilyl)-β-cyclodextrin in intermediate polarity polysiloxane	Chiral selective	Barbiturate enantiomers, ethosuximide enantiomers	

Many compounds of interest in the clinical laboratory are not volatilized easily at temperatures accessible in gas chromatography. As a result, they must be modified chemically to make them more volatile. Acylation, silylation, esterification, and oximation reactions have been used both to increase volatility and to improve detectability. Derivatization also improves separation characteristics. A chiral derivatizing agent, for example, allows separation of the d- and l-isomers of amphetamine on a nonchiral GC column. Many derivatization reactions have been reported (24).

Once the stationary phase is chosen, the column diameter, length, and phase thickness must be selected. Most separations using GC are performed on open-tubular fused silica columns with an internal diameter of 0.1–0.53 mm and an annulus of stationary phase cross-linked on the inner surface of the capillary. The β in open tubular capillary columns is determined by the radius of the column, r, and the film thickness, d_f:

$$\beta = \frac{r}{2d_f} \tag{19}$$

As a general rule, larger phase ratios result in lower elution temperatures. In contrast, a smaller amount of sample can be applied to the thinner films before overloaded peak shapes are observed. The column radius and film thickness also influence N. The van Deemter–Golay equation describes the relationship between H and mobile phase linear velocity, u:

$$H = A + \frac{B}{u} + (C_{mobile} + C_{stat})u \tag{20}$$

where A, B, C_{mobile}, and C_{stat} are terms that relate to various processes occurring as the molecules move through the column. For capillary GC, the eddy diffusion (A) term is negligible. The B term is the result of diffusion against the direction of mobile phase flow. C_{mobile} and C_{stat} are the result of diffusion of the analyte molecules in the mobile (gas) and stationary (liquid) phases. C_{mobile} is proportional to r^2 and inversely proportional to the diffusion coefficient of the molecule in the mobile phase gas. C_{stat} is proportional to the d_f^2. Columns with larger radii and thicker films have a lower N than a smaller diameter column with the same phase ratio and length. A good compromise for clinical and toxicological work is a 0.25-mm id 30-m column with a film thickness of 0.25 μm. If a smaller diameter column (e.g., 0.18 or 0.10 mm) can be used, the analysis time can be decreased. The use of short 0.10-mm id columns, which results in short analysis times, is often called "fast GC."

Permanent gases such as Ar, N_2, He, or H_2 have been used most commonly as the mobile phase in GC. Argon has not been shown to have any advantages in capillary GC and therefore is rarely used. Diffusion rates in nitrogen are the smallest, resulting in a small value for B and a larger value than the other gases for C_{mobile} in the van Deemter–Golay equation. Thus, while nitrogen gives the smallest value for H at the lowest flow rate, there is a strong dependence of H on flow rate (Figure 4). When the temperature increases, as is the case in temperature programming, the viscosity of any gas increases, resulting in decreasing flow rates at constant inlet pressure. Over the 50–350 °C range, the viscosity could increase by a factor of 1.5. For a constant pressure, temperature-programmed method, the decrease in flow rate with increasing temperature results in less than optimal H (moving from right to left along the N_2 curve in Figure 4) for peaks in some portion of the chromatogram. Diffusion rates are fastest in hydrogen since it is the least dense gas. Thus, hydrogen has the best combination of a small optimum value for H and a slowly

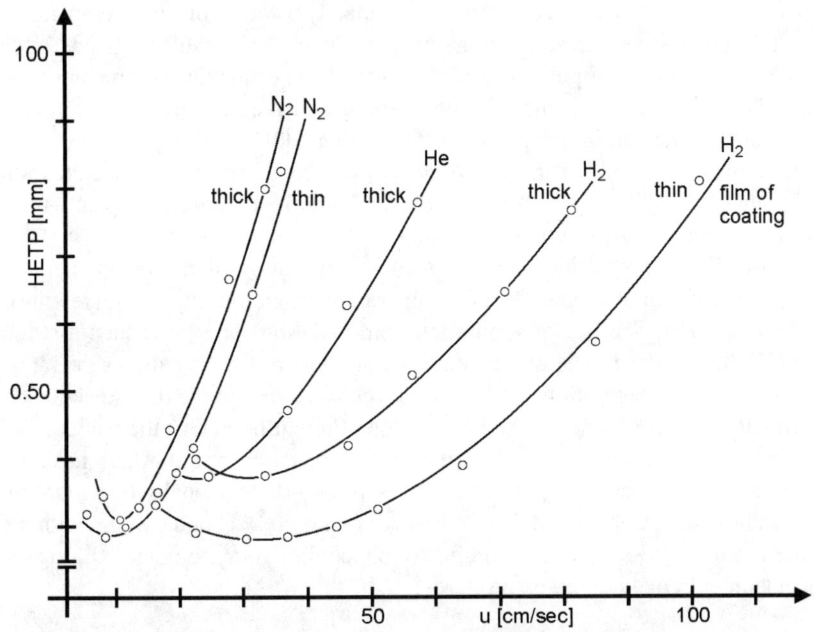

FIGURE 4. van Deemter–Golay plot for mobile phase gases commonly used in gas chromatography. Note that a thicker film of stationary phase alters both the minimum and the slope of the plot. (*From Gerhard Schomburg, Gas chromatography: a practical course. VCH, New York 1990. p. 48, with permission from Wiley-VCH*)

increasing H with increasing flow rate. There has been some reluctance to use hydrogen because of the potential for explosion. With the availability of hydrogen generators with relatively small storage reservoirs (thus reducing risk) and the relatively low flow rates in capillary GC, the use of hydrogen would appear to be an appealing alternative. The use of helium is a reasonable compromise since it has a moderate viscosity and is available in ultrahigh purity.

As a result of the compressibility of gases, the flow rate along the length of the column also varies. Longer columns or columns with smaller radii, which result in larger pressure drops, have larger changes in flow rate over the length of the column. In the past decade, the improvement of flow controllers and sensors has made constant flow methods practical. In these methods, the pressure on the head of the column is increased during the temperature program to maintain a constant flow rate. One final practical consideration is that the mobile phase must contain as few impurities as possible (e.g., helium purity >99.995%). The delivery system should be designed and constructed in such a way that oxygen and other impurities do not reenter the gas stream. Oxygen and water are particularly deleterious for immobilized phases.

The primary parameter that can be used to adjust retention behavior in GC is the separation temperature:

$$\ln k = \frac{\Delta H}{RT} - (\frac{\Delta S}{R} + \ln \beta) \tag{21}$$

where ΔH and ΔS are the enthalpy and entropy of vaporization of the analyte from the stationary into the gas phase, T is the temperature, and R is the gas constant. An increase in temperature of 30 °C decreases k by approximately a factor of two. Temperature programming is imperative for addressing the general elution problem. It has additional advantages such as cold trapping the analytes at the head of the GC column and thus concentrating them. In general, if the initial temperature of the program for compound(s) is 150 °C lower than the elution temperature, the compound will be trapped in a narrow band at the head of the column. The high temperature end of the program elutes strongly retained compounds that might otherwise contaminate the column or appear as a slowly increasing baseline signal in subsequent analyses.

Understanding the retention behavior of compounds allowed the development of computer programs that simulate the effect of temperature programming on both retention time and peak width (25). The use of simulation (extrapolation) programs such as Pro *ez*GC (26) and GC Simulation and Optimization Software (GC-SOS) (27) allows the rapid evaluation of a new set of separation conditions as well as assessing the robustness of the separation conditions. For a more detailed discussion of retention in GC, the reader is referred to Grob and Barry (28) and the fundamental review of Parcher (29). There has also been increased interest in recent years in comprehensive two-dimensional GC, which involves directing a chromatographic band from a first column onto a second column with a different separation factor (30, 31). This combination technique has the potential to resolve all components in extremely complex mixtures.

Chromatographic Systems

A gas chromatograph (*see* Figure 5) consists of a source of carrier gas, a system of flow regulation, a sample introduction system, a column contained within a temperature-controlled oven, and a detection system. Rood (32) published a useful monograph on the care and maintenance of capillary GC systems.

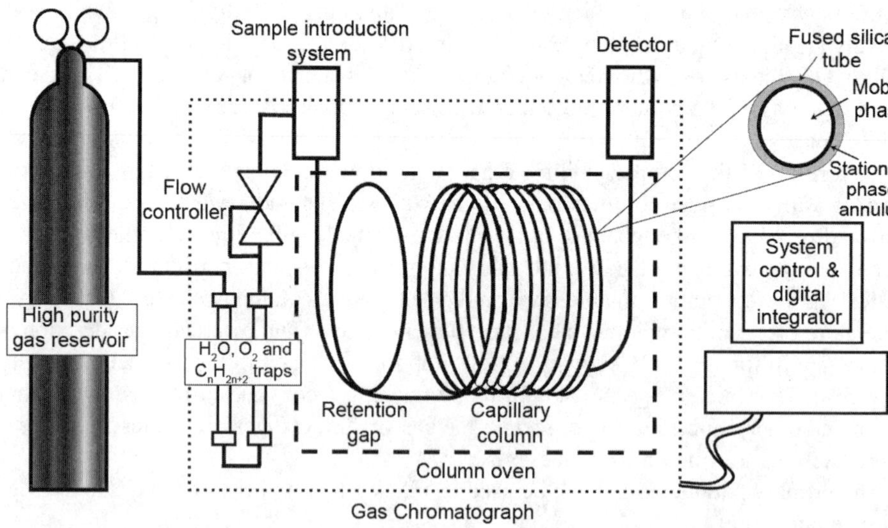

FIGURE 5. Schematic diagram of a gas chromatograph. A pressurized high purity gas mobile phase is delivered through a flow controller to the capillary column. The stationary phase is an ultra-thin annulus of material immobilized on the inner surface of the fused silica capillary tube. Trace amounts of oils, water, and oxygen should be removed to maximize column life. A retention gap can be used to improve peak shape with certain injection systems and to protect the column from strongly retained materials in the sample.

Sample Introduction Systems

The primary function of most GC injection systems is to volatilize the compounds in order to get them into the gas phase and quantitatively transfer them to the column. Due to the limited capacity of capillary GC columns, the injection system is a critical element to achieving accurate analytical results. The first injection system designed for use with open tubular capillary columns split the sample molecules; a portion went to the column and the remainder was discarded through the system split vent. The split ratio is calculated from the ratio of the column flow rate to the sum of the column and split vent flow rates. Thus, when 2 μL is injected into a system with a 1:100 split ratio, about 20 nL is directed onto the column.

While split injections are well suited for concentrated samples, they are not as useful for trace analysis. Splitless injection was developed to enable more analyte to be placed onto the column. In the splitless injection technique, all of the content of the injector, both solvent and analyte, is directed into the column for a period of time. The column temperature is held 10–20 °C below the boiling point of the injection solvent so that the solvent condenses onto the stationary phase. This process has the effect of dynamically increasing the volume of the stationary phase (solvent effect), which decreases β, which in turn increases k for the analyte. As the column temperature is increased, the solvent evaporates and is eluted from the column first. The analytes, having been concentrated in the initial portion of the column, can then be separated as narrow peaks.

All volatilization techniques suffer to some extent from discrimination between various components of the sample. For example, volatile components can boil out of the syringe needle as it is placed into the hot injection port and be lost. Depending on injector design, a cold spot could result in loss of nonvolatile components. Deactivation of the injection port may be a critical part of obtaining reproducible results. In summary, careful consideration of the preparation and maintenance of the injection port is critical to successful routine application of the method.

To achieve a larger and more quantitative transfer of sample components onto the column, several liquid injection techniques have been developed. Cold, on-column injection and direct injection place the liquid sample into the column or a 5- to 10-m segment of treated fused silica called a **retention gap**. The oven then is heated rapidly to elute the injection solvent, after which the components are separated. This results in more accurate and quantitative transfer of analytes onto the column. A number of drawbacks, however, include the need to use a needle that can be inserted inside a 0.25-mm column. This requirement makes the technique less robust and difficult to automate. An alternative is **programmable temperature volatilization** (PTV). In this approach, the sample is injected into a cool injector where the liquid microdroplets are held within a fused silica wool plug. The injector is heated to the point at which the solvent evaporates and the solvent vapor is discarded from the system through a vent. The injector is then ballistically heated to volatilize the sample components, which are quantitatively transferred to the column. One advantage of this technique is that large-volume injections are possible for trace analysis. The main disadvantage for routine operation is the increased hardware and supplies necessary to cool the injector rapidly between each run.

Column Oven

One of the most important parts of the GC instrument is the column oven. The oven must have a well-controlled, reproducible nominal temperature with minimal temperature gradients. For "fast GC," the ability of the oven to increase the temperature at a high rate

TABLE 2. Examples of gas chromatography detectors

Detector	Specificity	Dependence	Detection limit	Linearity
Thermal conductivity	Universal	Concentration	10^{-9} g/ml	10^3–10^4
Flame ionization	C	Mass flow	2×10^{-12} g C/s	$>10^7$
Photoionization	C	Mass flow	2×10^{-13} g C/s	$>10^7$
Thermionic specific	N, P	Mass flow	2×10^{-14} g N/s	$>10^6$
Electron capture	F, Cl, Br, I	Mass flow	10^{-14} g/s Lindane	$<10^4$
Flame photometric	S, P	Mass flow	3×10^{-13} g P/s	10^5
Mass spectrometric	Universal	Mass flow	10^{-9} g full scan	10^3

(>30 °C/minute) also is important. The ability to decrease the oven temperature rapidly at the end of a run is important for minimizing analysis time when temperature programming is used. The design of the column oven is important, since changing the GC column should be as convenient as possible. Column oven design is a critical consideration for two-dimensional GC.

Detectors

Both universal and selective detectors are available for GC (Table 2). The flame-ionization detector, with its nearly universal detection of carbon-containing compounds, has been particularly useful in clinical and bioanalytical methods. The thermionic-selective detector, which preferentially detects nitrogen- and phosphorous-containing compounds, has been used widely in drug analysis. The coupling of the gas chromatograph to the mass spectrometer has resulted in a system with tunable selectivity, sensitivity, and limits of detection.

LIQUID CHROMATOGRAPHY

Optimizing Resolution in High-Performance Liquid Chromatography

The primary parameters that can be used to optimize a separation by liquid chromatography and their effects on separation are:

Stationary phase	α
Particle size	N, pressure drop, sample capacity
Column diameter and length	N, pressure drop, sample capacity
Mobile phase composition	
% organic solvent	α, k, N
Type of organic solvent	α, k, N
Buffer	α, k
Mobile phase additives	α, k
Flow rate	N
Temperature	k, N, pressure drop, α

Although several modes of chromatography are available in high-performance liquid chromatography (HPLC), most water-soluble molecules found in biological fluids can be separated successfully by reversed-phase (RP) HPLC. In RP systems, the stationary phase is less polar than the mobile phase. This section will deal solely with RP separations of small molecules (<1000 daltons). An excellent book by Snyder et al. (33) describes development of methods based on other separation modes and provides more detail about RP methods.

Column Considerations

In HPLC, both the stationary phase and the mobile phase play important roles in determining k and α. Most RP-HPLC stationary phases consist of a layer of hydrocarbon immobilized on the surface of microparticulate, totally porous particles. The most common support particles are silica gel, but alumina, titanium oxide, zirconium oxide, and organic polymers such as polystyrene-divinylbenzene have been used. In the early days of HPLC, it was difficult to find columns from different manufacturers, or even different lots of support media prepared by the same manufacturer, that gave the same retention behavior. This was due to the differences in the underlying silica. Type A silica has three types of silanol (Si-OH) groups on the surface: free silanols, associated silanols, and geminal silanols. Free silanols are acidic and interact with basic compounds such as organic amines to give tailed peaks. In addition, impurities, such as aluminum, in the silica gel lattice further activate the free silanols. Finally, trace metal impurities such as iron, nickel, and zinc form complexes with certain analytes, again giving rise to asymmetrical peaks and unique separation factors. In the last decade, column manufacturers have prepared high purity silica gel (Type B silica) with fewer active free silanol groups. This has lead to less peak tailing with basic compounds and more reproducible and reliable columns.

Most stationary phases are chemically bonded to the surface. The most common bonding chemistries involve the use of octyl (C8)- or octadecyl (C18 or ODS)-dimethylchlorosilane, which form a single (monomeric) bond to the silanol groups on the surface of the silica gel. Due to steric considerations, only about 50% of the available surface silanols react. Many column packing materials are endcapped by further modifying the surface with trimethylchlorosilanes. In general, greater retention is observed with higher amounts of carbon on the surface. Higher amounts of carbon also protect the surface from being attacked by the water in the mobile phase, which can either remove the carbonaceous phase from the surface over time or dissolve the support particle. Degradation of column performance is accelerated at temperatures greater than 40 °C and pH values less than 3 or greater than 7. Several techniques have been used to extend the pH and temperature stability of the silica particles. Incorporation of an organic silane during the formation of the silica gel, stereochemical shielding of the surface silanols, and preparation of Type B silica have all improved column stability. Embedding polar amide or urea groups in the hydrocarbon chain or using polar endcapping reagents modifies retention behavior. Recently, a compilation of the characteristics of 300 columns was published along with an approach to compare column retention behavior (34).

The next decision regarding the column is the particle size diameter. The Kennedy–Knox equation describes the dependence of H on the flow velocity:

$$H = A'u^{1/3} + \frac{B'}{u} + C'u \tag{22}$$

The Kennedy–Knox equation is similar in form to the van Deemter–Golay equation, and they are sometimes used interchangeably. The coefficients A', B', and C' are slightly different than in the van Deemter–Golay equation, as is the effect of u on A'. The difference in the form of the two equations is due to the large difference in diffusion rates in a liquid mobile phase versus a gaseous mobile phase. Thus, at low flow rates in liquid chromatography, for example, the diffusion of the analyte against the mobile phase flow (B term) would have less influence on the peak width. In packed HPLC columns, the A' term is a function of the particle size and the homogeneity of the bed structure. The C' term is dependent on the square of the particle size and inversely proportional to the diffusion rate of the analyte in the mobile phase. The practical conclusion from the Kennedy–Knox equation is that smaller diameter particles result in smaller values of H at all values of u and in a slower rate of increase in H with increasing flow rate. The flow rate that results in the minimum value of H also is higher with smaller particles. Thus, column diameter and length can be decreased (*see* Equation 10) and u can be increased with a minimum loss of column performance, which results in improved detection limits (Equation 15) and faster analysis times (Equation 18).

There are two practical limits to the benefit of reducing particle diameter: column packing efficiency and the pressure drop across the column. The pressure drop across a column is inversely related to the square of the particle diameter and increases with increased solvent viscosity, flow velocity, and column length. Thus, at some point, the tradeoffs between decreased column length and particle diameter result in a column with such a high pressure drop that it is impractical to use the column. Fortunately, liquid mobile phases, unlike gases, are noncompressible, so the pressure drop does not affect the flow rate of the mobile phase across the length of the column and there is no reason to be concerned about an explosion if the pressure is suddenly released. State-of-the-art HPLC columns generally use 3.5- or 5-μm particle diameters with a column diameter of 2 or 4.6 mm and a length of 15 cm or less. The use of smaller volume columns makes the extra-column peak dispersion characteristics of the HPLC system much more important. Systems are commercially available that are optimized for use of columns packed with 1.7-μm diameter particles (ultrahigh-performance liquid chromatography).

The use of open tubular columns with an annulus of stationary phase does result in improvements in HPLC column efficiency. Interfacing HPLC with mass spectrometry, for example, benefits significantly from the use of open tubular columns and the resultant low solvent flow. The extremely low flow rates needed, the high pressure drops encountered with displacement pumps, the difficulty in generating reproducible solvent gradients, and the increased importance of extra-column peak broadening factors currently conspire to make the technique of limited practical value. The use of an electric field to drive solvent through the open tube (electroosmotic flow) works well to remove one of the difficulties.

Mobile Phase Selection

The mobile phase in RP-HPLC consists of a mixture of water and a miscible organic solvent such as methanol, acetonitrile, or tetrahydrofuran (THF). Larger percentages of water result in increased retention; a 10% increase in water results in approximately a threefold increase in k. Among the organic solvents, a 10% change in THF results in a larger decrease in k than a 10% change in acetonitrile or methanol. Thus, THF is termed a stronger solvent. In binary solvent systems, mixtures of water and acetonitrile have significant advantages and are thus usually the first solvent pair used in method development. Acetonitrile is relatively transparent at UV wavelengths below 210 nm and water–acetonitrile mixtures have the lowest viscosity which results in lower pressure drop across the column and higher N due to faster diffusion. The viscosity of water–organic solvent mixtures varies as a function of composition, with the highest viscosity occurring at about 40–50% organic content. In addition to differences in strength, the various solvents also may result in different separation factors. In some cases, the differences are large enough that peak elution order is reversed. These solvent differences can be exploited using mixtures of three solvents to obtain optimal peak resolution (35).

Since the ionization of organic acids and bases can be controlled as a function of pH, the use of buffers can alter retention and separation behavior significantly. The neutral form of the acid or base is retained better than the ionic form. The retention behavior of an acid or base changes most dramatically in the vicinity of its pK_a. A number of buffers have been used with HPLC including trifluoroacetate, phosphate, formate, acetate, and carbonate. It is important to use the buffers within ±1 pH unit of the pK_a of the acid. Acetate buffer, for example, is an effective buffer only in the pH range of 3.8 to 5.8. Measurement of pH with a glass electrode in buffer–organic solvent mixtures also is inaccurate, so the pH should be adjusted using only the aqueous portion of the mobile phase before mixing. The volatility of the buffer, its UV absorbance, and its solubility in the organic solvent should be considered when developing a method.

The use of **mobile phase additives** such as triethylamine in the mobile phase can have a dramatic effect on peak symmetry and to a lesser effect, retention when columns with active silanols are used. With the increasing use of Type B silica gels, this effect is becoming less important. Ion-pairing agents can be used to increase the retention of oppositely charged compounds. For example, alkylsulfonic acids (e.g., sodium octylsulfonate) can be used to increase the retention of basic amine compounds. In contradistinction, tetraalkylammonium salts (e.g., tetrabutylammonium bromide) can be used to increase the retention of acidic analytes. The ion-pair agent is strongly retained by the column and the separation of analyte molecules is the result of both hydrophobic and ion-exchange interactions with the stationary phase. Ion-pairing reagents containing more carbon atoms (e.g., octylsulfonates) are more retained than those with fewer carbon atoms (e.g., butylsulfonates). There is an asymptotic increase in retention with increasing ion-pairing reagent content of the mobile phase. The use of ion-pairing reagent concentration on the plateau generally results in a more robust separation system. In general, no improvement in α is achieved by changing the carbon content of the ion-pairing reagent. A column that has been used with ion-pairing agents should be labeled as such and not used for routine RP separations.

Temperature Effects

Temperature has a number of effects on the separation characteristics. First, increasing the temperature in general decreases k. A change in temperature also has an effect on α. This effect is more significant for ionic compounds than for nonionic ones. Unfortunately, changes in the separation factor are unpredictable and must be determined empirically. Nevertheless, temperature can be used as a tool to fine-tune the separation. Increasing the temperature also decreases solvent viscosity, which decreases pressure drop across the column and contributes, through increased diffusion rates, to an improvement in N. A 20 °C increase above ambient temperature reduces the viscosity by about 30%. Increasing the temperature to 150 °C results in a 65% decrease in viscosity. Ultrafast liquid chromatography separations have been achieved at temperatures as high as 200 °C using stable zirconium oxide support materials coated with polybutadiene (36).

Computer-based method development software programs such as Drylab (LC Resources), ChromSword, and ICOS (Agilent Technologies) make use of solvent selectivity to optimize separations and to locate robust separation conditions. The experiment-driven optimizations also model other conditions such as pH, temperature, and gradient elution.

In HPLC, programming solvent strength as a function of time, or gradient elution, has similar effects on the chromatography as temperature programming does in GC. One key concept in gradient elution is the "average value of k in gradient elution," defined as k*. The value of k* determines both the peak resolution and the peak width in gradient chromatography. For molecules with molecular weight less than 500 daltons, the value of k* is approximated by:

$$k^* \approx \frac{20 t_G F}{V_M (\Delta \% B)} \approx \frac{20F}{V_M (\% B/\min)} \tag{23}$$

where t_G is the length of the gradient in minutes and Δ%B is the difference in strong solvent percentage between the beginning and end of the gradient. These two terms can be combined to give a measure of gradient steepness as change in %B per minute. Note that the flow rate has an important role in determining the k*: increasing the flow rate effectively decreases the steepness of the gradient and increases k*. The column size also affects the elution of the compounds, with a decrease in either length or diameter of the column, through their effect on V_M, resulting in an increase in k*.The retention time and peak width of early eluting peaks can be influenced by the initial solvent strength of the mobile phase. If the initial solvent strength is weak, injecting a dilute sample has the same concentration effects as cold trapping in GC. Gradient elution also removes strongly retained components from the column that might otherwise elute as baseline drift in a subsequent injection or permanently alter the performance of the column. Snyder (37) and Snyder and Stadalius (38) provide a more detailed and unified discussion of gradient elution.

Chromatographic Systems

A schematic diagram of an HPLC system is shown in Figure 6. The purpose of the precolumn is to condition the solvent to achieve increased analytical column lifetime. For example, a RP column that no longer has the efficiency to achieve the separation might be used as a precolumn under elevated temperature conditions to saturate the mobile phase with silica so that the analytical column does not dissolve. The guard column functions to remove strongly retained compounds and any particulate matter in the sample, again to protect the analytical column from premature failure.

In general, positive displacement pumps have been used to move the mobile phase through the column. The use of dual piston pumps, with electronic and mechanical compensation to minimize the flow disruption when one piston is refilling and compressing solvent prior to delivery, has resulted in consistent performance with a variety of flow-sensitive detectors. For solvent gradient formation, both low-pressure (pump inlet side) and high-pressure (pump outlet side) mixing of the solvents have been used. Each approach has advantages and disadvantages. Any pumping system requires careful monitoring and a routine maintenance program to ensure consistent performance.

Sample introduction is performed almost exclusively by fixed-loop rotary valve systems. Either partial-loop or full-loop injection techniques can be used, although manual implementation of either requires a somewhat different technique in order to obtain precise results. Automated sample-handling systems generally are more reproducible than manual technique. The sample introduction valve also needs routine maintenance to function reliably.

A wide variety of **detection approaches** are available for use with HPLC, as summarized in Table 3. Detectors based on UV absorption are the most widely used. Initial

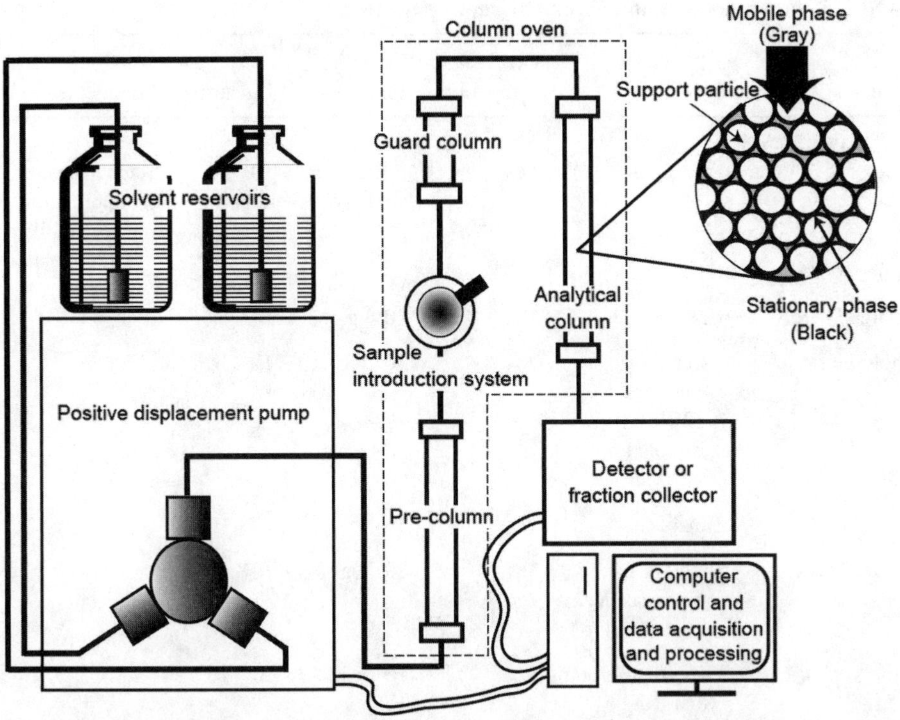

FIGURE 6. Schematic diagram of a high-performance liquid chromatograph. One or more solvents drawn from the solvent reservoirs are mixed and driven through the system under high pressure. The analytical column is usually packed with totally porous spherical support particles onto which the stationary phase is immobilized. The bulk mobile phase percolates through the column between the particles, while the molecules diffuse into and out of the pores in the support particles where the vast majority of the stationary phase is located. The precolumn is used to condition the mobile phase, while the guard column protects the analytical column from particulate or strongly retained materials in the sample. Temperature control is important for achieving reproducible retention behavior.

approaches involved fixed-wavelength detectors that were able to detect aromatic compounds at 254 nm or single double bonds (214 nm). The ability to obtain a UV spectrum while a peak is eluting using a photodiode-array (diode-array detector, DAD) is of significant value both in methods requiring identification of the analyte and in situations where the UV absorbance of the compound does not lend itself to fixed-wavelength detection.

Recently a number of detection approaches have begun to address the absence of a sensitive, universal detector in HPLC. The refractive index (RI) detector was for many years the only universal detector for HPLC. While RI works effectively in some applications, its relatively poor limit of detection and inability to be interfaced with gradient HPLC separations limited its utility. The **evaporative light-scattering detector** (ELSD) measures the amount of light scattered by particles remaining after evaporation of the mobile phase. Three steps are involved in the ELSD:

- Nebulization of eluent from the column
- Evaporation of the mobile phase in a heated drift tube
- Detection of light scattered by the dry particles carried through the detection cell by the flow of nebulizing gas.

TABLE 3. Examples of liquid chromatography detectors

Detector	Specificity	Gradient compatible	Detection limit	Linearity	Comments
Refractive index	Universal	No	10^{-7} g	10^{2}	
Evaporative light scattering	Universal	Yes	3×10^{-8} g	10^{2}–10^{3}	Temperature of vaporization affects ability to detect volatile compounds
Charged aerosol	Universal	Yes	10^{-8} g	10^{4}	
Photometric	Aromatic compounds (254 nm); double bonds (210 nm)	Yes	10^{-10} g	10^{2}–10^{3}	
Diode array	Tunable	Yes	10^{-9} g	10^{2}–10^{3}	
Fluorescence	Native fluorescence or derivative	Yes	10^{-11} g	10^{3}	
Amperometric	Functional group that can be oxidized or reduced; tunable	No	10^{-12} g	10^{2}–10^{3}	
Mass spectrometer	Tunable	Yes	10^{-11} g	10^{3}	

As a result of the mechanism of detection, the mobile phase cannot contain nonvolatile additives, and column bleed from loss of bonded phase and dissolution of the support particles will be detected. Since the mobile phase is removed prior to detection, the ELSD is fully compatible with gradient elution. The ELSD is a destructive detector, and thus it must be the last detector if sequential detection is used.

Another recent development is the **charged aerosol detector**. The column effluent is nebulized and the resulting droplets dry at ambient temperature, producing analyte particles. A second stream of positively charged gas is produced by a corona discharge. The charge is transferred to the analyte particles after collision between the gas and analyte streams. The analyte particles transfer their charges to a collector and the response is directly proportional to the analyte mass.

Several other solution phase detection techniques continue to be used for specific applications. **Fluorescence detection** has very low limits of detection if the compound exhibits native fluorescence or if a fluorescent derivative can be made. **Amperometric detectors**, particularly using potentials that result in oxidation such as for catecholamines, have very low detection limits. Two types of amperometric detectors, thin layer and coulometric, have been described. In the former, only a minute fraction of the compound is oxidized, whereas in the latter there is quantitative oxidation of the compound of interest. While intuitively there would seem to be an advantage to complete conversion, there is little difference in the performance of these approaches due to signal-to-noise considerations. Dual-electrode and multiple-electrode array systems also have been described. Additional specificity of detection or information about the eluting compound can be obtained from its electrochemical behavior, similar to that obtained from a DAD.

MASS SPECTROMETRY

Mass spectrometry is an analytical technique with both qualitative and quantitative capabilities. The mass spectrometer consists of a source of ions, a mass analyzer, and a detector. Mass analyzers separate ions according to their mass-to-charge (m/z) ratio. Mass analysis requires that the ion drift from its point of entry into the analyzer to the detector under specific conditions. Most mass spectrometer designs require a vacuum of sufficient magnitude to ensure that no collisions with other molecules (e.g., N_2, O_2, H_2O from the air) occur during the mass analysis process. The mass spectrometer is capable of providing structural information that can be used to identify an unknown compound. The combination of mass spectrometric detection with a separation technique such as GC or HPLC is a powerful tool for analysis of complex biological samples. If the mass of the analyte is known, mass-selective detection can be used to develop very sensitive and specific methods. Recently, mass spectrometric data were used to improve chromatographic resolution by deconvoluting the spectra of coeluting compounds (39).

Several different kinds of information are available from mass spectrometry. First, if the molecule is gently ionized and does not totally dissociate into fragments, the molecular weight of the molecule can be determined. If the mass of the molecular ion can be determined with sufficient accuracy, it can provide the exact molecular formula of the ion. This technique, called **accurate mass analysis**, can be applied because monoisotopic atomic weights are not whole numbers. For example, the exact mass of ^{16}O is 15.99491463. The exact mass of an ion from a molecule (or fragment) includes the "mass defect" (difference from the integer mass) from each of the constituent atoms. Thus, if the mass is determined with sufficient accuracy, only one possible combination of atoms can result in that mass. In some cases, a compound could be identified on this basis alone. The benefit of determining the elemental composition of an ion increases with the mass of the ion, since a more complex molecular formula can be revealed. The required accuracy of the mass determination at higher mass also increases as the possible combinations of atoms increase. A mass accuracy of 2 parts per million (ppm) is necessary to differentiate between the possible atomic compositions at a mass of 300 daltons (±0.006 daltons). High-resolution mass analyzers are capable of achieving these performance standards. Accurate mass monitoring also improves the detection limits for targeted analytes by disregarding signals from interfering compounds. However, this method cannot distinguish between isomers; in this case, one must augment accurate mass measurements with separations, e.g., chromatography.

The combination of selected ionization and mass analysis techniques results in additional structural information. In **electron ionization** (EI), interaction of the molecule of interest with a 70-eV electron beam transfers sufficient energy during formation of a radical cation that bonds are broken in a predictable way. In the open EI ion source design normally found in mass spectrometers, about 1 molecule in 10^5 is ionized. The positively charged fragments and any remaining molecular ion are directed into the mass analyzer, separated by m/z ratio, and detected. A **mass spectrum** (Figure 7) is obtained by plotting the relative abundance (%) of ion intensity as a function of ion m/z ratio (called the Thomson value or Th). If the ion has a single charge, the m/z ratio is equivalent to the mass of the ion. By plotting relative abundance, differences in absolute intensity due to different instruments or different concentrations can be minimized. The most abundant ion in the mass spectrum is called the **base peak**. In some cases, the highest mass ion is the molecular ion. By considering the mass and relative abundance of the various fragments, a hypothesis about the molecular structure can be formed (*see* Figure 8) (40). Alternatively, libraries of mass spectra have been collected [National Institutes of Health (NIH); National Institutes of Standards and Technology (NIST); Pfleger, Maurer, and Webber; American Academy of Forensic Toxicology—Toxicology Section Mass Spectrometry Database Committee (www.ualberta.ca/~gjones/mslib.htm); etc.] and the spectrum of the unknown compound can be compared to those in the library using computer-assisted library matching programs.

A **full spectrum** is generally obtained by scanning from 26 daltons to a mass well above the molecular weight of the compound(s) of interest. When derivatives are prepared for GC analysis or when chemical ionization is used, the spectrum could be dominated by

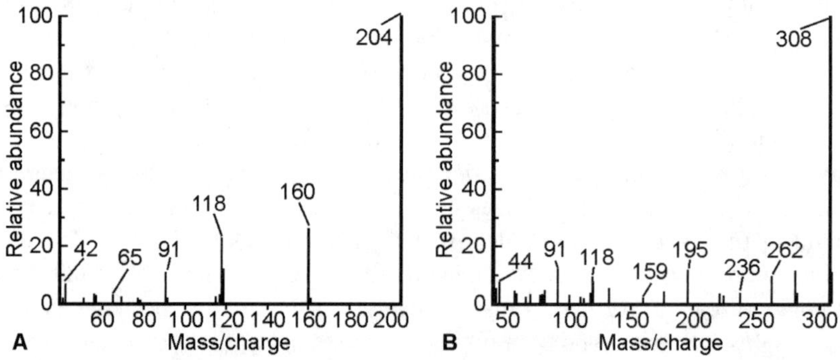

FIGURE 7. Mass spectrum of the (A) pentafluoropropionyl- and (B) carbethoxyhexafluorobutyryl-derivatives of methamphetamine. (*Reprinted from Tietz textbook of clinical chemistry, 3rd ed., Burtis CA, Ashwood ER, eds., p. 193, Copyright 1999, with permission from Elsevier*)

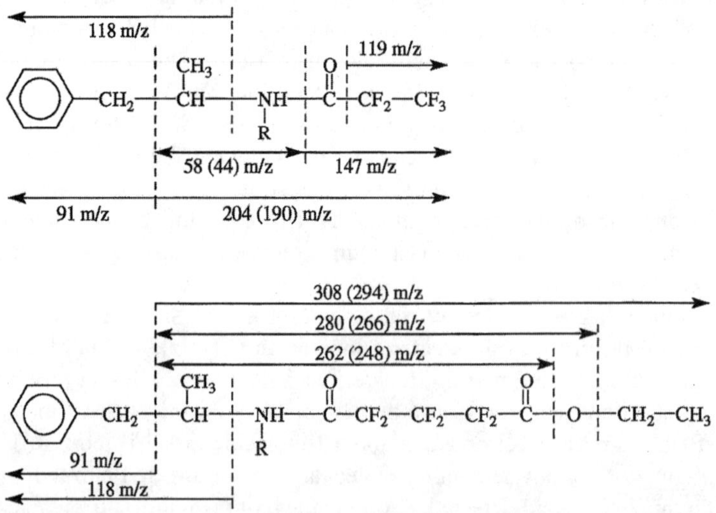

FIGURE 8. Fragmentation patterns of the pentafluoropropionyl- and carbethoxyhexafluorobutyryl-derivatives of methamphetamine (R = CH_3) and amphetamine (R = H). The mass of the fragments from amphetamine are shown in parenthesies. (*Reprinted from Tietz textbook of clinical chemistry, 3rd ed., Burtis CA, Ashwood ER, eds., p. 183, Copyright 1999, with permission from Elsevier*)

ions arising from the derivatization or chemical ionization reagent. When fit for the purpose of the assay, a **partial spectrum**, which begins above the mass of the derivatization reagent ions, may be obtained. In either case, background spectra, taken either before or after the chromatographic peak to minimize the effect of leaks, column bleed, or chemical background, should be subtracted from the spectrum before attempting to determine the structure. Because the concentration of compound eluting from the chromatographic column is continuously changing during the mass spectral acquisition process, it is important to collect sufficient spectra across the chromatographic peak to maintain both peak shape and mass spectral fidelity. Since spectra are obtained continuously across the peak, it is possible to reconstruct the mass spectral signal observed as a function of time. When the sum of all mass signals is displayed, the result is called a **total ion chromatogram** (TIC). Display of the signal at a specific mass is referred to as an **extracted ion chromatogram** (EIC).

A number of spectral search algorithms have been used to match unknown spectra with those in spectral libraries (41). The probability-based matching (PBM) and dot product approaches are commercially available. There are three types of searches: identity (or purity) search; similarity (or reverse fit) search; and reverse (or fit) search. The reverse search, which searches for the presence of ions and intensities from the library spectrum in the unknown spectrum, is the most frequently used in searches generated by GC–MS or LC–MS analysis. The reliability of mass spectral matching depends on several factors:

- the quality of the spectrum from the unknown
- the presence of the spectrum of the unknown compound in the library
- the quality of the library spectrum
- the use of condensed versus complete spectra in the library
- instrumental factors such as tuning and type of mass spectrometer used
- the search algorithm

In general, a confidence factor for the match is provided and a high value (1000 for dot product) is an indication of a perfect match. Depending on the factors affecting the spectral search algorithm, however, a lower confidence factor may still be consistent with a match between a compound in the library and the unknown. In either case, a competent scientist should evaluate the unknown spectra.

In methods for which the analyte(s) is known and the concentration is too low to obtain a full spectrum, a technique called **selected ion monitoring** (SIM) can be used. As described in subsequent sections, some mass analyzers selectively pass ions of a particular Thomson value to the detector for a specified period, usually called the dwell time. If one ion were to be selected, for example, rather than scanning ions from m/z 25 to 525, the detector would have about 500 times the signal acquisition time for that ion in the SIM mode relative to the scanning mode. Signal-to-noise ratio would be improved, and the resulting method would have a lower limit of detection. On the other hand, information related to the identification of the compound would have been sacrificed. Bethem et al. (42) addressed the issues of "fitness of purpose" of various approaches to the use of SIM for quantitative and qualitative analysis. In general, the monitoring of three or four characteristic ions and obtaining the same ratios of ion intensities as a contemporaneously assayed standard has been accepted as a criterion for identification (42), usually in conjunction with a consistent retention time from the chromatographic separation. Ion intensity ratios are generally obtained from integration of the chromatographic peak areas at each Thomson value. In general, larger dwell times result in better signal-to-noise ratios. There is a limit, however, to the number of ions that can be monitored simultaneously before sensitivity and chromatographic fidelity are lost (43). As a general rule, faster data acquisition speeds and data-handling methods result in better chromatographic–MS methods.

Ionization Techniques

Electron ionization is a very effective technique for obtaining structural data because of its ability to cause ionization and fragmentation of small organic molecules in the gas state. Because of the extent of bond cleavage observed, EI is often referred to as a "hard" ionization technique. Many advances in the application of mass spectrometry to bioanalytical systems have been the result of improved low energy or "soft" ionization techniques. These techniques have been developed to ionize compounds that are difficult to put into the gas phase such as thermally labile compounds, peptides, and proteins. With these techniques, it is also possible to obtain molecular mass information about compounds that fragment easily. The protonated molecular ions that are produced in high abundance also can be used in tandem mass spectrometry systems, which are described in a subsequent section. A wide variety of ionization mechanisms have been used "on-line" with chromatographic separations. With the rapid development of chromatography–MS interface technology in the last decade, some techniques, such as the moving belt, thermospray, and particle beam interfaces, have virtually disappeared after a period of popularity. Many other soft ionization techniques such as matrix-assisted laser desorption ionization (MALDI) are not routinely interfaced with chromatographic systems and thus are beyond the scope of this chapter. The interested reader is referred to texts on mass spectrometry.

Chemical Ionization

Chemical ionization (CI) is the result of proton transfer or proton abstraction reactions between a CI reagent gas and the molecule of interest. CI requires the use of a "tight" ion source where the electron beam ionizes the reagent gas. Methane, ammonia, isobutane, and water have been used frequently as reagent gases. Selection is determined by the proton-donating ability of the charged species. Higher pressure (0.1–1 torr) in the ion source results in collisions between the reagent gas ions and the molecules of interest that allows the reaction to proceed. Usually the reactions transfer little excess energy to the product, and thus there is little fragmentation. Different relative amounts of fragmentation are observed with different reagent gases. One interesting aspect of ion trap mass analyzers (discussed later) is that the reagent gas can be stored for much longer periods. As a result, much lower reagent gas pressures can be used. This makes it possible to use acetonitrile and methanol as CI reagents.

Negative ion chemical ionization (NICI) also can be performed. In this case, thermalized electrons are captured by electronegative substituents on the molecule of interest such as fluorine, chlorine, or bromine. Because a small fraction of organic molecules contain these substituents, the signal-to-noise ratio observed is very high, and detection limits are very low. As an example, Fitzgerald and Herold (44) reported on the use of NICI with the pentafluorobutyryl/trimethylsilyl-derivative of testosterone to determine low nanomole per liter (nmol/L) concentrations in the blood of females. NICI cannot be used in an internal ionization ion trap due to its inability to store thermalized electrons. Alternative negative ionization reagents have been investigated to provide a means to do NICI on the ion trap.

Atmospheric Pressure Chemical Ionization

In atmospheric pressure chemical ionization (APCI), electrons from either a radioactive source or a direct current corona discharge at atmospheric pressure ionize water molecules in the air to form $H_3O^+(H_2O)_n$ ions. Molecules of interest from the chromatographic effluent are ionized by proton exchange or charge transfer reactions with the hydronium ion. When coupled with HPLC, the liquid effluent is nebulized and the solvent removed by heating prior to interaction with the reactant gas. The interface also must incorporate a method for disrupting solvent clusters with the molecule of interest. In the negative ion mode, superoxide ion, $O_2^-(H_2O)_n$, is formed through an electron-capture mechanism. Charge-transfer reactions with electronegative species result in formation of negative ions. Although originally envisioned as a source of ions from either GC or HPLC separations, APCI has been used primarily in HPLC interfaces. It can be used effectively at flow rates compatible with routine HPLC. APCI has been shown to be particularly useful in ionizing nonpolar organic species (45).

Atmospheric Pressure Photoionization

Atmospheric pressure photoionization (APPI), like APCI, is particularly useful in ionizing molecules that are nonpolar. In APPI, the effluent from a high-performance liquid chromatograph is fully evaporated prior to entering the ionization region. A vacuum-UV lamp is used as a source of 10-eV photons for photoionization. Large quantities of an ionizable dopant are added to the liquid chromatography eluant, allowing for an excess of dopant photoions to be produced. The dopant photoions react with solvent and analyte molecules present in the ion source. Ionization using the dopant is 10–100 times as efficient as corona-discharge APCI. Charge-exchange reactions occur in low proton affinity solvents, whereas solvent-mediated proton transfer occurs in the presence of methanol and acetonitrile. In negative ion mode, the compounds with high electron affinity were ionized by electron capture or by charge exchange. The addition of buffers such as ammonium acetate, ammonium hydroxide, or acetic acid may suppress ionization in APPI.

Electrospray Ionization (ESI)

Electrospray ionization (ESI) is achieved by applying a large (3000–5000 volt) potential on a metal capillary containing a flowing liquid. The charge separation between the metal capillary and the liquid results in a series of charged microdroplets being expelled from the Taylor cone that forms at the capillary tip. As the droplets drift through a drying region, they evaporate and expel smaller charged droplets as the charge-to-volume ratio exceeds the Raleigh limit. Ions are thought to form from surface desorption from the highly charged liquid droplet surface. The protonated molecular ions formed, which may be associated with solvent molecules, are declustered before entering the mass spectrometer. One interesting aspect of ESI is the formation of multiply charged ions from proteins and peptides.

ESI is most effective at flow rates between 2 and 10 μL/min, although modifications of the interface have been used at flow rates as high as 200 μL/min. ESI is useful in ionizing polar organic molecules, and thus it compliments either the APCI or APPI technique. One on-going challenge in adapting both electrospray and APCI or APPI to RP-HPLC analysis has been the design of a source that efficiently accommodates the characteristics of both ionization techniques, since ESI works better on polar, early eluting compounds and APCI or APPI works better on nonpolar, late eluting compounds.

ESI is susceptible to suppression of formation of the ions of interest when other charged species are present (46). The ion suppression phenomenon is often sample specific. This could result in either underestimation of the concentration or the potential for a false negative in an assay screening for the presence of a substance. Incorporation of a deuterated or ^{13}C-containing internal standard for the compound of interest compensates for the suppression, or at least makes the analyst aware of the problem. Ion suppression may limit the use of ESI-LC–MS for screening purposes in complex sample matrices. The presence in the ion source of large amounts of an interferent might result in suppression of ionization or ion detection, even in EI-GC–MS (47).

Mass Analysis

Several approaches are available for separating ions based on their mass-to-charge ratio. Each type of mass analyzer has advantages and disadvantages to its separation and detection of ions. The most popular mass analyzers, based primarily on their cost-to-benefit ratio, are the quadrupole mass filter and the quadrupole ion trap. Due to advances in electronics and improvements in ion storage and focusing techniques, the time-of-flight mass analyzer has gained significant popularity. The impact of HPLC–MS on proteomics and metabonomics in the pharmaceutical industry has significantly changed the types of instruments that are available.

Tandem Mass Spectrometry

The increasing popularity of "soft" ionization techniques has resulted in increased reliance on mass analysis, and particularly sequential mass analysis, to provide structural and quantitative information in complex biological matrices. Tandem mass spectrometry, or MS–MS, was originally achieved by connecting two mass analyzers in tandem. Between the two mass analyzers was a collision cell that allowed the **precursor ion**[†] selected by the first mass analyzer to undergo collision-induced dissociation (CID) after collision(s) with neutral gas molecules passing through the collision cell. For low-ion-energy mass analyzers, such as the quadrupole, the fragmentation of the precursor ions to form product ions[†] can be controlled by the mass of the collision gas, the thickness of the collision gas, and the electric field strength controlling the precursor ion velocity in the collision cell. The product ions are then refocused for transmission into a second mass analyzer where they are analyzed to produce an MS–MS spectrum.

The fragmentation of "even electron ions," such as those produced with "soft" ionization techniques, is not the same as that observed for "odd electron ions" formed in EI. The ad initium interpretation of an MS–MS scan to identify the molecular structure is not nearly as advanced as that for MS. This is somewhat compensated for by the ability to perform "linked scans" between the first and second mass analyzer. For example, the second mass analyzer could be scanned while the first mass analyzer was held fixed at a constant mass to determine all product ions that arose from a particular precursor ion, termed a **product ion scan**. Unfortunately, differences in collision cell design make it very difficult to compare MS–MS spectral libraries from different instruments. Scanning the second mass analyzer while holding the first mass analyzer at a constant mass would detect all precursor ions giving rise to a particular product ion, termed a **precursor ion scan**. Finally, the two mass spectrometers could be scanned with a constant difference between

[†] The terms "parent," "daughter," and "grand-daughter" ions were commonly used for the precursor and product ions. The use of the former terms is discouraged.

the mass of ions transmitted, which would identify all precursor ions with the same loss of mass after CID (neutral loss scan). Finally, the mass of the precursor ion transmitted could be held constant while the second mass analyzer is stepped among several masses for specified dwell times, termed **selected reaction monitoring** (SRM). The SRM technique is analogous to SIM using a single mass analyzer and is frequently used for trace quantitation.

The application of tandem mass spectrometry to the analysis of dried blood spots taken from newborns for screening for metabolic disorders illustrates the power of the technique (48). For acylcarnitines, all of the various compounds give rise to a product ion of 85 Th. By fixing the second mass analyzer to detect only 85 Th and doing a precursor scan from about 270 Th to 500 Th, all of the acylcarnitines containing from three- to eighteen-carbon fatty acids can be detected. Inclusion of appropriately stable, isotope-labeled internal standards permits quantitative measurements of the various compounds. All butyl esters of α-amino acids lose a butyl formate fragment (102 daltons) with the charge retained on the amino portion of the ion. Thus, by performing a neutral loss scan with a constant difference of 102 between the mass analyzers, all α-amino acids can be identified by the mass of the ion in the first mass analyzer giving rise to the neutral loss signal. Thus, from a single dried blood spot, disorders of amino acid, fatty acid, and organic acid metabolism can be detected. Recent publications indicate that additional metabolic disorders, such as congenital adrenal hyperplasia, can be diagnosed in dried blood spots using tandem mass spectrometry.

Quadrupole Mass Filter

The most commonly used mass analyzer is the quadrupole mass filter (QMF). Ions from the ion source drift down the z-axis defined by four rods (Figure 9). A combination of radiofrequency (RF) and direct-current (DC) voltages are applied to the opposing pairs of rods. The resulting alternating electric field causes the ions to be alternately attracted to and repelled from the rods. The ions follow a corkscrew path as they drift toward the detector. Ions of particular m/z ratios have a stable trajectory to the detector at particular sets of DC and RF voltages. The RF frequency and quadrupole rod geometry and spacing, determined by the manufacturer, also influence the conditions under which particular ions are focused on the detector. A stability diagram (Figure 10) shows the RF and DC voltage amplitude pairs at which ions of a particular m/z ratio are transmitted through the rods. In the figure, any pairs of voltages that are within the triangle for a particular m/z ratio result in that ion being detected. For example, at point A the RF and DC voltage amplitudes result in both m/z 219 and 502 ions having a stable trajectory through the rods and being detected, while m/z 59 would be ejected laterally between the rods and would not be detected. The hatched area of the figure indicates a set of voltage pairs where m/z 219 ions would be transmitted but m/z 59 and 502 would not. It should be apparent that the set of voltage pairs that would result in a stable trajectory for m/z 219 ions but not for m/z 218 or 220 ions would be fairly small and would reside in the upper right apex of the stability diagram. The application of a pair of voltages that transmits only a single ion results in continuous monitoring of that selected ion. Continuously monitoring one m/z ion would provide the maximum sensitivity for that ion, since no instrument time is spent acquiring the signal from other ions. This is an advantage of a QMF operated in the SIM mode. It is relatively simple to step from one voltage pair to another, which allows rapid monitoring of multiple selected m/z ions. However, monitoring more ions results in decreased time spent detecting each ion (dwell time), which decreases sensitivity for each ion. Due to the

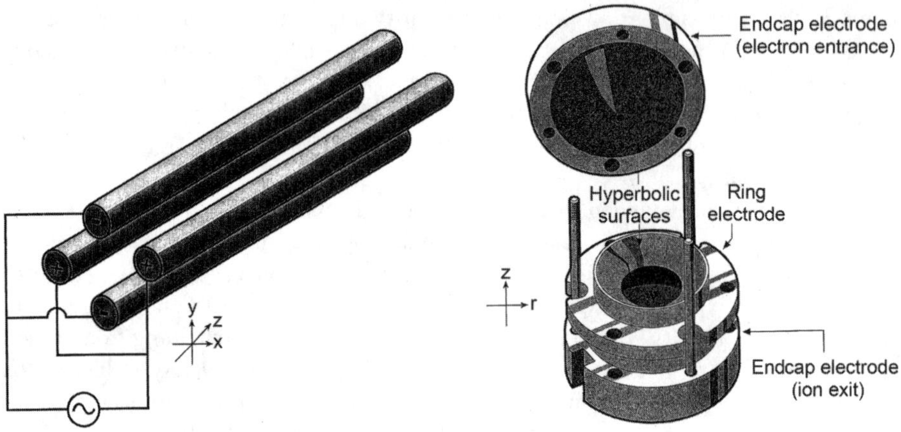

FIGURE 9. Schematic diagram of a quadrupole mass filter (left) and a quadrupole ion trap (right). (*Reprinted from Tietz textbook of clinical chemistry, 3rd ed., Burtis CA, Ashwood ER, eds., p. 197, Copyright 1999, with permission from Elsevier*)

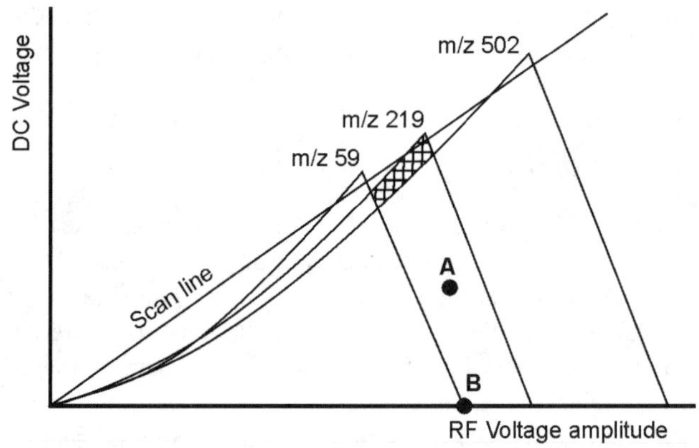

FIGURE 10. Stability diagram for trajectories of the m/z 59, 219, and 502 ions in a quadrupolar electric field. Any pair of DC and RF voltages falling within the stability "triangle" results in a stable trajectory of the ion within the quadrupole electrodes. (*Reprinted from Tietz textbook of clinical chemistry, 3rd ed., Burtis CA, Ashwood ER, eds., p. 197, Copyright 1999, with permission from Elsevier*)

time required for quadrupole settling after a change and associated computer/electronic response times, monitoring more than about six ions simultaneously in the SIM mode may become less efficient (43). In practice, it is a good idea to perform a "dynamic tune" to determine the optimal settings for monitoring a particular compound and ion. This consists of injecting the compound of interest into the gas chromatograph or liquid chromatograph and simultaneously monitoring masses in the area of the expected mass in 0.1-dalton increments (which is equivalent to making small changes in the RF–DC voltage pairs). The setting (e.g., m/z 219.4) that produces the largest peak height or peak area should then be used to achieve an analysis with maximum analytical sensitivity.

Obtaining a full scan on a QMF is somewhat more complex. From Figure 10, it would appear that changing the DC and RF voltages such that they just touch the upper right apex of each m/z stability "triangle" would result in a well-resolved mass spectrum. Unfortunately, the stability diagram is a representation of the probability of a particular ion being transmitted, and as the apex is approached, the number of ions transmitted decreases. In addition, any imperfections in the rod assembly or associated electronics could result in no ions at a particular mass being transmitted. As a result, a scan line is selected slightly below the apices and an asymmetrical triangular window is moved along the mass axis. This results in limited mass resolution. In addition, QMFs are "tuned" by adjusting the DC offset and slope of the RF voltage line to calibrate the mass axis and achieve acceptable ion intensity. Tuning also involves adjusting voltages in the ion source (e.g., repeller) and ion optics (e.g., lens stack) connecting the source to the QMF. Many laboratories use "autotune" programs provided by the manufacturer that systematically vary the tuning parameters to meet specific criteria. Experienced operators may choose to tune the system manually to achieve specific analytical objectives.

Although this discussion involved a quadrupole device, the same theoretical parameters apply to devices with more rods, such as an octopole. Both quadrupoles and octopoles can be used as ion focusing or storage devices. Note from Figure 10 that when a low RF-only voltage is applied to the rods, all ions are transmitted. Some critics suggest that an octopole device is not good as an m/z analyzer. It does not have a well-behaved stability diagram to make it amenable as a mass analyzer.

Quadrupole Ion Trap

The theoretical principles of the quadrupole ion trap (QIT) are the same as those of a QMF, that is, the stability of ion movement in a combined DC–RF field. The operating principles, however, result in significant differences between the two devices. Due to the three-dimensional nature of the QIT, ions can be trapped when no DC voltage and a low RF voltage are applied to the electrodes. Since the ion trajectories are stable within the trap, a different scan function was developed using mass instability ejection. By increasing the RF voltage amplitude, ions of a particular m/z become axially unstable (point B in Figure 10 for m/z 59) and are ejected from both endcaps of the QIT. An external continuous dynode multiplier can then detect the ions ejected from one of the endcaps. Operating the QIT at a higher pressure (10^{-3} Torr) than that used in the QMF improved the ion-trapping efficiency, which improved sensitivity and mass resolution. Additional improvement in the mass resolution and sensitivity was achieved by applying an axial modulation voltage to the endcaps, which increased ion ejection efficiency.

The initial approach to ion formation in the QIT was to use the trap itself as the ion source, called **internal ionization**. When interfaced to a GC system, entry of all components eluting from the column into the QIT resulted in two problems. If too many ions are present in the QIT, they shield each other from the electric field generated by the electrodes. This is called the space–charge effect and can result in mass misassignment. The problem has been addressed by performing a prescan. Based on the number of ions formed in the prescan, the ionization time for the analytical scan is adjusted to control the number of ions in the QIT.

The second problem is the potential for ion–neutral and ion–ion reactions such as proton transfer. This can result in a higher abundance of protonated molecular ion $(M+H)^+$ than would be observed in the spectrum from a QMF, for example. This can make manual interpretation of the mass spectrum more difficult (40) and result in lower matching factors in computer-assisted library searches, depending on the type of instrument(s) used to provide the library spectra. One way to address this problem is to form the ions outside of the trap and inject them into the QIT. This is termed **external ionization**, and has been used for interfacing both gas chromatograph and liquid chromatograph to the QIT.

External ionization–ion injection eliminates the potential for ion–neutral reactions but suffers from low trapping efficiencies (about 5%). Alternate trap geometries that improve the trapping efficiency, such as the rectilinear ion trap, have been reported.

The ion storage ability of the QIT also changes the approach to SIM. Rather than increasing the time monitoring an ion as occurs in the QMF, increased numbers of ions of a selected m/z can be stored in the trap while others are ejected. This is called **selected ion storage** (SIS). Ions of a particular m/z ratio oscillate radially and axially at specific, but different, frequencies, depending on the trap geometry and the RF frequency and amplitude. This is called the **secular frequency**. Applying a voltage waveform to the endcaps at the secular frequency causes ions of that m/z to exit the trap. Selective ejection of unwanted ions is achieved by applying various combinations of waveforms to the endcaps or a combination of various waveforms on the endcaps with a change in the RF voltage on the ring electrode. The variety of possible SIS approaches makes them difficult to compare (43). In any case, ejection of the selectively stored ions is accomplished by the mass instability scan function.

The ability to store ions in the QIT has additional advantages. First, MS–MS is relatively easy to accomplish. MS–MS on the QIT is the result of sequential trapping, collisional activation, and product ion formation steps. It is sometimes called MS–MS in time to distinguish it from MS–MS in space, which occurs with tandem QMF analyzers. Two approaches are available, one is application of a resonant or nonresonant waveform to increase the ion energy prior to collision. Since the product ions are stored in the trap, repeated sequences can be performed to achieve MS^n experiments. In the second approach using the mass instability scan, the mass resolution observed is inversely related to the scan rate. Thus, by slowing the scan rate, mass resolution comparable to that obtained on high-resolution sector instruments has been reported, although the accurate mass capability of most high-resolution mass spectrometers is not realized in this case. The versatility of the QIT and the advances made with trap geometries other than the hyperbolic ion trap initially described by Paul virtually ensure that ion traps will remain a major segment of the mass analyzer market.

Time of Flight

Time of flight (TOF) mass analyzers separate ions according to the length of time it takes for ions of a specific kinetic energy to move from the ion source to the detector. Assuming that all ions have the same kinetic energy and the same start time, the time (t) to traverse a flight path of length L is given by

$$t = L\sqrt{\frac{m}{z} \bullet \frac{1}{2V}} \tag{24}$$

where m/z is the mass-to-charge ratio, and V is the accelerating voltage. Because all of the ions must start simultaneously, TOF analyzers are particularly well suited to electronically gated ion pulses or ionization techniques that produce ions in a well-defined pulse, such as matrix-assisted laser desorption ionization (MALDI) in which ionization is initiated by a pulsed laser. In contrast to scanning instruments, all ions produced in the ion source are directed into the flight tube and detected. TOF instruments always produce full-scan spectra; there is no advantage to monitoring selected ions. The analyzer can be optimized to produce very fast scanning speeds, necessary to work with "fast GC," or to give high mass resolution and mass accuracy (2–5 ppm). In order to have instruments of reasonable size, reversing the direction of the ions, which also decreases ion spread and improves mass resolution, roughly doubles the ion flight path. Analyzers of this type are called **reflectrons**. Because of the relatively simple design, TOF analyzers are able to detect ions across a wide mass range and have excellent sensitivity. Improvements in the speed of detection electronics and computers and improved ion storage and gating techniques have made GC-TOF and LC-TOF instruments an important alternative to scanning mass spectrometers.

Other Mass Analyzers

In the original mass spectrometer design, ions accelerated from the ion source through a 1–10-kV field were deflected by a magnetic field (B) onto the detector. The m/z of the ion focused on the detector is a function of the radius of the trajectory of ions in a magnetic field, the field strength, and the ion accelerating voltage. In general, higher accelerating voltages result in better ion transmission and better analytical sensitivity. In contrast, decreasing the accelerating voltage extends the mass range of a magnetic sector instrument. Since both the ion accelerating voltage and the magnetic field strength affect the m/z of the ion detected, either can be varied as a function of time to sequentially focus ions of different m/z on the detector and produce a mass spectrum. The spectrum resulting from scanning the magnetic field provides a "classic" mass spectrum where the abundance of the ions detected is independent of the m/z ratio. The magnitude of the signal produced by scanning the accelerating voltage decreases with increasing m/z ratio, and thus the spectrum shows less relative abundance at high mass. For selected ion monitoring, the accelerating voltage is generally stepped to select specific m/z ions because more time is required to step and stabilize the magnetic field strength.

To improve mass resolution, an electric (E) sector that separates ions based on their kinetic energy-to-charge ratio can be added either before (E/B design) or after (B/E design) the magnetic sector. The electric sector cancels out trajectory differences in the magnetic field caused by energy variation. This instrumentation is often referred to as a double-focusing mass spectrometer and their design is somewhat analogous to achromatizing a lens in light optics. Designs incorporating additional electric sectors (e.g., E/B/E design) also are available. The advantage of double-focusing instruments is their ability to provide high mass resolution, which eliminates chemical noise and provides very high sensitivity. The disadvantages of the design are:

- a large instrument footprint and weight
- stringent site requirements for low frequency vibration
- the requirement for operator expertise for effective operation of the instrument

Accurate mass measurements are a good application for sector instruments.

A specific application of the magnetic sector design is the measurement of the isotopic content of gases such as H_2, CO_2, N_2, and O_2. In this case, the magnetic field is fixed and three characteristic m/z ions (e.g., m/z 44, 45, and 46 for CO_2) are focused continuously on individual Faraday cup detectors. To improve the accuracy of the measurement further, a reference gas of known composition and the unknown gas are alternately bled into the ion source. Atom excess on the order of 0.001% can be detected. This technique, called **isotope ratio mass spectrometry** (IRMS), has been used in the diagnosis of *Helicobacter pylori* infection, which is associated with gastrointestinal ulcers. The patient ingests a solution of ^{13}C-enriched urea. The patient's breath is then analyzed for increased $^{13}CO_2$

produced as a result of hydrolysis of the urea by the microorganism. The development of a combustion interface has allowed the technique to be used in conjunction with both GC (GC-C-IRMS) and LC (LC-C-IRMS). The effluent from the column is burned in a high temperature, oxidizing furnace to convert any carbon-containing compound into CO_2, which is then analyzed by IRMS. Using this technique, it can be determined whether testosterone in an athlete's urine came from physiological metabolism or from ingestion of a pharmaceutical compound since the two have slightly different ^{13}C-enrichment. While this is a very powerful technique, it is quite different from normal GC–MS operation and requires special skills.

In a **Fourier transform ion cyclotron resonance** (FT ICR) mass analyzer, ions are trapped in a circular cyclotron orbit by a very strong magnetic field. The orbital frequency of each ion is dependent on its mass-to-charge ratio while the amplitude of sine wave is a function of the number of ions. The frequencies of all ions in the cyclotron are measured simultaneously using a pair of electrodes on either side of the ion orbit. A Fourier transform of the frequencies and amplitudes provides a traditional mass spectrum. FT ICR instruments are capable of high mass resolution and high sensitivity since the ions are not ejected from the mass analyzer for detection. MS^n experiments are accomplished easily since the ions are trapped in the mass analyzer. The drawbacks of FT ICR instruments are the requirement for a superconducting magnet and very high vacuum.

REFERENCES

1. Ettre LS. Nomenclature for chromatography. Pure Appl Chem 1993;65:819–72.
2. Smith RM, Marton A. Classification and characterization of liquid chromatographic stationary phases. Pure Appl Chem 1997;69:1475–80.
3. Davankov VA. Analytical chiral separation methods. Pure Appl Chem 1997;69:1469–74.
4. Davankov VA. Retention parameters in gas chromatography. Pure Appl Chem 2000;73:982–92.
5. Domínguez JAG, Díez-Masa JC, Davankov VA. Retention parameters in chromatography. Pure Appl Chem 2001;73:969–92.
6. Ward TJ, Hamburg D-M. Chiral separations. Anal Chem 2004;76:4635–44.
7. Hennion MC, Pichon V. Immuno-based sample preparation for trace analysis. J Chromatogr A 2003;1000:29–52.
8. Raynie DE. Modern extraction techniques. Anal Chem 2004;76:4659–64.
9. Poole CF. Thin-layer chromatography: challenges and opportunities. J Chromatogr A 2003;1000:963–84.
10. Foley JP, Dorsey JG. Equations for calculation of chromatographic figures of merit for ideal and skewed peaks. Anal Chem 1983;55:730–7.
11. The fitness for purpose of analytical methods: a laboratory guide to method validation and related topics. EURACHEM, Internet version, 1998 (www.eurachem.ul.pt); Guides and Documents menu; accessed June 2004).
12. Thompson M, Ellefson SLR, Wood R. Harmonized guidelines for single-laboratory validation of methods of analysis. Pure Appl Chem 2002;74:835–55.
13. National Committee for Clinical Laboratory Standards. Gas chromatography/mass spectrometry (GC/MS) confirmation of drugs; approved guideline. NCCLS Document C43-A. Wayne, PA: NCCLS, 2002.
14. Felinger A. Data analysis and signal processing in chromatography. New York: Elsevier, 1998.
15. Snyder LR, Kirkland JJ, Glajch JL. Practical HPLC method development. 2nd ed. New York: Wiley, 1997:714–20.
16. Meyer VA. Errors in the area determination of incompletely resolved chromatographic peaks. J Chromatogr Sci 1995;33:26–33.

17. Foley JP. Systematic errors in the measurement of peak area and peak height for overlapping peaks. J Chromatogr 1987;384:301–13.
18. Williams A, Ellefson SLR, Roesslein M. Quantifying uncertainty in analytical measurements, 2nd ed. 2000. Available at http://www.eurachem.ul.pt/; Guides and Documents menu; accessed June 2004.
19. ISO/IEC/EN 17025:1999. General requirements for the competence of calibration and testing laboratories. Geneva: International Organization for Standardization, 1999.
20. Romero R, Garcia Bagur M, Gásquez D, et al. Estimation of the main sources of uncertainty in chromatographic analysis: determination of biogenic amines. LC/GC 2004;22:150–64.
21. Horwitz W. Uncertainty—a chemist's view. JAOAC 1998;81:785–94.
22. Ellison SLR. Uncertainties in qualitative testing and analysis. Accred Qual Assur 2000;5:346–8.
23. de Ruig WG, Dijkstra G, Stephany RW. Chemometric criteria for assessing the certainty of qualitative analytical methods. Anal Chim Acta 1989;223:277–82.
24. Blau K, Halket JM. Handbook of derivatives for chromatography. 2nd ed. New York: Wiley, 1993.
25. Dose EV. Simulation of gas chromatographic retention and peak width using thermodynamic retention indices. Anal Chem 1987;59:2414–9.
26. Dose EV. Simulating GC elution: *Pro ezGC*. Anal Chem 1995;67:476A–7A (software review).
27. Phillips JB. Reducing GC method development time: *GC-SOS*. Anal Chem 1995;67:360A–1A (software review).
28. Grob RL, Barry EF. Modern practice of gas chromatography. 4th ed. New York: Wiley, 2004.
29. Parcher JF. Fundamental relationships in gas chromatography. Chromatographia 1998; 47:570–4.
30. Bertsch W. Two-dimensional gas chromatography. Concepts, instrumentation, and applications – part 1: Fundamentals, conventional two-dimensional gas chromatography, selected applications. J High Resolut Chromatogr 1999;22:647–65.
31. Bertsch W. Two-dimensional gas chromatography. Concepts, instrumentation, and applications – part 2. Comprehensive two-dimensional gas chromatography. J High Resolut Chromatogr 2000;23:167–81.
32. Rood D. A practical guide to the care, maintenance, and troubleshooting of capillary gas chromatographic systems, 3rd rev ed. New York: Wiley-VCH, 1999.
33. Snyder LR, Kirkland JJ, Glajch JL. Practical HPLC method development. 2nd ed. New York: Wiley, 1997.
34. Snyder LR, Dolan JW, Carr PW. The hydrophobic-subtraction model of reversed-phase column selectivity. J Chromatogr 2004;1060:77–116.
35. Snyder LR, Kirkland JJ, Glajch JL. Practical HPLC method development. 2nd ed. New York: Wiley, 1997:257–60; 439–78.
36. Thompson JD, Carr PW. High-speed liquid chromatography by simultaneous optimization of temperature and eluent composition. Anal Chem 2002;74:4150–9.
37. Snyder LR. Gradient elution. In: Horvath C, ed. High-performance liquid chromatography: advances and perspectives. Vol. 1. San Diego: Academic Press, 1980:207–316.
38. Snyder LR, Stadalius MA. High-performance liquid chromatography separation of Lare molecules: a general model. In: Horvath C, ed. High-performance liquid chromatography: advances and perspectives. Vol. 4. San Diego: Academic Press, 1986:196–312.
39. Stein SE. An integrated method for spectrum extraction and compound identification from GC/MS data. J Am Soc Mass Spectrom 1999;10:770–781.
40. McLafferty FW, Turecek F. Interpretation of mass spectra. 4th ed. Mill Valley CA: University Science Books, 1993.
41. Stein SE, Scott DR. Optimization and testing of mass spectral library search algorithms for compound identification. J Am Soc Mass Spectrom 1994;5:859–66.
42. Bethem R, Boison J, Gale J, et al. Establishing the fitness for purpose of mass spectrometric methods. J Am Soc Mass Spectrom 2003;14:528–41.

43. Bowers LD, Borts DJ. Evaluation of selected-ion storage ion-trap mass spectrometry for detecting urinary anabolic agents. Clin Chem 1997;43:1033–9.
44. Fitzgerald RL, Herold DA. Serum total testosterone: immunoassay compared with negative chemical ionization-mass spectrometry. Clin Chem 1996;42:749–55.
45. Hayen H, Karst U. Strategies for the liquid chromatographic-mass spectrometric analysis of non-polar compounds. J Chromatogr A 2003;1000:549–65.
46. Annesley TM. Ion suppression in mass spectrometry. Clin Chem 2003;49:1041–4.
47. Ostheimer D, Cremese M, Wu AH, et al. Reduction in extraction efficiency of charged particles from the ion source as the cause of matrix effects in the GC-MS analysis of drugs. J Anal Toxicol 1997;21:17–22.
48. Chace DH, Kalas TA, Naylor EW. Use of tandem mass spectrometry for multianalyte screening of dried blood specimens from newborns. Clin Chem 2003;49:1797–817.

Chapter 6

Instrumentation in Immunoassay

Craig C. Foreback

Instrumentation in immunoassay began with the use of radioisotopes as labels to follow antigen–antibody reactions. This technique, known as radioimmunoassay (RIA), is a heterogeneous type of competitive immunoassay where labeled antigen is used. Yalow and Berson first reported the use of isotopes for labeling the antigen–antibody reaction (1) and set the standard for immunoassays. A competitive reaction is carried out in the presence of excess antigen from a sample where labeled antigen competes with unlabeled antigen (analyte) for binding sites on an antibody. When a labeled antibody is used, the assays are called immunoradiometric assays (IRMA). The ligand in the sample competes with the ligand attached to a solid surface for the binding sites of the labeled antibody. Early assays were developed for hormones such as insulin, cortisol, T_4, and some reproductive hormones. Procedures were automated to some extent but required separate equipment and thus separate steps for sample and reagent addition, separation of bound from unbound label, and isotope counting. Procedures could often encompass 8 hours or more. Laboratories were developed around these assays and focused more on research applications rather than service to the institution. For a number of reasons, availability and turnaround times were irregular. Because it was inefficient to set-up RIA or IRMA assays for just a few samples, specimens were accumulated until a sufficient number could be run in an efficient sized batch to justify the multiple standards and controls needed to validate the assay. Assays were run in duplicate and sometimes without benefit of quality control since adequate controls often were not available. Turnaround time could be as long as 30 days because the process was so labor-intensive due to lack of automation.

During the 1970s, a number of developments occurred that dramatically changed immunoassay. Reactions between antigens and antibodies were, in many instances, visualized by observing the produced turbidity. Initially, qualitative assessments could be made and were usually reported as titers. Attempts at spectrophotometric measurements of turbidity proved unsatisfactory. The use of antibodies bound to latex or Sephadex™ particles improved the uniformity of precipitation. Secondly, the process of measuring turbidity was enhanced by the development of **nephelometry** as a measuring tool.

Nephelometry utilized a fixed wavelength laser source at 600 nm or above directed on the sample. The other major difference as compared to a conventional absorbance measurement was to place the detector at an angle near forward of the light source, usually at 10–30°. This allowed light scattering to be measured rather than absorbance of particles in solution. This change in instrumentation revolutionized the analysis of specific proteins and even some therapeutic drugs. Evaluation of kinetic light scattering for the measurement of specific proteins was reported in 1975 (2) while assays for therapeutic drugs were reported in the late 1970s. Two instruments using near-forward light scattering with a laser source are included in this chapter. Improvements in optics and computer analysis of spectrophotometric readouts have facilitated the use of automated chemistry analyzers for monitoring of antigen–antibody reactions. These assays are not as sensitive and precise as nephelometric measurements but provide adequate performance for many analytes of clinical interest. Light scattering has limited applications because most antigen–antibody reactions do not form insoluble complexes.

ENZYME IMMUNOASSAYS

The introduction of enzyme immunoassays (EIA) in the 1970s has had an major impact on the laboratory and has added an incredible number of reliable and versatile assays, changing the nature of immunoassay. EIA uses enzyme activity to quantitate antigen–antibody complexes formed instead of radioactivity. EIA can be performed in any laboratory in any organization, not just those licensed for isotopes. EIA is a general term that includes all immunoassay methods that use enzymes such as horseradish peroxidase, alkaline phosphatase, or beta-D-galactosidase for detection. Various forms of EIA are in use, including enzyme-linked immunosorbent assays (ELISA), enzyme-multiplied immunoassay (EMIT), cloned enzyme donor immunoassay (CEDIA), immunoenzymometric assays, and chemiluminescence assays. Of the various EIAs, only the CEDIA and EMIT are homogeneous. Others require a separation step to remove excess reagents and sample that may interfere with quantitation. However, EMIT and CEDIA technology could be and were adapted to fully automated chemisty analyzers, thus beginning a revolution in immunoassays.

ELISA

ELISA, developed in 1971 (3), is a heterogeneous EIA technique that has many clinical applications. The ELISA format employs antigen or antibody bound to a solid surface such as the well of a microtiter plate. If the desired analyte is an antibody, e.g., antibody to an infectious agent such rubella, inactivated virus is coated on the solid surface. Antibody from the sample then attaches to the antigen. After a wash step, a second enzyme-labeled antibody which is specific to IgG or IgM is added and the measured enzyme activity is directly proportional to the antibody present in the sample. The technique also can be used to measure antigen in a sample by binding analyte-specific antibody to a solid surface. The analyte binds to the bound antibody. Following a wash step, a second enzyme-labeled antigen-specific antibody is added and enzyme activity is measured.

EMIT

EMIT was first described by Rubenstein et al. in 1972 (4). It is based on the competition between an antigen (Ag) (analyte) in a patient sample and an antigen that has been covalently bonded to an enzyme (*see* Figure 1). In the presence of an antibody (Ab) to the analyte, an antigen–antibody complex forms that blocks substrate access to the enzyme. Alternatively, the binding may change the conformation of the enzyme, altering its ability to catalyze a given substrate. As patient antigen increases, less antibody is available to bind to the enzyme–antigen complex and enzyme activity increases. When no patient antigen is present, enzyme activity is completely blocked.

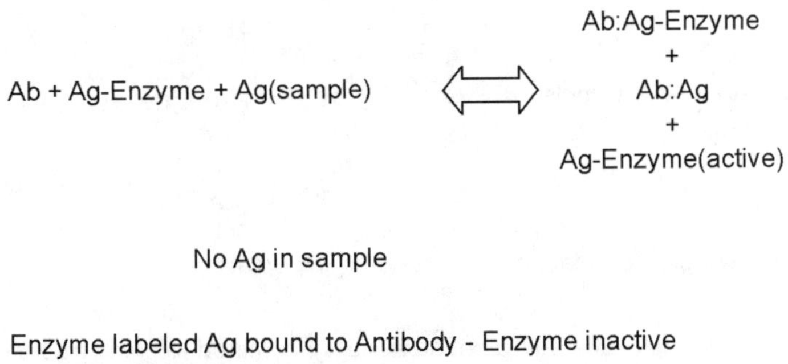

FIGURE 1. Principle of EMIT method.

CEDIA

CEDIA, introduced in 1986 (5), is based on the use of cloning techniques to prepare two inactive fragments of β-galactosidase that will spontaneously reassemble to form a fully active enzyme. The CEDIA technology has applications for drugs of abuse, therapeutic drugs, and thyroid hormones.

Fluorescence Immunoassays

Conjugating antigens or antibodies with a fluorescent label marked the beginning of a major breakthrough in clinical immunoassay testing. Many analytes that previously could only be analyzed by RIA or radioimmunometric assay could now be analyzed by fluorescent immunoassay (FIA). FIA has several advantages over RIA such as longer shelf life and faster assays, and it avoids the costs of radioactive disposal, licensing, and monitoring. Some disadvantages have been noted such as significant levels of background noise often found in biological systems. Use of ruthenium (I) or rhenium (I) in complex formation for the detection of high molecular weight analytes has overcome this problem (6, 7).

Another approach to eliminating background noise is Abbott's use of fluorescence-polarization immunoassay (FPIA). FPIA is a competitive assay using fluorescent-labeled antigen that competes with antigen in a sample for a limited number of binding sites on an antigen-specific antibody (8). When small fluorescent molecules are irradiated with plane polarized light, the emission radiation is totally random and lacks any direction since the molecule is constantly tumbling. However, if the small molecule is bound to a large molecule such as an antibody, its rate of tumbling is slowed. This means that the radiation of an antibody-bound fluorescent molecule with plane polarized light results in the emission of primarily plane polarized fluorescence. FPIA is a competitive assay in which fluorescent-labeled antigen (tracer) competes with antigen in a sample for antibody. If the targeted antigen is not present in the sample, the tracer binds to the antibody, its rotation is slowed, and the light emitted will be polarized. If analyte is present in the sample, the tracer will not bind to the antibody, it will continue to spin at a faster rate, and the level of polarized fluorescence will be diminished as shown in Figure 2. The amount of analyte is inversely proportional to the amount of fluorescence polarization. This technique was commercialized in 1981 in the form of the TDx (discussed later).

These advances in detection methods dramatically changed clinical immunoassay. Several totally new instruments were introduced into the clinical laboratory and existing chemistry analyzers were able to provide a much larger menu of clinically useful assays.

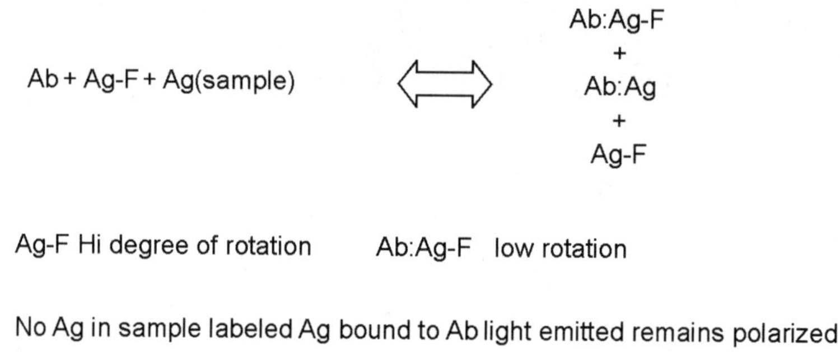

FIGURE 2. Principle of FPIA.

These developments allowed laboratories to switch from labor-intensive RIA assays to assays that were completely automated.

First-Generation Automation

The development of automated immunoassays began with early efforts to automate RIA systems. However, automation quickly focused on nonisotopic methods. Early instruments included the Dade Stratus (FIA) and the Abbott TDx (FPIA). Applications for EMIT assays were developed for Hitachi, Beckman, Olympus, and Dupont (Dade) chemistry analyzers. Applications for CEDIA assays were developed for Hitachi, Beckman, and Olympus systems. The Beckman Array, using nephelometric measurements, was introduced for specific proteins, including immunoglobulins, κ/λ ratio, transferrin, apolipoproteins, and many others.

The Abbott TDx was one of the most successful instruments introduced for performing immunoassays in clinical laboratories. It has been estimated that some 37,000 instruments were in use worldwide at its peak. A wide range of therapeutic drugs is available including one of the first immunoassays for immunosuppressants. Assays also include some for hormones that are in higher concentration in clinical samples; however, assays for large molecules and small molecules in low concentrations are not possible on the TDx.

The Dade Stratus was another important analyzer in the evolution of immunoassay. The Stratus was one of the first systems to employ a fully automated FIA. Using antibody bound to a fiber matrix, the Stratus uses a "sandwich" technique for analysis. The bound antibody was targeted to a specific antigen that would attach to the antibody. After washing, a second fluorescent-labeled antibody to the antigen was added, and the resulting fluorescence was directly proportional to the analyte present. The Stratus brought automation to a variety of analytes where faster turnaround time and stat capability were needed. The Stratus test menu included the first nonpretreatment digoxin assay, a full compliment of cardiac markers including the first commercially available troponin assay (in the United States) and hcG.

These analyzers along with the Abbott Imx, and the DPC Immunolite rapidly advanced the practice of immunoassay; they had one major disadvantage in that they were batch analyzers.

AVAILABLE INSTRUMENTS

Numerous automated analyzers are available with immunoassay capability. They can be grouped in five categories:

- Chemistry analyzers with homogeneous immunoassay tests
- Chemistry analyzers with homogeneous and heterogeneous immunoassay capability
- Completely automated stand-alone immunoassay instruments
- Immunoassay analyzers in which two or more steps are at separate workstations
- Immunoassay analyzers that can be combined with chemistry analyzers through common sampling and control systems

Typical immunoassay test menus are shown in Table 1. These systems are discussed in some detail; the list included is not meant to be comprehensive but an attempt has been made to include major manufacturers whose instruments offer multiple options. Also included are instruments that have nephelometric capability and may have somewhat limited test menus. The latter are often omitted from discussions of immunoassay instrumentation. The reader is also referred to publications such as *CAP Today* for up-to-date reviews on instrumentation. Much of the information for this section comes from the June 2004 issue (Vol. 18, pp 18–57). Readers are also encouraged to go to manufacturers' web sites for comprehensive, updated information (Table 2).

Progress toward Automation

Automation in immunoassay has progressed rapidly over the last 20 years. Homogeneous technology such as EMIT enabled traditional chemistry analyzers to offer expanded test menus that included therapeutic drugs, some hormones, and improved screening for drugs of abuse. Applications for the Syva EMIT methods were developed for numerous chemistry analyzers including the COBAS, Hitachi, Beckman CX, Olympus, and Dade Dimension systems. EMIT greatly improved the efficiency of several analytes by lowering costs, improving turnaround time, and providing around the clock stat capability. Newer generations of these same systems continue to provide this testing.

TABLE 1. Typical menus for immunoassay analyzers

Thyroid assays
Follicle-stimulating hormone
Luteinizing hormone
Prolactin
Cortisol
Human chorionic gonadotropin
Progesterone
Anemia markers
Therapeutic drugs
Drugs of abuse
Cardiac assesment
Creatine kinase-MB
Troponin T or I
Myoglobin
C-reactive protein
Homocysteine
B-Natriuretic peptide
Prostatic specific antigen
Hepatitis markers
Carcinoembryonic antigen

TABLE 2. Websites of manufacturers of instrumentation with immunoassay menus

Abbott Diagnostics	www.abbott.com
Bayer	www.bayer.com
Beckman–Coulter	www.beckmancoulter.com
The Binding Site	www.bindingsite.co.uk
bioMerieux	www.biomerieux-usa.com
Dade-Behring	www.dadebehring.com
Diagnostic Products Corporation	www.dpcweb.com
Luminex	www.luminexcorp.com
Olympus	www.olympus.com
Ortho Clinical Diagnostics	www.orthoclinical.com
Roche	www.roche.com
Tosoh	www.tosohbioscience.com

Immunoassay analyzers have lagged behind automation in clinical chemistry simply because the assays are much more complex than traditional chemistry. Advances in technology, particularly robotics and computerization, have brought the concept of total laboratory automation closer to reality and have broken down the traditional barriers that existed in the typical hospital laboratory for decades. Furthermore, the integration of clinical chemistry and immunoassay onto a single platform has been achieved. But the transition from the early developments has taken 30 years. Homogeneous assays were a big step toward integration because they could be run on any chemistry analyzer. Chemistry analyzers had already made the transition to random access, discrete sampling instruments in the late 1970s, enhancing their ability to provide immunoassays. While this development facilitated the ability of random access chemistry analyzers to test many common therapeutic drugs (TDM) and most classes of drugs of abuse (DAU), they could not offer assays for those tests required on a stat basis. Assays for cardiac markers, hcG, and digoxin were offered only on the early immunoassay analyzers which were batch analyzers with limited test menus and throughput. Fluorescent labels were an improvement in detection systems. Robotics and microprocessors improved these early systems, but they still suffered from the limitations of batch analyzers. The EMIT methods developed by Syva are still in use on modern instruments, even though the patents have expired. They continue to serve a useful purpose, but more sophisticated immunoassay instrumentation was needed.

Computers and robotics continued to improve to the point that immunoassay instruments could be made to function in a random access fashion much like a chemistry analyzer. Now all the tests on a patient could be run at once and results could be reported out in a single transaction. Pressure for random access came from the desire for shorter turnaround times of a growing list of stat immunoassays and from financial constraints by laboratory departments; reimbursement for laboratory testing continued to decline, and testing volume continued to increase.

A second major advance was the development of **chemiluminescence** as a label. Chemiluminescence was reported at the Oak Ridge Conference in 1979 (9). It would be more than 10 years before it was realized on commercial immunoassay instruments. Detection limits rivaled and even exceeded RIA. As with fluorescence, advantages of shelf life, assay speed, and cost were also possible with chemiluminescence. An additional advantage was that signal detection was done by photon counting in a manner similar to RIA. Standards were compared to the time it took to achieve a specified number of counts instead comparing to an absolute signal. Most of the few remaining RIA assays have been replaced by chemiluminescence detection. The majority of immunoassay analyzer instruments or modules use chemiluminescence in some form, particularly those introduced since 1994.

Early random access analyzers included the Abbott AxSYM, Ciba-Corning Chiron (now Bayer) ACS 180, the BMD (now Roche) Elecsys system, and the Sanofi (Beckman) Access. The AxSYM is a floor-standing model while the others are bench-top analyzers. The Access and the ACS 180 use chemiluminescence while the AxSYM uses FPIA and microparticle enzyme immunoassay (MEIA). More will be said about these analyzers later. None of these systems was able meet all the needs of the typical user. Even the latest available instruments have limitations in test menus or performance on certain tests. For example, AxSYM users still had to rely on the TDx's and Imx's for free drugs, immunosuppressants, and some low volume TDMs. The ACS 180, Access, and Elecsys lacked complete TDM menus when first introduced. All of them lacked a full complement of cardiac markers when first available, and they were all stand-alone systems requiring separate sample loading from the main chemistry analyzer. Throughput was limited and some were not compatible with the typical 24/7 operation of many chemistry laboratories. Most laboratories still required immunoassays with radioisotope labels for some esoteric tests and hepatitis and as well as for many other serological tests that are still performed on platforms that do not integrate sampling, reagent addition, washing, and reading steps.

Immunoassays Requiring Separation Steps

Enzyme immunoassays requiring complex separation steps are still in routine use. Examples include plastic or latex beads, coated tubes, magnetic and nonmagnetic particles, and microtiter plates. Plastic or latex beads are often used in the first step of an EIA. The bead may be coated with antibody or antigen. For example, when exposed to an infectious agent, animals and humans produce antibodies against the agent. Detection of antibody can be used to determine exposure to an infectious agent such as hepatitis. Patient antibodies react with inactivated or killed virus which is coated on the bead surface. After a mixing and washing step, the bead is incubated with enzyme-labeled antihuman immunoglobulin. The labeled-antibody binds to the antigen–antibody complex. The bound enzyme is incubated with substrate, and the measured enzyme activity is proportional to the antibody present in the sample. The Abbott Quantum II (Figure 3) is based on coated bead technology and is still used in many laboratories for hepatitis screening.

The coated tube concept is based on analyte being captured by immunogen impregnated on the inside of a plastic tube. This reactant could be antigen or antibody, depending on what is being measured. In many applications, the technique is used to measure antibody response to exposure to a specific virus, such as HIV or hepatitis. In many respects, the assay is similar to the assays described using beads. The disadvantage is that there is less surface area for the reactions to take place than with beads or microparticles.

Microparticles are suspended in the reaction mixture so that they can diffuse to the analytes and the analytes to the reactants. Their small size maximizes surface area. Separation is typically by filtration. The major problem with microparticle assays is that particulate materials other than the microparticles can be trapped and counted as bound.

To retain the advantages of microparticles but avoid the disadvantages of filtration, magnetic separations have been used. Separation of bound and free superparamagnetic particles is then achieved by having the binding agent attached to the magnetic particle. In the absence of an external magnetic field, these particles have no residual magnetic field. This technique can be automated and is the basis for several instruments discussed later.

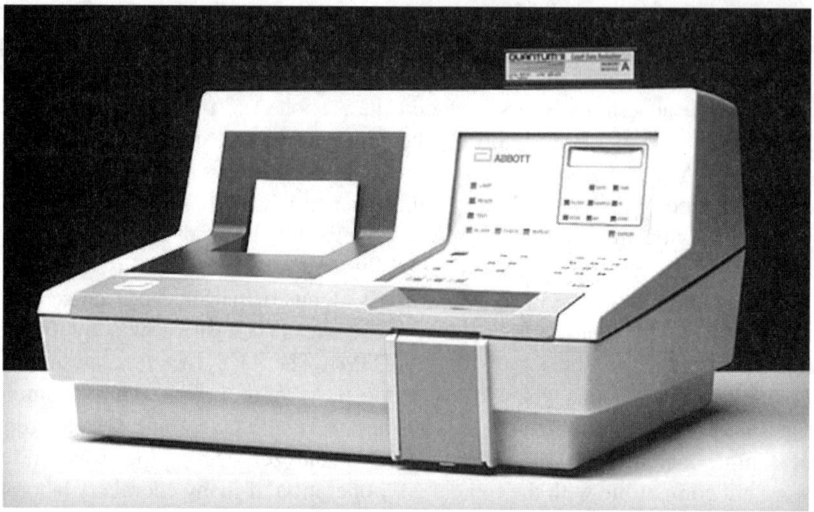

FIGURE 3. Abbott Quantum 2. (*Courtesy of Abbott Laboratories*)

The available surface area of the paramagnetic particles is 50 times higher than a well of a microtiter plate.

Manual Microtiter Plate Assays

With the multitude of fully automated random access immunoassay analyzers now available, it is usually more cost effective and faster to do most assays on an automated platform. However, for new assays involving only small numbers of samples, which may not be available on an automated system, microtiter plates offer a practical solution. Microtiter plates are available for a wide variety of low volume or emerging assays. Microtiter plates employ EIA for determination. Microtiter plate readers direct a beam of light down through the solution generated by the reaction of substrate with enzyme. The absorbance observed is converted into a standard curve to calculate analyte concentrations. Microtiter plate assays are for the most part batch assays. Each plate has to have a set of standards and controls. Tests are often run in duplicate; therefore, only about 40 samples can be done on the typical 96-well plate. Microtiter plates are slower than automated immunoassay analyzers and results may not be available for several hours. In the following sections, it will be apparent that modern automated equipment is much more efficient and timely.

CHEMISTRY PLATFORMS WITH IMMUNOASSAY CAPABILITY

Dade Dimension RxL

The Dade Dimension RxL evolved from the Dimension series of analyzers developed by Dupont. The RxL was one of the first analyzers to combine traditional chemistry with homogeneous assays and heterogeneous assays. Previous versions of the Dimension system incorporated homogeneous assays for TDMs and DAUs onto a chemistry platform. The RxL added fluorescent immunoassays so that tests such as hcG, digoxin, and cardiac markers could be integrated with routine clinical chemistry and therapeutic drug monitoring. The RxL Max is the most recent Dimension system (Figure 4). This instrument processes 168 tests per hour and it may be the only instrument needed in many smaller sites.

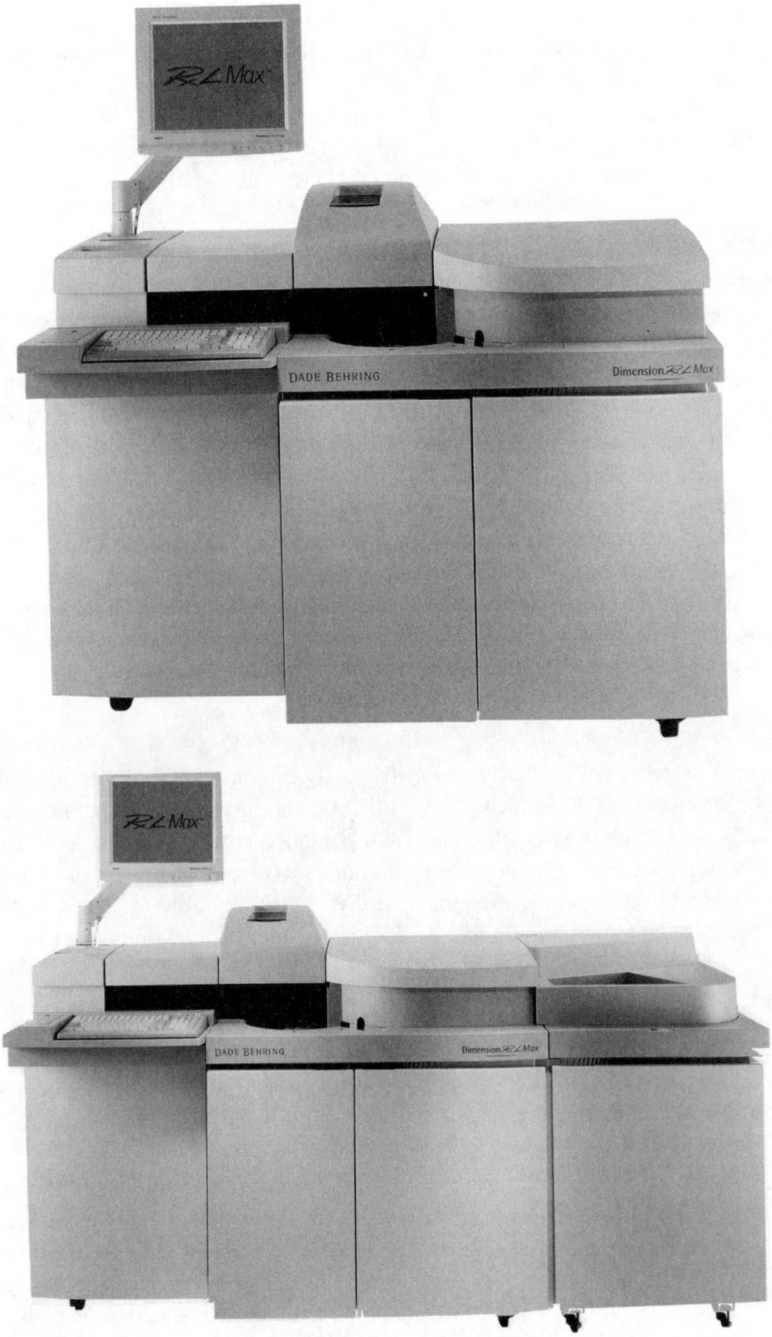

FIGURE 4. RxL Max. (*Courtesy of Dade Behring Inc.*)

VITROS 950

The VITROS 950 (Johnson and Johnson) is one of the families of analyzers originally developed by the Kodak Company. The analyzer is based on a dry-slide technology that includes potentiometric, colorimetric (reflectance), and immuno rate analyses. While the

VITROS 950 has an extensive chemistry menu, its immunoassay capability is quite limited. The dry-slide technology reduces analytical interferences and requires very small sample sizes, but it does not adapt well to immunoassays. The immunoassay test menu is limited to a small number of TDMs and C-reactive protein (CRP). The instrument performs up to 900 tests per hour and is complimented by the VITROS ECI system described later. The VITROS system lacks a complete menu of TDMs and had no capability for DAUs.

Beckman Synchron Systems

The Synchron systems are primarily chemistry analyzers on which homogeneous assays such as the EMIT and CEDIA have been adapted. In addition, Beckman–Coulter developed its own immunoassay for many TDMs and DAUs. The instruments are available in two series: the CX series and the LX series. The LX was designed for the high-volume laboratory while the CX series meets the needs of low- to mid-volume laboratories. Immunoassay test menus include specific proteins such as highly sensitive CRP, apolipoproteins, pancreatic amylase, DAUs, and TDMs. The LX 20 PRO includes the near-infrared particle immunoassay detection system. The LX 2000 PRO combines the LX 20 or LX 20 PRO with the Access 2. The LXi 725 system combines homogeneous and heterogeneous immunoassay with chemistry testing, including many assays from the Access 2 menu. It is the only system to perform heterogeneous immunoassays with general chemistry on a single platform using closed tube sampling. However, currently no systems are operating in the United States according to *CAP Today*.

Olympus Systems

The Olympus systems are primarily chemistry analyzers designed as open systems. They range in size from the AU 400 which can perform 400 photometric assays per hour to the AU 5400 which can do 5400 photometric and 1800 potentiometric assays per hour. They have the ability to run a variety of homogeneous immunoassays and as a result offer a complete menu of TDMs, DAUs, specific proteins, and thyroid testing. To complete a test menu, a clinical chemistry laboratory would require additional stand-alone immunoassay analyzers.

STAND-ALONE IMMUNOASSAY ANALYZERS

Many instrumentation platforms currently are available that perform only immunoassays. These instruments have more extensive menus than instruments with combined chemistry/immunoassay capabilities and often have superior throughput. Adding immunoassay to a chemistry analyzer often reduces its ability to process samples quickly. The ideal instrument would be one that performs all of the necessary assays on one platform. At the present time, none of the analyzers described here provides a comprehensive menu of robust assays on a fully automated platform capable of serving the entire immunoassay needs of the clinical laboratory. Some assays may not be performed satisfactorily on one instrument or some assays may not be available on another instrument, thus requiring two or more of the available platforms to complete the required menu. The instruments described include the most widely used systems. This chapter is not intended to be a complete and comprehensive listing of all available immunoassay analyzers.

Abbott AxSYM

The Abbott AxSYM (Figure 5) was introduced in 1993 and was one of the earliest random access immunoassay analyzers. It was the next step beyond the TDx and IMx systems and

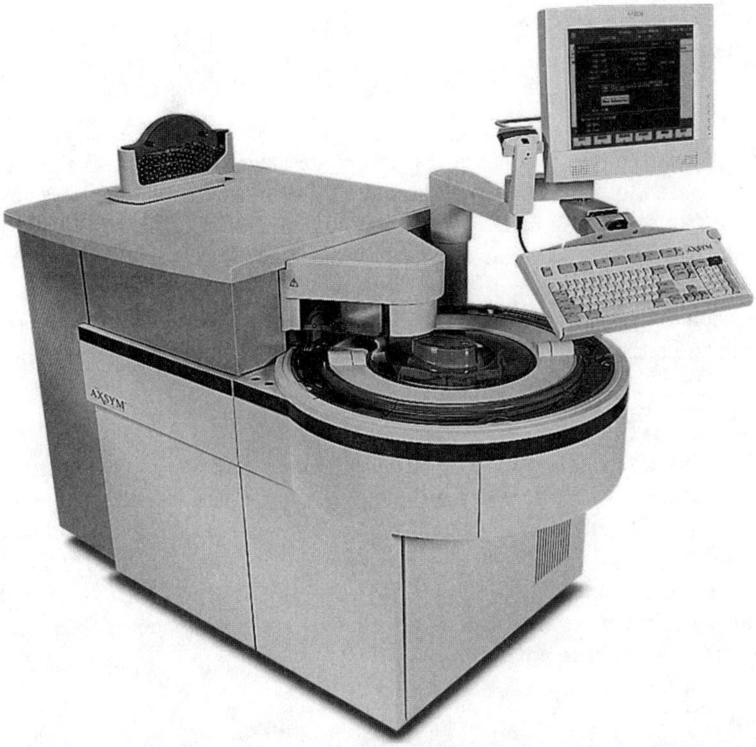

FIGURE 5. The Abbott Axsym. (*Courtesy of Abbott Laboratories*)

utilized the methods from those two systems including FPIA and MEIA. The MEIA technology is based on analytes binding to microparticles coated with antibody (capture antibody) to the analyte, creating an immune complex. The instrument transfers an aliquot of the immune complex to an inert glass fiber matrix in the reaction cell. The immune complex then binds to the glass fiber matrix. The matrix is washed to remove unbound materials and the immune complex is retained by the glass matrix. Alkaline-phosphatase-labeled conjugate is added to the matrix and the conjugate binds to the unbound antibody. After another wash cycle, fluorogenic phosphate substrate is added. The conjugate removes the phosphate, allowing the fluorogenic substrate to fluoresce. The rate of fluorescent product generation is a function of analyte concentraton in the test sample. It is a floor-standing system with a capacity of 80–120 tests per hour. It has an extensive list of assays including DAUs, TDMs, thyroids, fertility tests, cardiac markers, and serology tests. An extensive battery of hepatitis testing has recently been submitted to the FDA for approval.

Abbott ARCHITECT

The ARCHITECT system is Abbott's third generation immunoassay system and was released in 1999. It was designed as a modular system using chemiluminescence detection and magnetic microparticles. The base module is the i2000. It can be combined with another i2000 to form the i4000 or with the c8000 chemistry module to form the ci8200. Throughput of 200 tests per hour is possible with the i2000 and up to 400 tests per hour with i4000. Currently, the test menu in the United States is somewhat limited and has not expanded in the last three years. Thus, the ARCHITECT has had limited sales and has not displaced the AxSYM.

Bayer ACS 180 ADVIA Centaur

The ACS 180 was the first random access immunoassay instrument in the United States. It was also the first to use chemiluminescence detection and magnetic microparticles for separation of free and bound marker. The current version is the ACS 180 SE; it is capable of running up to 180 tests per hour. The ADVIA Centaur (Figure 6) is a more robust floor-standing model that can perform up to 240 tests per hour. Both instruments have extensive test menus including B-natriuretic peptide (BNP). There are more than 700 Centaur placements in the United States.

Beckman Immage

The Beckman Immage is intended to replace the Array for the analysis of specific proteins. The Immage employs new technology for light-scattering measurements in addition to rate nephelometry. Specific proteins or rate nephelometry is used. Rate inhibition nephelometry is used for therapeutic drugs. Near-infrared particle immunoassay (NIPIA) is used for high-sensitivity assays and rate inhibition NIPIA is used for low molecular weight therapeutic drugs. Beckman–Coulter has a proven track record in the analysis of specific proteins with nephelometric measurements.

Beckman Access

The Beckman Access was developed by Sanofi in Europe. Sanofi began selling the instrument in the United States in the mid-1990s. Beckman–Coulter acquired the instrument and its technology to establish a presence in the heterogeneous immunoassay market. The

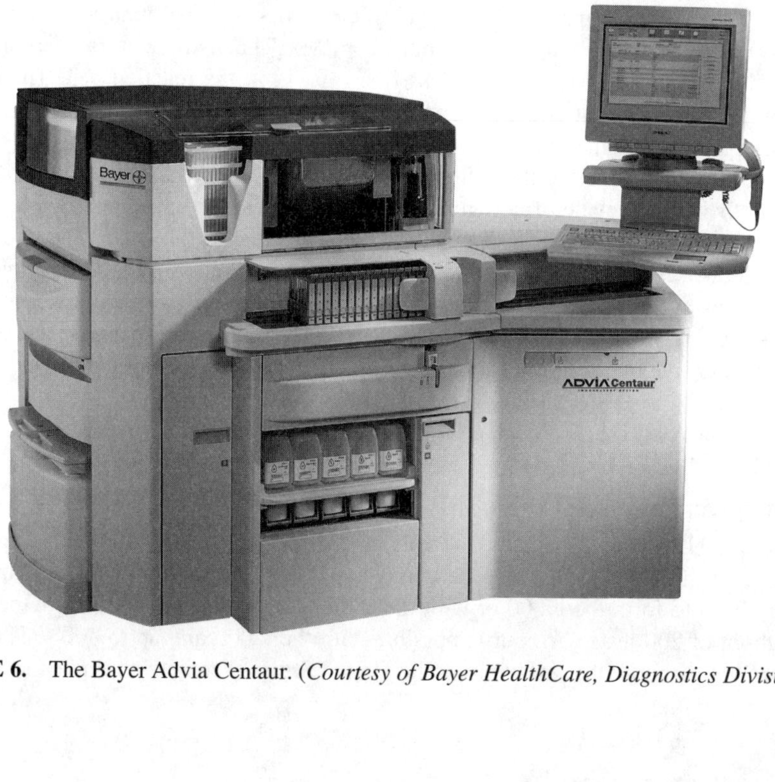

FIGURE 6. The Bayer Advia Centaur. (*Courtesy of Bayer HealthCare, Diagnostics Division*)

Access is a bench-top instrument and uses chemiluminescence detection with magnetic particles. The current version, the Access 2, analyzes up to 100 tests per hour. The instrument has a comprehensive menu of immunoassay tests. Beckman–Coulter introduced the UniCel DxI 800 system which is a high throughput floor-standing immunoassay analyzer and uses the same technology as Access. It has a maximum throughput of 400 tests per hour and, excluding chlamydia, has the same test menu as Access.

Dade Behring BN II

The BN II was developed by the Behring Corporation which was acquired by Dade. The BN II is based on light-scattering measurements using laser nephelometry and is an alternative to the Immage system for nonlabeled immunoassay. The BN II has some unique applications for nutritional assessment including retinol-binding protein and an assay for transferrin receptor which may be an effective anemia marker.

Diagnostic Products Corporation Immunolite Systems

The Immunolite system comes in several versions: Immunolite, Immunolite 1000, and Immunolite 2000. The Immunolite and Immunolite 1000 are bench-top models while the Immunolite 2000 is a floor-standing model. Immunolite and Immunolite 1000 are available with Turbo assays for cardiac markers, intact parathyroid hormone (PTH), and hcG. Turbo assays require special software and allow the user to obtain the first result for those assays in 15 minutes. The Immunolite and Immunolite 1000 systems can have 12 reagents on board at any one time and can process up to 120 tests per hour. The Immunolite 1000 and 2000 integrate the computer into the body of the analyzer while the Immunolite has a separate unit. The Immunolite 2000 has 24 tests in residence at any one time and processes up to 200 tests per hour. The test menus for both systems are extensive and for the most part identical. The Immunolite and Immunolite 1000 have a food allergy panel that is not available on the Immunolite 2000. The Immunolite systems have one of the largest test menus of any immunoassay analyzer and include several assays that were previously available only in an RIA format, e.g, androstenedione, DHEA –sulfate, and estriol. Both instruments utilize chemiluminescence detection using bead technology. Separation is done using a high-speed centrifuge to expel the wash solution.

Roche Elecsys

The Roche Elecsys system is available in two versions, the 1010 and 2010. Both are bench-top analyzers, but there are differences in performance. The 2010 performs up to 88 tests per hour and has 15 on-board tests, while the 1010 performs up to 55 tests per hour and has only six on-board tests. The Elecsys systems produces an hcG result in 9 minutes which is the best turnaround time of any currently available analyzer. The Elecsys systems are also the only analyzers with a troponin T assay. The Elecsys systems use electrochemiluminescence for detection with magnetic particle separation. Electrochemiluminescence enhances the sensitivity of the chemiluminescent compound by controlling the time delay of light emission until events such as immune or catalyzed reactions have taken place.

VITROS ECI

The VITROS ECI from Ortho Clinical Diagnostics is a floor-standing instrument which utilizes enhanced chemiluminescence with individually coated microwells. It has an extensive menu, including a significant number of hepatitis markers and a bone marker. Many new serological makers are under development. It processes 90 samples per hour. The combination of the VITROS 950 and the VITROS ECI covers many immunoassays. The notable deficiency of the VITROS systems is the lack of DAUs. The ECI has reagents for 20 assays on board at any one time.

IMMUNOASSAY SYSTEMS LINKED TO CHEMISTRY SYSTEMS THROUGH A COMMON SAMPLER AND OPERATOR INTERFACE

ARCHITECT ci8200

The ARCHITECT ci8200 (Figure 7) combines the ARCHITECT c8000 chemistry module with the i2000 immunoassay module through a unique retest sample handler that uses multidimensional sample handling. It produces 1200 chemistry results and 200 immunoassay results per hour. The current immunoassay test menu is limited; however, Abbott is aggressively pursuing FDA approval for more assays. The instrument was introduced in the U.S. market only recently and only a few have been placed. The immunoassay module, like the ARCHITECT 2000, is based on chemiluminescence with magnetic particles. The unique sample-handling system allows the two systems to act independently because samples can be placed on either module and tests can be done in any order, depending on priority. The ci8200 has the potential to integrate clinical chemistry with immunoassay, once its test menu is expanded.

Roche MODULAR

The Roche MODULAR system (Figure 8) uses several different types of modules connected with a common sampler. The D modules are used for high-volume chemistry, the P

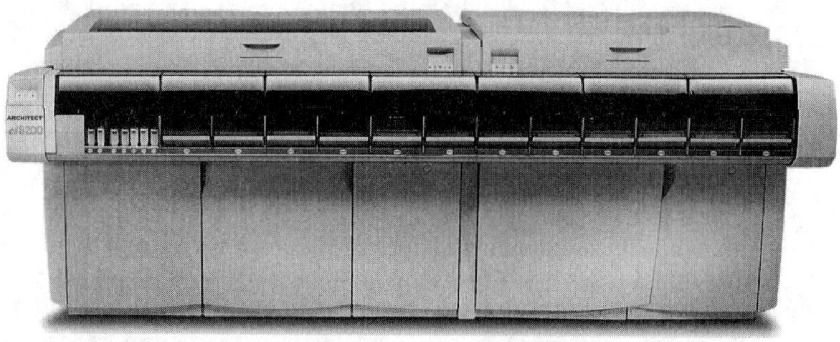

FIGURE 7. Abbott Architeck modular system. (*Courtesy of Abbott Laboratories*)

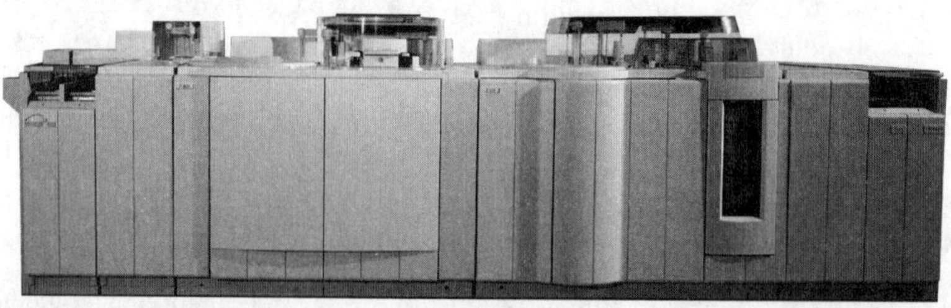

FIGURE 8. Roche Modular System with D, P, and E module. [*Courtesy of Roche Diagnostics Corporation. MODULAR (and design) is a trademark of a Member of the Roche Group*]

modules are used for low- to medium-volume chemistry and homogeneous immunoassay, and the E modules are used for heterogeneous immunoassay. The E module, known as the E170, mimics the test menu of the Elecsys system, but it is a floor-standing system that is integrated with the other modules through a three-way track on the back of the different modules. The E module performs up to 176 tests per hour.

Other Immunoassay Analyzers

Several other instruments should be mentioned. The **Vidas systems** from bioMerieux Inc have 1500 placements in the United States and more than 15,000 worldwide. Its test menu is more oriented toward serology. The Tosoh Bioscience AIA-600 enjoys some popularity. It can run 60 tests per hour and its menu includes the most common immunoassays. The reader is advised to check the manufacturers' web sites for more information.

AUTOMATED MICROTITER PLATE SYSTEMS

Luminex Systems

Luminex Corporation has developed a technique called xMAP technology for multiplexing. It can report up to 100 different analyte results from a single well on a microtiter plate. To put it another way, up to 100 different assays are available from a single drop of sample. The system starts with polystyrene microspheres internally dyed with red and infrared fluorophores. Different ratios of the two dyes allow for 100 xMAP microsphere sets and include cytokines, autoimmune, and kinases. The surface chemistry on the microspheres allows chemical coupling of capture molecules, such as oligonucleotides, peptides, antibodies, and receptors. The assays are carried out in a 96-well plate format with up to 100 assays per well. The reactions are read on an instrument such as the Luminex 100. A stream of suspended particles passes through a detection chamber. As a microsphere passes through the detection chamber, a red laser excites both the internal red and infrared dyes, allowing the proper classification of the microsphere to one of the 100 sets. A green laser excites any orange fluorescence associated with the binding of the desired analyte. Classification and reporter readings are made on each individual particle, allowing the Luminex 100 to determine precisely multiplexed assay results. The use of the microspheres allows three-dimensional exposure for reactions as compared to the single dimension of the well surface in conventional microtiter plates.

Applications include DNA, immunoassay, receptor ligand assays, and enzyme assays. The technology is useful for drug discovery, autoimmune assays, cytokines and chemokines, allergy screening, and pharmacogenetics. Luminex developed an extensive partner network for applications to the xMAP technology. This is a technology that readers with an interest in immunology and molecular biology will want to follow.

Other Automated Microtiter Plate Readers

While microtiter plate technology does not have the advantages of highly automated immunoassay analyzers, the technology has been improved in recent years as seen from the Luminex example. Microtiter plate technology has become much more automated in recent years and has integrated all of the steps onto a single platform. The Binding Site (San Diego) offers a full range of autoimmune and infectious disease ELISA kits with a fully automated four plate ELISA system. Trinity Biotech offers a fully automated microtiter plate system that is a completely open system. The fact that most microtiter systems are open systems gives them a significant advantage over most closed automated immunoassay systems (manufacturers' reagents only). It will be important for laboratorians to keep abreast of both technologies to ensure the highest efficiency for their laboratories.

REFERENCES

1. Yalow RS, Berson SA. Immunoassay of endogenous plasma insulin in man. J Clin Invest 1960;39:1157–75.
2. Buffone GJ, Savory J, Cross RE, et al. Evaluation of kinetic light scattering as an approach to the measurement of specific proteins with the centrifugal analyzer. I. Methodology. Clin Chem 1975; 21:1731–4.
3. Engual E, Perlman P. Enzyme linked immunosorbant assay (ELISA) quantitative assay of immunoglobulin G. Immunoassay 1971;8:871–4.
4. Rubenstein KE, Schneider RS, Ullman EF. Homogeneous enzyme immunoassay. A new immunochemical technique. Biochem Biophys Res Commun 1972;47:846–51.
5. Henderson DR, Friedman SB, Harris JB. CEDIA, a new homogeneous immunoassay system. Clin Chem 1986;32:1637–41.
6. Guo X-Q, Castellano FN, Li L, et al. A long-lifetime Ru(II) metal-ligand complex as a membrane probe. Biophys Chem 1998;71:51–6.
7. Reddington MV. New glycoconjugated cyanine dyes as fluorescent labeling reagents. J Chem Soc Perkin Trans 1998;1:143–8.
8. Jolley ME, Stroupe SD, Wang CJ. Fluorescence polarization immunoassay. I. Monitoring aminoglycoside antibodies in serum and plasma. Clin Chem 1981;27:1190–7.
9. Proceedings from the 11th annual Oak Ridge Conference; Section 3, Luminescence. Clin Chem 1979;25:1622–61.

SELECTED READING

Clinical chemistry, laboratory management and clinical correlations. Lewandrowski K, ed. Philadelphia: Lippincott Williams and Wilkins, 2002: chapter 15, integrated automation in the clinical laboratory; chapter 16, development of laboratory instrument platforms; chapter 23, the role of the diagnostics industry in the clinical laboratory; chapter 25, contemporary instruments in the clinical laboratory: a brief overview; chapter 28, an introduction to clinical laboratory immunodiagnostics: a perspective from the diagnostics industry; and chapter 29, immunoassay and immunoassay analyzers: a perspective from the clinical laboratory.

Clinical chemistry, theory, analysis, correlation, 4th ed. Kaplan LA, Pesce AJ, Kazmierczak S, eds, St Louis: Mosby, 2003; chapter 11, immunological reactions; chapter 12, immunochemical techniques; chapter 13, principles of competitive binding; and chapter 16, laboratory automation.

Chapter 7

Immunochemical Methods in Clinical Chemistry

William Clarke and Daniel W. Chan

Immunochemical methods can be defined as analytical methods that are based on the use of antibodies as reagents. The highly specific binding and large association constants (K_a) of antibodies make them useful for detection and quantitation of analytes in complex sample matrices such as body fluids. Methods based on immunochemical reactions are some of the most sensitive and specific assays available to laboratorians. Many immunochemical methods have been automated and are widely used in the clinical laboratory (1, 2).

SOME BASICS

Antibodies belong to a group of glycoproteins called immunoglobulins that demonstrate highly specific binding to both natural and synthetic analytes, also called **antigens**. The antibody-binding site on the antigen is known as the **epitope**; each antigen may have multiple epitopes, depending on its size and shape. Antibodies can be classified as either polyclonal or monoclonal. The term **polyclonal antibodies** refers to a group of antibodies derived from multiple cell lines that are all specific for the same antigen but bind to different epitopes on that antigen. **Monoclonal antibodies** are derived from a single cell line and are more specific in that they are not only directed toward a certain antigen but also a specific epitope on that antigen.

The five different types of immunoglobulins are characterized by their function and they are abbreviated as IgA, IgD, IgE, IgG, and IgM; only IgG is used for immunochemical analysis. Immunoglobulin G is a glycoprotein composed of multiple subunits with a molecular weight of approximately 160 kD. IgG consists of two identical heavy chains and two identical light chains that are joined by disulfide bonds (*see* Figure 1). The amino acid sequence at the carboxyl terminus is conserved regardless of the antibody specificity and is known as the constant region of the antibody. However, the amino acid sequence at the amino terminus is highly variable and is the portion that confers antigenic specificity to the antibody. The classic "Y" shape of the antibody gives it a single constant region with two variable regions that allow one antibody to bind two antigens, barring steric interference.

Antibody structure can be further characterized with respect to how it is cleaved by proteolytic enzymes. The enzyme papain cleaves IgG in the hinge region and divides the antibody into three sections (*see* Figure 1). The constant region, or "stem" of the Y, is one

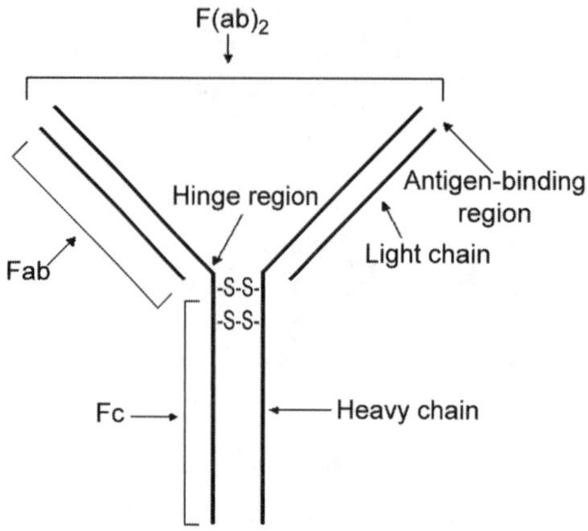

FIGURE 1. Basic antibody structure.

fragment and is known as the Fc fragment that has no antigen-binding properties. The remaining two fragments are the "arms" of the Y and are identical antigen-binding fragments known as Fab fragments that have one binding site each. Alternatively, pepsin can be used to digest antibodies, yielding a different fragmentation pattern. No Fc fragment is produced in this digestion because the constant region of IgG is digested completely. The fragment that remains after digestion consists of both binding sites and is known as an $F(ab)_2$ fragment (*see* Figure 1).

Antibodies are produced by the immune system when an **immunogen** is introduced into a foreign host. An immunogen can be a protein or sometimes an analyte of interest coupled to a large carrier molecule. In order for a substance to be immunogenic, it must possess randomness of structure while maintaining some areas of structural stability. In addition, it must have a molecular weight of at least 4–5 kD and be recognized as foreign by the host animal. An analyte/antigen that is unable to induce an immunogenic response on its own is called a **hapten** and must be coupled with a large carrier to stimulate a response.

Antiserum is the product of immunogenic stimulation that contains antibodies directed toward the antigen of interest. Polyclonal antiserum is derived by simple introduction of an immunogen to a normal animal host. This produces a heterogeneous mixture of antibodies from many cell clones directed against a wide variety of epitopes on the antigen of interest. The antibodies can then be isolated by using a chromatographic support containing immobilized antigen or immobilized protein A or protein G. Protein A and protein G are bacterial cell wall proteins that display a site-specific affinity for the Fc region of IgG and isolate all IgG molecules regardless of specificity. Use of immobilized antigen allows the isolation of only IgG that is specific for the analyte of interest.

Monoclonal antiserum is the product of a single clone or plasma cell line, so all the antibodies produced are identical and bind to the same epitope. The special technique for producing monoclonal antibodies begins by immunizing a host animal (usually mice) just as in polyclonal antibody production. Then sensitized lymphocytes from the spleen of the immunized animal are fused with an isolated murine myeloma cell line, which consists of immortalized B-cells. The myeloma cell line is deficient in the enzyme hypoxanthine guanine phosphoribosyl transferase (HGPRT), meaning they cannot synthesize purine bases from thymidine and hypoxanthine in the presence of aminopterin. The spleen cells, however, are not deficient in the enzyme so when the fusion mixture is cultured in a selective medium containing hypoxanthine, aminopterin, and thymidine (known as HAT medium), only the fused cells survive. The surviving cell lines are screened for binding to the antigen of interest, with the end product being immortal cell lines that produce antibodies of a single, known binding specificity.

Antibody–antigen binding can be described in terms of binding affinity and avidity. **Affinity** refers to the strength of binding for one site and can be described in terms of the energy of interaction for a single antibody-binding site and its corresponding epitope. **Avidity** refers to the overall binding of one antibody molecule to antigen, describing the sum of binding sites for the whole molecule (e.g., IgG has two binding sites while the IgM pentamer has 10 binding sites). For example, when comparing an IgG molecule versus an Fab obtained from the same clonal population, they would have identical affinities for the antigen of interest, but the IgG would have a higher avidity because it could bind two antigens and the Fab could only bind one. On the whole, affinity is characterized as a property of the antigen, while avidity is a property of the antibody.

Binding between an antibody and antigen is best described as an equilibrium process:

$$\mathrm{Ag} + \mathrm{Ab} <=======> \mathrm{AgAb}$$

where $k_1 >>> k_{-1}$; so, depending on the time frame of the experiment, the binding can sometimes be considered irreversible. These interactions are based on electrostatic (van der Waals) forces, hydrophobic forces, coulombic (ionic) forces, or a combination of the three. Antibody–antigen binding is pH and temperature dependent and can be affected by electrolyte concentration as well, depending on which types of interactions are prominent in binding. Cationic salts inhibit antibody binding with cationic haptens corresponding to decreasing ionic radius and increasing radius of hydration: $Cs^+ > Rb^+ > NH_4^+ > K^+ > Na^+ > Li^+$. The same effect is seen with anionic haptens and anionic salts: $CNS^- > NO_3^- > I^- > Br^- > Cl^- > F^-$.

If there is significant cross-linking of antigens during antigen–antibody binding, then precipitation can occur, but this is highly concentration dependent. If the number of antibody sites is much higher than antigen-binding sites, then the antigen-binding sites are quickly saturated and 1 : 1 complexes of antibody and antigen predominate. Alternatively, if the number of antibody-binding sites is limited with an excess of antigen binding sites, then the antibody sites are quickly saturated, 2 : 1 complexes of antigen to antibody predominate, and cross-linking does not occur. However, if the antibody is in moderate excess (two- to three-fold), then cross-linkage is more likely and large complexes can be formed that will precipitate; this is called the **precipitin reaction**. Addition of a linear polymer such as dextran, polyvinyl alcohol (PVA), or polyethylene glycol (PEG) will increase the rate of immune complex growth and enhance precipitation of the immune complex. Important characteristics of polymers used for this purpose are high molecular weight, minimal branching, and a high aqueous solubility.

QUALITATIVE METHODS

Gel Diffusion

Diffusion analyses are carried out in an agarose gel or agar to stabilize the diffusion process and minimize interferences derived from mixing by outside sources (e.g., convection, vibration, evaporation). The precipitin reaction occurs in solid gel matrices the same way it happens in the liquid phase. The same factors that influence liquid-phase immunoprecipitation including temperature, antibody–antigen ratio, salt concentration, and polymer enhancement demonstrate their effects in gel analyses as well. Another advantage of gel diffusion analysis is that the precipitate is trapped within the solid matrix, allowing convenient visualization of results for either quantitative or qualitative analysis.

Provided that the gel matrix is inert with respect to the analyte of interest, diffusion in the matrix is described by **Fick's equation**:

$$dQ/dt = -DA(dC/dx)$$

where dQ/dt = amount of analyte diffusing through area (A) over a fixed amount of time
dC/dx = concentration gradient
D = diffusion coefficient

The diffusion coefficient is directly proportional to the temperature of the analysis and inversely proportional to the hydrated radius of the analyte. Larger species migrate more slowly due to an increasing frictional coefficient, which decreases the diffusion coefficient and thus the diffusion rate. Increasing the temperature can increase the diffusion rate by increasing the rate of mass transfer, which increases the diffusion coefficient.

The success of gel diffusion analyses is dependent on the ability of the analyte and its corresponding antibody to form a precipitin line within the gel. In this technique, the initial concentration of antibody and antigen are of paramount importance as they help to determine the extent of distribution of analyte over a fixed time, which controls how quickly the precipitin line forms and at what distance from the application point. In **single immunodiffusion**, a concentration gradient is established only for one of the reactants (usually the antigen). The antigen is introduced into an antibody-impregnated agar and diffusion occurs until the precipitin line is formed.

Alternatively, a concentration gradient can be established for both antigen and antibody in a technique called **double immunodiffusion**. This approach is widespread in clinical laboratories and commonly known as the **Ouchterlony technique**. This method permits the direct comparison of two or more test materials and can determine whether the antigens in test specimens are identical, cross-reactive, or nonidentical. The antigens in question are placed in separate wells equidistant from a well containing the corresponding antibody. If the same antigen is present in adjacent wells, a continuous precipitin line forms (Figure 2A). If the test wells contain the same antigen in addition to different ones, then a partial identity line is formed (Figure 2B); and if the wells contain different antigens altogether, then two crossing precipitin lines—known as nonidentity—are formed (Figure 2C). This format can be used to test samples with several components because multiple bands are able to form due to differing diffusion rates for the components. It should be noted that this technique does not necessarily prove molecular identity, since it is possible that different antigens may share the same epitope.

Immunoelectrophoresis

Immunoelectrophoresis (IEP) is a technique used for both separation and identification of protein species in a solution such as serum, urine, or spinal fluid. IEP is accomplished in two distinct steps: separation and immunoprecipitation. The separation of proteins is achieved by gel electrophoresis. The second stage involves introduction of antiserum to the protein of interest in a trough that is parallel and adjacent to the separation lane. As both the antigen and antibodies diffuse in the gel, precipitin lines are formed in the gel next

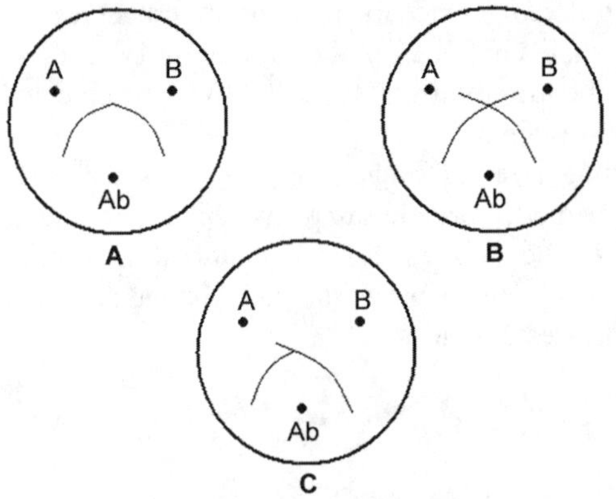

FIGURE 2. Immunodiffusion using Ouchterlony plates. A: identity reaction, B: non-identity reaction, and C: partial identity reaction.

to the analyte of interest. This technique is particularly useful in the characterization of human gammopathies and human myeloma proteins.

Alternative methods based on variations of IEP have been introduced that eliminate the diffusion step altogether. In **crossed immunoelectrophoresis** (CRIE), also known as **two-dimensional immunoelectrophoresis** (3), the separation is carried out as in IEP; but rather than allow diffusion to run its course, electrophoresis is performed in the perpendicular direction to drive the antibodies to the antigen and form a precipitin line. This produces a higher resolution for CRIE than possible with IEP, making it a more sensitive and rapid technique. **Counter immunoelectrophoresis** (CIE) is another variation of IEP used in clinical laboratories. In CIE, two parallel rows of wells are punched in the agar or gel; one row is filled with antigen solution, and the opposite row is filled with antibody solution. Constant voltage is applied across the gel to speed the migration of antibody and antigen toward each other to form the precipitin line. Using this technique, qualitative identification data useful for the detection of bacterial antigens in body fluids can be obtained in about 2 hours.

Immunofixation (IF) is another variation of IEP that has found widespread use in many laboratories (4). In this technique, electrophoresis is performed on an agarose gel to separate proteins in the sample. However, in this method antiserum is spread directly on the gel, causing the proteins of interest to precipitate and become trapped in the gel. The gel is then washed to remove any nonreactive proteins, followed by staining for visualization of the remaining proteins. In comparison, CRIE is a more sensitive technique than IF with the ability to detect closely related proteins with similar electrophoretic mobilities, but it is more labor intensive as well. The ease of use for IF is generally thought to offset any deficiencies in resolution, and it is used widely for the characterization of myeloma proteins.

Western Blotting

Western blotting is an alternative to immunoprecipitation when circumstances prevent that method of analysis. In some cases the concentration of antigen is low enough that a precipitin band cannot be formed, or separation must be carried out in polyacrylamide gel, which does not work well with immunoprecipitation. In this technique, electrophoresis is carried out to separate proteins, and then the separated bands are transferred to a nitrocellulose or nylon membrane by **electroblotting**. Once the proteins are transferred to the membrane, they can be detected using labeled antibody probes. By using isotope- or enzyme-labeled probes, detection limits can be lowered from 10 to 100 times when compared to direct immunoprecipitation or protein staining.

A simpler alternative to Western blotting is a technique that eliminates the electrophoresis step called **dot blotting**. In this method, a protein sample is applied, or dotted, to a membrane surface and dried. After drying the membrane, labeled antibodies specific for the antigen of interest are applied to the membrane. After washing, the bound antibody labels are detected in the same manner as the Western blot.

QUANTITATIVE METHODS

Radial Diffusion

Radial immunodiffusion (RID) is a quantitative technique based on passive diffusion. A concentration gradient is established for one reactant, usually the antigen, while the other reactant is dispersed uniformly throughout the gel (5). A well is formed in the gel where antigen is introduced and allowed to diffuse into the gel. Diffusion occurs until there is an excess of antibody with respect to antigen and a precipitin ring is formed. The ring diameter increases until the precipitin reaction reaches equilibrium. Calibrators are run along with the sample and the ring diameter plotted versus concentration to generate a calibration curve.

Rocket Immunoelectrophoresis (Electroimmunoassay)

Rocket immunoelectrophoresis, also known as an **electroimmunoassay**, uses an applied voltage to establish an antigen concentration gradient rather than passive diffusion (6). As with other immunoprecipitation techniques, the gradient is established in a gel containing a homogeneous suspension of antibody directed toward the antigen of interest. Electrophoresis results in a unidirectional migration of antigen that forms a "rocket" shaped precipitin line, with the height of the line proportional to initial antigen concentration. Quantitation is achieved using a set of calibrators run simultaneously with the unknown samples. One limitation of this technique is that the calibration curve is linear only over a narrow concentration range, so samples may have to be concentrated or diluted to fall within the linear range of the assay. In addition, the unidirectional migration results in decreased limits of detection for this technique.

Turbidimetry and Nephelometry

Turbidimetry and nephelometry are techniques used to measure the formation of immune complexes in solution. Turbidimetry measures light scatter based on a decrease in incident light intensity (I_s/I_0) due to formation of precipitin antibody–antigen complexes and is analogous to absorbance measurements. This is a straight-on measurement, with the detector in-line with the light source and sample container, and is useful when the concentration of antibody–antigen complex is relatively high and background interference from incident light is not a concern. Nephelometry measures light scatter from precipitin complexes directly by placing the detector at an angle from the sample and incident light so that background interference is minimized in a manner similar to fluorescence spectrometry. Less interference from the light source makes nephelometry a more sensitive technique, useful at lower analyte concentrations.

These techniques can be used quantitatively in both rate, or kinetic, assays and equilibrium-type assays. The antibody–antigen precipitin reaction begins within milliseconds after mixing and can continue for hours until it reaches equilibrium. Precipitation can be enhanced in both types of assays by the addition of water-soluble polymers. In rate-based assays, the change in intensity of scattered light (dI_s/dt) is measured in relation to calibrator concentration or unknown sample. This measurement is usually made early in the reaction because this is where the greatest change in intensity takes place. In theory, equilibrium assays are performed by allowing the reaction to reach equilibrium and measuring the total precipitate formed. In practice, however, this would take far too long to be practical, so pseudoequilibrium assays are performed by waiting for a fixed amount of time (30–60 minutes) until the rate of change in light scatter is small in relation to the time necessary to make the measurement.

Nephelometric methods are generally more sensitive than techniques based on turbidity measurements, with lower detection limits around 10–50 mg/L for proteins in serum. When body fluids such as CSF and urine are analyzed, even lower limits of detection are possible due to the lack of interference from lipid or protein content. In the case of lower molecular weight proteins, the limit of detection can be lowered further by using antibody-coated latex beads. Light-scattering immunoprecipitation techniques have also been adapted to measure small molecules in a competitive binding format. In this approach, the competition is between protein-labeled antigen, which has the ability to form immunoprecipitation complexes, and free antigen in the sample. If the analyte concentration is high, the antibody sites are saturated and immunoprecipitation complexes are not formed. This approach is compatible with both rate based and equilibrium assay formats. Light scattering is measured and plotted versus antigen concentration to produce a calibration curve, demonstrating an inversely proportional relationship.

Immunoassays

Immunoassays comprise the group of immunochemical methods that are most widely used in clinical diagnostics. By using chemical labels coupled to antibodies or antigens, much lower concentrations of analyte can be detected in samples without forming an immunoprecipitation complex. These assays can be performed in many different formats with a wide variety of detection methods and can be used to detect both large and small analytes. Immunoassays can be characterized with regard to whether a separation step is necessary, on the basis of whether the antigen or antibody is labeled, or by the type of label that is used for sample detection.

Homogeneous versus Heterogeneous Immunoassays

Heterogeneous immunoassays are assays that require physical separation of bound and free labels for analysis (7). During separations, heterogeneous assays assume that antibody–antigen binding is essentially irreversible during the separation step since k_1 is much greater than k_{-1} (the amount that dissociates is very small). One method of separation is to remove labeled antigen–antibody complex from solution by precipitation, either using a precipitating chemical or cross-linking with other antibodies and then reconstituting the precipitate to quantify the amount of bound label. In addition, adsorbents such as activated charcoal or other small particles can be added to solution to bind free antigen and then remove it by centrifugation. Another approach is to attach the antibodies to a solid support such as the interior of a microwell plate or magnetic beads and then remove the unbound molecules through various wash steps. Traditional separation techniques such as size-exclusion or ion-exchange chromatography as well as electrophoresis can also be used for heterogeneous immunoassays.

Homogeneous immunoassays are those that have the ability to distinguish between the free and bound label for detection without a physical separation step (7). This is accomplished by selecting a label that is modified by antibody binding, whether it results in an increase or decrease of signal. For this format to be useful, it is important that the change in signal due to antibody binding is proportional to the concentration of analyte under investigation. This technique allows a combination of the label incubation and detection of analyte into one simple step. This approach is useful because it eliminates the wash step and is very compatible with most automated chemistry analyzers.

Competitive Binding Immunoassays

Competitive binding immunoassays are based on immunochemical reactions in which the number of antigen-binding sites on the antibody is limited. Both the antigen of interest and a labeled analog are incubated with a known amount of the appropriate antibody and the signal produced is based on the competition between the analyte and corresponding label for the antibody binding sites (8). The amount of labeled antigen bound to the antibody is inversely proportional to the amount of analyte in the sample and can produce a calibration curve as seen in Figure 3A.

The most common approaches to a competitive binding immunoassay are the simultaneous or sequential addition techniques. In **simultaneous addition**, both the label and sample (or calibrator) are added to the reaction mixture at the same time. After a fixed period of time, the amount of bound label is determined and used to construct a calibration curve or determine the concentration of the unknown. For this method to be useful, the antibody should demonstrate the same binding affinity for both the sample antigen and the calibrator antigen. In addition, it is important for this approach that the probability of binding for both the labeled antigen and the sample antigen are similar. **Sequential addition** is a technique that proves to be of value when a lower limit of detection is needed; first the sample is incubated with the antibody to equilibrium, then the label is added and comes to equilibrium, followed by the detection of bound label. This sequential approach can lower the limit of detection up to fivefold and is also useful if there are slight differences in avidity for the analyte antigen and the labeled analog.

An alternative approach to the competitive binding immunoassay is the **displacement immunoassay**. In this technique, the antibody is saturated with labeled analog followed

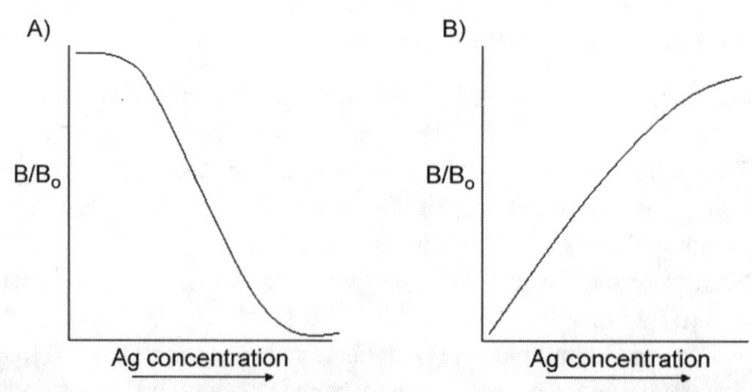

FIGURE 3. Immunoassay calibration curves. A: competitive binding assay; B: non-competitive binding assay.

by addition of sample. The analyte in the sample displaces the label and, contrary to other approaches, the displaced label is measured rather than bound label. This type of assay is dependent on local equilibria, so if $k_1 >> k_{-1}$, then less label is displaced in contrast to the situation where $k_1 \geq k_{-1}$. The signal for displacement immunoassays is directly proportional to the analyte concentration (Figure 3B), in contrast to the inversely proportional signals seen in the simultaneous and sequential addition immunoassays.

Noncompetitive (Immunometric) Immunoassays

Noncompetitive binding immunoassays, or immunometric assays, are based on immunochemical reaction where there is an excess of antigen-binding sites (8). In noncompetitive immunoassays, the signal is directly proportional to the amount of analyte in the sample producing a similar curve to that obtained with a displacement immunoassay (Figure 3B). The most common noncompetitive immunoassay format is the **sandwich immunoassay**, where two antibodies are used for analyte detection. Both polyclonal and monoclonal antibodies are suitable for use in sandwich immunoassays. However, in order to use this format, the antigen of interest must be sufficiently large to simultaneously bind two separate antibodies. The first antibody in the reaction is called the **capture antibody**, which is either adsorbed or covalently linked to a solid support and is used to extract the analyte from the sample matrix. A second labeled antibody, known as the **tracer** or **conjugate antibody**, reacts with the captured antigen at a separate and distinct epitope from the capture antibody and is used to detect the analyte when all other components have been washed away. This type of assay can be performed either in a sequential or simultaneous incubation format, although for simultaneous incubation two distinct monoclonal antibodies for different epitopes must be used to prevent competition.

A different approach to noncompetitive binding immunoassays is demonstrated in the one-site immunometric assay. The one-site immunometric assay involves incubation of an excess of labeled Fab fragments (for 1 : 1 binding) or antibodies (2 : 1 binding) with a sample containing the antigen of interest. The incubation mixture is then introduced to a solid support containing immobilized antigen of interest to remove unbound antibodies or Fab fragments from solution; the amount of label left in solution is directly proportional to the concentration of analyte in the sample. This format is particularly useful for automated flow injection or chromatographic immunoassays. Fab fragments are generally more useful than whole antibodies in this approach because the antibody can be bound to both the support and analyte, which would yield a falsely low signal.

Immunoassay Labels

There are many different types of labels, for both antigen and antibody, that can be used in immunoassays. The choice of label is dependent on the analytical sensitivity desired for the measurement as well as the immunoassay format. A list of label types along with typical detection limits associated with them can be seen in Table 1. The earliest immunoassays used isotopic labels such as ^{125}I, ^{131}I, ^{3}H, ^{57}Co, and ^{32}P for antigens in competitive binding immunoassays and for antibodies in sandwich immunoassays. The utility of radioactive labels is based on low limits of detection achievable due to very low background interference. Radioactive labels were also used to develop an early homogeneous assay (9) based on modulation of ^{3}H or ^{125}I labels by scintillant-laden microparticles. However, immunoassays using radiolabels are falling out of favor in clinical laboratories due to concerns regarding safe handling and disposal of radioactive materials as well as the inherent instability of radiolabels.

TABLE 1. Immunoassay label-detection limits

Label type	Detection limit (M)
Fluorescence	1×10^{-10}
Chemiluminescence	1×10^{-13}
Fluorescence polarization	1×10^{-14}
Radioactive	1×10^{-15}
Time-resolved fluorescence	1×10^{-17}
Electrochemiluminescence	2×10^{-20}
Enzyme-based:	
Photometric	1×10^{-16}
Fluorescence	1×10^{-19}
Coupled enzyme reaction	1×10^{-20}
Chemiluminescence	1×10^{-21}

Recently, there has been an emphasis on the development of nonisotopic labels in light of the drawbacks that come with handling radioactive labels. As early as the 1970s, enzyme labels for immunoassay were developed and since then a wide variety of nonisotopic labels have been established. These types of labels include enzyme-based, fluorescent, chemiluminescent, and even electrochemical labels as well as many other newly developed, unique labels. Some of these labels are able to achieve detection limits well below those possible with radiolabels, and none of them poses the problems of handling and disposal that occur when working with radioactive materials. Increased specificity can be gained in an immunoassay from incorporating a biotin–avidin interaction with the antibody–antigen interaction by using biotin-conjugated antibody or antigen and then introducing labeled avidin to the reaction mixture. In some instances, multiple labels are incorporated by taking advantage of the multiplicity of avidin–biotin binding. One avidin molecule can bind four biotin molecules so this complex scheme would involve a biotin conjugate, followed by addition of avidin, which could then bind three more labeled biotin molecules.

Fluorescence. Chemical labels that exhibit fluorescence are commonly used for competitive binding and sandwich immunoassays in much the same manner as radioisotope labels. The most commonly known label is fluorescein isothiocyanate (FITC), but dyes such as Lucifer Yellow or Rhodamine B can also be used as fluorescent labels. Typical detection limits using fluorescence range from 0.1 pM to 1 nM, which is sensitive enough to use for low concentration analytes, but avoids the handling and disposal issues that come with using radioactivity. However, a major problem with fluorescence detection is that many substances found in patient samples such as drugs and drug metabolites, proteins, and bilirubin exhibit fluorescence and can cause a high background and interference. One way to avoid this interference is the use of **time-resolved fluorescence (TRF)** with labels derived from lanthanide elements (i.e., europium, terbium, and samarium). The fluorescence lifetime for these lanthanide chelates is much longer than typical fluorescent molecules, so after excitation a delay time (400–800 ms) is introduced to let background fluorescence decay, and then the signal is measured (7).

Fluorescence detection can be used for homogeneous assays as well by employing a **fluorescence polarization immunoassay (FPIA)**. This technique uses a competitive binding format with a fluorescein-labeled antigen to compete with antigen in the sample for antibody-binding sites (7). An FPIA uses the polarization of fluorescence due to molecular rotation in solution to determine the extent of label–antibody binding. When the labeled antigen is unbound, it rotates very rapidly and therefore has a low degree of polarization; but when the label is bound to an antibody molecule that rotates at a much lower rate, the degree of polarization is increased (*see* Figure 4). The change in polarization is proportional to the concentration of antigen in the sample, and because the label behavior is modified by antibody binding, no separation step is needed.

Enzymes. Enzyme-based labels such as alkaline phosphatase, horseradish peroxidase, g-6-dehydrogenase, and β-galactosidase are also frequently used in quantitative immunoassays (7, 10). The big advantage for enzyme labels is the amplification aspect; one enzyme label can produce many reporter molecules, up to 100-fold amplification (using a fluorescent substrate can produce amplification up to 100,000-fold). The substrate for detection can be chosen to produce a colored product for photometric monitoring, a fluorescent product such as umbilliferone, or even to produce an intermediate substrate for a second enzymatic reaction to produce further amplification. The most common heterogeneous enzyme immunoassay is the **enzyme-linked immunosorbent assay (ELISA),** which is a sandwich immunoassay where the capture antibody is bound to a solid support and the tracer antibody is enzyme labeled (7). After the capture–antigen–tracer complex is formed, all other sample components are washed away and substrate is added; the amount of product formed is proportional to the concentration of antigen in the sample (Figure 5). The ELISA can be modified to detect antibodies of a given specificity by using antigen linked to the support, adding sample, and using labeled antibodies to IgG as the tracer (e.g., detection of anti-HCV antibodies).

As previously discussed, homogeneous immunoassays need a label that will be modified by binding and enzyme labels are particularly well suited for this role. There are two commonly used types of homogeneous enzyme immunoassays: the **enzyme-multiplied immunoassay technique (EMIT)** and the **cloned enzyme donor immunoassay (CEDIA)** (7, 11). In the EMIT assay, an aliquot of the patient sample or calibrator is incubated with an enzyme-labeled antigen and a fixed amount of antibody specific for the antigen of interest as well as enzyme substrate (Figure 6) (7, 11). The antigen in the sample and the labeled antigen compete for antibody-binding sites; when antibody is bound to the labeled antigen, the enzyme is inhibited because it is blocked from interaction with the substrate.

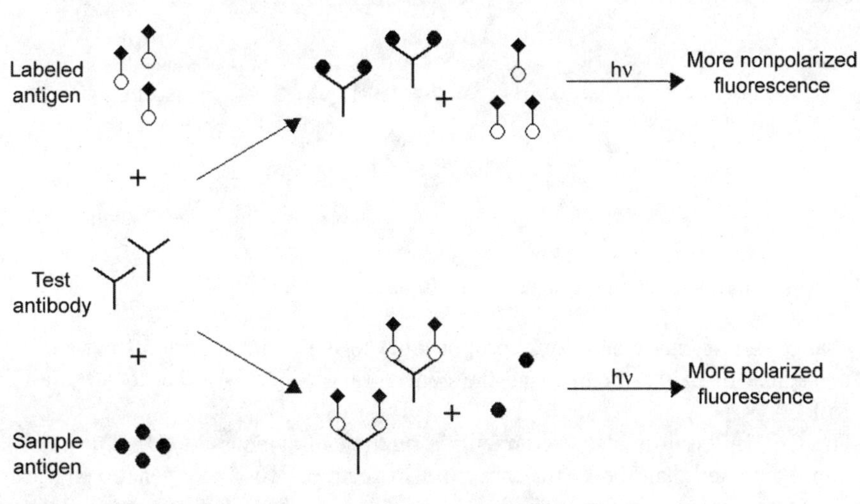

FIGURE 4. Fluorescence polarization immunoassay (FPIA).

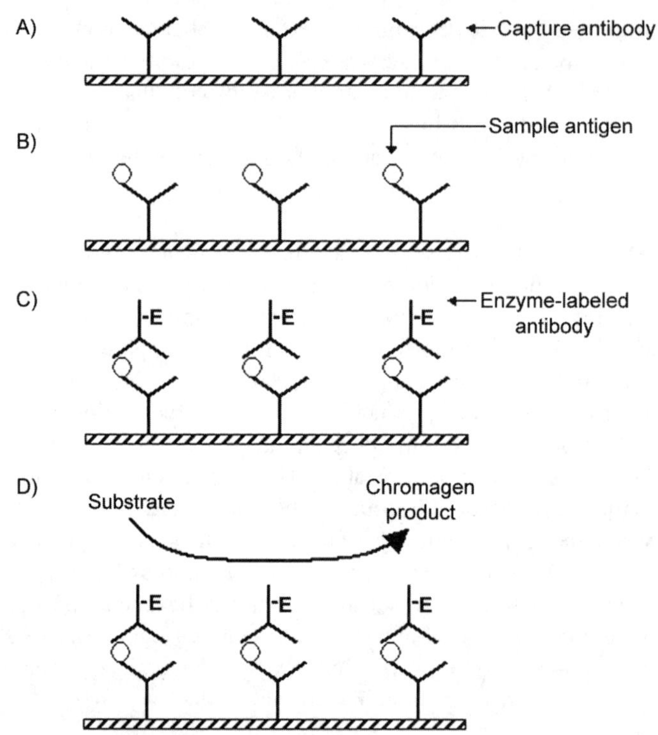

FIGURE 5. Enzyme-linked immunosorbent assay (ELISA).

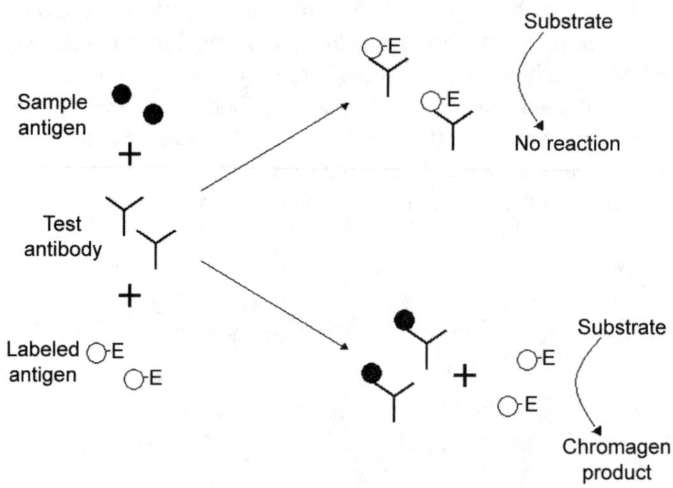

FIGURE 6. Enzyme-multiplied immunoassay technique (EMIT).

The change in enzymatic activity is proportional to the concentration of antigen in the patient sample or calibrator (e.g., as the concentration increases, so does the enzyme activity).

The CEDIA assay is also a competitive binding immunoassay (11, 12), but it is a little more complex than the EMIT assay in its execution. By using genetic engineering techniques, two inactive fragments of b-galactosidase are produced by manipulating the

Z gene of the *lac* operon of *Escherichia coli*. These two fragments are able to reassemble to form an active enzyme even if one of the fragments is covalently linked to another molecule. The competing antigen for the assay is labeled with one fragment of the enzyme and is incubated with patient sample, the second enzyme fragment, enzyme substrate, and a fixed amount of antibody directed toward the antigen of interest (Figure 7). Antibody that binds to labeled antigen prevents reassembly of the enzyme and no reporter molecule is produced; as the sample antigen concentration is increased, the enzyme activity is also increased. As with the EMIT assay, the change in enzymatic activity is directly proportional to the concentration of antigen in the sample.

Chemiluminescence. A chemiluminescent label is based on the emission of light produced during a chemical reaction. These labels are very useful because they offer very low limits of detection with little to no background interference; however, the complexity of the immunoassay is increased because the reaction conditions must be carefully controlled. Chemiluminescent labels can be found as both biologically derived and chemically manufactured. Biologically derived chemiluminescence labels include firefly luciferase (13) and apoaequorin, a protein derived from the bioluminescent jellyfish *Aequorin* (14). Firefly luciferase activates D-luciferin substrate by oxidation in the presence of ATP, molecular oxygen, and magnesium ions to emit light at 560 nm, while apoaequorin is activated by reaction with coelenterazin and calcium ions to emit light at 469 nm.

Other nonbiologic compounds can be used as chemiluminescent labels, including isoluminol and acridinium esters (15). Isoluminol is oxidized in the presence of a catalyst such as microperoxidase, producing a relatively long emission at 425 nm. Acridinium esters are commonly used, highly sensitive labels that are activated by oxidations using hydrogen peroxide in alkaline solution to give a brief flash of light at 429 nm. Chemiluminescence can be made even more sensitive when combined with other detection

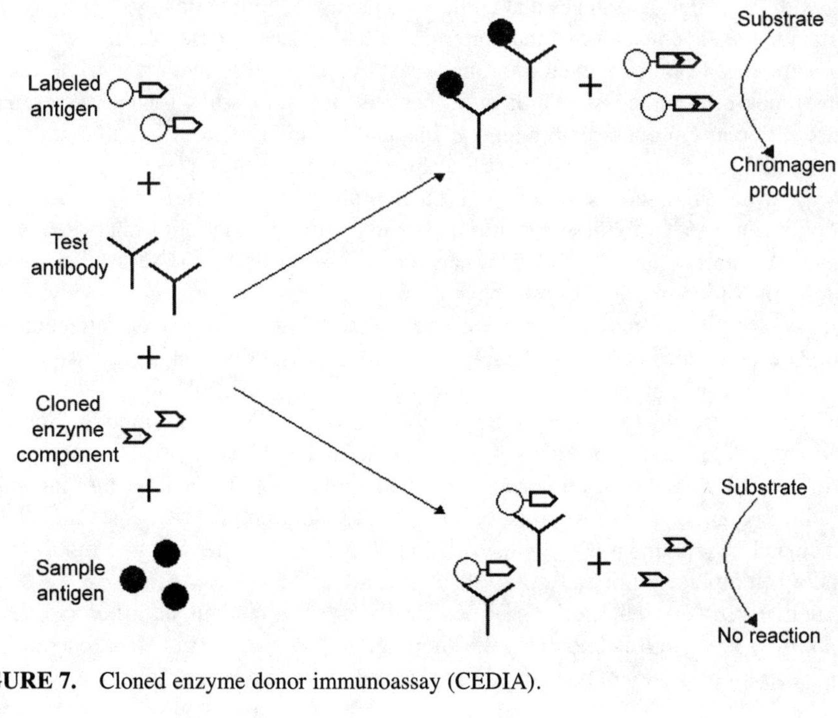

FIGURE 7. Cloned enzyme donor immunoassay (CEDIA).

methods. Electrochemiluminescence utilizes a molecule such as ruthenium (II) tris(bipyridyl) that undergoes chemiluminescence at a given redox potential, producing mass detection limits as low as 20×10^{-21} moles (14, 16). In addition, chemiluminescent substrates can be combined with enzymatic labels to take advantage of enzyme amplification effects along with the inherent sensitivity of chemiluminescence using a substrate known as AMPPD [disodium 3-(4-methylspiro-[1,2-dioxetane-3,2′-tricyclo-[3.3.1.1]decan]-4-yl) phenyl phosphate] to obtain mass detection limits as low as 1×10^{-21} mole (17, 18).

Alternative Labels. Many other alternative detection techniques for nonisotopic immunoassays have been developed in response to demands for lower detection limits, an increase in label specificity, or increased flexibility in applications. One example is the **enzyme channeling** immunoassay that combines the simplicity of a homogeneous immunoassay with the specificity of a sandwich immunoassay (19). In this approach, the antigen of interest binds two antibodies that are labeled with different enzymes; the enzyme reactions are coupled and more efficient when the enzymes are in close proximity due to binding within the immune complex. A similar approach is the **fluorescence excitation transfer immunoassay**, which is a competitive binding immunoassay utilizing a coupled fluorescence reaction (20). The labeled antigen contains a fluorophor donor while the antibody is labeled with a fluorescent acceptor; when the labeled antigen is antibody bound, a fluorescent signal occurs, and as the analyte concentration increases, the signal decreases. Various other methods have been introduced including those that incorporate PCR amplification with DNA or RNA labels, optical diffraction detection, and surface physiochemical detection techniques for biosensors (21–23).

Immunoassay Interferences

Along with the many advantages that come with the use of immunoassays, there are some important factors to consider that may interfere with the assay. These factors include interfering antibodies from the patient's serum, assay artifacts caused by large analyte concentrations (hook effect), and standardization between immunoassays for the same analyte that use different epitopes for binding. Each of these interferences has a characteristic effect that influences both immunoassay performance and utility.

In sandwich immunoassays, one particular problem is interference from circulating heterophilic human antibodies specific for animal immunoglobulins that are used as reagents. The most common type are human anti-mouse antibodies (HAMA) that are often present in the blood of patients who have been given mouse monoclonal antibody imaging or therapeutic agents or who have been exposed to other mouse antigens (24). Heterophile antibodies can cause false-positive results by cross-linking the capture and label antibodies in a manner similar to the analyte of interest, or they can cause false-negative results by blocking analyte binding to the capture of label antibody (Figure 8). The presence of HAMA or other heterophile antibodies can be confirmed through dilution experiments that do not give proportional results, or retesting of a sample after incubation with animal serum (e.g., mouse antisera for HAMA). Nonimmune animal serum is generally included in immunoassay kits using animal antibodies as reagents to minimize the effects of heterophile antibodies.

Another problem that can arise, specifically in simultaneous addition assays, and give a falsely low result is known as the "hook effect" (25, 26). This effect occurs when the concentration of the analyte is so high that both the capture and label antibodies are saturated. As a result, the assay response will decrease at high antigen concentrations, as demonstrated by a calibration curve including these concentrations; the response will drop off after a maximum response giving the curve a characteristic "hook" shape (*see* Figure 9). This situation can lead to falsely low patient results when the concentration of an analyte is elevated far above the analytical range of the assay and can be discovered by dilution followed by sample retesting. This type of error is avoided by using a large excess of capture and label antibodies with respect to the analytical range of the assay.

A different sort of problem arises when immunoassays are developed for the same analyte by different companies or researchers. Each developer uses a different antibody directed to a unique epitope that may exhibit varying binding properties, leading to different responses for the same concentration of analyte. In an isolated environment, this is not a problem so long as the institution uses only one type of assay; however, the establishment of a standard reference interval for the analyte becomes much more difficult because various institutions often use different assays for the same analyte. A prime example of this conundrum is demonstrated with the development of a cardiac troponin I assay. Cardiac troponin I (cTnI) is present in the circulation in three forms: as free cTnI, a two-unit complex with cardiac troponin C (cTnI-cTnC), and a three-unit complex with cTnC and cardiac troponin T (cTnI-cTnC-cTnT). The various assays fail to agree with each other because the reagent antibodies for each assay recognize different epitopes, making it difficult to develop a primary reference material (27, 28) for standardization of the method.

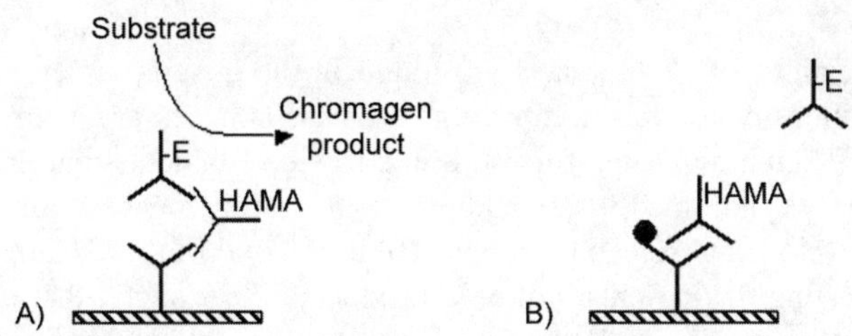

FIGURE 8. Heterophilic antibody interference (HAMA). A: positive interference and B: negative interference.

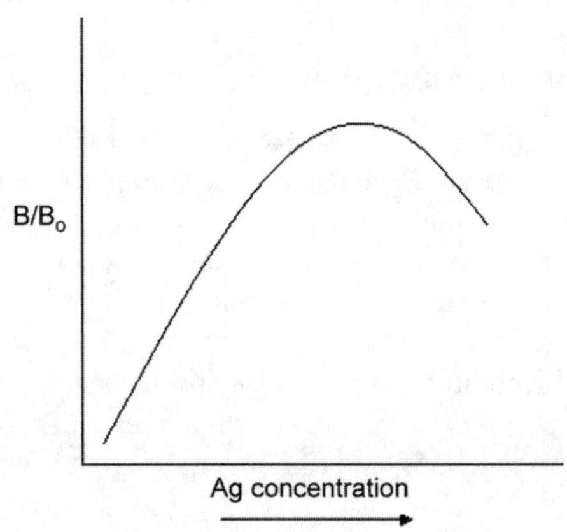

FIGURE 9. Calibration curve demonstrating the hook effect.

NEW APPROACHES TO IMMUNOCHEMICAL METHODS

Immunochemical methods are being adapted for alternative formats in order to expand their utility or perhaps to improve their precision by incorporating additional analytical methods. This allows immunoassays to be simplified for use outside the clinical laboratory, even for use as point-of-care (POC) testing devices. In addition, traditional laboratory methods are being modified to take advantage of the highly specific antibody–antigen interactions.

Point-of-Care Immunoassays

The most widely used POC immunoassay is used for the detection of hCG, more commonly known as a "home pregnancy test." Many different manufacturers produce these tests, but all the tests operate on the same basic principle. A urine specimen is applied to a porous membrane that draws the liquid from the application point to immobilized anti-hCG positioned further up the membrane. If hCG is present in the sample, it will be bound to the immobilized antibodies, followed by a detection step. Detection can be accomplished in a number of ways, depending on the manufacturer. One way is to add a second labeled antibody solution that will bind to the captured hCG, followed by a color development step (29). Another approach is to use colored microparticles for detection (Abbott). In this approach, the initial capture antibody is immobilized to colored beads, which are located at the point of application. As the sample and microbeads migrate up the membrane, they encounter a second capture antibody that will serve as a "detection zone"; if there is hCG present in a sample, a sandwich complex will be formed and a visible positive signal will occur.

Other applications of POC assays are found in the hospital emergency department (ED) and in locations where testing for drugs of abuse is necessary. Currently, POC tests for troponin I are being evaluated for use in the triage of patients that present to the ED with acute coronary syndrome (30). In addition, POC testing devices based on immunoassays are being developed to screen for drugs of abuse in oral fluids (31). In order to be useful, each POC testing device must not only produce a clear signal that makes it easy to distinguish between positive and negative, it must also contain a control mechanism to ensure that the device is working properly (e.g., the specimen moves up the membrane, all reagents are included in the reaction, the test detects the presence of interfering heterophilic antibodies).

Immunoaffinity Chromatography

Immunoaffinity chromatography (IAC) is a technique that utilizes antibodies or antibody fragments as ligands for chromatographic analyses. It couples the greater precision inherent in HPLC methods with the high selectivity derived from immunochemical methods of analysis. IAC is gaining consideration for use in the clinical laboratory due to the specificity of antibody–antigen interaction and the relative ease with which chromatography can be automated. This technique can be used for sample cleanup (immunoextraction) or can be adapted for the quantitative analysis of a specific analyte. HPLC-based IAC has been used to detect analytes such as human serum albumin (32, 33), tumor necrosis factor-a (34), parathyroid hormone (35), and fibrinogen (36), but it has yet to find use in routine clinical analyses.

REFERENCES

1. Chan DW, ed. Immunoassay automation: a practical guide. San Diego: Academic Press, 1992.
2. Chan DW, ed. Immunoassay automation: an updated guide to systems. San Diego: Academic Press, 1996.
3. Laurell CB. Antigen-antibody crossed electrophoresis. Anal Biochem 1965;10: 358–61.
4. Alper CA, Johnson AM. Immunofixation electrophoresis: a technique for the study of protein polymorphism. Vox Sang 1969;17:445–52.
5. Mancini G, Carbonara AO, Heremans JF. Immunochemical quantitation of antigens by single radial immunodiffusion. Immunochemistry 1965;2(3):235–54.
6. Weeke B. Rocket immunoelectrophoresis. Scand J Immunol 1973;1(Suppl):37–46.
7. Chan DW, ed. Immunoassay: a practical guide. San Diego: Academic Press, 1987.
8. Ekins R. Toward immunoassays of greater sensitivity, specificity and speed: an overview. In: Albertini A, Ekins R, eds. Monoclonal antibodies and developments in immunoassay. New York: Elsevier/North-Holland Biomedical Press, 1981:3–21.
9. Picardo M, Hughes KT. Scintillation proximity assays. In: Devlin JP, ed. High throughput screening. New York: Marcel Dekker, 1997:307–16.
10. Porstmann T, Kiessig ST. Enzyme immunoassay techniques: an overview. J Immunol Methods 1992;150:5–21.
11. Jenkins SH. Homogeneous enzyme immunoassay. J Immunol Methods 1992;150:91–7.
12. Engel WD, Khanna, PL. CEDIA® in vitro diagnostics with a novel homogeneous immunoassay technique: current status and future prospects. J Immunol Methods 1992;150:99–102.
13. Seto Y, Iba T, Abe K. Development of ultra-high sensitivity bioluminescent enzyme immunoassay for prostate-specific antigen (PSA) using firefly luciferase. Luminescence 2001;16:285–90.
14. Siddiqi AM, Jennings VM, Kidd MR, Actor JK, Hunter RL. Evaluation of electrochemiluminescence- and bioluminescence-based assays for quantitating specific DNA. J Clin Lab Anal 1996;10(6):423–31.
15. Kricka LJ. Chemiluminescent and bioluminescent techniques. Clin Chem 1991;37(9):1472–81.
16. Grimshaw C, Gleason C, Chojnicki E, Young J. Development of an equilibrium immunoassay using electrochemiluminescent detection for a novel recombinant protein product and its application to pre-clinical product development. J Pharm Biomed Anal 1997;16:605–12.
17. Bronstein I, Edwards B, Voyta JC. 1,2-Dioxetanes: novel chemiluminescent enzyme substrates. Applications to immunoassays. J Biolumin Chemilumin 1989;4(1):99–111.
18. Janda I, Jaensch H, Braun J, Wood WG. A comparison of four immunometric assays for myeloperoxidase using luminescent and colorimetric signal detection. J Clin Chem Clin Biochem 1990;28(7):475–80.
19. Litman DJ, Hanlon TM, Ullman EF. Enzyme channeling immunoassay: a new homogeneous enzyme immunoassay technique. Anal Biochem 1980;106(1):223–9.
20. Ullman EF, Schwarzberg M, Rubenstein KE. Fluorescent excitation transfer immunoassay. A general method for determination of antigens. J Biol Chem 1976;251(14):4172–8.
21. Sano T, Smith CL, Canto CR. Immuno-PCR: very sensitive antigen detection by means of specific antibody-DNA conjugates. Science 1992;258(5079):120–2.
22. Tsay YG, Lin CI, Lee J, Gustafson EK, Appelqvist R, Magginetti P, et al. Optical biosensor assay (OBA). Clin Chem 1991;37(9):1502–5.
23. Attridge JW, Daniels PB, Deacon JK, Robinson GA, Davidson GP. Sensitivity enhancement of optical immunosensors by the use of a surface plasmon resonance fluoroimmunoassay. Biosens Bioelectron 1991;6(3):201–14.
24. Klee GG. Human anti-mouse antibodies. Arch Pathol Lab Med 2000;124:921–3.
25. Miles LE. Properties, variants, and applications of the immunoradiometric assay method. Ric Clin Lab 1975;5(1):59–72.
26. Wu JT, Christensen SE. Effect of different test designs of immunoassays on "hook effect" of CA 19-9 measurement. J Clin Lab Anal 1991;5:228–32.

27. Apple FS. Clinical and analytical standardization issues confronting cardiac troponin I. Clin Chem 1999;45:18–20.
28. Wu AH, Feng YJ, Moore R, Apple FS, McPherson PH, Buechler KF, et al. Characterization of cardiac troponin subunit release into serum after acute myocardial infarction and comparison of assays for troponin T and I. American Association for Clinical Chemistry Subcommittee on cTnI Standardization. Clin Chem 1998;44: 1198–208.
29. Price CP, Newman DJ, eds. Principles and practice of immunoassay, 2nd ed. New York: Stockton Press, 1997.
30. Pagani F, Serena C, Bosio C, Cuccia C, Panteghini M. Evaluation of a rapid bedside immunochromatographic assay for detection of cardiac troponin I in whole blood. Clin Chem Lab Med 2007;39(5):458–9.
31. Barrett C, Good C, Moore C. Comparison of point-of-collection screening of drugs of abuse in oral fluid with a laboratory-based urine screen. Forensic Sci Int 2001; 122:163–6.
32. Hage DS, Walters RR. Dual-column determination of albumin and immunoglobulin G in serum by high-performance affinity chromatography. J Chromatogr 1987; 386:37–49.
33. Ruhn PF, Taylor JD, Hage DS. Determination of urinary albumin using high-performance immunoaffinity chromatography and flow injection analysis. Anal Chem 1994; 66:4265–71.
34. Phillips TM, Krum JM. Recycling immunoaffinity chromatography for multiple analyte analysis on biological samples. J Chromatogr B 1998;715:55–63.
35. Hage DS, Taylor B, Kao PC. Intact parathyroid hormone: performance and clinical utility of an automated assay based on high-performance immunoaffinity chromatography and chemiluminescence detection. Clin Chem 1992;38:1494–500.
36. McConnell JP, Anderson DJ. Determination of fibrinogen in plasma by high-performance immunoaffinity chromatography. J Chromatogr 1993;615:67–75.

Chapter 8

Electrophoresis

Christine N. Papadea

The separation of particles by an electric current passed through a liquid or solid field is called electrophoresis. This basic definition may give the impression that electrophoresis is a simple technique. While most familiar applications of electrophoresis are readily performed, the ease of running these procedures belies the technical complexities associated with the wide variety of configurations and the lack of a complete theoretical understanding of some of them. Electrophoresis works because a particle given an electric charge is made to move in a viscous medium (liquid or gel) by the force of an electric field. The driving force is counterbalanced by the frictional resistance which the macromolecule must overcome to migrate in the support medium.

The "ideal" electrophoretic system has the following desirable features:

- Rapid and complete resolution of the solutes of interest
- No heat generation
- No diffusion
- A stable buffer (pH and chemical)
- No interaction between solute and solid (stabilizing) support

Many but not all of these features can be achieved simultaneously through various modifications and adaptations of the basic components of electrophoresis. This chapter covers these basic elements as they apply to commonly used electrophoretic methods. The focus will be on the uses of electrophoretic methods in clinical laboratories. The reader is referred to the references at the end of this chapter for uses in other settings and for detailed theoretical discussions.

BACKGROUND

History

When electrophoresis is carried out in a liquid environment, the proteins have minimal interaction and their movement is not impeded in a free or moving boundary mode. In 1937, Tiselius constructed such a moving boundary electrophoresis apparatus (1), using a room-size U-tube filled with a buffer that surrounded the electrodes connected to a direct current power supply. Although impractical due to its size and the amount of the sample itself (approximately 1 liter of serum), it was the first device designed to separate proteins in such a complex sample. In this early apparatus, the boundaries between the solutes were not clear-cut and only four components (albumin, alpha-globulin, beta-globulin, and gamma-globulin) were separated (2). The boundaries were determined using complex Schlierin interference optics that detected differences in light refraction caused by concentration changes. This early system was based on the use of a liquid medium that was eventually replaced by a variety of diversified and practical types of solid supports.

Solid Support Techniques

One of the earliest solid matrix separation techniques was described by the term "zone" which was coined in the 1940s when electrophoresis of plasma was performed on filter paper to separate the protein fractions into five zones. A decade later, cellulose acetate was introduced and became popular for its advantages compared to paper: resolution was better and the time for separation decreased from several hours to 40 minutes or less (3). Solid supports control undesirable solute diffusion or distortions that occur in liquid, permit rapid migration, and even can act as sieves that separate by molecular size. Additional gains in resolution and time were later achieved with gels prepared from agar or its purified derivative, agarose. With the introduction of starch slabs in the 1950s (4) and polyacrylamide gels (5), the separation of particles could be achieved by principles based not only on charge differences but also on molecular mass differences.

Polyacrylamide gels and agarose media are more versatile than cellulose acetate for the separation of macromolecules and smaller classes of proteins. Starch, agarose, and polyacrylamide rapidly gained acceptance because of improved resolution, matrix clarity, reproducibility, efficiency, and reduced costs. Further advantages of the stabilizing media included ease of staining and destaining, visualization, and quantification of the identified solutes. These features stimulated interest in using electrophoresis in clinical laboratories in addition to the traditional uses in research laboratories.

Theory of Separation

Separation by electrophoresis occurs as a result of interactions and influences of numerous variables in the system:

- Net charge on the molecules in the sample mixture
- The molecular size (mass) of the particles (solutes)
- The mobility of the particles
- The applied voltage driving the current between the electrodes
- Heat production
- Electroendosmosis
- The pore size of the supporting matrix
- The composition and ionic strength of the buffer system (6)

The net charge and mobility of the solutes to be separated depend on the properties of the surrounding buffer. In an electric current, proteins, amphoteric solutes with acidic and basic functional groups, will migrate according to the net charges that are conferred by the pH of the buffer. At the pH that is greater or less than that of the isoelectric (neutral) point of the particle, the particle has a net charge that is either negative or positive. At the point of its neutrality where positive and negative charges are balanced, the amphoteric particle stops moving.

Two forces cause the migration to occur (2, 6, 7). The **first force** is the driving force (F) that accelerates the particles and can be expressed as:

$$F = QE \tag{1}$$

where F is the force of electrostatic attraction, Q is the charge on the sample particles, and E is the electrical potential (expressed in volts per centimeter) applied to the electrophoresis compartment.

The **second force** is an opposing or retarding force (Fs) caused by the viscosity of the medium through which the sample particles are moving. This force is defined by the radius (r) of the particle, the viscosity (n) of the medium, and the velocity of the particle (v) as shown in the following expression (where $\pi = 3.1416$):

$$Fs = (r \bullet n \bullet v)\ 6\pi \tag{2}$$

which predicts the opposing force will increase with increasing sample velocity. At some point, the two forces, F and Fs, will be equal:

$$F = Fs \quad \text{or} \quad QE = (r \bullet n \bullet v)\ 6\pi \tag{3}$$

and the velocity along the electrophoresis support medium will be constant and not influenced by the distance from the electrode attracting the charged particle.

The mobility (U) of a particle is a term used to express the ability of the charged particle to move. It is defined as the ratio of the velocity to the electrical potential. Mobility can be expressed by:

$$U = v/E \tag{4}$$

and has units of cm^2/vol sec. Substituting the terms of Equation 3 into Equation 4 gives:

$$U = Q/([r \bullet n]\ 6\pi) \tag{5}$$

which becomes the basic expression of electrophoresis and describes the mobility of the charged particle in relation to its size and the viscosity of the medium. Thus, it is clear how several variables, in addition to the charge and size of particles affect separation by electrophoresis. The electrophoretic force and the viscosity become opposing forces such that the velocity ([v], rate of movement) of a particle in a given electric field is determined by the charge, size, and the shape of the particle together with the viscosity of the solvent. Mobility of the particle is influenced by pH and is proportional to its charge properties.

The voltage causes the charged particles to migrate in the direction of either the anode ([+], the electrode attracting anions or negatively charged particles) or the cathode ([–], the electrode attracting cations or positively charged particles). The anode and cathode wires are submerged in separate compartments filled with buffer (Figure 1). When a voltage is impressed across the support matrix, current flows through the closed circuit (8). If the applied current is held constant, voltage decreases and migration stays constant. If voltage is held constant, the current increases as the resistance decreases, heat production increases, and the migration rate increases. Resistance to the movement is encountered due to the viscosity, as already discussed, and to electroendosmotic effects.

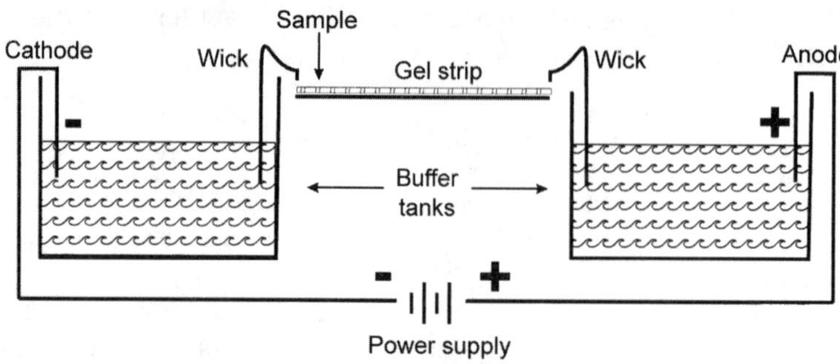

FIGURE 1. Schematic of a conventional electrophoresis chamber. Solutes are separated on the gel strip and buffer-saturated wicks complete the electrical circuit. The anode (+) attracts the negatively charges solutes; the cathode (–) attracts the positively charged solutes. The electromotive force is supplied by the power supply. The system, excluding the power supply, is covered by a safety lid (not shown) during operation.

Electroendosmosis is due to the interaction between the negative charges on the solid support and positively charged cations in the buffer that move toward the cathode of the system carrying the solvent (water) with them (7, 8). Most proteins are negatively charged in electrophoresis at alkaline pH and are attracted to the anode. Uncharged or weakly negatively charged molecules such as immunoglobulins are carried toward the cathode with the electroendosmotic movement. The ultimate effect is that proteins with slow mobilities are swept toward the cathode.

In addition to differences in electrical charge of various proteins in the mixture, separation occurs due to differences in molecular sizes in a "molecular sieve" effect using polyacrylamide or starch gels. The spaces or pores within the gel matrix are determined by the percentage of substance, e.g., in a 5% agarose gel, the average space is approximately 50 Å (2). Polyacrylamide is a network of linear polymers of acrylamide cross-linked by methylene bridges (9). The pore size is controlled by varying the amounts of acrylamide and the polymerizing agent that make up the gel. Advantages of polyacrylamide over starch gels include the following:

- The gel structure is more easily reproduced.
- Electroendosmosis is negligible.
- The gel is easier to handle and it can be dried, made transparent, and stored for a permanent record.
- Separation time is less.

Electrophoresis must be controlled by buffers to optimize the pH for best resolution of the particle of interest (10, 11). Buffer composition influences separation due to the interaction with the support medium (contributing to electroendosmosis) and to determining the net charge the proteins will acquire. Alkaline buffers will confer a negative charge to most of the proteins in the sample, thereby causing them to move toward the anode. The addition of calcium or ethylenediaminetetraacetate (EDTA) to buffer has been shown to sharpen the separation of the numerous components migrating into the beta-globulin zone at alkaline pH. Most buffers are continuous, i.e., consisting of a single composition, versus discontinuous meaning the use of different buffer compositions as is often preferred in polyacrylamide "stacked" gel systems (*see* Separation Techniques later).

The ionic strength of the buffer also has an effect on resolution. Increasing the ionic strength can improve separation, but it will also increase heat production. Increasing temperature causes increased evaporation which further increases the ionic strength of the buffer. High ionic strength decreases resistance, which in turn, causes the current to increase and heat production to rise. To offset this circular series of problems, heat sinks (Peltier devices) or other methods of dissipating heat (e.g., circulating cold water jacket) are used to keep migration time to a minimum, control heat production, minimize distortions in the gel, reduce diffusion of the solutes, and other serious problems that cause artifacts and failures in the separation process.

Specimen Types

Proteins represent approximately 50% of the dry weight of cells and comprise one of the major classes of biochemical macromolecules. They function in all processes of cellular activity and serve as a depot of amino acids (12). Separation of proteins by electrophoresis provides a quick, efficient way to view various fractions and their alterations of clinical significance. In clinical laboratory medicine, the most common specimen types for protein electrophoresis are serum, urine, cerebrospinal fluid, nasopharyngeal fluid, and peritoneal fluid. Disease conditions are associated with increased, decreased, or absent levels of one or more different types and classes of proteins in these sample types.

Types of Electrophoresis in Clinical Laboratories

Zone Electrophoresis

Because of the diffusion and relatively poor separation of solutes in a moving boundary electrophoresis in liquid, filter paper was the first anticonvective and was used widely in the 1940s (13). This solid support permitted the separation of protein fractions into five zones, namely albumin and the four globulin components, alpha-1, alpha-2, beta, and gamma (*see* Figure 2). Filter paper was replaced with the introduction of materials such as cellulose acetate, agar, and agarose (14). Separation in zone electrophoresis is determined by charge differences of the solutes in a single continuous buffer system.

Isoelectric Focusing (IEF)

In this technique, separation of solutes occurs across a pH gradient formed from a heterogeneous mixture of small, charged, synthetic oligopeptides called **carrier ampholytes**. The ampholytes migrate to a pH at which they have a zero net charge, i.e., positive and negative charges are equal. This pH is the isoelectric point (pI) of the respective amphoteric molecule. Being amphoteric, proteins applied in the same field with carrier ampholytes also migrate to the pH point at which the positive and negative charges on the protein are balanced. The migrating protein becomes stationary at its pI. In this way, individual components of heterogeneous mixtures become separated into dense, tightly resolved, narrow bands, representing the array of pIs of the components in the starting sample mixture.

Capillary Electrophoresis (CE)

This technique is reminiscent of the separation in liquid in the moving-boundary method. Separation occurs in a free liquid medium in a narrow (20–200 μm) capillary under high-voltage conditions (7, 15, 16). The CE instrumentation consists of two buffer chambers connected by a long, narrow capillary tube that has a negatively charged inner surface. When the electric field is activated, cations migrate along the negatively charged inner surface.

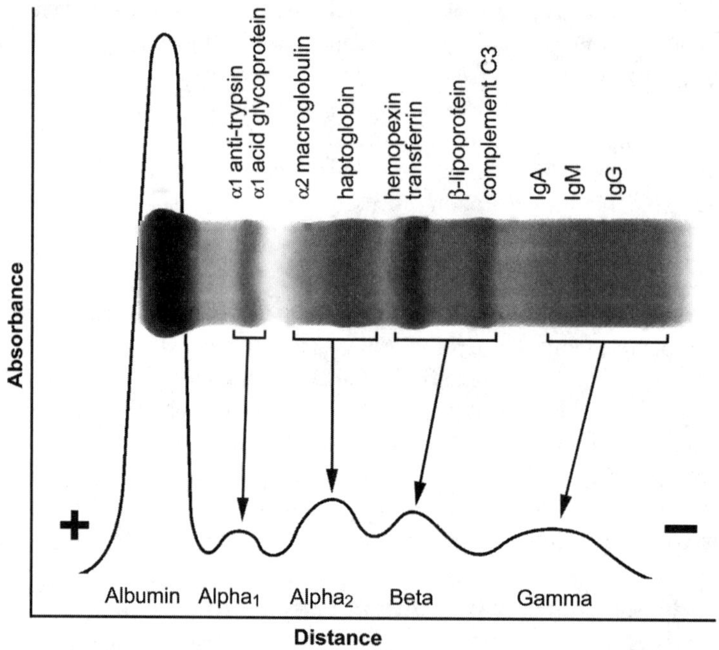

FIGURE 2. Total protein in serum separated on an agarose gel at pH 8.4, a zone electrophoresis procedure. The distance (horizontal axis) traveled by the proteins in each stained fraction—albumin, $alpha_1$ globulin, $alpha_2$ globulin, beta globulin, and gamma globulin—are determined by the differences in their net charges and can be delineated easily by scanning densitometry. Subfractions of the four major globulin fractions are labeled above to indicate the slight differences of charges among the heterogeneous population which cannot be resolved by this method. Absorbance (vertical axis) is the response to the signal received by the photodetector of the scanning densitometer and is directly related to the concentration of each fraction detected.

Electroosmotic flow exceeds the electrophoretic mobilities of the proteins, resulting in the movement of positively charged molecules toward the cathode, followed by neutral molecules, and then by negatively charged substances. Resolution depends on the amount of sample applied and by the applied electric field. The column length influences the analysis time; thus the shortest possible length with the highest voltage possible are combined to obtain the greatest possible resolution in the shortest time. The high surface-to-volume ratio in the column is highly efficient in dissipating heat and permits high-voltage operation.

Applications in Clinical Laboratories

Electrophoresis is one of the most important diagnostic tools in clinical laboratory medicine. It is a relatively inexpensive and efficient technique for studying protein patterns in biological fluids, especially serum, urine, and cerebrospinal fluid. Electrophoretic techniques have been used to study specific classes of proteins including isoenzymes, lipoproteins, glycoproteins, and genetic variants of proteins including hemoglobins. These analyses of proteins in serum, urine, and cerebrospinal fluid or other biological fluid provide valuable supportive pathological and therapeutic information for the diagnosis and management of diseases.

Zone electrophoresis is the technique most often performed for clinical laboratory applications but is considered to be semiquantitative due to the incomplete resolution of individual proteins, differences in dye-binding affinities among various proteins, differences among gel compositions and sample volume applied, and other factors (2). The separation of serum proteins according to differences in their electric charge into between five and 10 zones, as typically seen in conventional zone methods, oversimplifies the highly complex pattern of the highly heterogeneous mixture of components in serum. However, current understanding of how the myriad of different protein constituents contribute to the diagnostic utility of serum protein electrophoresis is incomplete, thus the value of greater resolution (i.e., >10 fractions in serum) by zone electrophoresis for routine clinical laboratory examination is controversial (17).

SEPARATION TECHNIQUES

Electrophoretic separation of proteins in clinical applications is related to three molecular properties of these solutes: (1) net charge at the pH of the environment; (2) molecular mass (size); and (3) isoelectric point (6). These properties can be discussed as associated with two different media: liquid and semisolid states (gels). Gels used in electrophoresis are three-dimensional networks of dense barriers of polymer fiber interspersed with air pockets that will be filled with buffer.

Solid Support, One Dimension

In zone electrophoresis, separation is primarily based on net electrical charge of the constituents in the sample mixture and only minimally related to molecular mass. It is the most widely used technique in clinical laboratories and is based on the separation of molecules according to charge in an electric field. The buffer system controlling the pH of the environment is continuous to maintain the environment at one pH, and the support is uniform with respect to composition and pore size. Media widely used for zone electrophoresis include cellulose acetate, agarose, and starch gel as discussed in the following paragraphs.

Cellulose acetate is formed by combining cellulose and acetic anhydride to produce an opaque slurry that is applied in a thin film onto a plastic backing (18). Cellulose acetate gels are supplied as dry, somewhat brittle strips and must be soaked in buffer prior to use to fill the large proportion (~80%) of air spaces within the network of cellulose acetate fibers on the support. Electrophoresis of <3 µL of serum on the wetted pliable strips is rapid (~30 minutes at 100 V) and the electropherogram can be fixed, stained, and cleared quickly for analysis. Cellulose acetate strips are known to differ among commercial suppliers as a result of the variables in the manufacturing processes that include acetylation, additives used, and the uniformity of the thickness of the coating applied to the plastic support. This technique has largely been replaced for clinical applications by ready-to-use agarose for better resolution and minimal electroendosmotic and adsorption properties.

Agarose, a natural polysaccharide isolated from agar, forms a gel in a neutral matrix held together by hydrogen bond formation (8, 9). It exists as random distribution of polymers and spaces (pores). The pore sizes of the gel are best defined by the sieving effect they create that limits or allows various sizes and shapes of charged molecules to migrate through the spaces. Agarose is preferred over cellulose acetate because:

- It contains relatively few ionizable groups, making it essentially free of electroendosmotic effects.
- The natural clarity of the gel after staining and drying facilitates the visual and densitometric interpretation of the detected solutes.

Sample volume, electrophoresis conditions, running time, and subsequent processing (staining, destaining, and drying) steps are similar to those used for cellulose acetate strips.

To achieve the separation of serum proteins into 10 or more zones on agarose gels, a high ionic strength buffer is added to the agarose, usually by incorporating a calcium salt. This modification leads to so-called "high" resolution agarose gels. The high ionic buffer increases the resolution of the constituents of the alpha- and beta-globulin fractions having similar mobilities, a property that is recommended for the laboratory detection and quantification of monoclonal immunoglobulins (17). High resolution has also been achieved by using a discontinuous buffer system which involves use of a different buffer for the electrodes than for the gels. Buffer salts moving during electrophoresis produce a pH front that differs from that within the gel such that the migrating solutes encounter two different pHs. As movement proceeds into the pores containing a different buffer, the mobility changes as determined by the charges at the different pHs.

Starch gels separate molecules according to their surface charge and molecular size. Hydrolyzed starch is used to form a horizontal or a vertical slab of uniform dimensions. An advantage of starch gel electrophoresis is the resolution of as many as 20 fractions of proteins in serum or red blood cell hemolysates. This matrix is useful for studying isoenzymes or globin chains of hemoglobin variants, respectively.

Polyacrylamide gel (PAG) is the product of acrylamide (CH_2=CH–CO–NH_2) and a cross-linking co-monomer, N, N′-methylenebisacrylamide (bis) (8, 9). Cross-linking agents are bifunctional acrylic agents which covalently link polyacrylamide chains. Polymerization is catalyzed by a free radical-producing reaction using an initiator, ammonium persulfate, and an accelerator, tetramethylethylenediamine (TEMED). The cross-linking of polyacrylamide at an alkaline pH forms a three-dimensional charge-free lattice.

PAG has several advantages: it has no electroendosmotic effects; it forms a clear, strong matrix which is compatible with densitometric scanning; and the pore size of the cross-linkages may be varied by changing the amounts of acrylamide and bis. Disadvantages include the following: (1) hazards are associated with the handling of the potentially toxic chemicals; (2) the by-products of polymerization, e.g., sulfate, can change the electrical properties and, consequently, the separation properties of the gel. Use of proper handling procedures to avoid personal exposure and the highest quality of impurity-free chemical reagents will ensure personal safety, reproducible gels, and satisfactory results.

The pore size of PAG is described in two terms: the weight percentage of total monomer (%T), which includes the monomer and the co-monomer cross-linking agent, and the percentage of the cross-linker (%C) in the total monomer. Pore size is inversely related to the total concentrations of the monomer and the cross-linker (8). The higher the %T, the smaller the pore size. The pore size is also controlled by the %C in a biphasic function; pore size decreases to a minimum with the cross-linker as high as 5%, and then with further increases of %C, the pore size begins to increase. The average pore size in the typical 7.5% PAG matrix is about 50 Å (2).

The gels can be constructed as tubes or slabs which are stacked in two layers. In this modification of PAG, the two layers differ in pore size and composition, a configuration that was introduced in 1964 (5, 19) to improve the separation of a mixture of proteins having the same mobility in zone electrophoresis. The small-pore separating gel is poured first and allowed to solidify in the bottom of the tube and then is followed by a large-pore polymer, the spacer gel, which forms the upper layer. In this configuration, the smaller molecular weight constituents in the sample are able to stack in a narrow zone above the small-pore separating gel. The effect is to concentrate the proteins and enhance zone-sharpening as the proteins enter the separating gel. Proteins of molecular size less than the average pore size of the PAG will migrate freely while those that exceed the pore size will be retarded.

In another variation of PAG, a detergent such as sodium dodecyl sulfate (SDS) is added to the sample to facilitate the separation of proteins according to their molecular weight (11, 18, 20). SDS binds to individual proteins in a mixture in proportion to the molecular weight of the individual proteins and eliminates the differences in charge. The charge-to-mass ratio of the native protein thus having being altered, the separation of the proteins is determined by molecular mass and not by charge.

IEF is a high-resolution technique in which a pH gradient is established by carrier ampholytes (having both positive and negative charges) within the gel to effect the separation of proteins based on differences in their pIs (2). This concept is easily understood by first considering the amphoteric nature of proteins, i.e., they have both positive and negative charges. The net charge on a protein is the sum of its negative and positive charges as determined by its constituent amino acids. The pH at which the protein has a zero net charge is the pI. If the number of acidic amino acids or side chains is greater than the number of basic groups, the pI of the protein will be at a low pH and conversely, if the basic groups exceed the number of acidic groups, the pI of the protein will be at a high pH. The pI values of proteins occur in a pH range from 3 to 10, with the majority being between pH 4 and 7 (8).

The pH gradient is developed by carrier ampholytes, which are polyaminocarboxylic acid peptides. Ampholytes with molecular weights of 300–1000 are added to the gel in carefully selected mixtures to create a pH gradient across a narrow range between the electrodes. IEF can separate proteins with pI differences as small as 0.02 pH unit if the mixture of carrier ampholytes is carefully selected to obtain very narrow zones of pH. During electrophoresis the ampholytes become arranged according to their respective charges and create the continuum of tightly spaced zones between the anode and cathode (Figure 3). Proteins applied as samples will migrate according to their net charge within the gradient determined by the carrier ampholytes. During its migration toward the electrode, the individual protein component will arrive at the point in the pH gradient that is equal to its pI, and its net charge is zero, thus its migration stops. The result is that the protein components in the original mixture become focused into sharply restricted bands, reflecting the small variations among pIs of the various proteins. From an apparent single band of protein by zone electrophoresis, IEF separates discrete individual bands of a heterogeneous but closely related population of proteins. A high-voltage (up to 2000 V) power supply is required for IEF. As a result, heat is produced and the gel must be cooled during IEF by placing the support platform on a Peltier heat trap or surrounding it with a cold water jacket.

Two-dimensional (2D) electrophoresis has the greatest resolving ability for separating complex mixtures of proteins into their fractional components (3, 11). This method uses two different high-resolution techniques in tandem to resolve hundreds of proteins in a single gel. The first dimension electrophoresis is performed by IEF, and it separates the solutes according to pI. This step is followed, in the second dimension, by SDS-PAG electrophoresis for further separation by molecular weight (*see* Figure 4). The IEF phase uses either carrier ampholytes in tube gels or in ready-to-use immobilized pH gradient (IPG) strips obtained as a commercial product, e.g., the ReadyStrip™ (BioRad Laboratories, Life Science Group, Hercules, CA). The IPG strip in the first dimension is not only convenient but also provides the advantages over tube gels of enhanced reproducibility, stability, and predictability of the pH gradient incorporated into acrylamide. In addition, IPG strips enable the application of large loads of protein and, because they are very thin, they are able to dissipate heat and withstand high-voltage fields. The applied electrical field

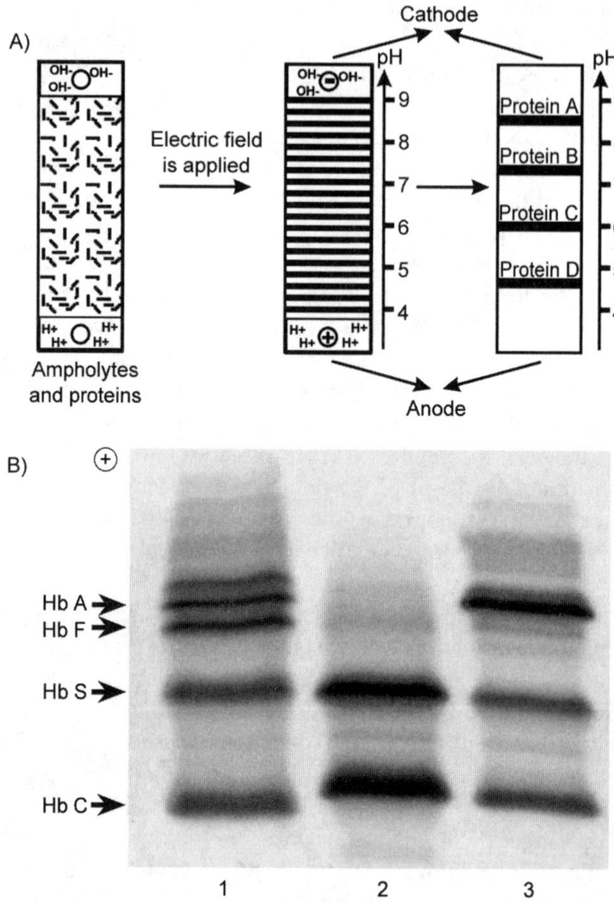

FIGURE 3. Isoelectric focusing electrophoresis (IEF). Panel A: diagram of the three stages of IEF. First, a sample containing various proteins (A, B, C, D) is applied to the gel constructed with a mixture of ampholytes carrying negative and positive charges. A dilute acid (H^+) and a dilute base (OH^-) are placed in contact with the IEF gel at the anode and cathode, respectively. Next, when electric current is applied, the ampholytes form a ladder-like gradient across a pH range, e.g., between pH 4 and 9, according to the mixture of ampholytes. Finally, proteins A, B, C, and D migrate to the pH where the charge on the respective protein is zero. This pH is the isoelectric point (pI). The individual proteins separate into tight, discrete bands as determined by the differences in their pIs. Panel B: separation of hemoglobin (Hb) variants in three samples on an IEF gel (pH 6–8). The proteins are separated in tightly packed bands as a result of the different pIs of the globin chains in the pH gradient.

strength has a key role in the resolution in the IEF phase and must be considered since the high voltage is accompanied by potentially damaging heat. External methods of rapid, efficient cooling must be provided.

After the initial separation, the first dimension IEF medium is equilibrated with SDS, and then mercaptoethanol denaturing solutions are placed adjoining the top of the PAG for continued electrophoresis for 2–3 hours controlled at constant voltage (~150 V). After final separation, detection of the proteins can be visualized by stains (e.g., Coomassie Blue R250, fluorescent stains, silver staining) or by immunoblotting.

Conducting 2D electrophoresis requires labor-intensive attention to several technical aspects including the properties of the solute, the equilibration of the media, the power

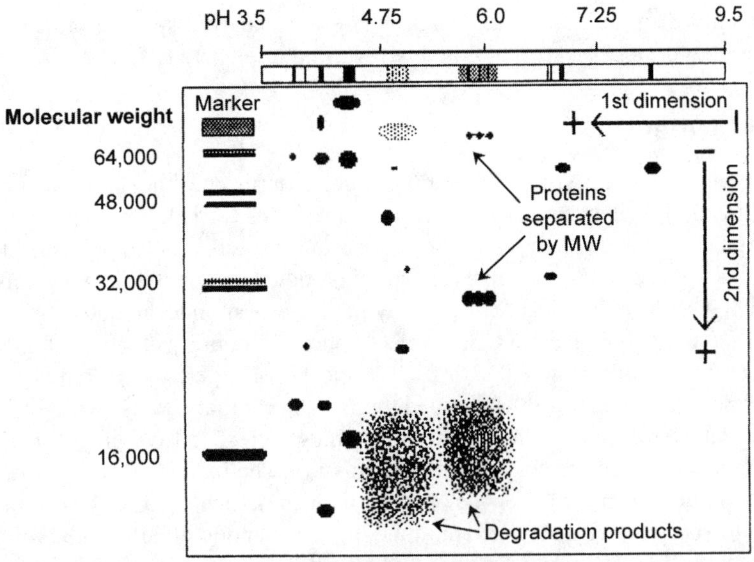

FIGURE 4. Principle of two-dimensional (2D) electrophoresis. Separation in the first dimension is based on the isoelectric point of each protein in the sample mixture (*see* Figure 3). The pH gradient and the direction of migration are indicated at the top of the illustration. In the second dimension in SDS-PAG, electrophoretic separation becomes a function of molecular mass. A mixture of proteins (Marker) having known molecular weights (MW) is placed at the top of the gel to serve as a guide after the completion of the separation. (*Courtesy of Helena Laboratories, Beaumont, TX*)

supply, the detection of the protein products after the second dimension is completed, and the analysis of large amounts of data generated in the experiment. Reducing the complexity of the sample by extraction or by preparative prefocusing, before loading the first dimension IEF gel, can facilitate the detection of minor proteins. The amount loaded on the gel must be sufficient to detect low-abundance proteins yet not excessive such that high-abundance proteins could obscure the low-level solutes of interest.

Some limitations of 2D electrophoresis are (1) the difficulty in visually assessing variations in protein (spot) size and intensity; (2) inability to detect slight modifications of normal spots that can indicate abnormality; and (3) high degree of sensitivity to minor alterations which may not necessarily mean an abnormality or be related to a particular disease (21, 22). Imaging and image analysis through software designed for this purpose are available in commercial packages. These enable the collection, cataloging, and unbiased comparison of vast amounts of data. Highly reproducible methods are required to identify protein maps that may be associated with disease. Since 2D electrophoresis can resolve hundreds of proteins in a single gel with good reproducibility, the power it has to examine protein changes at the molecular level is unparalleled at the present.

Two-dimensional electrophoresis is not well suited for routine clinical laboratory use because samples as complex as serum and urine contain hundreds of different proteins at different concentrations that produce patterns that are difficult to interpret. On the other hand, 2D electrophoresis has gained prominence in the field of proteomics for characterizing the vast assortment of protein mixtures in the highly complex network of cell regulation. Indeed, Anderson and Anderson (22) accurately predicted that 2D electrophoresis maps would make a major contribution in the development of molecular physiology and the analysis of the function of gene products and all cell proteins (the proteome). The potential clinical usefulness of 2D electrophoresis to analyze specific proteins in serum and other body fluids has been thoroughly reviewed elsewhere (21, 22).

Liquid Medium

Capillary electrophoresis (CE) separations were described in the 1960s using 300-mm glass tubes and UV light to detect the separated proteins (7, 16). Electrophoresis in tubes was recognized as a new technique when Jorgenson and Lukacs (15) published their findings on this high-resolution capillary electrophoretic technique. CE is now considered to have the highest resolution capability of any liquid separation technique (16).

Two forces are dominant in CE: the electrophoretic mobility of the solutes themselves and the electroosmotic flow (EOF) of the liquid (7). The latter term refers to the flow resulting from interactions of the charged ions on the capillary walls. With CE, the capillary has a large surface area and the negative charge effect of EOF plays a major role in the separation of the solute constituents in a mixture. The individual solutes are driven in the direction determined by their net charge, their mass, and to a lesser extent, by their shape and hydrophobicity. At the same time, the endosmotic effect of the buffer moving toward the cathode has a greater magnitude ("pull") than the individual electrophoretic mobilities of individual mobilities of the solutes (8). Ultimately the solutes all move toward the cathode because the EOF is usually sufficient to force the movement in one direction. A representation of CE is shown in Figure 5.

EOF depends on the net charge of the protein, buffer conditions, and the strength of the electrical field. EOF increases as the pH and field strength increase (8). At pH >3, the inner wall of the capillary becomes highly negatively charged, attracting positively charged cations in the buffer. In a high-voltage electric field at this pH, migration proceeds toward the cathode and positively charged molecules migrate toward the anode, dragging the water of hydration along. Reproducibility of separation is affected by EOF which must be controlled for clinical applications and to minimize the potentially untenable effect of nonreproducibility.

The basic type of commercial CE apparatus in current usage includes multiple fused silica capillaries (~50 cm length) with internal diameters of 20–200 μm, a high-voltage power supply, and on-column UV detection (185–200 nm) for the solute bands as they migrate past the detector windows (7). (Multiple capillaries and detectors provide rapid throughput capability in high-volume testing settings.) Capillaries are coated on the exterior with a layer of polyamide to add flexibility and mechanical strength to the otherwise fragile narrow-bore tubing. Samples are introduced (volumes in commercial systems are in the nanoliter range) into the capillary by injection either electrokinetically (low voltage) or hydrodynamically (pressure or suction). Highly controlled electrokinetic injection is preferred for its ability to achieve a solute-concentrating effect.

Resolution in CE depends on the charge and the mass of the solutes in the mixture and on the voltage that is applied. Detection limits are dependent on the type of detector, the matrix of the sample, and the injection method used.

Biological fluids usually consist of very complex mixtures of solutes in a matrix which makes CE measurement of the specific analytes in them difficult. Depending of its physicochemical properties, the matrix can affect reproducibility, quantitation, and peak shape due to interactions among the constituents. CE provides high-efficiency separation of such mixtures by various related specialized techniques such as capillary zone electrophoresis (CZE); capillary isoelectric focusing; micellar electrokinetic capillary chromatography; and capillary gel electrophoresis (CGE). The principles of separation are

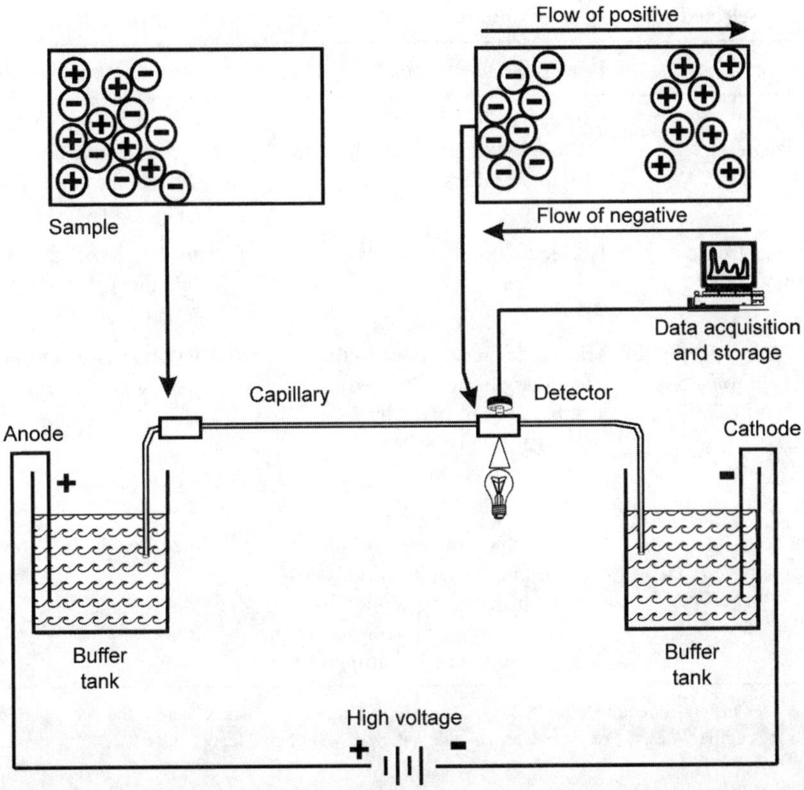

FIGURE 5. Principle of capillary electrophoresis (CE). The individual charged components of the sample mixture are driven in the direction of the electrode that attracts the oppositely charged analytes. Two forces effect the separation: the electrophoretic mobility of the charged solutes and the electrosmotic flow of the buffer. The latter force dominates resulting in the cations moving past the detector toward the cathode first, followed by the neutral ions, and finally by the anions. (*From reference 7 with permission*)

summarized in Table 1. While these CE assays can be labor-intensive due to the possible requirement of a manually performed sample preparation prior to the CE analysis, the assays are useful in the analyses of ligands, ions, and other small substances in body fluids (Table 1).

CE is utilized in various major fields of study such as clinical chemistry, pharmaceutical chemistry, molecular biology, forensic analysis, and others (7, 16, 23). One of the most successful methods has been CZE for the separation of peptides. In this mode, the capillary and electrode reservoirs are filled with a single buffer. Constituents of the samples are resolved by differences in their electrophoretic mobilities. Similarly, gel-filled capillaries are used for the resolution of nucleic acids in the CGE mode. Separation of proteins by size has been obtained by using hydrophilic polymers that are analogous to cross-linked gels such that the mobility of macromolecules is based on size differences.

Recent commercially developed automated electrokinetic capillary instrumentation is gaining acceptance in clinical laboratories. Instruments for serum protein electrophoresis or DNA analysis include the Paragon CCE 2000 Clinical Capillary Electrophoresis System (Beckman Coulter, Brea, CA), the ABI PRISM 310 Genetic Analyzer (Perkin Elmer Applied Biosystems Division, Foster City, CA), and Capillarys Capillary Electrophoresis

TABLE 1. Selected capillary electrophoresis modes and applications (7, 16, 23)

Mode	Principles of separation*	Examples of applications
Capillary zone electrophoresis (CZE)	Differences in mass-to-charge ratio. Low ionic strength buffer in the capillary.	Small molecules such as drugs, amino acids, catecholamines, peptides, protein macro-molecules
Capillary isoelectric focusing (CIEF)	Isoelectric point. Ampholytes in the capillary form the gradient.	Peptides, proteins such as globin chains of hemoglobin variants
Micellar electrokinetic capillary chromatography (MECC, MEKC)	Micelle detergent added to the capillary buffer. Charged substances resolved by charge-to-mass differences, uncharged species by hydrophobicity.	Bile acids, homocysteine, cortisone, cortisol, DNA
Capillary gel electrophoresis (CGE)	Sieving in polymerized gel matrix (PAG) in the capillary. In non-denaturing gel, separation by mass to charge, in SDS-denaturing gel, separation by hydrophobicity.	Nucleic acids, PCR products

*Analyses generally require sample preparation, depending on the matrix, before the substance is introduced into the capillary. Key: PAG = polyacrylamide gel, SDS = sodium dodecyl sulfate.

System (Sebia, Issy-les-Moulineaux, France). The Sebia system features a patented "bubble" capillary that has an enlarged area at the detector allowing a large sample volume to be measured directly, thereby improving sensitivity and reproducibility.

Commercial CE systems offer several advantages over gel-based techniques including:

- Efficient autosampling
- Nanoliter amounts of sample
- Microliter amounts of buffer
- Rapid (4 minutes) protein separation with high-resolving power, i.e., multiple capillaries in parallel for multiple analyses simultaneously
- Ease of operation for the inexperienced analyst
- Less labor-intensive
- Discrete separation between protein zones
- Highly reproducible peak heights and areas
- High surface-to-volume ratio to promote heat dissipation
- On-line direct detection

Disadvantages include:

- Distance between beta and gamma zones in serum protein separation is shortened, causing an asymmetrical distortion of the gamma peak.
- EOF must be controlled carefully to achieve reproducible results.
- Expensive apparatus may not be feasible for low-volume testing (<40 tests/day).

Although no gel is involved in CE technology, a recording is produced from the continuum of UV absorbances measured. This record or "tracing" is analogous to the densitometer tracings of bands stained in a gel-based electrophoresis system. Commercial software is available to convert the absorbance recordings to a virtual gel image, simulating the familiar banding pattern in solid support electrophoresis methods.

ANALYTICAL COMPONENTS

Apparatus

The chamber (cell) for solid support electrophoresis is usually a plastic or glass box containing two compartments, one each for an anode and a cathode wire. The solid support, with or without additional wicks according to the matrix and chamber size, makes a bridge between the electrodes (Figure 1). The electrodes are usually made of platinum wire, submerged in the buffer-containing compartments, and lead into jacks in the power supply to make electrical contact. As a safety feature, an electrical switch is activated only after a lid is correctly positioned to seal the system.

Gels are cast most often as slabs but also may be poured in tubes. Slabs are run in either vertical or horizontal flat-bed positions (8). Long gels (>20 cm) may be used for complex samples, as in SDS-PAG electrophoresis. Conventional polyacrylamide slabs are usually 15–20 cm in length, but so-called minigels, about 8-cm square or less, are easier to handle and permit rapid analysis.

The gel thickness of the slab configuration varies. Approximately 1-mm thickness allows adequate sufficient sample load and voltage to be applied without excessive heating. Agarose gels are typically approximately 8-cm square or less and quite thin (<1 cm), the thickness being determined by the percentage dry weight (grams) of agarose in the volume of buffer poured to make the gel.

Power Supply

The power supply sends the electromotor force through the electrophoresis system which causes the solute to become charged. The electrophoresis apparatus and the power supply comprise a closed circuit in which the apparatus creates electrical resistance associated with the production of heat. Ohm's law describes this electrical circuit:

$$V = R \bullet I \tag{6}$$

where V is the electromotive force in volts, I is the current in amperes, and R is the resistance in ohms (8). In addition, power (P, in watts) can be expressed as:

$$P = V \bullet R \tag{7}$$

Power supplies are available for electrophoresis that are designed to control all the electrophoresis operating parameters and to maintain constant power, constant current, or constant voltage modes. Many power supplies have automatic timers or integrators to terminate the electrophoresis automatically after a set period of time or other accumulated variable. The separation of proteins in a mixture is more rapid in high-voltage electrophoresis, and the distance of migration is directly related to the voltage and time and inversely related to the length of the support matrix (11). To minimize the time of electrophoresis without sacrificing resolution, voltage must be increased. However, with increased voltage, current will also be increased, adding to heat production.

The major limitation in electrophoresis is the heat generated by the electrical current. Heat causes diffusion of the separated zones, evaporation of water, increased ion concentration, and accelerated migration of solutes. It can be partially controlled by decreasing the ionic strength of the buffer and by cooling the support medium. If heat is controlled, the migration rate is held constant. Constant current is preferred to keep heat and solute diffusion to a minimum and to complete adequate separation in the shortest time. Constant power is preferred for IEF due to the continual decrease in current as a result of lower conductivity as the ampholytes reach their isoelectric points. Constant power or constant voltage is used with a cooling system to perform the separations in a minimum time period. The best way to regulate excessive heat production while maintaining good resolution is to use constant power so that current and voltage automatically become adjusted (refer to Equation 6) (8).

Buffers

Continuous Buffer System

The choice of buffer components, ionic strength, and pH are key elements in determining the buffering capacity and controlling the pH at which the separation will be carried out (2, 8, 11). In addition, the buffer system should not interact with the sample solutes. The ionic strength determines the electrokinetic potential (buffer and nonbuffer ions) and the effective final charges on the migrating solutes. Low ionic strength buffers allow high-migration velocities with little heat generated. High ionic strengths tend to produce lower migration velocities and sharper zone separation but also greater heat.

The most commonly used buffers for protein separation are univalent Tris-boric acid-ethylenediamine-tetraacetic acid (Tris-borate-EDTA) and barbital buffers at alkaline pH between 8 and 9. The ionic strength of a monovalent/divalent buffer system such as Tris-sulfate is three times the molar concentration of a univalent buffer, while univalent/trivalent buffers such as Tris-phosphate have an ionic strength six times that of a univalent buffer.

Multiphasic Buffer System

This type of buffer system, sometimes referred to as **discontinuous** (5, 11, 19), involves different buffers and/or gels and is used in techniques such as IEF and discontinuous electrophoresis. In discontinuous electrophoresis, slabs or tubes are stacked on each other to create a separation of solutes in two phases. In the first phase (top), a stacking or spacer gel is used in which sample components are first concentrated into narrow starting zones before they enter the lower gel. After stacking, electrophoresis continues in the second phase in a "small pore" or running gel in which separation is determined by charge and molecular mass. This system of stacked gels is able to achieve sharp zones and enhanced resolution of the components produced by the different properties of the gels and buffer discontinuities. The ionic activities are the same in the stacking and the running gels but the pH is different in each gel phase. The buffer in the electrode compartments is different from that in the gel phases. For example, a Tris-HCl buffer may be used in the gels while Tris-glycine buffer may surround the electrodes. By selecting the pH of each buffer, the mobilities of the chloride ions advance ahead of the sample components which are followed by the glycinate ions. Because the sample components have mobilities intermediate between the leading and trailing ions, the samples stack in layers in order of their respective mobilities based on their electric properties. When this moving boundary reaches the juncture between the stacking and the running gels, the sudden change in pH and pore size causes an "unstacking" so that the sample molecules move into a uniform voltage gradient at constant pH and then separate according to molecular weight.

Support Media

Agarose

Agarose is a polysaccharide derived from agar in seaweed with repeating units of 1→4 linked 3,6-anhydro-∀-L-galactopyranose and 1→3 linked ∃-D-pyranose (9). With the removal of the highly charged carboxylic acid and sulfate groups of agar that contribute to endosmotic effects, the resulting derivative, agarose, has a lower content of charged groups that contribute to undesirable endosmotic effects. Agarose is most often used as 1%–2% (w/v) solutions in barbital or Tris-borate-EDTA buffer at pH 8.6. Calcium salts may be added to increase ionic strength and improve resolution; however, the resolution by agarose gel electrophoresis is less than that of polyacrylamide since agarose has no sieving effects for separation of solutes by the differences in molecular sizes.

PAG

PAG is formed by combining the monomer acrylamide (CH_2=CH–CO–NH_2) with a monomeric cross-linking agent N, N′-methylenebisacrylamide (bis). As a result of the reaction, a network lattice of polyacrylamide units (CH_2=CH–CO–NH–CH_2–NH–CO–CH=CH_2) forms (9). The porosity or density of the lattice is determined by the concentrations of the acrylamide and bis. The polymerization of the monomers is initiated by the catalyst ammonium persulfate and accelerated by TEMED (as discussed previously in Separation Techniques).

Variations of acrylamide gel electrophoresis have been developed, most notably discontinuous electrophoresis and SDS electrophoresis. The original configuration used two rod-like gels stacked one above the other having different acrylamide concentrations and buffer systems. Various modifications of the original design have been developed, but the basic principle is unchanged. By this stacking arrangement, the constituents of the sample being electrophoresed can be separated in sharp zones. SDS, an anionic detergent that induces conformational changes of the proteins to which it binds, is added in PAG to estimate the molecular sizes of the separated components.

Starch Gel

Hydrolyzed starch was first used as an electrophoretic support in the 1950s and gave a major improvement in resolution over the filter paper medium that had been widely used up to that time. The disadvantage of starch is the unpredictable variability in the proportions of amylose and amylopectin in its hydrolyzed products. The pore size, gelling properties, and resolution of separated sample components are difficult to control due to the inconsistency of the pore sizes, which determine the molecular sieving properties of starch gels. Another disadvantage is the difficulty in scanning the semitransparent gel with an optical densitometer. For these reasons, the use of starch gels has declined in recent years and PAG electrophoresis has become the conventional electrophoresis method for molecular sizing applications. Starch gel electrophoresis is performed on horizontal slabs and is still used in some reference laboratories for abnormal hemoglobin classification and for isoenzyme studies.

Sample Loading

For applications using zone electrophoresis, samples are typically applied in microliter amounts directly onto the support matrix. The amount applied is determined by the concentration of solute. Commercial kits provide application aids that consist of precut applicators designed to assist, facilitate, and limit the manual or automatic application of sample through slotted, grooved, or dentated disposable templates. A dye is sometimes added to the sample as a visible indicator of sample application and the subsequent separation during electrophoresis. Preanalytical treatments of the sample such as dilution, concentration, or dialysis appropriate for certain types of samples, e.g., urine, whole blood, and cerebrospinal fluid, or for certain electrophoresis techniques, such as SDS-PAG electrophoresis may be required as determined by the specific application.

Visualization

Following the separation procedure, the components of interest must be detected, identified, and, as needed, quantitated. Proteins in solid supports are usually immobilized ("fixed") or precipitated in the gel matrix to minimize band-broadening (diffusion) by transferring the gel to a dilute solution of acid such as acetic, sulfosalicylic, or trichloroacetic, or an aqueous alcohol solution before proceeding to the staining steps. Modifications of the immobilization phase must be used if the functional activity of isoenzymes needs to be preserved for detection or if a detergent such as SDS, which interferes with some stains, is in the gel.

Various stains, dyes, and detector substances are used to localize the solute of interest following electrophoretic separation. A range of agents from all-purpose to highly specific can be used, depending on the purpose and the information expected from the electrophoretic technique. A list of stains commonly used with specific groups of substances is given in Table 2.

Amido Black 10B, Coomassie Blue 250, Ponceau S, and silver stain are among the most widely used protein stains (6, 11). Most proteins can be detected by a red color imparted by the all-purpose nucleic acid stain, Stains-All, the abbreviated name for 1-ethyl-2, 3-(1-ethylnaphtho-[1,2d]-thiazolin-2-ylidene)-2-methylpropenyl-naphth-[1,2d]-thiazolium bromide (11). Lipoproteins, glycoproteins, and phosphoproteins can be treated with agents that react specifically with the chemical group that is unique for that class of proteins. For example, the carbohydrates in glycoproteins can be localized by periodic-Schiff stain in an oxidation reaction that forms aldehydes that react with fuchsin dye. Lipoproteins can be detected with lipophilic (fat-binding) dyes. Isoforms of enzymes separated by electrophoresis can be localized in the gel strip by applying specific substrates that are converted to products that, in turn, can be coupled with color-forming reactions for detection. Stains-All is useful for detecting phosphoproteins which are stained blue, differentiating them from many other proteins which are colored red by this stain.

Another technique for localizing proteins and nucleic acids takes advantage of radioactive labels such as ^{125}I and ^{131}I which can be incorporated into the molecules. A piece of x-ray film is placed in contact with the electropherogram and then developed to reveal the position of the radioactively tagged molecule.

Problem Solving

The condition and maintenance of each component of the apparatus and the supplies (components of the gels and buffers) and the sample itself must be monitored carefully.

TABLE 2. Common stains for various electrophoresis applications

Analysis	Stain	Solid medium	Comment*
Protein	Amido Black 10B	Agarose	Widely used. One of the earliest protein stains for qualitative work. Detection = 1 µg/band.
	Coomassie Blue G250/R250	Agarose, PAG	10 times more sensitive than Amido Black. Can be used with SDS and ampholyte gels.
	Anilinonaphthalene sulfonate		Detection limit = 20 µg/band.
	Silver staining	PAG	Up to 50 times more sensitive than Coomassie Blue.
	Ponceau S	CA	General sensitivity. Specific for proteins.
Phosphoprotein	Stains—All	PAG	Stains most proteins red. Forms blue color with phosphoproteins. General sensitivity.
Hemoglobin	Ortho-dianisidine	PAG	Heme-specific stain.
	Ponceau S	CA	Protein-specific stain.
Lipoprotein	Oil Red O Sudan Black B	Agarose	
Isoenzymes			Enzyme activity measured as a product of hydrolyzed substrate.
Alkaline phosphatase	1-Naphtholphosphate and Fast Blue BB, at alkaline pH	PAG	
Amylase	Blue starch	CA, PAG	
Creatine kinase	NADP coupled with creatinine phosphate or nitroblue tetrazolium	Agarose	Fluorogenic product visualized with UV light or visible if tetrazolium is part of substrate mixture.
Glycoprotein	Periodic-Schiff	Agarose	Detection limit = 2–3 µg of carbohydrate.

*Detection limits and sensitivities are approximations, provided for comparison purposes only.
Key: PAG = polyacrylamide gel; CA = cellulose acetate. Sources: references 6 and 11 (p. 29).

Manufacturers of commercial systems provide problem-solving guides to assist the analyst in preventative monitoring and troubleshooting when adverse events interrupt the electrophoresis run. Some recommendations and suggestions are provided in Table 3.

QUANTITATION

The position, density, and width of each stained band on the gel are transformed to quantitatively interpretable information by densitometry or image analysis of the medium. The density and width of the individual bands stained represent the fraction of the total stained area in a specific lane as the matrix strip is moved through the optical path of the densitometer or image analyzer. The position of the band relative to other positions is determined by its mobility in the specific medium, as previously discussed.

TABLE 3. Frequently encountered technical problems* in electrophoresis (6)

Symptom	Cause	Suggested remedy
Little or no migration or current	Faulty power supply, bad electrical connections, electrodes incorrectly connected	Check the cables, connections, and polarity of the electrodes; clean the electrodes.
Current increasing with time	Electrode wicks incorrectly applied, incorrect electrode solutions	Check electrode polarity, check pH of electrode solutions.
Sparking or burning under or along edges of the gel	Faulty cooling plate, incorrect power on voltage setting, insufficient liquid between cooling plate and gel, electrode strips overhanging the edges of the gel	Check temperature of the system, check all power supply settings in advance.
Bands uneven, diffused, or streaked	Salt concentration in the sample too high, dirty electrodes, old electrode solution, overapplication (overloading) of sample onto gel, electrode wicks not unevenly wetted, gel too wet	Remove salts by dialysis or dilute the sample, clean the electrodes, prepare/use fresh buffer solutions, apply smaller sample volume or dilute the sample, wet the strips evenly, blot the gel as recommended.
Apparent loss of bands	Protein not fixed after separation and before staining, sample unstable at the application site	Use the correct or recommended fixative procedure, check that the pH is compatible with the sample.
Unstained spots in the stained pattern	Sample too concentrated in the application volume	Dilute the sample with a compatible diluent or apply less sample.

*Additional source: Laboratory manual, LKB 2117 Multiphor II electrophoresis system, LKB Produkter AAB, Bromma, Sweden, 1986.

Densitometry refers to the method of measurement performed by an instrument that determines the amount of light absorbed by the stained bands in relation to the distance traversed along the horizontal axis of the tracing (2). The absorbance value of the separated components is transformed into interpretable values (percentage and concentration units) by a microprocessor or computer by scaled integration of the area under each peak of the tracing.

Information about the separated components in samples analyzed by electrophoresis for clinical interpretation is usually expressed as the individual percentages of the total protein and as concentrations (Figure 6). In the examples depicted in Figure 6 for the quantified fractions of total protein in serum, the concentration of each fraction in concentration units (grams per deciliter) was derived from the percentage value of the respective fraction.

The densitometer includes the basic components of a photometer: light source, monochromator, photodetector, and a motor-driven stage to support the medium while the mechanical stage moves it through the beam of light. Integrating the area under each peak, which corresponds to the stained band, is directly related to its proportion of the total stained areas. The support medium must have a clear background for the optical system to differentiate between nonspecific staining and the stain that is protein-bound.

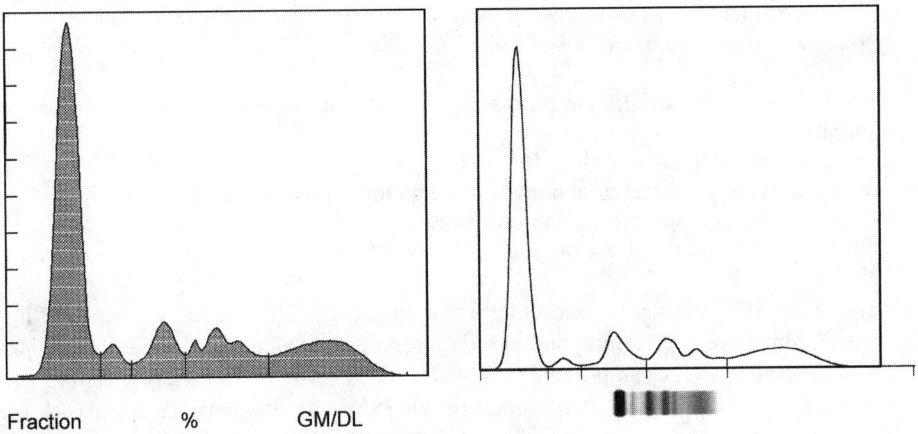

Fraction	%	GM/DL
Albumin	54.27	3.96
Alpha 1	4.25	0.31
Alpha 2	10.07	0.74
Beta	14.58	1.06
Gamma	16.82	1.23
Total protein		7.30

Fractions	%	g/dl
Albumin	58.1	4.13
Alpha 1	2.4	0.17
Alpha 2	10.9	0.77
Beta	13.2	0.94
Gamma	15.4	1.09
Total protein		7.10

FIGURE 6. Serum protein electrophoresis tracing and report produced by a conventional densitometer (left panel) compared with the enhanced tracing and report generated by a digital image analyzer (right panel). The digital analyzer is capable of inserting an image of the gel pattern on the report.

Important features for a clinical laboratory densitometer used for quantitative interpretation of zone electrophoresis gels include the following (2):

- Ability to scan patterns on gels up to 150 mm in length
- Automatic and manual gain control to allow the instrument or the operator to adjust the most intensely stained band (scanned peak) from going off-scale
- Automatic and manual zeroing of absorbance for nonspecific background correction, which allows the lowest amount of stain in the electrophoretogram to be set as the baseline, preventing minor peaks from being cut-off and lost
- Variable wavelength control, either by a continuously variable monochromator or by selectable interference filters, to allow operation in the 400–700-nm range
- Variable slits to allow adjustment of the width of the light beam
- Computerized integration and printed report

The digital image analyzer, employed for complex DNA analysis, has been introduced successfully in recent years into clinical laboratories for routine electrophoresis applications. This type of gel analyzer stores images collected by a flat-bed scanner as two-dimensional accumulations of picture elements (pixels) (24). The image of the pattern is obtained by light transmission and converted to absorbance scale. Depending on the software and hardware utilized, the image analyzer can scan multiple gels simultaneously and process the data in minutes for high-efficiency throughput. Like modern automated densitometers, flat-bed scanners and image analyzers require compatible computers to store, manage, and manipulate the large amounts of data extracted from the analysis of stained patterns. The tasks performed by the software created for the specific electrophoresis application may include various options such as:

- Specific algorithms, depending on the application, for quantitative analysis of patient samples
- Data analysis for quality control
- Ability to overlay normal or abnormal tracings for comparison
- Ability to enlarge, enhance, or sharpen images
- Ability to delete minimal or nonspecific fractions

Additional capabilities such as recording, displaying, recalling records, storing, labeling, inserting interpretive comments, and printing reports are valuable features. A printed report of the pattern of the sample acquired by a conventional densitometer compared with an enhanced (the inserted gel pattern) report provided by a digital image analyzer is shown in Figure 6.

In the selection of an automated densitometer or image analysis equipment, the user must consider the sample identification information and degree of enhancement that will be required. Unless a moderate-to-high number of samples (>30/day) will be processed, costs may outweigh the benefits of commercial digital image analyzer systems that include the compatible flat-bed scanner, desktop computer, and software for analysis.

CLINICAL CONSIDERATIONS USING ELECTROPHORETIC METHODS

Analytes

The most valuable clinical use of electrophoresis is for the detection and quantitation of abnormal gamma globulins in serum and urine. Other important applications of electrophoresis in laboratory medicine for diagnosis and management of clinical disorders include the detection and/or quantitation of the following substances: hemoglobin variants in blood; isoenzymes of alkaline phosphatase, lactate dehydrogenase, and creatine kinase in serum; alpha-1-antitrypsin (an alpha-1-globulin) in serum; lipoproteins in serum; and oligoclonal bands of gamma globulin in cerebrospinal fluid. The significance of these analytes in health and disease are discussed in other chapters of this publication.

Immunofixation electrophoresis (IFE) and **immunoblotting** are two special techniques widely used for the identification of specific proteins having clinical relevance. These techniques are described briefly in the following paragraphs.

IFE is an immunochemical method based on direct immunoprecipitation of proteins in a thin agarose gel matrix. It is used to identify the class of heavy and light chains of discrete bands observed on electropherograms of gels or CE. IFE has superceded immunoelectrophoresis for laboratory evaluation of monoclonal proteins in the diagnosis and management of plasma cell dyscrasias such as multiple myeloma.

This technique is performed in two phases. First, the serum or urine sample, after appropriate dilution or concentration, is applied on the agarose gel at the origin of six lanes marked TP (or other convenient designation for total protein), G, A, M, kappa, and lambda. The proteins are then separated by electrophoresis. In the second phase, a protein fixative is applied to the TP lane to immobilize the proteins at the positions where they migrated. To each of the other lanes, a heavy-chain- or light-chain-specific antiserum is applied over the designated lane to react with and precipitate the immunoglobin antigen, in an antigen–antibody complex. After the excess protein is washed away, the immune complex in the matrix is stained. Interpretation is made by comparing the immunofixed precipitate with the discrete band seen on the sample in the TP lane (Figure 7).

The advantages of IFE include the technical ease, sensitivity, and speed of the procedure that allows specific identification of monoclonal immunoglobulin heavy and/or light chains. The disadvantage of IFE is the need for optimizing the amount of antigen by dilution or concentration of the original sample. Another disadvantage is that no control is run on the same gel for comparison with the patient sample.

Immunoblots are immunoreactions in which a protein is immobilized on a synthetic membrane and probed for the antigen of interest with a specific antibody conjugated with a reporter molecule, e.g., an enzyme. Immunoblotting takes advantage of the high-resolution property of PAG. It is particularly useful for applications involving the nucleic acids DNA and RNA, where there is insufficient antigen in the sample to produce an easily detectable immunoprecipitate. High-sensitivity detection methods that can be used with immunoblotting include ligand probes as well as antigen–antibody reactions that can be visualized by protein stains and by enzymatic reactions using appropriate substrates that produce a detectable chromagen.

Immunoblotting consists of at least five steps (25), which are summarized briefly:

1. Antigen is immobilized onto a synthetic membrane after being transferred from the original electrophoresis gel or after direct application.
2. Unoccupied binding sites on the membrane are blocked to prevent nonspecific binding.
3. The blot is probed with a specific antibody for the antigen of interest.
4. Another antibody conjugated with a label that can be detected is added.
5. The labeled antigen–antibody–antibody complex is made visible.

A solid material such as nitrocellulose or charged nylon-based membrane is the typical surface, and transfer is carried out by applying an electric current or by capillary action. The original pattern of separated proteins is thus replicated on the receiving material, then immobilized, and probed in steps following the application or transfer. Depending on the

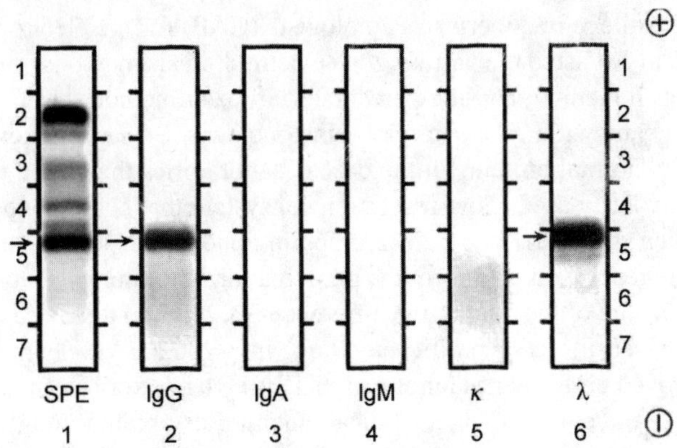

FIGURE 7. Immunofixation electrophoresis (IFE) of serum performed on an agarose gel. IFE is one of the most valuable applications of zone electrophoresis in clinical laboratory medicine for the detection of monoclonal proteins. Separation of total protein in the serum is shown in lane 1 (SPE) with albumin at the top closest to the anode (+) followed by the globulin fractions alpha-1, alpha-2, beta-1, beta-2, and gamma. A discrete abnormal protein, indicated by the arrow just below the beta-2 fraction, is identified as immunoglobulin (Ig)G-lambda by an immunoprecipitation reaction with specific antisera for immunoglobulin heavy (G, A, M) and light (kappa and lambda) chains.

apparatus used, as many as 800 different reactions can be performed on a single membrane. A detailed stepwise account of the immunoblotting procedure which requires a high level of skill and involves several labor-intensive steps, special blotting supplies, and apparatus is given elsewhere (25).

Quality Control

Quality control criteria apply to electrophoresis just as they do for other laboratory testing methods in the same category of high complexity. Quality control materials for various electrophoresis techniques can be purchased from commercial suppliers in a variety of stabilized forms including liquid, frozen, or lyophilized. Alternatively or in addition to commercial materials, controls may be prepared from a pool of samples accumulated within the laboratory, filtered, divided into small portions, tightly sealed, and frozen at –70 °C or below for long-term stability. Stable controls or other mixtures of known composition (markers), regardless of the source, should be included with electrophoretic separations of test samples to detect systematic errors or changes in running conditions that would affect the results of the test sample. One exception in the clinical laboratory is the IFE procedure in which no controls are included on the same gel. The concern is a valid one: if there is no precipitate in the patient sample, one cannot be certain that the correct antiserum or dilution was applied.

In addition to internal quality control procedures for electrophoresis, external quality assessment programs are available which are sponsored by the manufacturers of control materials and by professional laboratory organizations. Such programs periodically distribute sets of samples to the participating laboratories to be analyzed with the routine daily workloads that include controls and patient samples. The results are returned to the sponsoring agent and data analysis summaries are subsequently returned to the participating laboratories. The quality of the performance of individual laboratories can be compared within laboratory peer groups, categorized by methods and instrumentation.

Summary reports of the proficiency testing programs frequently provide informative and practical discussions related to the clinical significance of the analytes, the methods of analyses, and analytical problems and ways to solve them. For example, a summary report published by the College of American Pathologists (CAP) for the electrophoresis surveys conducted in 2001 (26) listed the various zone electrophoresis methods, the number of laboratories using each method, and the percentages of each method that failed to detect an abnormal protein band within the beta-globulin zone. Only 36% of participating laboratories detected the abnormal protein. Of the 64% of laboratories that failed to see the abnormal protein, the majority used a low-resolution gel system that could not provide a distinct separation between the beta-1 and beta-2 globulin zones. The purpose of the discussion accompanying the report was to inform the participating laboratories using gel-based electrophoresis to be aware of the qualitative differences of gels and to advise them of relevant information published in the scientific literature. In a 2002 CAP electrophoresis survey report (27), improved performance among participating laboratories can be extracted from the data provided, reflecting the value clinical laboratories obtain through participation in professionally sponsored external control programs.

Current Trends

Gel-Based Systems

The distinction between low-resolution (LR) and high-resolution (HR) techniques is defined operationally. LR gels are those such as cellulose acetate and some agarose gels that produce only five-band patterns without a crisp separation of beta-1 and beta-2 bands, referred to in the preceding paragraph. Such gels were considered a poor choice for clinical laboratories (17). Improved separation can be achieved on the so-called HR gels that provide six-band separation for a sharp delineation of beta-1 and beta-2 globulins. Such systems generally include a temperature control along with modifications of the agarose buffer and the stain. Even higher resolution (10–12 bands) can be obtained on special formulations of agarose gels electrophoresed with temperature control. Electrophoresis performed in small-bore capillaries, e.g., capillary electrophoresis is considered to be a HR system.

Automated Electrophoresis Systems

Since the mid-1990s, the U.S. Food and Drug Administration (FDA) has cleared for marketing commercial semiautomated electrophoresis systems from two vendors, Sebia (Issy-les-Moulineaux, France) and Helena Laboratories (Beaumont, TX) using agarose gels for zone electrophoresis. In addition, automated CE systems manufactured by Beckman Coulter (Brea, CA), and Sebia are currently FDA-approved for clinical laboratories. Each system uses the respective manufacturer's kits (gels or capillaries, buffers, stains, and other supplies), procedures, software, and hardware. A choice of gels for quality of resolution, either low resolution or high resolution as already defined is available from the respective manufacturer.

The semiautomated systems perform the processing of the gels under software-controlled conditions. Once the operator loads the samples according to the manufacturer's instructions for the electrophoresis, staining, destaining, and drying of the gels are automatically carried out under the conditions specified by the hardware and software. Transfer of the stained gel to a densitometer or digital image analyzer for quantitation is done manually. Editing of the pattern tracing, which can include adjustment of the baseline and making decisions about marking bands that may or may not be abnormal, require the operator's judgment and intervention. Thus an experienced reviewer must examine and interpret the patterns on the gel in conjunction with the quantified tracings.

Semiautomated systems provide several advantages including minimal training and technical skill, user-friendly operation of equipment, reproducibility and quality of results independent of operator skill, and the convenience of disposable supplies. Disadvantages include manual preparation of samples and expensive equipment and supplies. These systems are designed for high-volume testing and may not be feasible in small laboratory settings. The notable disadvantages for the use of CE in clinical laboratories concerns the sample type. Only serum can be used; urine cannot be conveniently assayed due to interfering urinary salts and other metabolites. In addition, CE may not be cost-efficient for laboratories performing less than 40 serum samples a day (17, 28).

Despite many recent improvements such as the quality of gels (resolution) and labor-saving automation, questions and practical concerns unique to electrophoresis will probably continue to require the interpretation and judgment by experienced, well-informed laboratorians.

ACKNOWLEDGMENT

The author gratefully acknowledges Mr. James Nicholson, Research Image Core Facility, Department of Pathology and Laboratory Medicine, Medical University of South Carolina, for expert assistance with the production of the figures in this chapter.

REFERENCES

1. Tiselius A. A new apparatus for electrophoretic analysis of colloidal mixtures. Trans Faraday Soc 1937;33:524–31.
2. Karcher RE, Nuttall KL. Electrophoresis. In: Burtis CA, Ashwood ER, eds. Tietz textbook of clinical chemistry, 3rd ed. Philadelphia: WB Saunders, 1999:150–63.
3. Wians FH Jr, Baskin LB. Electrophoretic methods for the evaluation of proteins in human body fluids. Diagnostic endocrinology and metabolism. 1998:16(12):371–83. American Association for Clinical Chemistry, Inc.
4. Smithies O. Zone electrophoresis in starch gels: group variations in serum proteins of normal human adults. Biochem J 1955;61:629–41.
5. Davis BJ. Disc electrophoresis II. Method and application to human serum proteins. Ann NY Acad Sci 1964;121:404–27.
6. Brewer JM. Electrophoresis. In: Kaplan LA, Pesce AJ, eds. Clinical chemistry: theory, analysis, and correlation, 3rd ed. St. Louis: Mosby-Year Book, 1996:199–212.
7. Landers JP. Clinical capillary electrophoresis. Clin Chem 1995;41:495–509.
8. Garfin DE. Electrophoretic methods. In: Glasel JA, Deutscher MP, eds. Introduction to biophysical methods for protein and nucleic acid research. San Diego: Academic Press, 1995:53–109.
9. Allen RC, Sarvis CA, Maurer HR. Gel electrophoresis and isoelectric focusing of proteins: selected techniques. New York: de Gryter, 1984.
10. Cawley LP, Minard B, Penn GM. Electrophoresis and immunochemical reactions in gels: techniques and interpretations, 2nd ed. Chicago: American Society of Clinical Pathologists, 1978:1–5.
11. Andrews AT. Electrophoresis: theory, techniques, and biochemical and clinical applications, 2nd ed. New York: Oxford University Press, 1986.
12. Papadea C. Amino acids and proteins. In: Christenson RH, Gregory LC, Johnson LJ, eds. Appleton & Lange's outline review clinical chemistry. New York: McGraw-Hill, 2001:51–70.
13. Wunderly CH. Paper electrophoresis. In: Bier M, ed. Electrophoresis, theory, methods, and applications. New York: Academic Press, 1959:179–223.
14. Kunkel HB, Trautman R. Zone electrophoresis in various types of supporting media. In: Bier M, ed. Electrophoresis, theory, methods, and applications. New York: Academic Press, 1959: 225–62.
15. Jorgenson JW, Lukacs KD. Free zone electrophoresis in glass capillaries. Clin Chem 1981;27:1551–3.
16. Issaq HJ. A decade of capillary electrophoresis. Electrophoresis 2000;21:1921–39.
17. Keren DF. Procedures for the evaluation of monoclonal immunoglobulins. Arch Pathol Lab Med 1999;123:126–32.
18. Christenson RH, Anderson FP. Separation techniques. In: Christenson RH, Gregory L, Johnson L, eds. Appleton & Lange's outline review clinical chemistry. New York: McGraw-Hill, 2001: 323–35.
19. Ornstein L. Disc electrophoresis I. Background and theory. Ann NY Acad Sci 1964;121:321–49.
20. Hrkal Z, Gel-type techniques. In: Deyl Z, Everaerts FM, Prusik Z, Svendsend PJ, eds. Electrophoresis: a survey of techniques and applications (Journal of Chromatography Library, vol 18, part A, Techniques). New York: Elsevier, 1979:113–31.
21. Hockstrasser DF, Tissat J-D. Clinical applications of high-resolution two-dimensional polyacrylamide gel electrophoresis. Adv Electrophoresis 1993;6:270–375.
22. Anderson NG, Anderson NL. Twenty years of two-dimensional electrophoresis: past, present, and future. Electrophoresis 1996;17:443–53.
23. Thormann W, Wey AB, Lurie IS, Gerber H, Byland C, Malik N, et al. Capillary electrophoresis in clinical and forensic analysis: recent advances and breakthrough to routine applications. Electrophoresis 1999;20:3203–36.
24. Horgan G, Glasby CA. Uses of digital image analysis in electrophoresis. Electrophoresis 1995;16:298–305.

25. Ledue TB, Garfin DE. Immunofixation and immunoblotting. In: Rose NR, deMacario EC, Fold JD, Lane HC, Nakamura RM, eds. Manual of clinical laboratory immunology, 5th ed. Washington DC: ASM Press, 1997:54–74.
26. College of American Pathologists Survey Report, Electrophoresis, ELP-B, Northfield, Ill: College of American Pathologists, 2001.
27. College of American Pathologists Survey Report, Electrophoresis, ELP-A, Northfield, Ill: College of American Pathologists, 2002.
28. Keren DF. Capillary zone electrophoresis in the evaluation of serum protein abnormalities. Am J Clin Pathol 1998;110:248–52.

Chapter 9

Chemistry Analyzers

William L. Roberts

Great advances have been made in replacing many manual tasks performed in the process of clinical chemistry testing with instrumentation commonly referred to as clinical chemistry analyzers. The International Union of Pure and Applied Chemistry (IUPAC) has defined **automation** as the replacement of human manipulative effort and facilities in the performance of a given process by mechanical and instrumental devices that are regulated by feedback of information so that an apparatus is self-monitoring or self-adjusting (1). Based on this definition, no current clinical chemistry analyzer can be considered truly automated. However, many parts of the analytical process performed by clinical chemistry analyzers do meet the definition of automation. A number of terms can be used to describe more specifically different parts of the analytical process and the operation of instrumentation. Many of these terms are defined in the following section.

DEFINITION OF TERMS

The **analyzer configuration** is the format in which the analytical instrument is configured. In practice, an automated analyzer can be configured by the manufacturer as either an integrated or a modular system (2). Both **open** and **closed** systems are available. Open systems have operator-modifiable assay parameters and reagents can be purchased from more than one source. Closed systems have parameters set by the manufacturer and reagents are in a unique format or container and are generally only available from the instrument manufacturer.

Several terms can be used to describe how samples are analyzed. **Batch analysis** specifies a type of analysis in which a number of specimens are processed in the same analytical session or **run** (3). **Single-channel analysis** is a type of analysis in which each specimen is subjected to a single process so that only results for a single analyte are produced. In contrast, **multiple-channel analysis** is a type of analysis in which each specimen is subjected to multiple analytical processes so that a set of test results is obtained on a single specimen. **Continuous-flow analysis** indicates that each specimen in the batch passes through the same continuous stream and is subjected to the same analytical reactions as every other specimen and at the same rate. **Discrete analysis** indicates that each specimen in a batch has its own physical and chemical space separate from every other specimen. In contrast to continuous-flow analysis, **discretionary multiple-channel analysis** indicates that each specimen can be analyzed by any one or by more than one of the available processes, referred to as methods or channels, as a result of specimen-specific commands from the processing system. **Random-access analysis** specifies that any specimen, by a command to the processing system, can be analyzed by any available process in or out of sequence with other specimens and without regard to their initial order. **Parallel analysis** indicates that all specimens are subjected to a series of analytical processes at the same time in a parallel fashion.

The **dwell time** is the amount of time from when sample is first aspirated until the final measurement cycle is completed for a specimen. The **specimen throughput rate** is the rate at which an analytical system processes specimens. In most multiple-channel, random-access systems, this parameter is independent of the reaction times of the chemistry procedures; instead, it depends on a fixed sequence of events involving mechanical operations and optical measurement cycles (2).

HISTORY OF AUTOMATED CHEMISTRY ANALYZERS

At the start of the twentieth century, the discipline of clinical chemistry emerged into its own in American medical practice (4). Two individuals dominated this period: Otto Folin and Donald Van Slyke. They developed practical and clinically useful manual methods for the analysis of blood and urine. Some of the early quantitative assays included a colorimetric urine creatinine assay employing a Duboscq-type visual colorimeter, a volumetric carbon dioxide gas analysis apparatus, and a protein-free ultrafiltrate method for blood glucose determinations. The Duboscq-type colorimeter was the mainstay of the clinical chemistry laboratory for nearly five decades and in 1939 was described as "still the most versatile and useful instrument" for colorimetric chemical analysis (5). By the early 1960s, a photometer was used for all colorimetric methods.

As a result of concerns over the quality of results, Skeggs (6) began to design an automated single-channel analyzer that would perform analyses without error. The first automated analyzer for a single colorimetric method was described in 1957 (7). A multichannel analyzer was described in 1964 that was capable of analyzing 20 samples per hour (8). The introduction of the SMA 12/60 analyzer a short time later revolutionized the clinical chemistry laboratory. It was capable of analyzing 60 samples per hour for 12 analytes. The introduction of this analyzer meant that one person could perform most of the routine chemistry testing for a large hospital in one shift (6). The major limitation of these early sequential automated analyzers was that every sample was analyzed for every analyte, even if the physician only needed a result for one of them. The first commercial centrifugal analyzer was introduced in 1970 as an alternative to continuous-flow technology, which had significant carry-over problems and wasted reagents (9). One of the first published papers on this technology measured alkaline phosphatase (10). The second generation of these instruments was available in 1975 and was much improved over the earlier generation in terms of both computer miniaturization and high-grade polymer cuvets. Another major advance in clinical chemistry analyzers occurred in 1970 with the introduction of the DuPont Automated Clinical Chemistry Analyzer (aca®). It was a discrete analyzer with random-access capabilities that permitted stat specimen testing (9).

Many improvements have been made since the first automated analyzers. These developments have been reviewed (11). The remainder of this chapter describes the current state of the art for commercial clinical chemistry analyzers. Recent consolidation of in vitro diagnostics companies has resulted in fewer vendors to choose from. Currently there are seven companies manufacturing automated, medium-to-high volume clinical chemistry analyzers for the U.S. market. It is noteworthy that Abbott Aeroset® and

ARCHITECT® analyzers are manufactured jointly with Toshiba Corp., the Bayer ADVIA® chemistry analyzers are manufactured jointly with JEOL, Ltd., and the Roche MODULAR® chemistry analyzers are manufactured jointly with Hitachi.

BASIC ANALYZER OPERATIONS

The analytical process can be divided into four distinct operations: sampling, processing, reaction, and computation (12, 13). Fifty years ago, all of these operations were performed manually. Over time more and more of these operations have been mechanized by refinements in analyzer design. Chemistry analyzers developed since 1990 perform most if not all of these operations. A survey of features of clinical chemistry analyzers designed for medium- and high-volume laboratories was recently performed and results from this article are summarized in Table 1 (14). A list of vendors and contact information is presented in Table 2. When evaluating current commercial analyzers, some unique features of individual analyzers are apparent. These unique features will be highlighted in the following sections as the basic operating features are described. A picture of an Olympus chemistry analyzer is shown in Figure 1 to illustrate the overall layout of the component parts and how they can be spatially related to one another.

Sample Handling

When the process of sample handling is examined in more detail, a number of operations can be defined. First, the sample is placed on the analyzer in a loading zone. The sample can be held in a variety of carriers including five- or 10-position racks or in a large carousel that can hold 100 or more samples. The use of five- or 10-position sample racks provides a more convenient method to load samples as they arrive at the analyzer. Several analyzers can hold a maximum of 200–300 samples using these racks. The carousel sample rack can be more convenient for large batches of samples that are run infrequently. Another feature found on most analyzers is the ability to insert new samples ahead of samples already loaded. This can be accomplished through a dedicated entry port or by a special rack. These samples are given priority over samples already on the analyzer for sampling and analysis so that the results can be reported more rapidly.

A sample can be identified either by its position on the analyzer or by a specimen bar code. Nearly all contemporary chemistry analyzers read the specimen bar-code label, if present, close to the time sample is aspirated. This permits positive sample identification and allows the analyzer to query the laboratory information system (LIS) about what testing to perform. Most chemistry analyzers are designed to work with primary blood collection tubes. Typically, these tubes contain a polymeric gel layer that separates the serum or plasma layer from the cellular components during centrifugation. The cap from the primary tube is removed prior to placing the sample on the analyzer and the analyzer removes an aliquot directly from the primary tube. For "short" samples from adults or pediatric samples, disposable sample cups designed to minimize dead volume, analyte absorption, and sample evaporation can be used. Calcium has been shown to absorb onto the walls of some polystyrene cups, causing clinically significant lowering of the calcium result (15). Evaporation of specimen from cups on the analyzer that are waiting to be sampled may cause analytical errors as great as 50% over 4 hours (16). Covers that minimize both sample and reagent evaporation have been described (17). In addition to sample absorption and evaporation, certain sample components can undergo degradation. Photolabile components such as bilirubin are destroyed by exposure to light. Photodegradation can be

TABLE 1. Features for selected clinical chemistry analyzers*

Vendor	Abbott Diagnostics Aeroset	Abbott Diagnostics ARCHITECT c8000	Bayer ADVIA 1650	Beckman Coulter SYNCHRON LX20 Pro	Dade Behring Dimension RxL	Olympus America AU640e	Ortho-Clinical Diagnostics VITROS 950	Roche COBAS INTEGRA 800	Roche Diagnostics P module
First year sold in U.S.	1998	2002	1999	2001	1997	2002	1995	2001	1998
Number of assays onboard simultaneously	59	68	49	41/71	48/95	51	75	72	47
Number of open channels	100	220	62	41/71	10	95	Closed system	Utility channels available	5
Number of ion-selective electrode channels	3	3	3	5	4	3	3	4	3
Requires DI water system connection	Yes	Yes	Yes	Yes	Yes	Yes	No	Yes	Yes
Minimum sample volume aspirated	2 µL	2 µL	2 µL	3 µL	2 µL	1 µL	6 µL	2 µL	2 µL
Pediatric sample cup dead volume	50 µL	50 µL	50 µL	40 µL	20 µL	Not available	30 µL	50 µL	50 µL

Primary tube cap piercing	No	No	No	Yes	No	No	No	No	No
Minimum final reaction volume	160 µL	160 µL	80 µL	210 µL	350 µL	150 µL	Not applicable	200 µL	180 µL
Short sample detection	Yes	Yes	Yes	Yes	Yes	Yes	Yes	Yes	Yes
Clot detection	No	Yes	Yes	Yes	Yes	Yes	Yes	Yes	No
Index measurements	Yes	Yes	Yes	Yes	No	Yes	No	No	Yes
Automatic patient sample dilution and retest	Yes	Yes	Yes	Yes	Yes	Yes	No	Yes	Yes
Uses LOINC codes to transmit orders and results	No	No	Yes	No	No	No	No	No	No
Onboard test automatic inventory	Yes	Yes	Yes	Yes	Yes	Yes	Yes	Yes	Yes
Automatic startup programmable	Yes	Yes	Yes	Not required	Yes	Yes	No	Yes	Yes
Remote trouble-shooting by modem	No	Yes	Yes	Yes	Yes	Yes	No	Yes	Yes

*Information obtained from reference 14 and directly from vendors.

TABLE 2. Contact information for vendors of mid- and high-volume clinical chemistry analyzers*

Vendor	Abbott Diagnostics	Bayer Corp., Diagnostics Div.	Beckman Coulter Inc.	Dade Behring Inc.	Olympus America Inc.	Ortho Clinical Diagnostics	Roche Diagnostics
Street address*	100 Abbott Park Rd.	511 Benedict Ave.	200 South Kraemer Blvd.	P.O. Box 6101	Two Corporate Center Dr.	1001 U.S. Highway 202	9115 Hague Road
City, state,	Abbott Park IL	Tarrytown NY	Brea CA	Newark DE	Melville NY	Raritan NJ	Indianapolis IN
zip code	60031	10591	92822-8000	19714-6101	11747	08869	46250
Phone	(800) 323-9100	(914) 333-6122	(800) 526-3821	(302) 631-6000	(800) 223-0125	(800) 828-6316	(800) 428-5074
E-mail	www.abbott.com	www.bayerds.com	www.beckmancoulter.com	www.dadebehring.com	www.olympus.com	www.orthoclinical.com	us.labsystems.roche.com
Analyzers	i-Stat Aeroset ARCHITECT c8000	ADVIA 1650 ADVIA 2400	SYNCHRON CX4 SYNCHRON CX5 SYNCHRON CX9 SYNCHRON LX20 SYNCHRON LX4201 Regular and "Pro" lines are available	Dimension AR Dimension ARx Dimension Xpand Dimension RxL	AU400e AU640e AU2700 AU5400	VITROS DT60 VITROS 250 VITROS 950	COBAS Mira Plus COBAS INTEGRA 400 VITROS 800 Hitachi 902 Hitachi 912 P Module D Module

*Information obtained from references 14 and 32.

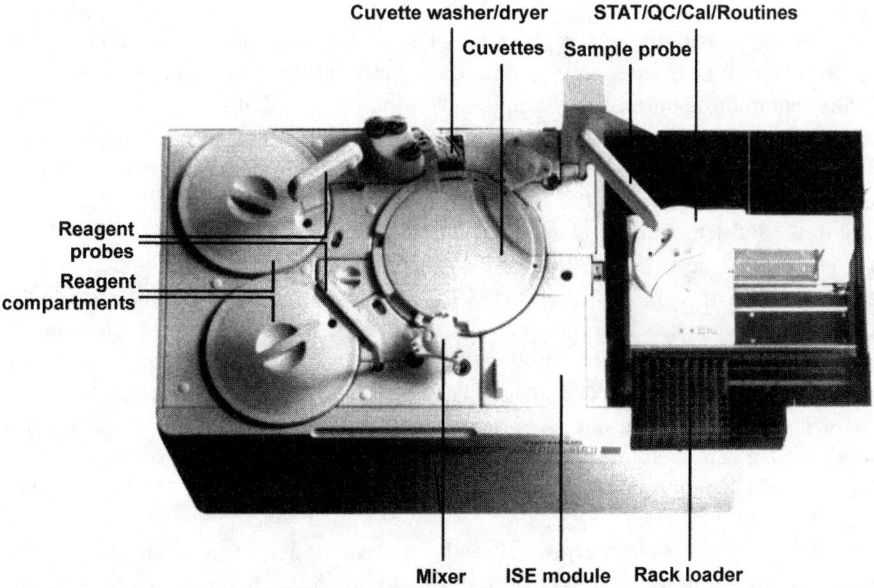

FIGURE 1. Schematic of Olympus analyzer. (*Courtesy of Olympus America*)

reduced by the use of smoke-colored plastic covers over the specimens. Some smaller specialized analyzers are designed to use whole blood specimens without centrifugation for certain analytes such as electrolytes for which very rapid result reporting is required (18). These analytes, which include sodium, potassium, and unbound calcium, are generally measured with ion-selective electrodes.

A positive-displacement pipet is used for sample handling. It consists of a glass or plastic syringe with a Teflon®-tipped plunger. Careful control of the speed with which the pipet plunger is moved is required for both aspiration and delivery. When liquid is used as the displacement medium, liquid-displacement pipets are capable of highly reproducible measurement of serum. Pipets may be categorized as fixed, variable, or selectable volume. Variable systems are most commonly used and can allow as many as one hundred 1-μL increments to be used in a pipet with a maximum delivery volume of 100 μL. The size of the sample in part determines the reagent volume that may be used in a system since the ratio of sample to reagent typically determines the analytic measurement range for a particular analyte. Inaccuracy and imprecision in the delivery of sample should not exceed 1%. Reagent delivery pipets require similar precision and accuracy (2).

Most analyzers use a permanent sample probe that is washed between samples. Obviously, carry-over between samples should be minimized. This is an even greater concern for analytes whose concentrations vary over several orders of magnitude such as C-reactive protein. Carry-over can be quantified by the procedure described in the National Committee for Clinical Laboratory Standards guideline (19). Carry-over studies have been performed on the Bayer ADVIA 1650 analyzer (20). Sample probe carry-over and predilution tray carry-over were not detectable under the conditions used (<20 ppm). High-speed video analysis has been used on the ARCHITECT c8000 analyzer to optimize the sample probe wash. The most significant variables that influence carry-over are sample volume and the wash sequence and duration of the internal and external sample probe washes. After balancing critical system variables, the between-sample carry-over was less than 0.1 ppm with minimal compromise to specimen throughput (21). The VITROS®

system uses a disposable sample probe tip that is changed after each sample. This feature minimizes the possibility of sample carry-over and eliminates the possibility of a probe clogged by a clot from one sample affecting aspiration from subsequent samples.

One common feature of the sample aspiration process that many analyzers utilize is clot detection. If clots are present in the sample, they may clog the sample probe, decrease the amount of sample aspirated, and lead to erroneously low results. It is noteworthy that two contemporary analyzers, the Abbott Aeroset and the Roche MODULAR, do not currently have clot detection but the ARCHITECT c8000 and COBAS INTEGRA® analyzers from these same vendors do have clot detection capabilities. The clot detection and pressure-monitoring capabilities of the ARCHITECT c8000 analyzer have been described (22). The c8000 analyzes aspirations and internal probe wash functions for clots and semi-obstructions within the sample probe. Pressure in the sample probe is measured by a piezoresistive pressure transducer that converts mechanical energy to electric voltage. The electrical output of the transducer is processed by electronic circuitry to evaluate the pressure within the sample tubing and determine if the aspirated sample would cause a probe obstruction and possible test result error. This system was optimized to allow aspirations of samples with a viscosity of ≤5 centipoises to be "good" unclotted samples. In laboratory simulations, this system performed well. Final validation in the clinical laboratory is still necessary. However, this subsystem should improve the integrity of sample test results.

Transmission of infectious agents by automated analyzers is a concern for clinical laboratories (23). Serum can splatter during the acquisition of sample from rapidly moving specimen probes (24). One unique feature of a few chemistry analyzers is the option of **closed tube sampling**. Although this sampling technique is commonly found on hematology analyzers, the Beckman SYNCHRON LX®20 Pro and LX4201 Pro are the only current chemistry analyzers that have this feature. Historically, the Dade Paramax, which is no longer manufactured, also had this feature. There are two major advantages of closed tube sampling. First, labor is reduced since the need for both decapping and recapping is eliminated. Second, the likelihood of a sample spill is greatly reduced. Since this feature has only recently been introduced, little information is available about what problems, if any, may occur using this approach in the high-volume production setting of a clinical laboratory.

Another unique feature of some analyzers is the **predilution** of a relatively large amount of sample and then distribution of the diluted sample for multiple tests. This feature is found on the Bayer ADVIA 1650 and 2400 analyzers. Basically, a patient sample is diluted 1:5 with saline (30-μL sample plus 120-μL of saline). This provides enough diluted sample for up to 15 test results. The predilution tray holds 120 dilution cups. The advantages of this approach include the ability to perform repeat testing without additional sampling from the primary tube and reduced reagent usage by analyzing smaller volumes of diluted sample while maintaining accurate pipetting. In fact the ADVIA 1650 has a minimum final reaction volume that is 47% less than its nearest competitor (Table 1). The associated reduction in reagent usage can decrease reagent costs substantially.

Chemical Analysis

After sample is aspirated from the primary tube or sample cup, it is introduced into the analyzer for analysis. A number of assay methodologies can be employed, depending on the analyte. Potentiometry can be performed using ion-selective electrodes for either direct or indirect analysis of several ions including sodium, potassium, chloride, calcium, total carbon dioxide, and lithium. Valinomycin and monensin derivatives are commonly used ionophores for potassium and sodium, respectively. Photometric assays for divalent cations such as calcium and magnesium, albumin and total protein, and a number of enzymes and drugs using enzyme immunoassay can also be performed. Turbidimetry can be used to quantify a number of serum proteins. Fluorescent polarization immunoassay can be used for therapeutic drug monitoring, clinical toxicology, and drugs of abuse testing. These latter three classes of assays typically use liquid reagents and require one or two reagents per analyte. Manufacturers use single reagents for test procedures whenever possible.

A large number of different assays, referred to as discrete channels, can be run concurrently on modern clinical chemistry analyzers. The minimum is around 40 and the maximum approaches 100. This has permitted consolidation of routine chemistry, serum protein assays, therapeutic drug monitoring, and clinical toxicology all on one platform with the concomitant elimination of several other platforms, enhancing efficiency. Reagent packs are typically labeled with bar codes to facilitate reagent management by the analyzer and are often stored in refrigerated compartments onboard the analyzer. The analyzer typically pipets one reagent and combines it with an aliquot of the patient's sample in a cuvet, mixes the two together, incubates at a fixed temperature, and makes spectrophotometric readings. As noted in Table 1, two current systems, the VITROS and COBAS INTEGRA lines of analyzers, are closed, i.e., they can only use reagents from one manufacturer. The COBAS INTEGRA uses liquid reagents while the VITROS analyzers use dry slides that will be discussed in detail later. The COBAS INTEGRA system can in theory have open channels programmed by the manufacturer. Whether users will take advantage of this potential increase in flexibility remains to be seen. Several vendors have liquid reagents that are premixed and bar-code labeled that can be loaded directly on the analyzer. The inventory of reagents onboard the analyzer is determined automatically. One feature present on the COBAS INTEGRA analyzer is the ability to predict the amount of reagent necessary based on a history of previous usage.

Carry-over from one sample to the next is limited to the sample aspiration probe in systems with disposable cuvets or dry slides. Most analyzers use reusable plastic or glass cuvets and liquid reagents. The cuvets must be optically transparent to below 340 nm, a wavelength monitored for many enzymatic assays. One exception to the use of reusable cuvets is the Dimension line of analyzers from Dade Behring. The analyzer forms a new plastic cuvet with an optical pathlength of 5 mm for each test. Each cuvet is sealed by the analyzer after testing is complete for disposal (Figure 2). With reusable cuvets, carry-over can arise anywhere that sample comes in contact with the analyzer. Reusable cuvets are washed extensively between samples to minimize carry-over of either sample or reagent from one assay to another. Typically, the previous reaction mixture is aspirated, detergent, and acid and/or base solutions are repeatedly dispensed into and aspirated from the cuvet, and finally the cuvet is extensively rinsed with water. The optical integrity of the cuvet is usually checked after washing and prior to use with a new sample. Reagent probes are also washed extensively to minimize contamination of reaction cuvets and reagent bottles.

After sample and reagent are dispensed, the reaction mixture must be mixed to ensure homogeneity. This can be accomplished by a variety of techniques including forceful dispensing of reagent, magnetic stirring, a spinning paddle, or by ultrasonic energy from a piezoelectric element. Dry slide systems do not require mixing as the liquid component of serum interacts with the dry chemicals as it flows through slide. The reaction mixture is incubated at a constant temperature. Several methods are used to maintain temperature including water baths, oil baths, and circulated air. Kinetic methods have been described for measuring the temperature of the reaction cuvets in automated analyzers (25, 26). Reaction times for colorimetric assays typically range between about 3 and 20 minutes.

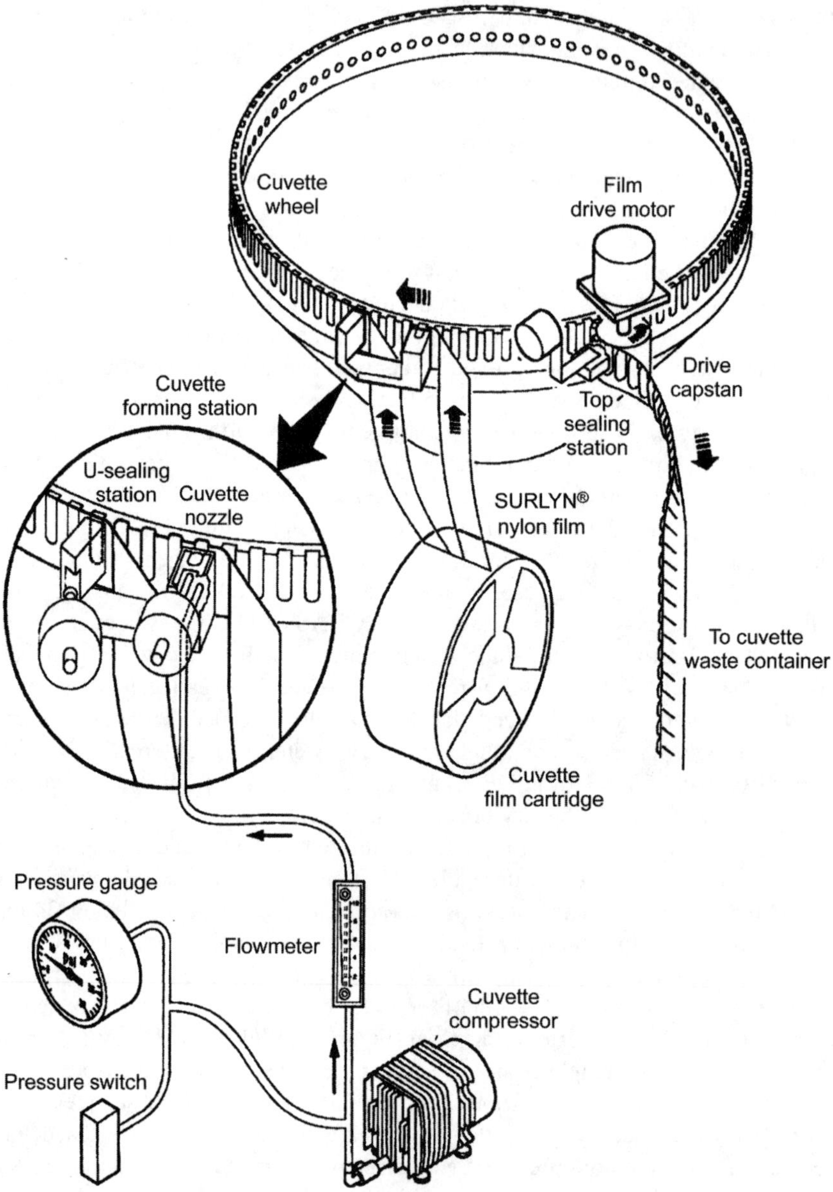

FIGURE 2. Schematic of Dimension sealed cuvets. (*Courtesy of Dade Behring*)

Some analyzers have a single fixed read time of 10 min (Roche D MODULAR) whereas others have six choices over that range of times (Bayer ADVIA 1650 with choices of 3, 4, 5, 10, 15, and 20 minutes).

One of the truly unique reagent systems for clinical chemistry is the layered coating or **dry slide technology** developed by Eastman Kodak in the 1970s (27). One of the major challenges of this approach was to evenly spread the test sample over the dry film. The preferred composition of the spreading or metering layer was based on cellulose acetate pigmented with titanium dioxide. A schematic cross-section is shown in Figure 3. The spreading layer reduces interferences by removing small particulates and large molecules.

Because the spreading layer is opaque, the colored reaction products must be quantified by reflection densitometry. Light of the appropriate wavelength is passed through the transparent support into the reagent layers at a 45° angle and the back-reflected light is detected at 90°, thereby minimizing specular reflection (Figure 4). The sensitivity and specificity of clinical chemistry assays can be enhanced by the flexibility afforded by the choices available in coating design (28). Multiple layers in a coating, typically three to seven of which contain reagent, provide multiple environments in which sequential chemical reactions can occur. Some of the operative mechanisms available include filtration, selective absorption, reactant and/or product immobilization, and the ability to control reaction kinetics via diffusion rates, layer proximities, and intralayer environments. The development of ion-selective electrodes in the dry film format was another challenging project. The measurement of chloride was a relatively straightforward proposition, but to measure sodium and potassium more complex electrodes had to be developed. A reference layer was

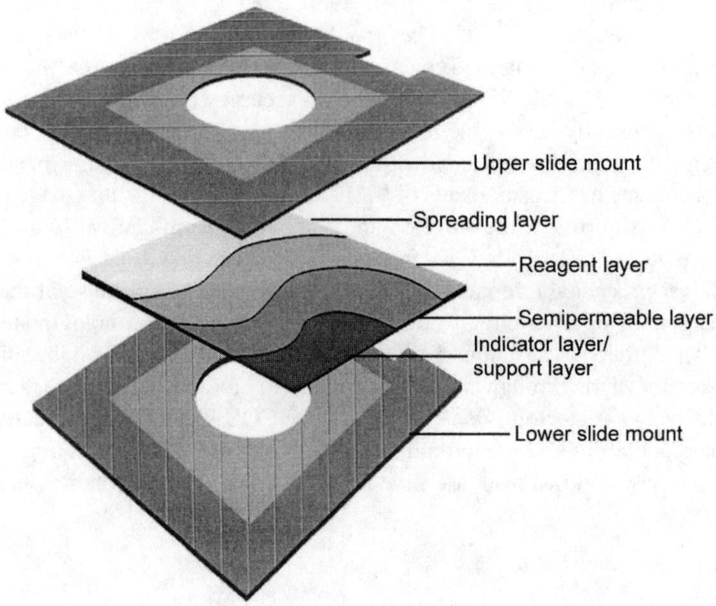

FIGURE 3. Schematic of VITROS dry slide. (*Courtesy of Ortho Clinical Diagnostics*)

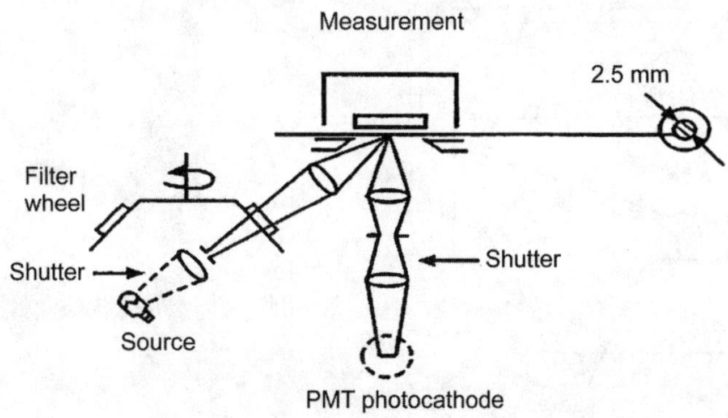

FIGURE 4. Schematic of VITROS reflection densitometer. [*Reprinted with permission (27)*]

coated over the silver–silver chloride electrode and an appropriate ion-selective layer coated over the reference layer. Producing electrodes that worked well required creative organic chemistry to obtain the required ionophores, electrochemistry, and clinical systems engineering. A schematic of an ion-selective electrode slide is shown in Figure 5. The design and fabrication of a sensitive and stable potentiometer were difficult and required several years of work. The first five clinical assays were cleared by the FDA in 1980 and the Ektachem 400 analyzer with 12 analytes became commercially available in 1981 (27). Today the analyzers are named VITROS and sold by Ortho Clinical Diagnostics.

For colorimetric tests the measurement of absorbance requires three basic components: a light source, some means of selecting the wavelength of light, and a detector. The light source is typically an incandescent quartz-halogen lamp that produces light with wavelengths from 300 to 700 nm. Some analyzers may employ a pulsed xenon lamp that provides a high-intensity source. Some means of obtaining light with a narrow range of wavelengths, referred to as spectral isolation, is necessary for many assays. One way to achieve this goal is to use interference filters. Only a few are needed to cover the range of wavelengths that are routinely used. They can be mounted in a wheel that rotates to provide the desired spectral isolation. Typical interference filters transmit 30%–80% of light in a narrow bandwidth of 5–15 nm (2). A spectral accuracy of 10 nm and a bandwidth of 20 nm or less are usually acceptable for most assays. Several methods have been devised for measurement of the spectral bandwidth (29). The effect of spectral bandwidth and wavelength accuracy on measurements of NAD and alkaline phosphatase have been investigated (30, 31). An error in the wavelength as small as 3 nm can cause alkaline phosphatase results to be 23% too low when measured by a method that is very sensitive to wavelength inaccuracy (31). Monochromators can also be used. Because of the relatively few wavelengths of light required, a fixed monochromator with a holographically ruled grating is often coupled to a stationary diode array detector. Fiber optic light guides can be used to direct the light through moveable cuvets. Photodiode array detectors are used almost exclusively as detectors. One exception is the COBAS INTEGRA that incorporates both a photodiode array and a photomultiplier detector. The latter is required to provide adequate sensitivity and fast response time for fluorescent polarization measurements.

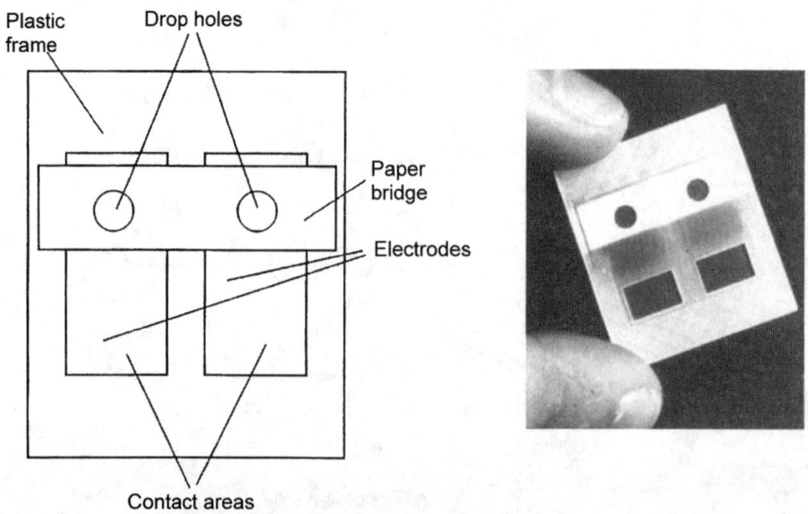

FIGURE 5. Schematic of VITROS ion-selective electrode slide. [*Reprinted with permission (27)*]

The **sample throughput** of chemistry analyzers varies widely and depends primarily on the cycle time for the electromechanical operations of pipetting and making spectrophotometric measurements. The mix of potentiometric and colorimetric/turbidimetric assays can also affect the sample throughput. Each diagnostic vendor usually offers more than one analyzer with differing rates of sample throughput to fit small, medium, and large laboratory applications. For example, the Olympus line starts with the AU400 analyzer that is rated at 400 colorimetric and 400 potentiometric tests per hour for a total of 800 results per hour. There are analyzers with intermediate rates of sample throughput, the AU 640 and AU 2700, and the AU5400 is rated at up to 6600 tests per hour. Table 2 indicates the range of different analyzers that are available for mid- and high-volume laboratories. Other vendors offer smaller chemistry analyzers that are designed for lower volume settings. Some of these are handheld units for use in point-of-care settings and others are tabletop analyzers suitable for physician office laboratories. A review of these smaller analyzers has been published recently (32).

Detecting and Minimizing Common Interferences

Analysis of sample integrity is used to evaluate specimen quality and to determine whether analytical interference can occur. The effects of interferences on test results can be determined by the procedure described by NCCLS (33). Visual assessment of these interferences is subjective and operator dependent. The degree of hemolysis, lipemia (turbidity), and icterus can be quantified by spectrophotometric measurements made at multiple wavelengths and reported as sample indices. Most contemporary clinical chemistry analyzers are capable of performing these measurements. The three exceptions are the COBAS INTEGRA, Dimension, and VITROS analyzers. The VITROS analyzers are generally more resistant to interference from these substances due to the design of their dry slide reagents. However, the ability to detect and quantify interferences, particularly hemolysis, in an automated fashion is desirable. A VITROS system under development will have this feature (34). Open channels on the Dimension and COBAS INTEGRA analyzers can be used for checking sample integrity.

One commonly used approach to minimize spectral interferences is the use of **bichromatic measurements**. Basically, a spectrophotometric reading for the analyte is made at one wavelength, referred to as the primary wavelength, and a blank reading is made at a second wavelength, referred to as the secondary wavelength. The blank reading permits correction of the result for the presence of interfering substances. Bichromatic methods require multiple wavelength measurements by the analyzer over a broad range of wavelengths. This technique has been applied to a number of analytes, albumin and bilirubin methods providing some early examples of this approach (35, 36). A bichromatic measurement of triglycerides has been demonstrated to be less subject to interference from turbidity (37). However, bichromatic measurements are not perfect. One example of their shortcomings is the negative bias observed for glucose measurement on red blood cell hemolysates (38). This process has been carried one step farther on the SYNCHRON CX7 analyzer using polychromatic correction. Up to five wavelengths can be measured simultaneously by this analyzer. A polychromatic correction matrix was developed to reduce spectral interference from hemoglobin, bilirubin, and lipemia for several assays including glucose, phosphate, total protein, and uric acid (39).

Signal Processing

Analysis of data generated by a spectrophotometer for colorimetric methods can be divided into two general categories called **equilibrium methods** and **kinetic methods** (40). Nearly all enzymes are measured using a kinetic method while equilibrium methods can be used to measure a variety of other analytes. In a kinetic method, either the enzyme activity or substrate concentration determines the rate of product formation. In an equilibrium method, only the substrate concentration determines the amount of product formed. In kinetic methods most frequently used on automated analyzers, a sensor signal that is typically a spectrophotometer reading varies with time as a reactant or product concentration changes. The objective of measurement is usually the sensor signal at preselected time points. The measurements are often blanked. The purpose of blank measurements is to compensate for unexpected interactions among different reagent and sample components. Blanks can be measured on reagent alone, sample plus saline, sample plus selected reagent components, sample plus inactivated reagent, and sample plus complete reagent. The latter has the best chance of compensating for unexpected interactions (40). Most of the common kinetic methods use one or more discrete values of sensor signal measured at selected time points to compute enzyme activity or analyte concentration. The number of data points used in computations is an important consideration. The information content of a data set increases as the number of data points is increased. The counting of data points is made only on measurements made on the complete reaction mixture. Procedures can be based on one, two, and three or more data points. One data point provides no information on either sample or reagent blank or the shape of the response curve. Two data points provide no information on the shape of the response curve. Three or more data points can provide information related to both blanks and the shape of the response curve if used properly. In multipoint methods, two approaches can be identified. In one, discrete differences, referred to as deltas, between signals at different points of equal time intervals along a response curve are computed and used to determine both degrees of nonlinearity and to calculate analyte concentration. In the second approach, some form of curve fitting or regression analysis is used to obtain the "best fit" of the data to an expected shape that can be either linear or nonlinear. Parameters are obtained that can be used to calculate the analyte concentration.

A feature that has been developed by Abbott Laboratories for its Aeroset and ARCHITECT c8000 analyzers to increase the analytic measurement range for a number of enzymatic assays is referred to as FlexRate (Figure 6). Bichromatic absorbance reading are made every 18 seconds. The assay's main read time is between 6.3 and 9.9 minutes. Enzyme activity is calculated based on the rate of change during this main read period. With elevated enzyme activities, the number of absorbance values within the main read time that pass substrate depletion and linearity quality control checks drops below three. The analyzer reflexes to use absorbance readings made between 5.1 and 6.6 minutes (flex read time). These readings are also subjected to quality control checks and acceptable values are used to calculate the enzyme rate. Absorbance results below the lower limit suggest either substrate depletion or a highly colored sample. A linearity check confirms a linear reaction curve by comparing the slope of the first three points to the slope of the last three points. A minimum of three absorbance values is required to calculate a final result. These samples typically require manual intervention with dilution, reanalysis, and the calculation of a final result. Data from a tertiary hospital laboratory demonstrated that 0.56% of samples required manual dilutions with an analyzer from another vendor. The use of FlexRate on the Aeroset reduced the need for manual dilutions ninefold to 0.06% (41). The potential benefits of this approach are reduced reruns, faster sample turnaround times, and reduced reagent costs.

Data Handling

Analytical results from the analyzer are transmitted to the LIS. Some systems use standard LOINC codes to transmit results unambiguously to the LIS (*see* Table 1). If the result is

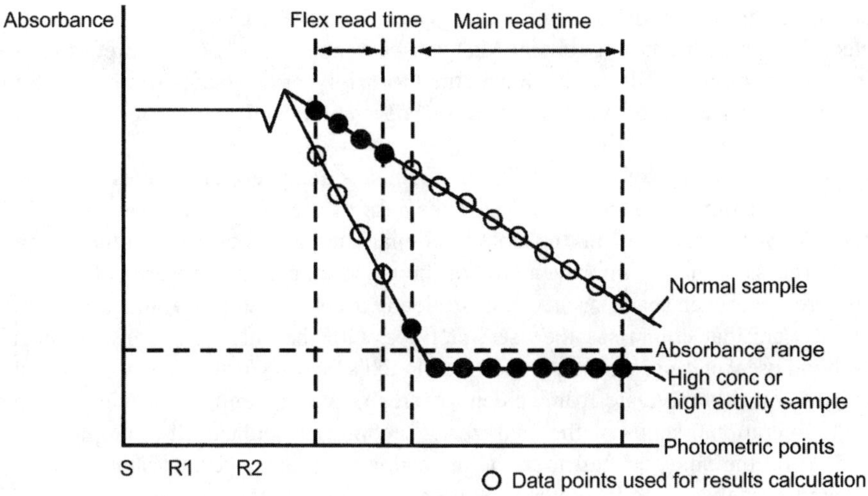

FIGURE 6. Abbott Flex-Rate schematic. (*Reproduction of Figure 1 from poster #558 presented at the AACC annual meeting, July 23–27, 2000, San Francisco, CA, has been granted with approval from Abbott Laboratories, Inc. All rights reserved by Abbott Laboratories, Inc.*)

outside of the analytic measurement range of the assay, most analyzers can be programmed to repeat the analysis if the result was low and repeat the analysis on a smaller sample volume or after dilution if the result is high. In addition, a reflexive test can be ordered either through the LIS or automatically by some analyzers based on the results of another analyte. The ability to order tests reflexively provides many advantages to patients and their physicians (42). This capability may be increasingly important in the future to improve the quality of patient care while minimizing costs.

One area of analyzer development that has lagged many of the other areas mentioned thus far is the ability to use a **rules-based system** to verify that results are valid and can be released to the LIS. Many LIS do have rules-based systems for autoverification of analyzer results but these capabilities can be quite limited. For example, it might be desirable to have the index results for hemolysis, lipemia, and icterus reviewed prior to verifying the results for other tests. Most LIS can use the index result to add a comment to another test. For example, if a sample is mildly hemolyzed, then a hemolyzed sample comment can be added to tests like potassium and lactate dehydrogenase if ordered. However, in the case of lipemia, where ultracentrifugation should be performed and the sample reanalyzed, most LIS do not have adequate rules-based systems to accomplish this task and very few automated chemistry analyzers have a rules-based system to deal with this situation. Recently, Data Innovations (Burlington, VT) developed a system called Instrument Manager that links the analyzer to the LIS and serves to fill gaps between the two systems. This product contains a versatile rules-based system that can be used to add comments to one test result based on results from another test, to initiate reflex testing, and to determine which test results should not be released to the LIS based on the results of another test performed on the same sample. This latter function is unique and provides the option of autoverification of all analyzer results with a user-definable set of rules. This system is currently available with the Roche MODULAR system. For example, it permits one to define which samples require ultracentrifugation prior to analysis when lipemia thresholds tailored to the individual tests that were ordered are exceeded. In addition, with the Roche triglycerides reagent, a very high triglycerides concentration can produce a normal triglycerides result. Using the lipemic index to detect this situation, the Instrument Manager can automatically order a retest on a 1 : 10 dilution, providing a truly automated method for triglycerides that permits the LIS to perform autoverification on the diluted result after automated review and release by the rules-based system.

A general feature of current clinical chemistry analyzers that represents a substantial improvement over earlier systems is the ease of use of the **software** controlling the analyzer. With increases in the computational and graphics capabilities of modern microprocessors, many improvements in the performance and features of the analyzer software have been made. Vendors have devoted considerable resources to enhancing the software that comprises the user interface with the analyzer. Many systems have graphical user interfaces and several utilize touch screens. Current software provides the ability to quickly navigate from screen to screen. One screen may provide information on the operational status of the analyzer, a second may indicate the samples currently residing on the analyzer and their status, a third may provide information on how to operate the analyzer, while another one provides access to the instrument manual. These important and commonly available features simplify analyzer operation and enhance productivity. One particularly useful help feature is the availability of schematic diagrams and step-by-step procedures on the analyzer data system when performing maintenance and troubleshooting operations. The ability to use similar software for multiple analyzers from the same vendor also facilitates training and enhances competency of laboratory staff.

Another data-handling feature available on most analyzers is a **quality control (QC) package**. The instrument is able to track the results of QC testing over a period of time. This package may also be able to track the lot numbers of reagent, calibrator, and QC material being used to generate each QC result. Some instruments may also be able to apply complicated algorithms for assessment of QC results including Westgard rules. These tools facilitate a careful assessment of the operating performance of an analyzer by the individual at the bench who is responsible for its operation. The advantages of having a QC package included in the analyzer software is that all samples run as QC can automatically be captured and included in the data displayed and analyzed. Second, the QC packages on many analyzers are more flexible and user friendly than the QC programs available with the LIS.

BENEFITS OF INCREASED AUTOMATION

Some of the benefits of the increased degree of automation found on contemporary clinical chemistry analyzers include decreases in imprecision and turnaround time. Another major benefit is enhanced productivity for the operator. During the past decade the job vacancy rate for medical technologists has steadily increased and is now between 7% and 20% (43). More effective utilization of staff through increased automation is essential for hospitals and other clinical laboratories to continue to provide adequate levels of service. Additional instrumentation enhancements including the combination of multiple modular chemistry analyzers into one system and the combination of chemistry and immunoassay modular analyzers into single systems will be necessary for an industry that will continue to see staff shortages into the foreseeable future. As routine data-handling tasks become more automated through enhancements to the analyzer, the LIS, and any gap-filler between the two, the clinical laboratory will likely see additional benefits in both labor savings and increased accuracy.

MODULAR Systems

The combination of multiple chemistry analyzers into one modular system has been most fully developed to date by Roche in their MODULAR Analytics systems. This concept consists of a core unit which manages the entire testing process and shuttles samples to the preanalytical and analytical modules. MODULAR processing allows sample transport in three directions (Figure 7). The core unit provides high efficiency advanced process management by separating rack transport from rack processing within each module. The maximum rack transport speed is 1200 samples per hour. The core unit also facilitates automatic rerun and reflex testing. These systems can be reconfigured in the field by connecting additional modules. This allows for scalable increases in analyzer throughput.

Chemistry and Immunoassay Analyzer Combinations

Three vendors currently offer modular systems with both chemistry and immunoassay modules. The benefits of this approach include additional consolidation of testing onto a single platform, decreased sample splitting, and faster turnaround times. These combined chemistry–immunoassay analyzers are depicted in Figure 8. The Dimension RxL with a heterogeneous module was the industry's first high-volume general chemistry analyzer to combine sensitive, heterogeneous immunoassays with routine chemistries. The ARCHITECT ci8200 is the more recent addition to this group of analyzers and provides a somewhat higher throughput than the Dimension RxL. Only the MODULAR Analytics system from Roche is scalable, i.e., it permits more than one chemistry or immunoassay module to be operational in a single system and a total of four chemistry and immunoassay modules may be operated in a single system.

The other emerging trend in chemistry analyzers is the ability to connect with laboratory automation systems so that samples are delivered to an analyzer by means of a track without human intervention. Two general types of systems can be used. In one system the instrument vendor also supplies the automation system. These systems generally permit equipment from only one vendor to be connected to the track. The second alternative is to have automation provided by a third party and analyzers from different vendors can be connected. This approach, although it provides more flexibility, can potentially be more expensive and troubleshooting a bit more difficult. Not all chemistry analyzers are compatible with automation systems. The analyzers that function well with third-party automation systems usually are capable of specimen sampling direct from the track, i.e., the

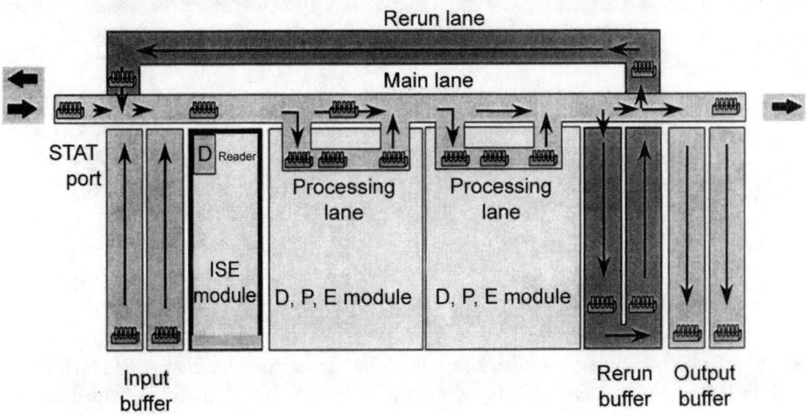

FIGURE 7. Schematic of sample routing on Roche MODULAR. (*Courtesy of Roche Diagnostics*)

analyzer sample probe articulates to a position on the automation track and aspirates sample while the specimen is on the track. This configuration provides the most flexibility. It also requires an analyzer designed for this task.

Choosing a Clinical Chemistry Analyzer

When it comes time to choose a clinical chemistry analyzer for a specific laboratory environment, the information provided in Tables 1 and 2 can serve as a basis. Defining the requirements based on the laboratory requirements is a key part of the decision process. One laboratory may need an analyzer capable of providing sample results in the shortest time possible, while another may need a high throughput analyzer for routine samples. Another major concern is the analytic performance of analyzers in terms of accuracy,

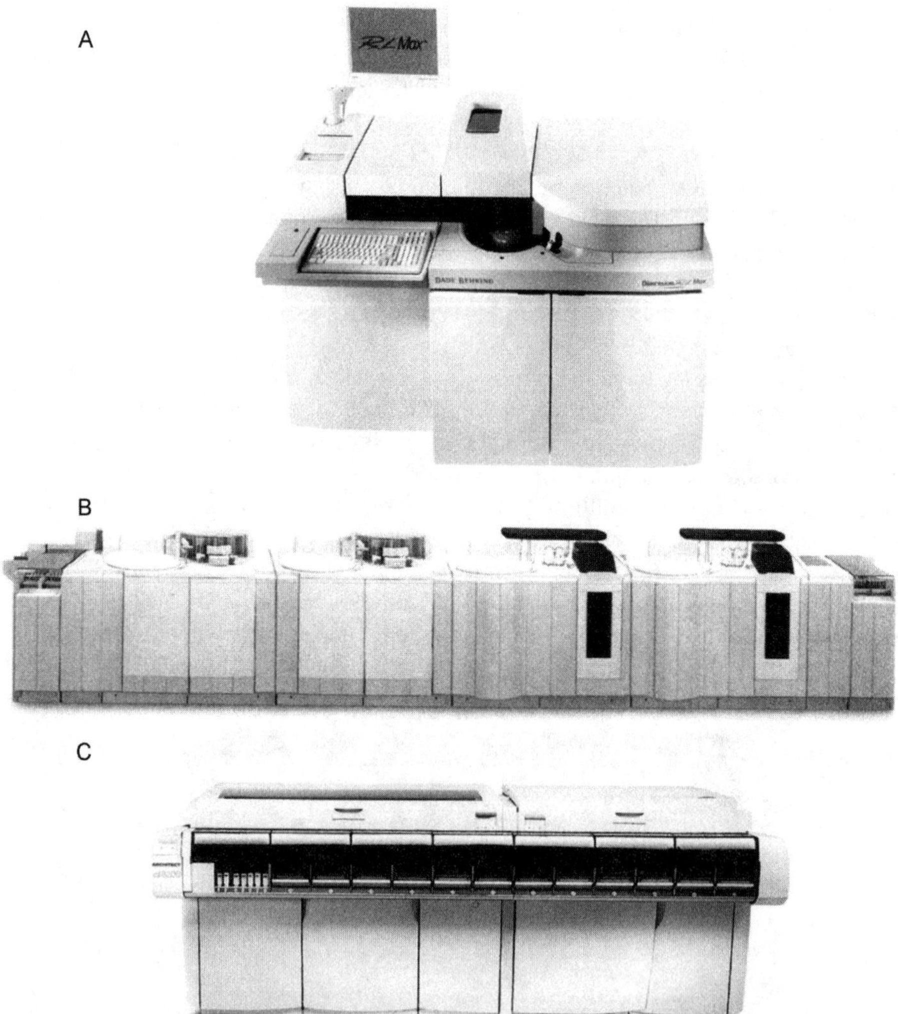

FIGURE 8. Three combined chemistry/immunoassay systems: Dimension RxL with Heterogeneous Module [*Courtesy of Dade Behring* (panel A)]; MODULAR Analytics with two P and two E modules [*Courtesy of Roche Diagnostics* (panel B)]; ARCHITECT ci8200 system. [*Courtesy of Abbott Diagnostics* (panel C)]

precision, linearity, and freedom from interference. The ability to use reagents from more than one supplier may be important but so may calibration stability and reagent stability, both on the shelf and on the analyzer. The labor component of analyzer operation may also be an important factor. This includes hands-on running time, walk-away time, calibration time, and routine maintenance requirements. Ease of use of the analyzer's software is another important consideration. Ideally, an analyzer would be evaluated for a trial period in the actual laboratory environment, but this is often impractical. Evaluation studies of some specific analyzers have been published and may also be useful in the decision process. The most recent article published on a Beckman SYNCHRON CX system appeared in 1990 and was written about the CX4 analyzer (44). The most recent evaluation of an Hitachi analyzer was also written in 1990 on the Hitachi 717 system (45). The Dimension RxL and Olympus AU 400 analyzers have been evaluated recently (46, 47). Three articles have been published on COBAS INTEGRA analyzers (48–50). Numerous additional articles evaluating specific methods on automated analyzers are also available and may be useful for specific applications. One particularly useful example of this type of article is the evaluation of 14 immunoturbidimetric assays for human serum proteins on the Hitachi 912 analyzer (51).

REFERENCES

1. International Union of Pure and Applied Chemistry: Nomenclature for automated and mechanised analysis (Recommendation 1989). Pure Appl Chem 1989;61:1657–64.
2. Boyd JC, Young DS. Automation in the clinical laboratory. In: Burtis CA, Ashwood ER, eds. Tietz textbook of clinical chemistry, 3rd ed. Philadelphia: WB Saunders, 1999:226–61.
3. Maclin E, Young DS. Automation in the clinical laboratory. In: Burtis CA, Ashwood ER, eds. Tietz textbook of clinical chemistry, 2nd ed. Philadelphia: WB Saunders, 1994:313–73.
4. Rosenfeld L. Clinical chemistry since 1800: growth and development. Clin Chem 2002;48:186–97.
5. Muller RH. Photoelectric methods in analytical chemistry. Ind Eng Chem Anal Ed 1939;11:1–17.
6. Skeggs LT Jr. Persistence... and prayer: from the artificial kidney to the AutoAnalyzer. Clin Chem 2000;46:1425–36.
7. Skeggs LT Jr. An automatic method for colorimetric analysis. Am J Clin Pathol 1957;28:311–22.
8. Skeggs LT Jr, Hochstrasser H. Multiple automatic sequential analysis. Clin Chem 1964; 10:918–36.
9. Schoeff L. Principles of clinical chemistry automation. In: Bishop M, Duben-Englekirk J, Fody E, eds. Clinical chemistry: principles, procedures, and correlations, 4th ed. Philadelphia: Lippincott Williams & Wilkins, 2000:124–41.
10. Statland BE, Nishi HH, Young DS. Serum alkaline phosphatase: total activity and isoenzyme determinations made by use of the centrifugal fast analyzer. Clin Chem 1972;18:1468–74.
11. Schoeff LE. Clinical analyzers. General chemistry. Anal Chem 1999;71:351–5R.
12. Burtis CA, Painter PC. Analytical systems for the clinical laboratory. Am Clin Lab 1989;8:14–9.
13. Burtis CA, Painter PC. Analytical systems for the clinical laboratory. Am Clin Lab 1989;8:43–9.
14. Aller RD. Chemistry analyzers branching out. CAP Today, 2002a;July:84–106.
15. Hall RA, Whitehead TP. Absorption of serum calcium by sample plastic cups. J Clin Pathol 1970;23:323–6.
16. Burtis CA, Begovich JM, Watson JS. Factors influencing evaporation from sample cups and assessment of their effect on analytical error. Clin Chem 1975;21:1907–17.
17. Burtis CA, Watson JS. Design and evaluation of an anti-evaporative cover for use with liquid containers. Clin Chem 1992;38:768–75.
18. Kost GJ. New whole blood analyzers and their impact on cardiac and critical care. Crit Rev Clin Lab Sci 1993;30:153–202.

19. National Committee for Clinical Laboratory Standards. Preliminary evaluation of quantitative clinical laboratory methods; approved guideline. EP10-A. Wayne, PA: NCCLS, 1998.
20. Harff GA, van den Bosch MJ. Evaluation of carry-over on the (Bayer) ADVIA 1650 clinical chemistry analyzer. Clin Chem 2002;48:A58–59.
21. Ravalico TH, Wilson CW, Ingram HX, Alonzo DM. Optimized sample probe wash on the Abbott ARCHITECT® ci8200™ analyzer to minimize between sample carryover on an integrated clinical chemistry and immunoassay platform. Clin Chem 2002;48:A59.
22. Ford GO, Blackwell GA. Evaluation of clot detection/pressure monitoring in the Abbott Architect® c8000™ clinical chemistry analyzer. Clin Chem 2002;48:A9–10.
23. Sewell DL. Laboratory-associated infections and biosafety. Clin Microbiol Rev 1995;8: 389–405.
24. Evans MR, Henderson DK, Bennett JE. Potential for laboratory exposures to biohazardous agents found in blood. Am J Public Health 1990;80:423–7.
25. Adams PC, Berman MC. A kinetic standard for precise calibration of spectrophotometer cell temperature. Clin Chem 1981;27:753–5.
26. Armitage EK, Miller WG. Optical kinetic method for calibration of spectrophotometer temperature: demonstration with the Cobas-Bio analyzer. Clin Chem 1987;33:1891–5.
27. Curme H, Rand RN. Early history of Eastman Kodak Ektachem slides and instrumentation. Clin Chem 1997;43:1647–52.
28. Shirey TL. Development of a layered-coating technology for clinical chemistry. Clin Biochem 1983;16:147–55.
29. Passey RB, Gillum RL, Fuller JB. Measurement of spectral bandwidth, as exemplified with the Beckman "Enzyme Analyzer System TR spectrophotometer." Clin Chem 1975;21:1582–4.
30. Rains S. Effect of spectral bandwidth and wavelength accuracy on the measurement of reduced NAD. Clin Chem 1973;19:647.
31. Lott JA, Turner K, Scott J. Factors affecting measurement of total alkaline phosphatase activity in human serum, especially wavelength accuracy. Clin Chem 1978;24:938–41.
32. Aller RD. Don't leave patient safety to the roll of the dice. CAP Today, 2002b;June:60–84.
33. National Committee for Clinical Laboratory Standards. Interference testing in clinical chemistry; proposed guideline. EP7-P. Wayne, PA: NCCLS, 1986.
34. Warren KL, Sawyer B, Stearns S, Cheehan T, Merrill G, Mehalek G, et al. Interference evaluation of the VITROS 5,1 FS chemistry system MicroSensor™ (sample integrity) module. Clin Chem 2002;48:A55–56.
35. Kelly A, McKenna JP, McLelland A, Percy RA, Spooner RJ. A bichromatic method for total bilirubin with a CentrifiChem 400. Clin Chem 1979;25:1482–4.
36. Maguire GA. Bichromatic blanking in the bromcresol purple method for albumin in serum and plasma. Clin Chem 1984;30:1886–7.
37. Sampson M, Ruddel M, Elin RJ. Effects of specimen turbidity and glycerol concentration on nine enzymatic methods for triglyceride determination. Clin Chem 1994;40:221–6.
38. da Fonseca-Wollheim F. Haemoglobin interference in the bichromatic spectrophotometry of NAD(P)H at 340/380 nm. Eur J Clin Chem Clin Biochem 1993;31:595–601.
39. Pierre K, Metzler M, Dewberry T, Shui R, Vogt D, Leyva P. Polychromatic correction for serum bilirubin, hemoglobin, and lipemia interferents on the Beckman Synchron CX7 system. Clin Chem 1992;30:1024.
40. Pardue HL. A comprehensive classification of kinetic methods of analysis used in clinical chemistry. Clin Chem 1977;23:2189–2201.
41. George PM, Kennedy LA, Southby SJ, Robertson JM, Ahern K. An evaluation of extended linearity enzyme assays with FlexRate on the Abbott AEROSET analyzer. Clin Chem 2000;46(Suppl):A144.
42. MacMillan DH, Soderberg BL, Laposata M. Regulations regarding reflexive testing and narrative interpretations in laboratory medicine. Am J Clin Pathol 2001;116(Suppl):S129–32.
43. Ward-Cook K, Tannar S. 2000 wage and vacancy survey of medical laboratories. Lab Med 2001;32:124–38.

44. Ambus T, Korogyi N, DeCampos F, Groom B, Innanen VT. Evaluation of the Beckman Synchron CX4 clinical chemistry analyzer in a hospital laboratory. J Clin Lab Anal 1990;4:120–5.
45. Flood J, Kiedtke R, Mattenheimer H, Rothouse L, Trundle D, Vroon D, et al. A multicenter evaluation of the Boehringer Mannheim/Hitachi 717 system. Clin Biochem 1990;23:477–88.
46. Cuka S, Dvornik S, Drzenovic K, Mihic J. Evaluation of the Dade Behring Dimension RxL clinical chemistry analyzer. Clin Lab 2001;47:35–40.
47. Bilic A, Alpeza I, Rukavine AS. Evaluation of the Olympus AU 400 clinical chemistry analyzer. Clin Lab 2000;46:1–6.
48. Palmer SM, Kaufman RA, Salamone SJ, Blake-Courtney J, Bette W, Wahl HP, et al. Cobas Integra: clinical laboratory instrument with continuous and random-access capabilities. Clin Chem 1995;41:1751–60.
49. Brombacher PJ, Marell GJ, Westerhuis LW. Laboratory work flow analysis and introduction of a multifunctional analyser. Eur J Clin Chem Clin Biochem 1996;34:287–92.
50. Muser J, Bienvenu J, Blanckaert N, Brandslund I, Delattre J, Soffiati G, et al. Inter-laboratory evaluation of the COBAS INTEGRA 400 analytical system. Clin Chem Lab Med 2001; 39:539–59.
51. Ledue TB, Collins MF, Ritchie RF. Development of immunoturbidimetric assays for fourteen human serum proteins on the Hitachi 912. Clin Chem Lab Med 2002;40:520–8.

Chapter 10

Electrochemistry

Anthony O. Okorodudu

The physiologic well-being of living organisms depends on a balanced control of the activity of several critical ions (and gases). These ions and gases include Na^+, K^+, Ca^{2+}, H^+, Mg^{2+}, NH_4^+, Cl^-, HCO_3^-, pCO_2, and pO_2. The cellular and extracellular levels of these ions and gases are maintained within defined physiologic ranges that correlate with normal homeostatic control. Alterations in their levels are corrected by one of several regulatory processes, i.e., regulation of Na^+ and K^+ by the renin–angiotensin–aldosterone system (refer to a textbook on physiology and/or pathophysiology for details). Other ions that are used therapeutically (i.e., Li^+) may require maintenance within narrow ranges for optimum patient care. The measurement of their concentrations is an important analytic function in clinical laboratory medicine. Since these analytes are in solutions of the different intracellular and extracellular (blood, cerebrospinal fluid, urine) compartments, they can be measured in terms of molar concentration or activity. The activity of the ionic form of the analyte is directly proportional to its concentration. Concentration of an analyte can be calculated from the obtained activity using:

$$a = \gamma c \qquad (1)$$

where a = activity
γ = the activity coefficient (the activity coefficient of each species in a solution is inversely related to the ionic strength, μ)
$\mu = 0.5(\Sigma c_i z_i^2)$; c_i = concentration and z = charge number for each species in solution
c = concentration (mmol/L)

The activity coefficient of each ion in a solution is dependent on its ionic strength and temperature. It is a difficult coefficient to calculate for complex fluids such as blood or plasma because of variations in the contribution of macromolecular ions to the ionic strength. At 37 °C and an ionic strength of 160 mmol/kg, the calculated activity coefficients for selected ions are 0.75, 0.74, and 0.31 for Na^+, K^+, and Ca^{2+}, respectively. These coefficients are calculated using the Debye–Huckel equation:

$$\log \gamma = -(Az^2I^{1/2})/(1 + B\alpha I^{1/2}) \qquad (2)$$

where A = 0.5213 at 37 °C (temperature-dependent constant)
B = 3.305 at 37 °C (temperature-dependent constant)
z = charge of the ion
I = ionic strength

The activity of each ion in solution is directly proportional to changes in generated current or voltage. The electrochemical principles involved with the measurement of current or voltage generated because of the **activity** of specific ion species in an electrochemical cell have been used extensively for the quantitation of these essential analytes. These electrochemical reactions for determining activity of ions were first applied to pH measurement and thereafter the technology was extended to include measurement of various of electrolytes and gases. Electroanalysis has made it possible to use very small sample volumes (microliters) for the measurement of analytes that exist in the concentration range of 10^{-8} to 10^{-3} mol/L. Instruments that use this technique exhibit an unprecedented degree of precision, ease of operation, and a remarkably short analysis time.

This chapter provides a general review of electrochemical principles widely applicable to clinical chemistry laboratory measurements. Specifically, potentiometric, voltammetric (polarographic and anodic stripping), conductometric, amperometric, and coulometric techniques are reviewed and illustrated with selected analytes. Following this general review, characteristics of some analyzers that use electroanalytic principles are presented. The chapter concludes with a review of new and emerging instruments in the field of electrochemistry.

POTENTIOMETRIC MEASUREMENTS

Potentiometry is the measurement of voltage or electrical potential difference that is developed between two electrodes (indicator and reference electrodes) in proportion to a specific analyte in solution with no flow of current. It is used for the measurement of H^+, Na^+, K^+, Ca^{2+}, Mg^{2+}, Li^+, NH_4^+, and Cl^- in biological fluids.

Nearly all conductors of electricity are metals or electrolytes with the current being carried by either electrons or ions. When current passes from metal to electrolyte or from electrolyte to metal, the type of carrier usually changes suddenly and certain interesting phenomena occur. Whenever there is an interface between the metal and ions of that metal in a solution, an electrode potential is produced. This potential is called the electric potential of that metal. An electrode potential is also produced when different concentrations of an ion are separated by a membrane that is semipermeable to that ion. Nonmetallic elements such as hydrogen also have electrode potentials. It is impossible to assign a specific value to the potential of each substance because it depends on such factors as concentration, complexity, and temperature of the solution. Thus, in practice, each may be assigned a relative electrode potential using the hydrogen half-cell as 0.0 V.

$$\tfrac{1}{2} H \rightleftharpoons H^+ + e^-$$
$$E^\circ = 0.00 \text{ V}$$

Thus, the calcium half-cell has an electrode potential of –2.87 V, and mercury has an electrode potential of +0.789 V.

$$Ca \rightleftharpoons Ca^{2+} + 2e^-$$
$$E^\circ = -2.87 \text{ V}$$

To measure an electrode potential, a second voltage source (such as another metal–solution interface) is needed to be used as a reference for measurements by the first electrode. Each of the electrodes is called a half-cell. The two half-cells arranged together constitute an electrochemical cell in which one of the half-cells maintains a constant voltage. The electrode in the half-cell with constant voltage is called the reference electrode, whereas the variable voltage portion is termed the indicator electrode. It is possible to measure the potential difference between these two electrodes and calculate the concentration of ions in the solution of the indicator (measuring) electrode (Figure 1).

This concept is illustrated using two silver half-cells in a specific measuring system. If a silver wire is immersed in a solution of silver chloride, ionization of the silver metal occurs with the formation of silver ions (Ag^+) and electrons. An electric potential now exists between the wire and the solution. If two half-cells are used, each with a silver wire or foil immersed in a different silver solution and the two solutions are connected through a meter, a difference in potential can be detected between them (Figure 2). Because the potential of each solution depends on the concentration of silver ions in it, the concentration of ions in one solution can be predicted if the value for the other and the difference in potential between them are known. In practice, such a system can be set up and, by calibrating it against known standards, a workable measuring system can be designed. A temperature difference between the two half-cells would affect the reproducibility of measurement. Other minor technical factors such as coating (e.g., protein deposit when using biologic fluids) will affect the measurements.

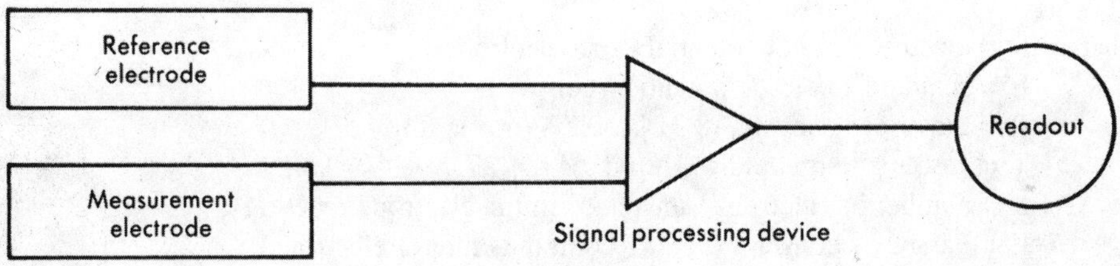

FIGURE 1. Basic functional units of electrode system. (*Reprinted from Okorodudu AO. Electrochemistry, In: Schoeff LE, Williams RH, eds., Principles of laboratory instruments, Copyright 1993, with permission from Elsevier*)

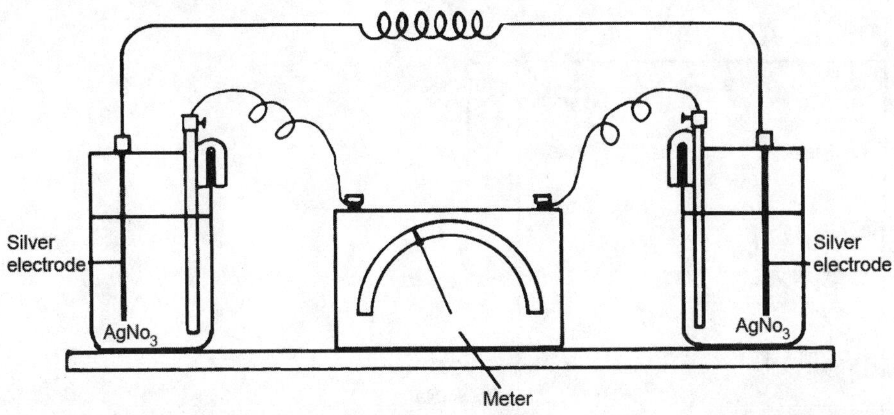

FIGURE 2. Two silver half-cells connected through a meter. If one knows the potential difference and the concentration of silver nitrate in one half-cell, the concentration in the test solution can be calculated. (*Reprinted from Okorodudu AO. Electrochemistry, In: Schoeff LE, Williams RH, eds., Principles of laboratory instruments, Copyright 1993, with permission from Elsevier*)

It is not necessary that the two half-cells contain the same materials as long as two similar potentials are produced. In fact, it is possible to devise a reference electrode that will give a very precise and reproducible potential. Using this reference electrode with a highly reliable potential, it is possible to calibrate the system with known standards and measure the concentration of the ion in question on a precalibrated scale. Figure 3 illustrates a calibration scheme in which two standards are used for the calibration, and the electrode slope is determined.

Potentiometric methods are based on the quantitative relationship between the potential of a cell as given by the following distribution of potential:

$$E_{cell} = E_{reference} + E_{indicator} + E_{junction} \quad (3)$$

Because the reference and junction potentials are constant, the indicator potential can be determined. The potential of the indicator (measuring electrode) is therefore directly related to concentration of the specific ion.

Electrode systems used in the clinical laboratory have precalibrated readout devices that give results in concentration units. The **cell potential** is related to concentration through the Nernst equation:

$$E = E° + (2.303\ RT/zF)\ \log a_i \quad (4)$$

where E = electrochemical potential of an electrode
$E°$= standard electrode potential (constant)
R = molar gas constant (8.314 joules)/(mol)(°K)
T = absolute temperature (Kelvin or K) (273° + °C = °K)
z = number of electrons transferred in the electrode reaction
F = Faraday's constant (96,487 coulombs/mol of electrons)
a_i = activity of ion of interest

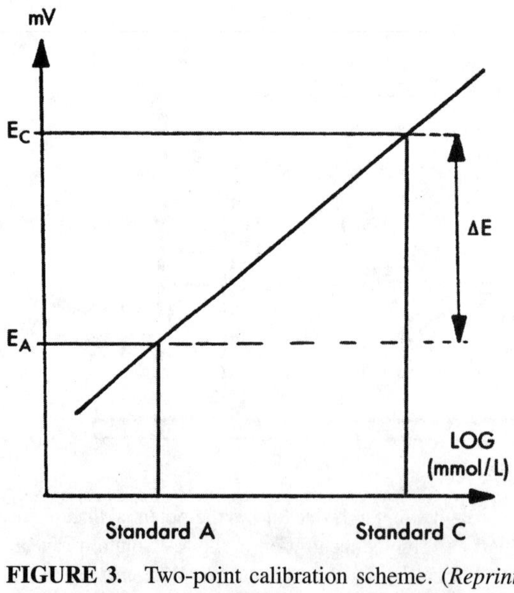

FIGURE 3. Two-point calibration scheme. (*Reprinted from Okorodudu AO. Electrochemistry, In: Schoeff LE, Williams RH, eds., Principles of laboratory instruments, Copyright 1993, with permission from Elsevier*)

To simplify Equation 4, the voltage developed between the reference and measuring electrodes will be:

$$E = KT \log (C_1/C_2) \quad (5)$$

where K = constant $2.3(R/zF)$
(C_1/C_2) = If either C_1 or C_2 is known, the concentration of the unknown can be calculated from the measurement of the potential developed.

In summary, the reference electrode has a constant potential. An indicator electrode is sensitive to the concentration of a specific component of the solution being analyzed. The potential resulting from the ion to be measured is obtained by finding the difference between the reference and measured potentials. By using the Nernst relationship, the concentration of the ion is calculated. The principles of the different types of reference and indicator electrodes used in clinical laboratory instruments are described in this chapter.

Liquid–Liquid Junction Potential

In making an electrical connection between the reference electrode and the sample solution via a salt bridge, a negligible but reproducible potential is produced. This potential develops at the interface between two nonidentical solutions and is called the **liquid–liquid junction potential**. A concentrated or saturated potassium chloride salt bridge is commonly used because it provides several advantages.

Figure 4 is a conceptual diagram of an enlarged section of a liquid–liquid junction. Consider the A^+ ions and the B^- ions. Initially there are none of these in the sample solution, but there is a large concentration of them in the salt bridge. These ions, following the laws of thermodynamics, will diffuse from the region of higher concentration to the region of lower concentration. Because the A^+ ions are smaller, they diffuse more quickly than the larger B^- ions and the result is that a small positive–negative charge difference (or potential) is established. The same process happens with the C^+ and D^{2-} ions in the sample diffusing into the salt bridge. The cumulative result, which is the liquid–liquid junction

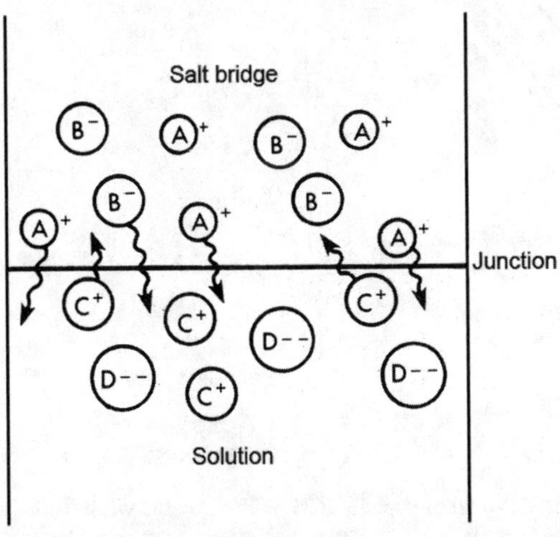

FIGURE 4. Liquid–liquid junction. (*Reprinted from Okorodudu AO. Electrochemistry, In: Schoeff LE, Williams RH, eds., Principles of laboratory instruments, Copyright 1993, with permission from Elsevier*)

potential, can be 20 to 30 mV as calculated by the Henderson equation. This is a large value when measuring electrode potentials to a few tenths of a millivolt. The impact of this liquid–liquid potential is minimized by using calibrators that match the samples containing the analyte of interest in terms of ionic content and ionic strength. An equitransferant electrolyte reference solution at high concentration (> 2 molar) also is used to decrease the liquid junction potential.

Figure 5 shows examples of reference electrodes using potassium chloride as the reference solution. If the hydrated positive ion and the negative ion were the same size, they would diffuse at the same rate and no potential would be established. Because potassium ions and chloride ions have about the same mobility, potassium chloride is a good compound for use as a salt bridge. This similarity in mobility of the ions reduces the junction potential considerably. In routine clinical analyses there is no such choice of ions in the sample solution and no control of this kind to reduce the diffusion of ions from the sample. Therefore, diffusion is controlled by having a saturated potassium chloride solution in the reference electrode. This results in many ions diffusing from the salt bridge against which the sample ions must diffuse. Diffusion of ions from the sample to the junction is thus relatively negligible so that the junction potential is 1 mV or less and reproducible. Now electrode potentials can be measured to fractions of millivolts more accurately.

Reference Electrodes

A reference electrode is an electrochemical half-cell with a known constant potential against which the potential of the indicator half-cell is measured. Electrodes that generate a constant potential and can be used as a reference include the standard hydrogen electrode, the saturated calomel electrode, and the silver–silver chloride electrode. These

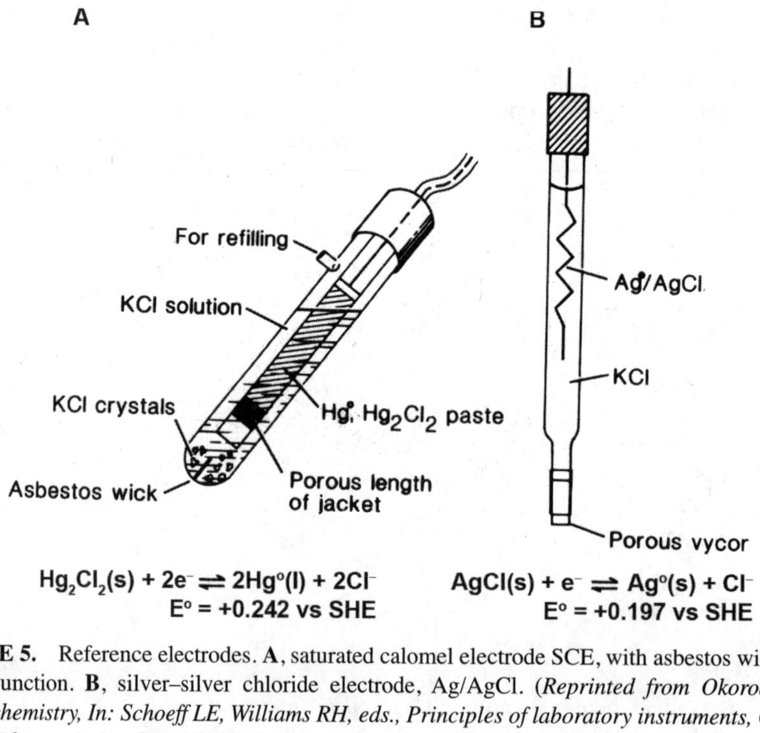

$Hg_2Cl_2(s) + 2e^- \rightleftharpoons 2Hg^\circ(l) + 2Cl^-$ $E^\circ = +0.242$ vs SHE

$AgCl(s) + e^- \rightleftharpoons Ag^\circ(s) + Cl^-$ $E^\circ = +0.197$ vs SHE

FIGURE 5. Reference electrodes. **A**, saturated calomel electrode SCE, with asbestos wick for salt bridge junction. **B**, silver–silver chloride electrode, Ag/AgCl. (*Reprinted from Okorodudu AO. Electrochemistry, In: Schoeff LE, Williams RH, eds., Principles of laboratory instruments, Copyright 1993, with permission from Elsevier*)

electrodes are stable with easily reproducible half-cell potentials and have chemically stable components.

Standard Hydrogen Electrode

The standard hydrogen electrode is the international standard but is seldom used for routine work because more convenient types with reliable calibration buffers are available. Hydrogen electrodes are produced by coating a platinum electrode with platinum black (finely divided particles of platinum). Hydrogen gas at a pressure of 1 atmosphere is then bubbled around the coated platinum that is immersed in an acidic solution with H^+ activity set at unity. Although this type of electrode is quite accurate, it is unstable and very awkward to use. This standard hydrogen electrode, by definition, has a potential of 0.00 **volts (V)** at all temperatures. It is the absolute reference half-cell used for the standardization of other reference electrodes that are part of routine clinical chemistry instruments.

Saturated Calomel Electrode

The saturated calomel electrode is a widely used reference electrode. As shown in Figure 5A, its function is based on the reversible reaction:

$$Hg_2Cl_2 + 2e^- ==== 2Hg^\circ + 2Cl^-$$

The calomel electrode contains an inert element (e.g., platinum) in contact with mercury, mercurous chloride (calomel), and a solution of potassium chloride of known concentration. The saturated calomel electrode in which the solution is saturated with potassium chloride (4.2 M at 25 °C) is commonly used because it is easy to prepare and maintain. If the salt concentration around the electrode is different from the salt bridge concentration, another liquid–liquid junction potential is established. For this reason, the salt solution in a calomel electrode is usually saturated.

When a high degree of accuracy is desired, a 0.1 M or 1.0 M potassium chloride solution electrode is preferred because it reaches its equilibrium potential quicker and its potential depends less on temperature than does the saturated type. Calomel electrodes become unstable at temperatures above 80 °C and should be replaced with silver–silver electrodes.

Silver–Silver Chloride Electrode

The silver–silver chloride electrode is a very reproducible electrode. Its operation is based on the reversible reaction:

$$AgCl + e^- ====== Ag^+ + Cl^-$$

The electrode is prepared by electroplating a layer of silver on a platinum wire and then converting the surface silver to silver chloride by electrolysis in hydrochloric acid (Figure 5B). The solution surrounding the electrode should be saturated with potassium chloride and silver chloride.

Indicator Electrodes

The indicator electrode system is a half-cell whose potential varies as the concentration of a specific ion in the solution changes. This change in potential is governed by the Nernst equation. The term ion-selective electrode (ISE) is increasingly used to describe electrodes used for measurement of ions. The ion-selective electrode unit simply consists of a membrane separating a reference solution and reference electrode from a solution to be analyzed (Figure 6). The complexity of ISE design is in the membrane formulation that determines its ionic selectivity. Several types of ion-selective indicator electrodes are described in the following section.

Glass Electrode

The glass electrode was the first and is still the most commonly used ion-selective electrode for measuring hydrogen ion activity. With certain types or compositions of glass, an electrical potential develops across a thin film of the glass when solutions of different hydrogen ion activities (concentrations) are on the opposite sides of the film. A glass electrode consists of a small bulb of special glass that contains a solution of known hydrogen ion concentration (e.g., 0.1 N HCl) and an internal reference electrode, usually calomel or silver–silver chloride. The special composition of hydrated glass containing Na_2O, CaO, SiO_2, and perhaps small amounts of other ions makes the ion-exchange reaction of hydrogen at the surface of the glass possible. As a hydrogen ion combines with an oxygen ion within the lattice on the outer glass surface, a hydrogen ion leaves a binding site on the opposite surface. This combined activity on the glass surface maintains the electrical neutrality of the glass while establishing a hydrogen equilibrium and thus producing a potential. Because of the high resistance of the glass, electronic amplification is necessary for measurement of the potential.

When the glass measuring electrode and the calomel electrode (silver–silver chloride electrode) are immersed in a solution containing hydrogen ions, the small potential difference between these two half-cells is measured on a very sensitive voltmeter. When the instrument is calibrated against standards and adjusted for temperature effect, the activity of hydrogen ion (pH or negative log of the hydrogen ion activity) can be read very accurately. A very sophisticated, stable, and sensitive measuring device is required. This combination of parts is a pH meter. For convenience, both the glass measuring electrode and the reference electrode are sometimes built into a single glass housing and called a combination electrode. Combination electrodes are convenient to handle and can be used where a very small amount of fluid sample is available. No significant accuracy is lost.

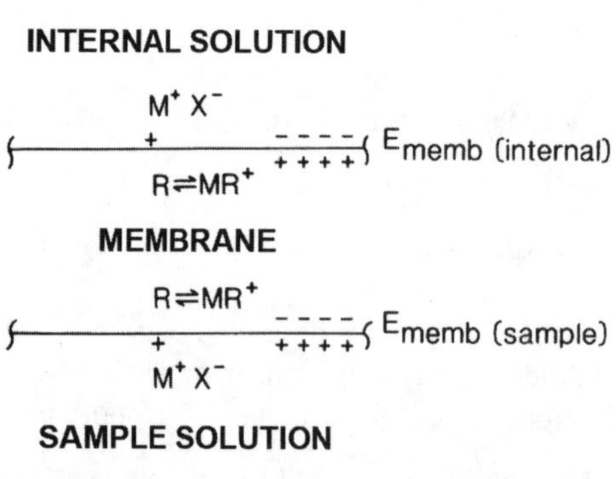

FIGURE 6. Schematic illustration of liquid membrane ISE, where M^+ represents analyte cation and R represents neutral carrier ionophore. (*Reprinted from Okorodudu AO. Electrochemistry, In: Schoeff LE, Williams RH, eds., Principles of laboratory instruments, Copyright 1993, with permission from Elsevier*)

The pH meter is designed to measure the effective concentration of hydrogen ions in a solution. In general, three parameters are involved in the effective concentration. The first of these is the actual molar concentration of hydrogen ions. The second is the dissociation constant of the acid, or the pK_a. The third is the temperature.

Since the early twentieth century, various technicians have reported that a difference in electric potential could be measured between two solutions of different pH separated by a thin glass membrane. All the measuring devices available however, had such a high internal resistance that the amplitude of the current produced could not be measured. Around 1930, an amplifier system was devised that allowed the pH meter, as it is now known, to be developed.

When a calomel reference electrode is used, the potential produced by hydrogen ions is quite constant, amounting to 59.15 mV per pH unit when measured at 25 °C. Temperature has considerable effect; each degree of temperature increase raises the cell's output by about 0.2 mV.

It is immediately apparent that there are a number of interfaces in this total pH-measuring system. The technician must assume that the potential at each of these interfaces is constant in all situations when making measurements. If a difference in potential of 59.15 mV represents one pH unit, then a device that can measure a voltage change of 1.2 mV to indicate a change of 0.02 pH unit must be used. The complexity of the process is appreciated when the many variables, such as the phase junctions in the measuring system, the temperature effect on each of these, and variables in electrical components are considered.

Resistance of this circuit is between 50,000 and 200,000,000 Ω. The tiny potential discussed is extremely hard to measure. For this reason a device similar to a vacuum tube voltmeter is used. Because of the high resistance of the electrode system, a circuit that will measure very high impedance is required.

When very alkaline solutions were tested with glass electrodes, it was found that pH measurements were strongly affected by the presence of sodium and other alkali metal ions. By changing the composition of the glass, this type of error could be minimized. At the same time it was found that glass electrodes could be developed that could actually measure sodium ion activity under proper conditions. When measuring very high pH values, some small sodium correction may be necessary. This correction is usually stated by the manufacturer.

Modern pH meters are, of course, quite different instruments. Electrode design has progressed to the point that nearly any type of configuration for any sort of use can be obtained. Very small, trouble-free combination electrodes are now available for routine laboratory measurements in nearly any sort of container or condition.

Liquid Membrane Ion-Selective Electrode

Liquid membrane ion-selective electrodes have been developed that use liquid ion-exchange resins or neutral carrier electroactive substances called ionophores that react selectively with specific ions. Figure 6 illustrates a portion of a liquid ISE membrane. The membrane is composed of an ionophore (1–3% wt), plasticizer (~64% wt), additives that enhance selectivity for a specific ion (<1% wt), and an appropriate water-insoluble, non-volatile organic solvent–polyvinyl chloride (~30% wt). The liquid electroactive substances are allowed to fill the pores of a porous membrane by capillary action or are bound by other forces, such as electrostatic action, in a membrane. The external (sample) and internal solutions then develop potentials on the surface of the electroactive substances in the membrane in much the same way as with the glass membrane in a glass electrode. The choice of ionophore is an important factor in determining the ionic selectivity of the electrode. Table 1 lists the composition of membrane, linearity characteristics, and possible interferences in clinical laboratory instruments. Neutral ion-carriers such as nonactin or valinomycin are used in ISEs for K^+ (Figure 7), Ba^{2+}, Na^+, Ca^{2+}, and NH_4^+. The Ca^{2+}- and Mg^{2+}-sensitive ISEs use phosphoric acid esters; NO_3^-, Cl^-, and other anion determinations are obtained with ISEs using membranes with electroactive substances of substituted arsonium, phosphonium, and ammonium salts.

Precipitate-Impregnated Membrane Electrode

Once the ion-exchange mechanism of the glass electrode was established, electrochemists started to investigate ion-exchange membranes with the hope of devising an anion-sensitive

TABLE 1. ISEs used in clinical chemistry

	Analytes	Membrane composition	Linear response range (mol/L)	Possible interferences
Glass	H^+	72.17% SiO_2, 6.44% CaO, 21.39% Na_2O (mol %)	$10^{-12} - 10^{-2}$	Na^+
	Na^+	11% Na_2O, 18% Al_2O_3, 71% SiO_2	$10^{-6} - 10^{-1}$	K^+, Ag^+
Solid-state liquid or polymer membrane	F^-	LaF_3 crystal	10^{-6} – sat'd	OH^-
	Na^+	Na^+ ionophore (ETH 227) 2-nitrophenyloctyl ether, sodium tetraphenylborate	$10^{-3} - 10^{-1}$	Li^+, K^+, Ca^{2+}
	Cl^-	Tri-n-octylpropylammonium chloride, decanol	$10^{-3} - 10^{-1}$	OH^-, Br^-, F^-
	K^+	Valinomycin, dioctyladipate, PVC	$3 \times 10^{-5} - 1$	NH_4^+
	Ca^{2+}	Ca^{2+} ionophore (ETH 1001), 2-nitrophenyloctyl ether, sodium tetraphenylborate	$10^{-7} - 10^{-2}$	
	Ca^{2+}	Calcium di-(n-decyl)phosphate, di-(n-octylphenyl)-phosphate, PVC	$3 \times 10^{-5} - 1$	Mg^{2+}
	Li^+	Dodecyl methyl-14-crown-4 (ETH 1810)	$10^{-7} - 5 \times 10^{-2}$	Na^+
Gas sensors	CO_2	Combination glass pH electrode, 0.01–0.1 M $NaHCO_3$–NaCl filling solution behind silicone rubber membrane	$10^{-4} - 10^{-1}$	Organic acids
	NH_3	Combination glass pH electrode, 0.1 M NH_4Cl filling solution; behind porous Teflon gas-permeable membrane	$10^{-5} - 5 \times 10^{-2}$	Volatile amines

(Reprinted from Okorodudu AO. Electrochemistry, In: Schoeff LE, Williams RH, eds., Principles of laboratory instruments, Copyright 1993, with permission from Elsevier)

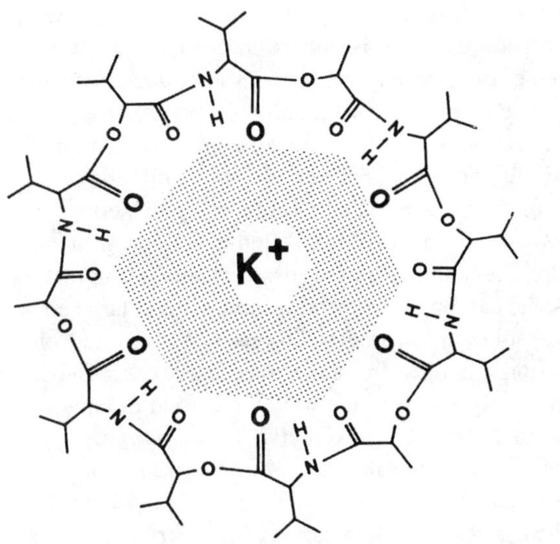

FIGURE 7. Model of valinomycin with a hydrated K^+ in the cavity surrounded by oxygen atoms. (*Reprinted from Okorodudu AO. Electrochemistry, In: Schoeff LE, Williams RH, eds., Principles of laboratory instruments, Copyright 1993, with permission from Elsevier*)

electrode. In this type of electrode, a slightly soluble salt containing the anion to be measured is immobilized in a silicone rubber matrix. For example, an electrode that is to be chloride-sensitive would be constructed by forming a silicone rubber membrane that contains about 50% weight-to-weight silver chloride and silicone rubber. The silver chloride particles are generally about 5–10 μm in diameter and are in actual physical contact throughout the silicone rubber. Such an electrode functions because of the selective permeability of the membrane. This type of electrode can be used for measurement of anions such as chloride, bromide, and iodide.

Solid-State Electrode

The solid-state electrode is another type of anion-sensitive electrode that functions on the same principle as the precipitate-impregnated electrode. The active membrane portion of the solid-state electrode consists of an inorganic single crystal doped with a rare earth metal. For example, the solid-state fluoride electrode has a crystalline lanthanum fluoride membrane that has been doped with europium (II) to lower its electrical resistance and facilitate ionic charge transport. This type of electrode has been commercially produced for Br^-, Cd^{2+}, Cl^-, Cu^{2+}, CN^-, F^-, I^-, Pb^{2+}, Ag^+, S^{2-}, Na^+, and SCN^- ion measurements.

A membrane produced by Beckman Instruments appears to be solid but is actually lipid-based in structure. The true solid membranes are crystallographic in structure, whereas the firm lipid structure is due to close spatial orientation of molecules. Lipids provide a medium in which electrostatic forces function. An ISE for K^+ consists of diphenyl ether, valinomycin, lecithin, and Nujol (mineral oil), and an NH_4^+-sensitive electrode is prepared with bromodiphenyl ether, nonactin, lecithin, and Nujol.

Gas Electrode

In the oxygen-sensing amperometric electrode, the anode and cathode are separated from the sample by a polyethylene gas-permeable membrane. A small applied potential between the anode and cathode causes an oxidation–reduction reaction with the oxygen diffusing through the membrane. A current is generated proportionately to the partial pressure of oxygen in the sample. Because oxygen diffuses instantaneously, sensor response is fast.

A pCO_2-sensing electrode is a standard glass pH electrode that has been modified to measure the concentration of carbon dioxide in aqueous solution. The electrode is placed in contact with the solution being analyzed for carbon dioxide content. Carbon dioxide can pass through a Teflon membrane because Teflon is highly permeable to the gas. After a few seconds, the solution on the inside of the Teflon membrane is at equilibrium with the solution on the outside. The solution on the inside of the Teflon membrane contains sodium bicarbonate. Thus, the carbon dioxide concentration has a large effect on the concentration of hydrogen ions in solution. Hydrogen ions easily permeate a cellophane membrane that separates the reaction chamber from the glass electrode. The hydrogen ions are then detected by the glass electrode. In this way, the carbon dioxide concentration affects the pH and the pH can then be measured directly.

The technique of measuring pH has been previously discussed. Measuring pCO_2 is accomplished in the same manner, but the details of the electrode require some explanation (Figure 8). The blood sample is separated from a combination pH electrode system by a membrane. Carbon dioxide passes through this membrane from the blood sample into an electrolyte solution that perfuses the sensing tip of the electrode. As the carbon dioxide is absorbed by the electrolyte, carbonic acid is formed, altering the pH. This pH change is a linear function of the carbon dioxide content of the blood, and it obviously can be measured by the electronics of the pH meter on an appropriate scale. This arrangement may be called a Severinghous electrode (Figure 9). The electrolyte solution perfusing its tip makes contact with both measuring and reference electrode elements. The carbon dioxide electrode in various systems may differ in physical arrangement from the electrode illustration in Figure 9 but will function in the same way.

Enzyme Electrode

Enzyme electrodes have been developed to extend the application of ISEs to the measurement of nonionic compounds. In enzyme ISEs, an intermediary reaction is used to generate ions that can be related directly to the concentration of the compounds of interest. Enzymes are perfectly suited to catalyze the production of ions from compounds such as glucose or urea. Enzyme electrodes have been used specifically for glucose and blood urea nitrogen (BUN) analysis; therefore, these two applications are described.

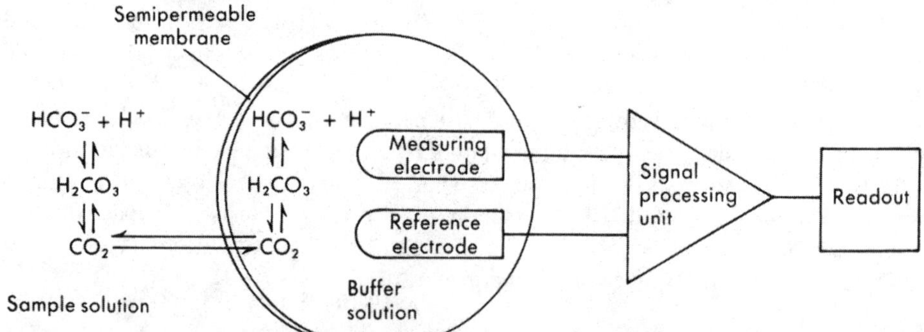

FIGURE 8. Principle of pCO_2 electrode system. (*Reprinted from Okorodudu AO. Electrochemistry, In: Schoeff LE, Williams RH, eds., Principles of laboratory instruments, Copyright 1993, with permission from Elsevier*)

In general, an enzyme electrode is made by polymerizing a gelatinous membrane of immobilized enzyme directly over an ISE. A glucose-specific enzyme electrode (Figure 10) is made by polymerizing a gelatinous membrane of immobilized glucose oxidase over a polarographic oxygen electrode. When the enzyme electrode is in contact with a glucose-containing solution, the glucose and oxygen diffuse into the immobilized glucose oxidase layer. Oxygen diffuses through a plastic membrane to the oxygen electrode where it is detected. The polarographic electrode is used to measure the oxygen consumed when glucose oxidase reacts with glucose in the sample solution. Therefore, the decrease in the amount of oxygen detected by the oxygen electrode is related to an increase in the amount

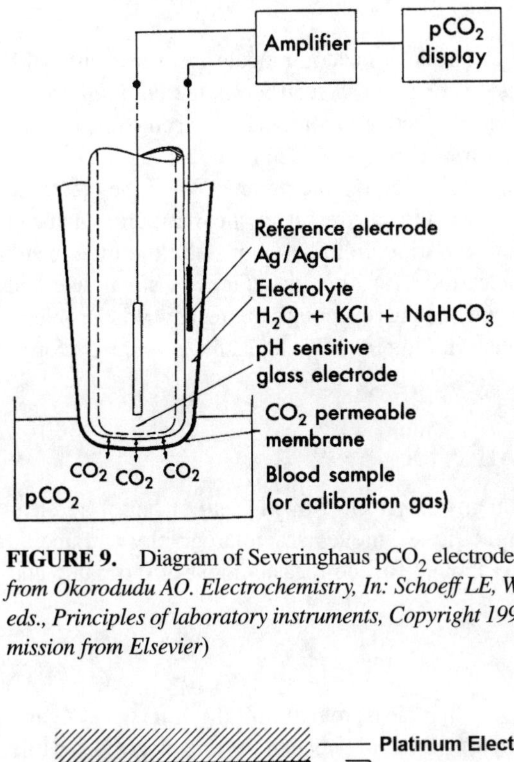

FIGURE 9. Diagram of Severinghaus pCO_2 electrode. (*Reprinted from Okorodudu AO. Electrochemistry, In: Schoeff LE, Williams RH, eds., Principles of laboratory instruments, Copyright 1993, with permission from Elsevier*)

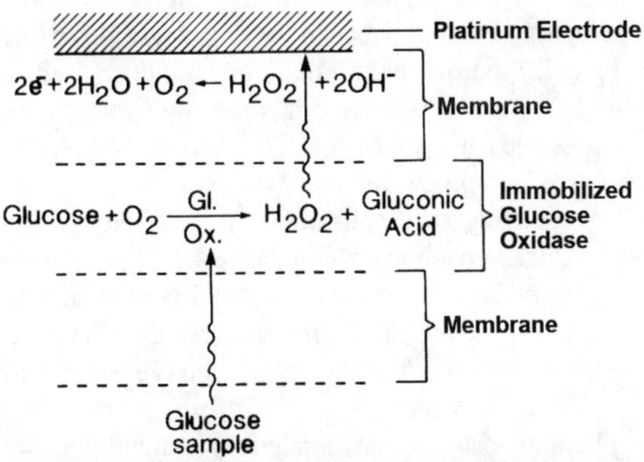

FIGURE 10. Schematic diagram of glucose electrode. (*Reprinted from Okorodudu AO. Electrochemistry, In: Schoeff LE, Williams RH, eds., Principles of laboratory instruments, Copyright 1993, with permission from Elsevier*)

of glucose present. This type of electrode also can be used to detect the rate of reduction of oxygen rather than the absolute reduction and to relate it to glucose concentration.

In another approach to glucose analysis, glucose oxidase acting on the glucose produces hydrogen peroxide, which is measured by a polarographic electrode. It is the level of peroxide production, rather than the reaction rate, that is proportional to glucose concentration.

An enzyme electrode also can be used for the determination of urea. The electrode consists of a membrane containing immobilized urease over a NH_4^+-selective glass electrode. The urea in the sample diffuses into the enzyme-containing membrane where it is hydrolyzed to NH_4^+. NH_4^+ is measured by the glass electrode and is related directly to urea concentration.

Microelectrodes

Efforts are being directed to miniaturize electrodes to accommodate measurements with small amounts of solution. A creative design for a microelectrode is the combination of ISEs with transistors. In one approach, an ion-selective membrane is placed over the gate of a metal oxide-semiconductor field effect transistor (MOSFET). Such a microelectrode has been constructed with MOSFET using a K^+-selective membrane. When the electrode is in contact with the test solution, K^+ activity at the gate results in a current drain that can be monitored and related directly to K^+ concentration. Initially, poor stability of the measured signal limited the use of this microelectrode, but the advantages of small size and direct electronic handling of the signal are incentive enough to rectify this problem. Microelectrodes are becoming more popular with improved designs that give the performance required for quantitative analysis.

VOLTAMMETRIC MEASUREMENTS

Voltammetric measurements are measurements of current flowing into or out of an electrode in solution. Two varieties of voltammetric techniques are polarography and anodic stripping voltammetry. The techniques are applied for the measurement of inorganic and organic species and trace metals.

Polarography

The **polarographic** technique is based on the measurement of the **current** flowing through an electrochemical cell and the electric potential between the two electrodes while a constant external voltage is being applied. Polarographic apparatus is widely used in analytical chemistry but has seldom been employed in clinical laboratory methods until recently. Measurement of the partial pressure of oxygen (pO_2) required a different approach. The pO_2 electrode works on a polarographic principle.

Nearly all conductors are metallic or electrolytic in nature. When electricity passes from a metal to a solution of electrolyte or vice versa, the type of carrier changes abruptly and either an oxidation or a reduction takes place. In the case of oxygen in solution, oxygen is reduced with the release of electrons and the current increases as a direct function of the electrons released. Hence the change in current is an analog of the oxygen concentration in the solution.

The pO_2 electrode consists of a platinum cathode surrounded by a tubular silver anode. The two electrodes are insulated from each other and make contact only through a drop of electrolyte at the electrode tip. A gas-permeable membrane holds this drop at the tip of the electrode and separates it from the blood to be measured. Oxygen in the blood diffuses across the membrane into the electrolyte where it is reduced and measured as a change in current that is directly proportional to the pO_2 (Figure 11).

The very tiny change in current sensed by the pO_2 electrode is amplified and measured by a sensitive electrometer against a reference current provided by a reference cell or Zener source. The pH meter's ammeter can be used for reading this signal on an appropriate scale. A polarographic electrode, often referred to as the Clark electrode, is the usual means of measuring pO_2 in the systems described here. A cross-sectional view of a pO_2 electrode is shown in Figure 12.

Anodic Stripping Voltammetry

The anodic stripping voltammetric technique consists of the analyte preconcentration on the electrode followed by stripping from the electrode. A negative potential (plating

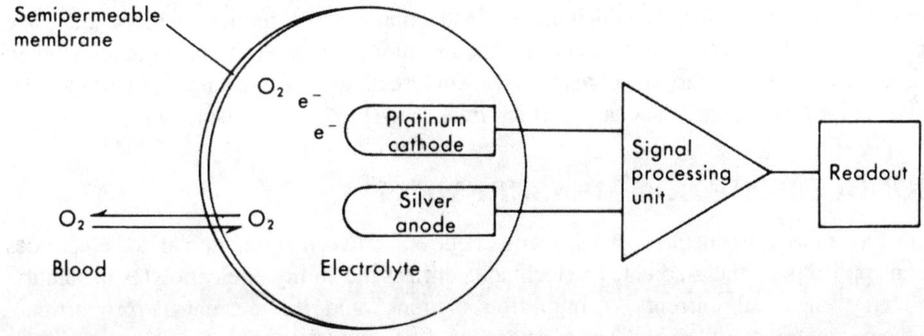

FIGURE 11. Principle of pO_2 electrode system. (*Reprinted from Okorodudu AO. Electrochemistry, In: Schoeff LE, Williams RH, eds., Principles of laboratory instruments, Copyright 1993, with permission from Elsevier*)

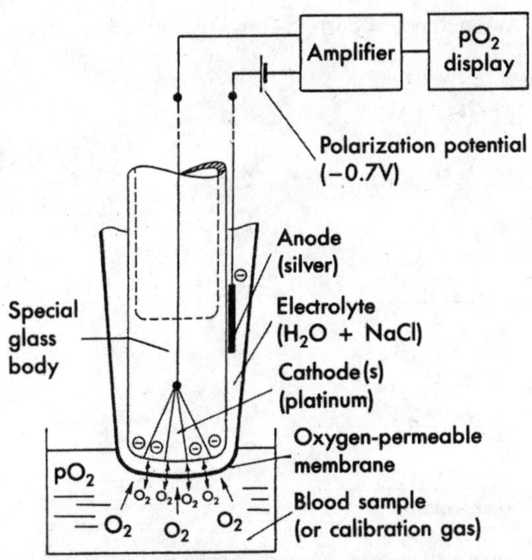

FIGURE 12. Diagram of polarographic oxygen electrode used by Instrumentation Laboratory in its blood gas system. (*Reprinted from Okorodudu AO. Electrochemistry, In: Schoeff LE, Williams RH, eds., Principles of laboratory instruments, Copyright 1993, with permission from Elsevier*)

voltage) is applied for a fixed period, usually 30 seconds to 30 minutes, to plate the electroactive metal ions onto the mercury electrode (Figure 13, upper panel). Only a fraction of the analyte is deposited on the mercury electrode during the fixed time of electroplating. Complete electroplating is time-consuming and unnecessary because the amount deposited on the mercury electrode is directly proportional to the concentration of the analyte. This preconcentration step makes it possible to measure analytes as low as 10^{-10} M using this technique.

After plating, the deposited metal ions are removed from the electrode by application of increasingly positive potential. As each ion returns to solution, a sharp current peak occurs at a potential level that is characteristic for each metal. Figure 13 (lower panel) shows the current peak generated for some metals. The peak height or area is directly proportional to the analyte's concentration. By assaying standards and unknowns under identical conditions, the unknown can be identified and quantitated by peak height or area comparison.

The anodic stripping voltammetric technique is used in the clinical laboratory for the quantitation of heavy metals, which include lead, copper, and chromium in blood and urine specimens. These metals can be freed from association with other biologic components of blood and urine by various digestion reagents such as Metexchange® (marketed by Environmental Science Associates), which frees lead (Pb^{2+}) for measurement.

CONDUCTOMETRIC MEASUREMENT

This type of measurement involves electrical current between two nonpolarized electrodes at an applied potential gradient. The technique utilizes the ability of electrolytes in solution to carry electrical current by migration of ions, and the current is proportional to the concentration of the ion. The resistance to the flow of the ions is the reciprocal of the conductance and from Ohm's law, these parameters can be calculated from the following:

$$\text{Resistance} = \text{applied voltage/current flowing} \tag{6}$$

$$\text{Conductance} = \text{current flowing/applied voltage} \tag{7}$$

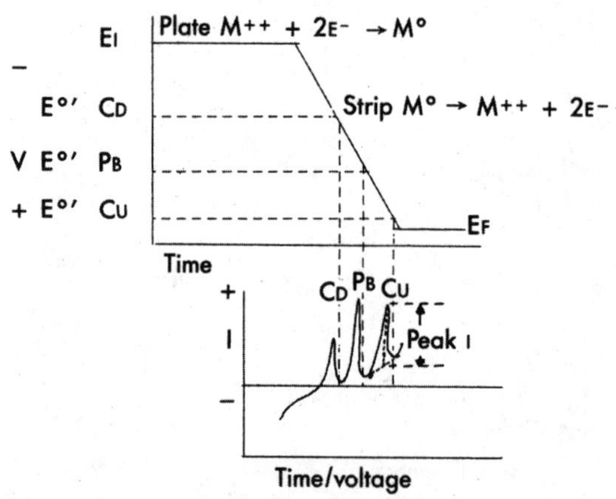

FIGURE 13. Basic sequence of events in anodic stripping voltammetry. (*Reprinted from Okorodudu AO. Electrochemistry, In: Schoeff LE, Williams RH, eds., Principles of laboratory instruments, Copyright 1993, with permission from Elsevier*)

Thus, an increase in resistance of the solution causes a decrease in conductivity with a resultant decrease in current. Their applications in clinical laboratories include the measurement of erythrocyte volume fraction (hematocrit) and for analysis of analytes that include urea and creatinine.

Conductometric measurement is illustrated by the measurement of hematocrit (HCT) in blood gas analyzers. It is based on the measurement of electrical resistance across an aperture as particles in a solution (blood) pass through the aperture. This electrical impedance is due to the electrical insulating properties of the erythrocytes (RBCs). This electrophysical characteristic of the erythrocytes is due to the lipid content in the membrane that makes it essentially nonconducting. The voltage pulse generated as the RBCs pass through the aperture is proportional to the cell size and the number of pulses is directly proportional to the cell count. Based on erythrocyte size and the number of voltage pulses counted in a given volume of blood, the HCT is calculated as follows:

$$\text{HCT} = (\text{volume of RBCs in the sample/volume of sample})100\% \quad (8)$$

Factors that cause false elevation in HCT measured by conductometry include increased Na^+ and K^+, while a decrease in their concentrations causes a false decrease in HCT. Other causes of erroneous HCT results by this method are volume fraction and shape of the RBCs, abnormal protein levels, and preanalytical errors such as inadequate mixing of samples prior to measurement.

The conductometric technique has been applied to the measurement of other analytes such as urea in blood. In this application, ions generated from the hydrolysis of urea result in increased conductivity in the sample. The net increase in conductivity is proportional to the concentration of urea:

$$\text{Urea} \xrightarrow{\text{Urease}} (NH_4)_2CO_3 \longrightarrow 2NH_4^+ + CO_3^{2-}$$

Thermal conductivity detection is used for analysis of carbon dioxide in an instrument that is designated Model E 100 (Ericsen Instruments). This ingenious instrument is designed to detect only carbon dioxide by using an analytic principle. When an electric current is passed through a resistance wire, some electrical energy is lost as heat energy and thus the temperature of the wire increases. As the wire gets hotter, resistance, in turn, increases. The heat produced is radiated into the air or surrounding gas and dissipates at a rate determined by the composition of the gas. Heat would dissipate more quickly in carbon dioxide than in helium. As the heat dissipates, the temperature and hence the resistance of the wire decrease. A thermal conductivity (TC) detector is a measuring device set up to sense the resistance change that occurs when the gas surrounding the resistance element changes. In most configurations the sensor is one arm of a Wheatstone bridge, which is a configuration of four resistors set up to measure resistance accurately.

In the carbon dioxide analyzer, carbon dioxide is displaced from the serum sample using lactic acid. The released gas is then forced from the reaction chamber by fluid displacement into the sensing chamber. Here the displaced carbon dioxide serves to change the relative percentage of carbon dioxide in room air, and this is sensed by the thermal conductivity detector.

The instrument is semiautomated. A 100-μL sample is required, and the test cycle requires less than a minute. The sample is injected into the reaction chamber and the cover closed. The start button is depressed, initiating a mixing sequence. Reagent fills the chamber, forcing the carbon dioxide into the TC detector. The electronic circuit converts the sensed change in resistance to millimoles per liter, and the result is displayed. Recycling the instrument flushes the sample and prepares the instrument for a new sample.

AMPEROMETRIC AND COULOMETRIC MEASUREMENTS

Amperometry is the measurement of current between two electrodes at a fixed potential. The resulting current is directly proportional to the amount of redox species. The change in current is sensitive to concentration of the species and not to the activity generated in the electrode.

Coulometry is the measurement of the amount of charge (coulombs) passing between two electrodes at a fixed potential. The amount of charge is directly proportional to the quantitative oxidation or reduction of an electroactive species at one of the electrodes.

Amperometry deals with measurement of current at a single applied potential, whereas coulometry is concerned with measurement of charge. These techniques will be illustrated here by the coulometric method because their chemical basis is similar.

Several chloride titrators have been produced that work on the principle of coulometry. If a carefully controlled current is passed between two silver electrodes in an ionic solution, silver ions will be released by ionization at one electrode. If chloride ions are in the solution, these combine with released silver ions to produce insoluble silver chloride:

$$\text{Anode electrode: } Ag \rightarrow Ag^+ + e^-$$

$$\text{Solution reaction: } Ag^+ + Cl^- \rightarrow AgCl \text{ (solid)}$$

The chloride titrator makes use of this principle. A silver-detecting electrode and reference half-cell are included in the system to sense the excess of free silver ions when the chloride is used up. When silver is detected, the current to the silver-releasing electrode is discontinued. If the amperage of the ionizing current and the time it was flowing are known, the coulombs that passed can be calculated. Faraday's law states that ionization produced when an electric current is passed from a metal into an electrolyte depends only on the coulombs passing through the current:

$$Q = It = znF \tag{9}$$

where Q = charge passed for a finite time (t) at a constant current (I)
z = the number of electrons involved in the electrochemical reaction
F = Faraday's constant
n = the number of moles of analyte in the sample

Hence, the ions of silver released by ionization, which will exactly equal the ions of chloride that were present in the solution, can be calculated.

In the clinical chemistry laboratory, a constant current coulometric assay is used for the determination of serum chloride in a fixed volume of sample. In this approach, the concentration of the unknown is calculated from the titration times for the blank (T_{blk}), standard (T_{std}), and unknown (T_{unk}) using:

$$[Cl^-]_{unk}\ \text{mmol/L} = (T_{unk} - T_{blk})/(T_{std} - T_{blk}) \times [STD]\ \text{mmol/L} \quad (10)$$

CHARACTERISTICS OF ELECTROCHEMICAL ANALYZERS

During the 1980s, clinical chemistry laboratories experienced a rapid change of instrumentation from flame photometric and colorimetric to electrochemical-based analyzers. A search for safer, accurate, more precise, and less cumbersome ways of quantitation were among the factors that aided the rapid conversion to the electrochemical systems. Analytes such as sodium, potassium, and lithium routinely had been quantitated using the flame photometer, which is labor intensive, technologist dependent, cumbersome, and dangerous. These problems prompted many instrument manufacturers toward the use of electrochemistry. These manufacturers sought methods of combining clinically relevant analytes that are measurable by electrochemical techniques with the formation of automated multichannel analyzers. Table 2 lists some characteristics of the major instruments that use electrochemical methods. These are usually multichannel systems for measurement of electrolytes or electrolytes and blood gases with or without other chemistries. Table 3 focuses on technical factors that have been documented to cause errors in ISE measurements. Strict adherence to the manufacturer's operation and maintenance protocol is intended to eliminate some of these factors. The analytic difference between direct ISE and flame atomic emission spectroscopy (i.e., indirect ISE) is usually handled through software manipulation in the measurement system.

Because these systems are very similar technically, the Bayer Rapidpoint 400 system is presented here to illustrate the features of an electrochemical analyzer designed for patient care.

The Rapidpoint 400 is a fully automated, desktop microanalyzer that has a single measurement cartridge containing sensors, reagents, and electronic and fluidic components. The sensors are for measuring pH, pO_2, pCO_2, Na^+, K^+, Ca^{2+}, Cl^-, glucose, and hematocrit. The test menu in the Rapidpoint 405 is designed to include measurement of total hemoglobin, oxyhemoglobin, deoxyhemoglobin, methemoglobin, and carboxyhemoglobin. The cartridges are available in 400- and 750-sample analyses sizes that are stable for 28 days from installation on the analyzer. It is a maintenance-free system that reports results within 60 seconds of sample introduction.

The measurement principle in the Rapidpoint is based on electrochemical phenomena. The sensors for the pH and electrolyte measurements are based on ion-selective electrode technology, while pO_2 and glucose sensors are electrochemical cells that use amperometric principles. Other measurement principles for the Rapidpoint include conductometry for hematocrit and an indirect potentiometric method based on the principles described by Bradley and Severinghaus for bicarbonate measurement.

TABLE 2. Representative analyzers that use electrochemical principles

Company	Product[a]	Analytes[b]
Bayer Diagnostics, United States	Rapidpoint	Blood gases, electrolytes, glucose, lactate, hematocrit
Beckman Instruments, United States	LabLyte, E, and Synchron	Blood gases, electrolytes, glucose, lactate, hematocrit
Dr Lange, Germany	LEA	Electrolytes
DuPont, United States	Dimension and Lye systems	Electrolytes, lithium
Leschweiler & Company, Germany	S2000 and ECO 2000	Blood gases, electrolytes
Fresenius Ag Fr, Germany	Ionometer	pH, electrolytes
Horiba, Japan	Sera-200 series	pH, electrolytes
Instrumentation Laboratories, United States	Synthesis 1745 & GEM Premier 3000	Blood gases, electrolytes, glucose, lactate, hematocrit
Ionetics, United States	Ionetics	pH, electrolytes
Kodak, United States	VITROS and Fusion series	Electrolytes, other chemistries
Kone, Finland	Microlyte	pH, electrolytes, lithium
Medica, United States	Easylyte	Blood gases, electrolytes, glucose, hematocrit
Nova Biomedical, United States	Stat Profile CCX 6	Blood gases, electrolytes, hematocrit, hemoglobin
Osmetech Inc., United States	Osmetech CCA Opti	Blood gases, electrolytes, glucose, hematocrit
Radiometer, United States	ABL Series	Blood gases, electrolytes, glucose, lactate, hematocrit
Roche Diagnostics, United States	OMNI Series	Blood gases, electrolytes, glucose, lactate, hematocrit

[a]Each manufacturer has several models with different combinations of analytes. [b]Sample volume ranges from 10 μL to several hundred microliters. (*Reprinted from Okorodudu AO. Electrochemistry, In: Schoeff LE, Williams RH, eds., Principles of laboratory instruments, Copyright 1993, with permission from Elsevier*)

FUTURE DEVELOPMENTS

Clinically acceptable ion-selective electrodes have been successfully developed for physiologically important alkali and alkaline earth cations (K^+, Na^+, Ca^{2+}, Li^+, H^+). The only relevant cation for which an acceptable ISE is yet to be introduced in the clinical laboratory is magnesium. It is anticipated that the substantial efforts by various manufacturers will result in the introduction of a Mg^{2+} ISE system with acceptable selectivity by 2010.

To date, this technology has not been readily applied to measurement of anions due to the problems associated with developing ionophore-like species and electrodes with unique selectivity interactions. The inorganic anions of main interest include sulfate and phosphate. Significant effort is currently in progress to improve the analytic performance of the anion-selective membrane to meet clinical requirements.

TABLE 3. General technical considerations in the use of potentiometric systems

Cause of error	Explanation
Temperature	Determination of electrode potential according to the Nernst equation is temperature-dependent. Thus, maintenance of a fixed and constant temperature is required in potentiometric measurement.
Interferent ions	High selectivity of an electrode for a specific ion is usually attained by modification of the ionophore and addition of various additives that reduce the electrode's selectivity for other ions. In some situations, it is essential to measure the concentration of the interferent ion concurrently and correct for its effect.
Protein and miscellaneous coat on electrode	Miscellaneous components in biologic fluids change the sensitivity and selectivity by binding to an electrode surface. This problem is usually limited or eliminated by scheduled electrode cleaning (or deproteinizing) and conditioning steps recommended by manufacturers.
Loss of CO_2 and change in pH	Some ions (e.g., ionized calcium) are particularly sensitive to pH changes because of competitive binding to proteins and other complex molecules. This problem indicates a preanalytic factor that must be taken into consideration in the interpretation of results.
Ionic strength	Equation 1 shows that the activity coefficient (γ) of an ion depends on the ionic strength of the solution. Thus, extreme changes in ionic strength (e.g., severe hyper- or hyponatremia) can affect the potentiometric measurement.
Direct versus indirect potentiometry	Direct (undiluted) measurement by ISE is concerned with ion activity in only the fluid compartment of the sample. Increasing the protein and/or lipid concentration introduces methodologic differences between direct ISE and indirect (diluted) ISE or the flame atomic emission spectroscopy.

(Reprinted from Okorodudu AO. Electrochemistry, In: Schoeff LE, Williams RH, eds., Principles of laboratory instruments, Copyright 1993, with permission from Elsevier)

SUGGESTED READING

Bates RG, Robinson RA. An approach to conventional scales of ionic activity for standardization of ion-selective electrodes. Pure Appl Chem 1973;37:575.

Czaban JD, Cormier AD, Legg KD. Establishing the direct-potentiometric "normal" range for Na/K: residual liquid junction potential and activity coefficient effects. Clin Chem 1982;28: 1936–45.

Guilbault GG. Analytical uses of immobilized enzymes. Biotechnol Bioeng 1972;3:361.

Heyrovsky J, Kuta J. Principles of polarography, Prague: Publishing House of Czechoslovak Academy of Science, 1965.

Lunte CE, Heineman WR. Electrochemical techniques in bioanalysis. Top Curr Chem 1988;143:1.

Oesch U, Ammann D, Simon W. Ion-selective membrane electrodes for clinical use. Clin Chem 1986;32:1448–59.

Okorodudu AO, Burnett RW, McComb RB, et al. Evaluation of three first-generation ion-selective electrode analyzers for lithium: systematic errors, frequency of random interferences, and recommendations based on comparison with flame atomic emission spectrometry. Clin Chem 1990;36:104–10.

Rehak N, Cecco SA, Niemela JE, et al. Linearity and stability of the AVL and Nova magnesium and calcium ion-selective electrodes. Clin Chem 1996;42:880–7.

Salling N, Siggaard-Andersen O. Liquid junction potentials between plasma or erythrolysate and KCl solutions. Scand J Clin Lab Invest 1971;28:33–40.

Siggaard-Andersen O. The acid-base status of the blood, 4th ed. Baltimore: Williams & Wilkins, 1974.

Chapter 11

Hematology, Coagulation, and Urinalysis

Kathleen Finnegan and Donna D. Castellone

Clinical tests on blood and urine samples are among the most common and routine tests patients and laboratorians encounter. Automation of hematology testing has resulted in a substantial increase in the number of samples analyzed and in a greater level of accuracy compared to manual methods. Coagulation testing dates back to the 1780s with automation being introduced in the 1960s. Urinalysis has been around for many years with its scope increasing as automation improved to now include chemical composition and microscopic examination. Various aspects of the automation and instrumentation related to these important clinical tests will be detailed. Additional reading for the three areas is included at the end of the chapter.

HEMATOLOGY AUTOMATION

Automation in the hematology laboratory has under gone many changes in the last 30–40 years. Prior to the introduction of automation, most hematology testing was done manually, which is time consuming and introduced many analytical variables. Hematology testing had many variations in standardization of technique from counting cells to the differential. With the introduction of automation, results from these hematology analyzers provide greater reliability, accuracy, and precision than the levels achieved with manual methods.

Hematology automation first focused on the enumeration of white blood cells (WBCs), red blood cells (RBCs), and platelets (PLTs). Wallace Coulter introduced the first method of counting cells in the 1950s. The method described is called electrical resistance or electrical impedance. Counting cells by electrical impedance is based on the principle of an increased resistance that occurs when a cell passes through an electrical field. In the 1960s, Technicon Instruments introduced darkfield optical scanning, and in the 1970s Ortho Diagnostics followed with a laser-based optical instrument. In addition to providing a complete blood count (CBC), other parameters are now provided. RBC indices, red cell distribution width (RDW), platelet distribution width (PDW), and mean platelet volume (MPV) are some examples. The automated differential analysis is based on the evaluation

Kathleen Finnegan wrote the hematology and urinalysis sections, and Donna Castellone wrote the coagulation section.

of cell volume, light scatter, and cytochemistry. This analysis provides information about enumeration of the different populations and subpopulations of WBCs. More recently, some advanced hematology analyzers perform automated reticulocyte counting with the addition of fluorescent light scatter.

Operation

The automation of hematology testing is based on three principles. These principles are electrical impedance, radiofrequency, and optical scatter. Each will be discussed in the following sections with the relevant methodology.

Electrical Impedance

The electrical impedance principle of counting cells is based on the detection and measurement of changes in electrical resistance produced by cells as they pass through an electrical field. A blood sample is diluted in saline, which is a good conductor of electrical current. The cells then are pulled through an aperture by creating a vacuum. Two electrodes establish an electrical current. The external electrode is located in the blood cell suspension. The second electrode is the internal electrode and is located in the glass hollow tube, which contains the aperture or orifice. Low-frequency electrical current is applied to the external electrode and the internal electrode. Direct current (DC) is applied between the two electrodes. Electrical resistance or impedance occurs as the cells pass through the aperture, causing a change in voltage. This change in voltage generates a pulse (Figure 1).

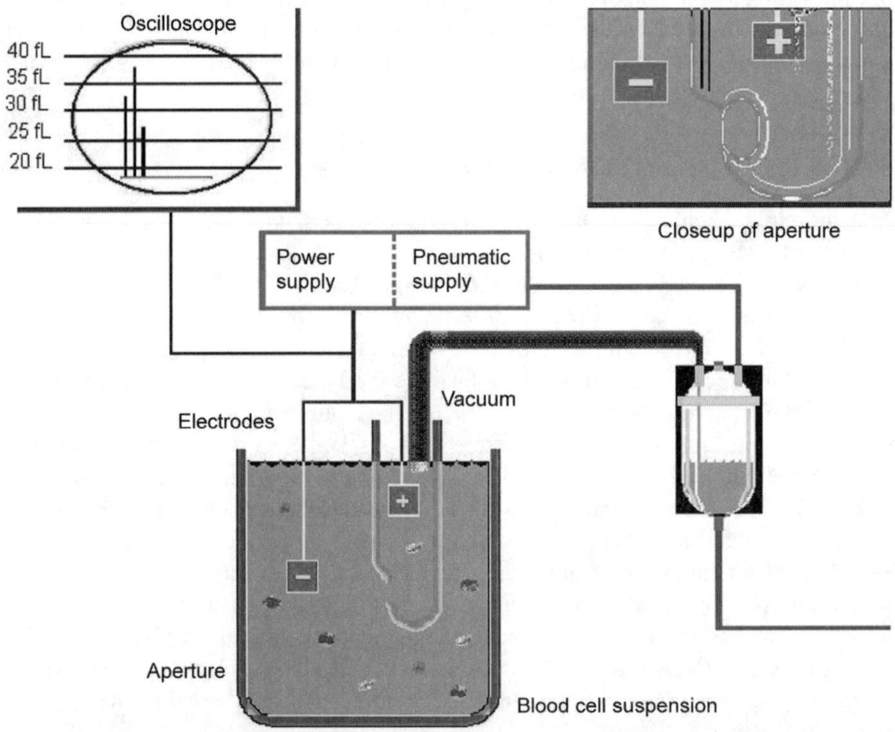

FIGURE 1. Coulter principle impedance. (*From Coulter Electronics GEN.S System: Book of Knowledge 1997, Courtesy of Beckman Coulter, Inc.*)

The number of pulses is proportional to the number of cells counted. The size of the voltage pulse is also directly proportional to the volume or size of the cell. Threshold limits are established for the enumeration of each cell population based on the cell volume (Figure 2). Pulses are channelized by their height or amplitude. The data are collected and plotted on a volume/frequency distribution histogram. The relative number is on the y-axis and the size or volume is on the x-axis. Histograms are created for the erythrocyte or RBC, leukocyte or WBC, and PLT populations based on cell volume measured in femtoliters (fL) and relative number (Figure 3). Particles in the red cell bath greater than 36 fL are counted as RBCs. Particles between 2 and 20 fL are counted as PLTs. In the white cell bath, the red cells are lysed and particles greater than 35 fL are counted as WBCs.

Histograms. Histograms are graphic representations of cell frequencies versus size. The histogram provides information about RBCs, WBCs, and PLT frequency; distribution about the mean; and the presence of subpopulations. The x-axis reflects the size of cells and the y-axis reflects the relative number (Figure 4).

Hydrodynamic Focusing. Hydrodynamic focusing is a process to generate a narrow channel through which cells separate and align in a single file in front of a detection system, one at a time. Laminar flow allows cells to flow in parallel lines through the flow cell without mixing with the sheath fluid. The hydrodynamic focusing allows greater accuracy and resolution of blood cells. Diluted cells are surrounded by a sheath fluid, which lines up the cells in a single file while passing through the detection aperture. After passing through

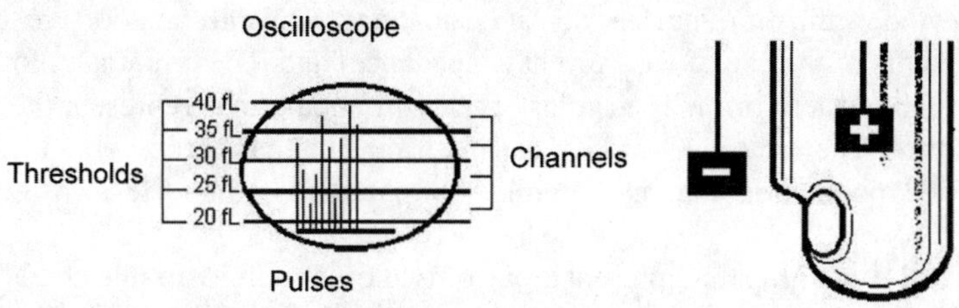

FIGURE 2. Oscilloscope pulse and histogram. (*From Coulter Electronics GEN.S System: Book of Knowledge 1997, Courtesy of Beckman Coulter, Inc.*)

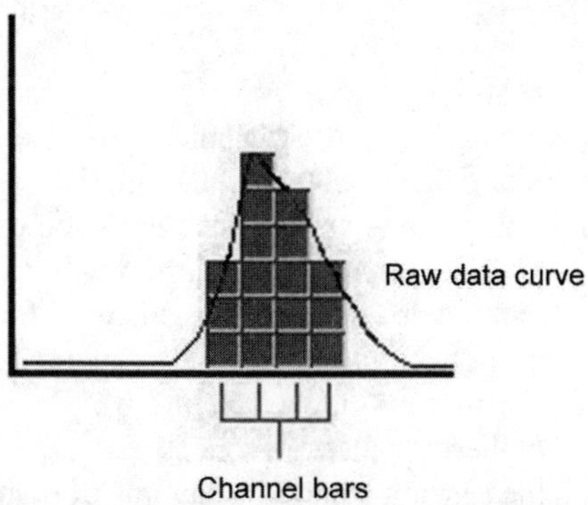

FIGURE 3. Histogram. (*From Coulter Electronics GEN.S System: Book of Knowledge 1997, Courtesy of Beckman Coulter, Inc.*)

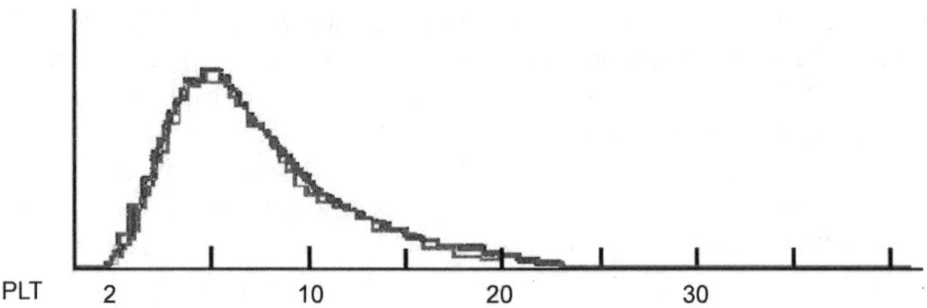

FIGURE 4. Platelet histogram. (*From Coulter Electronics GEN.S System: Book of Knowledge 1997, Courtesy of Beckman Coulter, Inc.*)

the aperture, the cells are then directed away from the back of the aperture. This process eliminates the recirculation of cells and the counting of cells twice (Figure 5).

Radiofrequency

Radiofrequency or RF resistance is a high-voltage electromagnetic current flowing between the electrodes that is used to detect the size of cells based on the cellular density. Radiofrequency is a high-frequency pulsating sine wave. Conductivity or radiofrequency measurements provide information about the internal characteristics of the cell. The cell wall acts as a conductor when exposed to high-frequency current (Figure 6). As the current passes through the cell, measurable changes are detected. The cell interior density or nuclear volume is directly proportional to pulse size or a change in RF resistance. The nuclear to cytoplasmic ratio, nuclear density, and cytoplasmic granulation are determined. When the results of the use of DC current (impedance) and RF current are plotted against each other, cell clusters form. These clusters or cell populations represent the concentration of cell type. The use of DC and RF can determine cell properties, which can separate the white cell population into neutrophils, lymphocytes, monocytes, eosinophils, and basophils.

Scatterplots are graphic representations of two or more measurable characteristics of cells. These three-dimensional plots visualize and analyze cellular data. The scatterplot provides information about abnormalities of populations and subpopulations of cells. The plots use conductivity and light scatter. Lymphocytes, granulocytes, and monocytes are the prominent populations viewed (Figure 7).

Optical Scatter

A sample of blood is diluted with an isotonic diluent and then hydrodynamically focused through a quartz flow cell. Cells pass through a flow cell on which a bean of light is focused. The light source is a laser light that is light amplified by stimulated emission of radiation. Laser light or monochromatic light is emitted as a single wavelength. A helium-neon light source is used for RBCs and PLTs. A tungsten-halogen light source is used for WBCs. As the cell passes through the sensing zone, light is scattered in all directions. Photodetectors sense and collect the scattered rays at different angles (Figure 8). These data are then converted to an electric pulse. The number of pulses generated is directly proportional to the number of cells passing through the sensing zone. The patterns of light are measured at various angles, forward light scatter at 180° and right angle scatter at 90°. Cell counts, size, cell structure, shape, and reflectivity are determined by the analysis of the light scatter data.

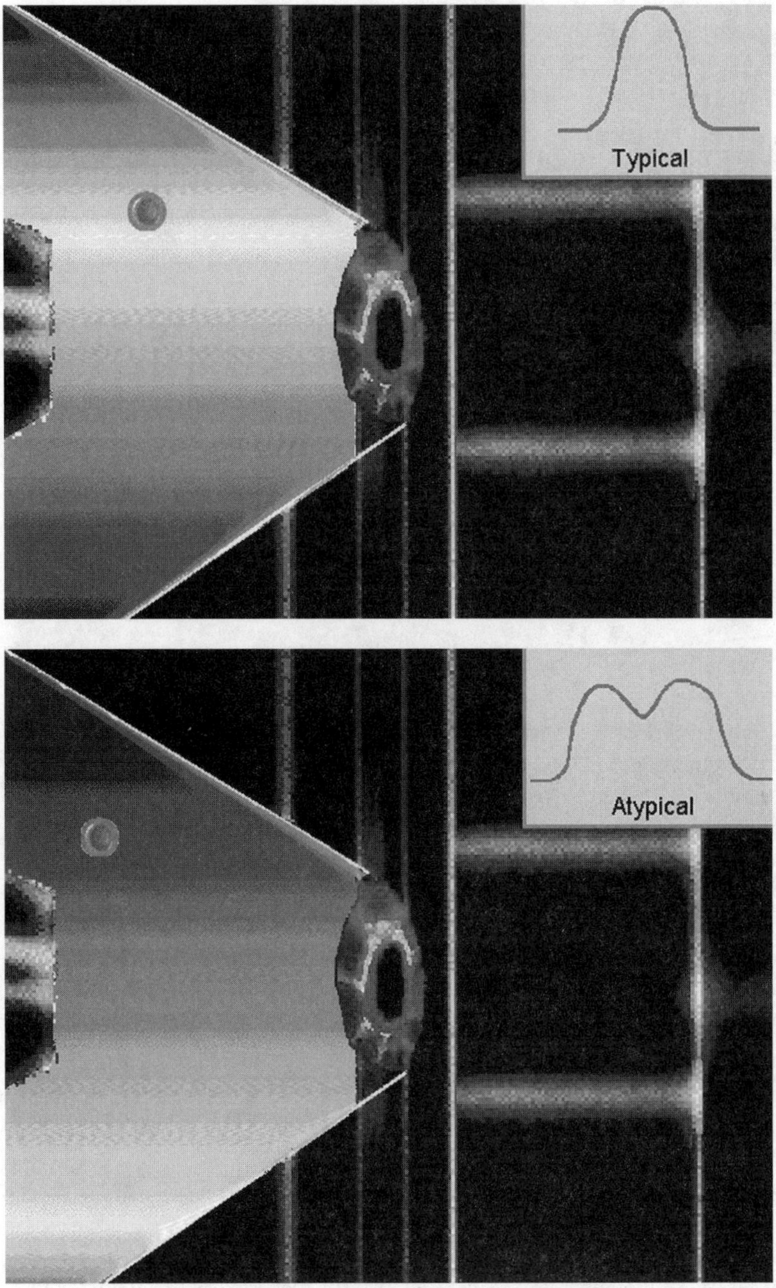

FIGURE 5. Coulter hydrofocusing. (*From Coulter Electronics GEN.S System: Book of Knowledge 1997, Courtesy of Beckman Coulter, Inc.*)

Light scatter results from independent processes. The processes are:

- Diffraction or the bending of light around corners with the use of small angles
- Refraction or the bending of light because of a change in speed with the use of intermediate angles
- Reflection or light waves turned back by an obstruction with the use of large angles

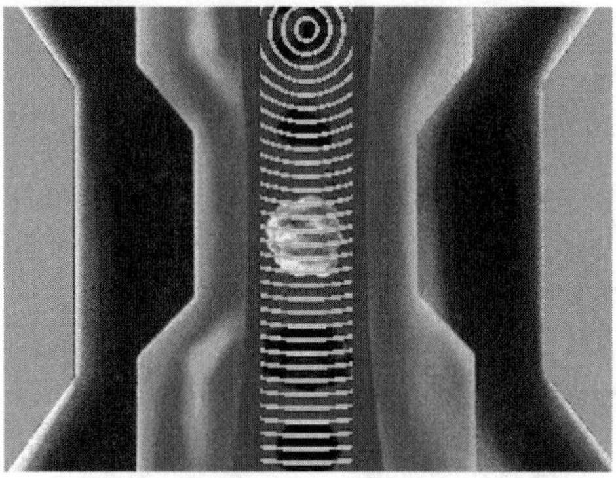

FIGURE 6. Conductivity. (*From Coulter Electronics GEN.S System: Book of Knowledge 1997, Courtesy of Beckman Coulter, Inc.*)

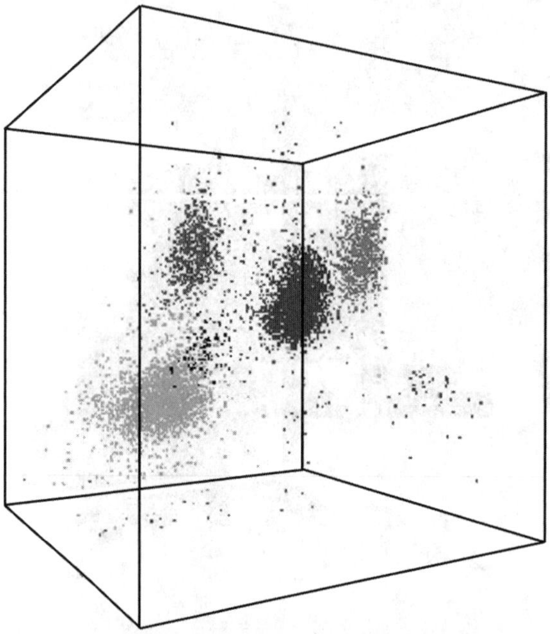

FIGURE 7. Coulter scatterplot. (*From Coulter Electronics GEN.S System: Book of Knowledge 1997, Courtesy of Beckman Coulter, Inc.*)

Forward angle light scatter (0°) is diffracted light that relates to volume. Forward low-angle light scatter (2–3°) relates to cell size or volume. Forward high-angle scatter (5–15°) relates to the internal complexity or refractive index of cellular components. Orthogonal light scatter (90°) or side scatter is a combination of reflection and refraction related to internal components.

Flow cytometry is the measurement of the physical or antigenic characteristics of cells with the use of a laser light source. Each cell can be measured for the intensity of scattered light, which includes cell size, cell density, nuclear complexity, cell granularity, and the staining capacity of dye in each cell. Other cellular characteristics can also be evaluated which

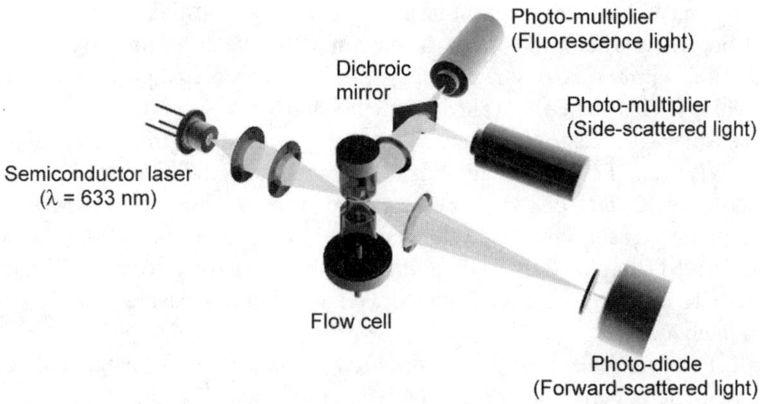

FIGURE 8. Sysmex fluorescence flow cytometry. (*Courtesy of Roche Diagnostics, Sysmex XE-2100, 1999*)

include nuclear DNA content, surface antigens, and cytoplasmic antigens. With flow cytometry, multiparameter analysis of cells can be done as they pass through a beam of laser light.

Light scatter is measured as forward light scatter (FALS) at 2–10° and orthogonal or side scatter (SSC) at 70–90°. FALS evaluates cell size and SSC evaluates cytoplasmic and nuclear complexity. Light scatter signals are amplified and converted to digital signals. FALS and SSC are plotted to form a scattergram to separate the cells into cell clusters. These clusters are separated into granulocytes, monocytes, and lymphocytes. The cells of interest can be selected for specific analysis.

With the addition of antibodies, ligands, and molecular probes that are conjugated to fluorochromes (fluorescent dyes) that fluoresce when excited by light, the flow cytometer can measure the fluorescence of each cell. Each cell can be analyzed for the presence or absence of various surface antigens, receptors, or enzymes. The newer generation of analyzers uses fluorescent flow cytometry to stain nuclear DNA, which permits the differentiation of nucleated RBCs (NRBCs) from WBCs.

Instruments

Basic automated hematology analyzers provide electronically measured RBC, WBC, and PLT counts; mean PLT volume (MPV); hemoglobin concentration (Hb); and the mean red cell volume (MCV). From these measured quantities, the hematocrit (Hct), mean cell hemoglobin (MCH), mean cell hemoglobin concentration (MCHC), and the RDW are calculated. The newer analyzers include white cell differential counts, relative (or percent) and absolute number, and reticulocyte analysis. The differential may be a three-part differential which includes granulocytes, lymphocytes, and monocytes or a five-part differential which includes neutrophils, lymphocytes, monocytes, eosinophils, and basophils. The new generation of analyzers now offers a sixth parameter, which is the enumeration of NRBCs. Hematology instruments also include verification systems. The verification system utilizes review of past results or delta checks and instrument flagging, e.g., R flags, population flags, suspect flags, definitive or quantitative flags.

Beckman Coulter Instrumentation (http://www.beckmancoulter.com)

Coulter® STKS™, Coulter GEN S™, and Coulter LH 750 series uses VCS technology, which is an acronym for volume (V), conductivity (C), and laser light scatter (S). The simultaneous measurement of cell volume, conductivity, and light scatter provides high statistical accuracy. The cell volume is measured by electrical impedance using low-frequency direct current. To ensure accuracy, Coulter incorporated pulse editing and sweep flow technology. This technology allows the cells that are being counted to line up in a single file to ensure size measurement integrity and to prevent cells from being counted twice. The RBC, WBC, and PLT counts are obtained by analyzing the number of pulses generated. The RBC, WBC, and PLT data are then plotted in the form of a histogram. The cell number is plotted on the y-axis and the cell size is plotted on the x-axis. The MCV and RDW are derived from the RBC histogram. The MPV is derived from the PLT histogram. The Hct, MCH, and MCHC are calculated. Hemoglobin is measured by the cyanmethemoglobin method.

Conductivity is measured by using high-frequency electromagnetic current for nuclear and granular constituents. Conductivity is influenced by the internal structures of the cell such as the nuclear–cytoplasm ratio and the cytoplasmic granular content. A monochromatic helium-neon laser is the light source to measure light scatter for surface structure, shape, and granularity. Forward angle light scatter is affected by cell shape, surface characteristics, and cytoplasmic granular content. The enumeration of relative percentage and the absolute number are displayed in a scatterplot (Figure 9).

Coulter GEN S uses AccuGate™ software technology to isolate subpopulations of WBCs. This technology increases the precision of results and the reliability of the flagging system. This system also uses Intellikinetics, which ensures continuous monitoring and the control of the cell measurement environment.

Reticulocyte counting is fully automated on the GEN S. Blood is mixed with new methylene blue. An acidic hypoosmotic solution is then added to clear the hemoglobin while preserving the stained RNA within the reticulocyte. The cells are then passed

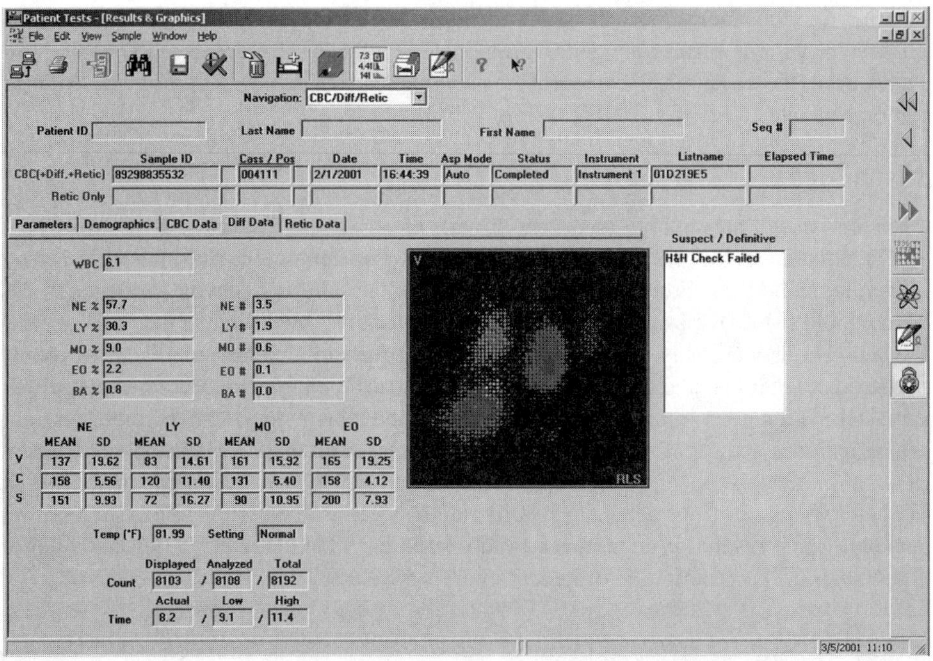

FIGURE 9. GENS scatterplot. (*From Beckman Coulter Electronics. The LH 755 Hematology Workcell Bulletin 9224, 2001, Courtesy of Beckman Coulter, Inc.*)

through a laser light beam at angles of 0° to 90°. The reticulocytes are identified and classified by simultaneous three-dimensional analysis using volume, conductivity, and light scatter. Red cells containing residual RNA scatter more light than mature red cells. Light scatter is displayed on the x-axis and volume on the y-axis (Figure 10). Parameters derived from light scatter are the reticulocyte percent (RET%), reticulocyte absolute number (RET#), and the immature reticulocyte fraction (IRF). The IRF is defined as the ratio of young or immature reticulocytes to the total number of reticulocytes. The IRF provides additional red cell information in the classification of anemias, monitoring bone marrow recovery, and related therapies.

The Coulter LH 750 is a high-volume system. This system features NRBC enumeration, flagging efficiency, and automated workflow management. The AccuCount cell enumeration technology provides better linearity and accuracy for WBCs and PLTs. Interferences from substances such as NRBCs, unlysed RBCs, and PLT clumps have been minimized. The AccuCount technology reduces the number of false-positive results. It also can identify and enumerate NRBCs and automatically corrects the WBC count.

The LH series features random access and the Aqueduct™ hematology workflow management (Orchard Software, Carmel, IN). This is a type of data management software that offers onboard decision rules. The system can interface up to four Coulter instruments and allows the user to view the information from multiple instruments in a common database. The Coulter LH 755 is the hematology analyzer that integrates a slide preparation platform, which consists of a slide maker and slide stainer, to form a single trackless automation workstation. The LH 755 offers automatic reflex slide making based on user-defined protocols.

Abbott Diagnostics Instrumentation (CELL-DYN, http://www.abbott.com)

Abbott Diagnostics offers smaller automated instruments that include the CELL-DYN 1200 and 1700. These smaller analyzers provide an 18-parameter CBC with a three-part differential. The CELL-DYN 3200 and 3700 series provide a 25-parameter CBC, a five-part differential, and a semiautomated reticulocyte count. The CELL-DYN 4000 provides

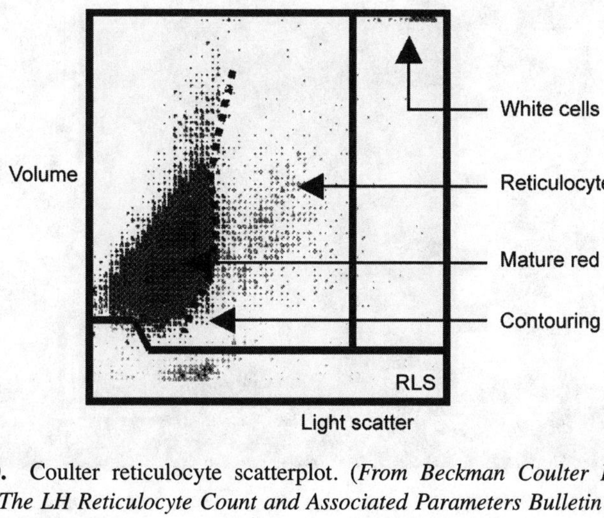

FIGURE 10. Coulter reticulocyte scatterplot. (*From Beckman Coulter Electronics Technical Information. The LH Reticulocyte Count and Associated Parameters Bulletin 9231 2001, Courtesy of Beckman Coulter, Inc.*)

a fully automated reticulocyte count with random access, a 25-parameter CBC, and a five-part leukocyte differential.

The CELL-DYN system uses three independent measurement technologies:

- An optical channel for the white count and differential
- An impedance channel for the red count and PLTs
- A hemoglobin channel for hemoglobin determination

A unique design of CELL-DYN is the technology of multiangle polarized scatter separation (MAPSS). The WBC count and differential are derived from this patented optical channel. A hydrodynamically focused sample stream is directed through a high-resolution flow cytometer. A cell suspension is prepared with a diluent that maintains the WBCs in their native state, and this suspension is then passed through an air-cooled argon ion laser light source. Scattered light is measured at multiple angles. Low-angle (1–3°) forward light scatter represents the cell size. Wide-angle (3–11°) forward light measures the cell complexity. Orthogonal light scatter (90°) determines cell lobularity; 90° depolarized (90D) is for the evaluation of cellular granularity. Various combinations of these four angle measurements are used to differentiate the white cell populations. Neutrophils and eosinophils are separated from mononuclear cells by plotting 90° light scatter data which are on the y-axis and wide-angle forward light scatter data which are on the x-axis. Eosinophils are separated from the neutrophil population by the eosinophils' ability to depolarize the polarized light scatter. The lymphocyte, monocyte, and basophil populations can be separated by plotting low-angle forward light scatter on the y-axis and wide-angle forward light scatter on the x-axis (Figure 11).

The RBCs, WBCs, and PLTs are counted and sized by electrical impedance. The MCV is the average volume of the red cells derived from the RBC size distribution plot. A 3–D MVC measurement ensures accurate RBC analysis. Hemoglobin is measured directly using the cyanmethemoglobin method at absorbance 540 nm. The hematocrit, MCH, and MCHC are calculated from the directly measured parameters.

The CELL-DYN 4000 has added fluorescent detection technology. Fluorescent detection of RNA allows for fully automated, random-access reticulocyte testing. Fluorescent

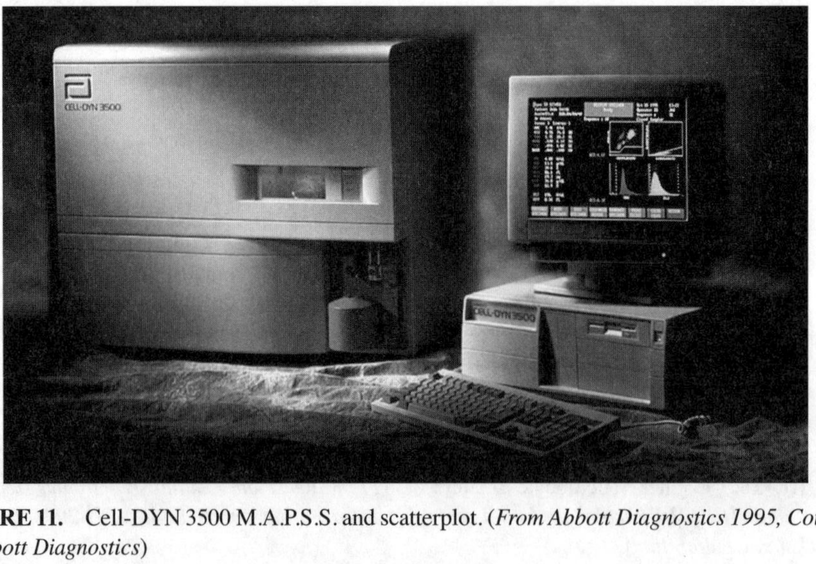

FIGURE 11. Cell-DYN 3500 M.A.P.S.S. and scatterplot. (*From Abbott Diagnostics 1995, Courtesy of Abbott Diagnostics*)

detection of DNA staining of NRBCs allows direct NRBC counting which is gated out of the WBC count. The NRBCs are enumerated in relative percent and absolute number, and WBC count is automatically corrected for the NRBCs present. Two-dimensional optical PLT analysis with automatic verification by focused flow impedance provides enhanced information for PLT analysis.

Roche Diagnostics Corp. (Sysmex Instrumentation, http://www.roche.com)

Sysmex manufactures a full line of hematology analyzers that include the K-4500, which provides WBC, RBC, and PLT counts and a three-part differential. The SE series and SF-3000 perform a CBC with a five-part differential. The newest analyzer added to the line is the XE-2100, which provides a CBC, five-part differential, and a fully automated reticulocyte count.

The SE series measures WBCs, RBCs, and PLTs using DC electrical impedance for counting and sizing of cells, hydrodynamic focusing, and automatic discrimination for accuracy and precision. The SE series generates the standard hematology parameters and the added parameters of RDW-SD (red cell distribution width by standard deviation), RDW-CV (red cell distribution width by coefficient), and MPV. Hemoglobin values are determined by the use of a cyanide-free, nontoxic reagent and are measured at 555 nm. The white cell count uses a separate channel and utilizes DC electrical impedance.

The white cell five-part differential includes simultaneous measurements using RF and DC detection methods for separating the white cell populations. There are four separate detection channels for the determination of each white cell type. A plot of low-frequency DC impedance plotted on the x-axis and high-frequency current RF on the y-axis determines lymphocytes, monocytes, and granulocytes. This channel is called the DIFF channel. The second channel is used with a special reagent for detecting the presence of immature cells. This channel is called the IMI channel. This channel also allows for abnormal morphology findings. The last two channels are the EO and the BASO chambers. Eosinophils and basophils are enumerated by impedance after the sample has been treated with specific lysing or buffer reagents (Figure 12).

The Sysmex XE-2100 is the latest analyzer. This system utilizes a combination of impedance technology, light scattering, and fluorescent staining to obtain information to

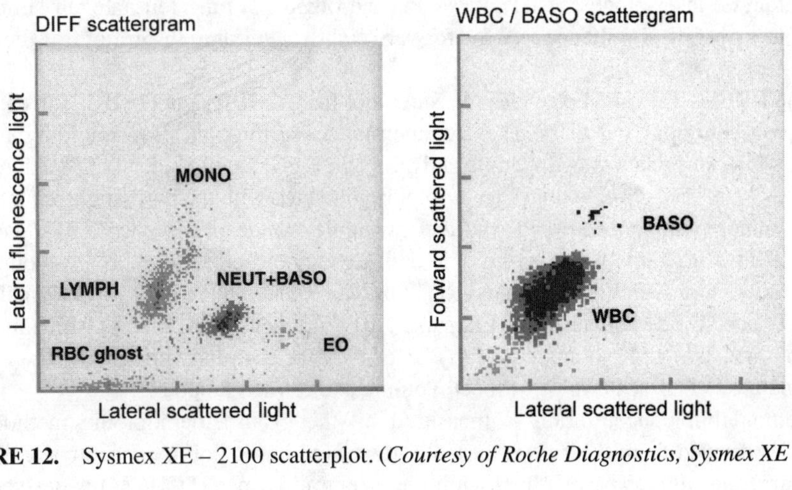

FIGURE 12. Sysmex XE – 2100 scatterplot. (*Courtesy of Roche Diagnostics, Sysmex XE – 2100, 1995*)

classify white cells. This analyzer has introduced new diagnostic parameters that include: reporting NRBCs, fluorescent optical PLT counts, fluorescent enhanced differential leukocyte counts, fluorescent reticulocyte count with a immature reticulocyte fraction (IRF), and human progenitor cell counts (HPC). The IRF parameter is used in monitoring erythropoietic marrow activity. The HPC parameter is used for managing cancer patients undergoing stem cell transplantation. Side scatter light (x-axis) is plotted against fluorescence (y-axis) generated data from the DIFF channel which allows the separation of lymphocytes, monocytes, eosinophils, and other granulocytes. Side scatter light (x-axis) is plotted against forward light scatter generated data from the WBC/BASO channel, which separates basophils from the rest of the white cell population. This channel also provides the WBC count. A plot of impedance on the x-axis against the RF impedance on the y-axis generates data from the IMI channel that provides information about immature cells and the HPC parameter. Side fluorescence on the x-axis plotted against forward light scatter on the y-axis allows the enumeration of NRBCs with automatic correction of the WBC count.

Bayer Instrumentation (ADVIA®, http://www.bayerdiag.com)

The ADVIA 120 hematology analyzer is a whole blood cell analyzer from Bayer Diagnostics that uses Unifluidics™ technology. This technology of the ADVIA 120 has evolved from the Technicon H-1, H-2, and H-3 systems. Unifluidics technology consists of an acrylic block with eight layers. Pathways for the fluids and air flow are machined within these acrylic layers for blood analysis. This eliminates most tubing and pinch values. There are five reaction chambers:

- Hemoglobin chamber
- Basophil–lobularity (BASO) chamber
- RBC/PLT chamber
- Reticulocyte chamber
- Peroxidase (PEROX) chamber

The ADVIA 120 analyzer uses flow cytometry for the analysis of cells. Aperture impedance counting is not used in this analyzer. The only parameter not derived from flow cytometry is hemoglobin, which is determined by the classical colorimetric method and read at 546 nm. The ADVIA 120 incorporates two independent flow cytometers. One cytometer is a laser-diode crystal source and the other is a tungsten-halogen lamp. Both cytometers operate simultaneously for forward light scatter and absorption for the counting and sorting of cells.

The RBC/PLT channel provides measurement for the RBC count, RBC indices, hemoglobin concentration, and PLTs. The specimen is passed through a low-angle light scatter (2–3°), which correlates to cell volume and size, and high angle (5–15°) light scatter, which correlates to internal complexity. A scatterplot is generated with the high-angle scatter on the x-axis (hemoglobin concentration) and the low-angle scatter on the y-axis (RBC volume). Independent histograms for RBC volume and hemoglobin concentration are plotted. The RBC histogram provides the MCV and RDW measurements. Then HCT, MCH, and MCHC are calculated. The system analyzes PLTs using a two-dimensional analysis which measures PLT volume (size) and refractive index (PLT density) of each individual PLT. The ADVIA 120 generates a PLT scatterplot with cell volume and refractive index.

Hemoglobin concentration is measured by the cyanmethemoglobin method. The MCHC is derived from the colorimetrically measured hemoglobin concentration, the red cell count, and MCV. The cell hemoglobin concentration mean (CHCM) is derived from the directly measured red cell hemoglobin concentration histogram. Interferences in the hemoglobin colorimetric method such as lipemia or icterus affect the calculated MCHC but not the CHCM parameter.

The white cell count is measured from two reaction chambers, the peroxidase channel and BASO-lobularity channel. They are measured by cytochemistry or myeloperoxidase activity and light scatter. In the peroxidase chamber, the WBCs are stained for myeloperoxidase activity and then passed through an optical chamber that measures light scatter or cell size and light absorption or stain intensity. These two measurements allow enumeration and classification of leukocytes into neutrophils, monocytes, lymphocytes, and eosinophils. Only those cells with peroxidase activity are stained. Neutrophils and eosinophils contain the most peroxidase. Monocytes stain weak. Lymphocytes, basophils, and large unstained cells (LUC) contain no peroxidase staining. Each cell passing the focused beam will be counted, light absorbed will relate to peroxidase staining, and the light scatter in the forward direction (1–3°) relates to size (Figure 13). In the BASO-lobularity channel, the leukocytes are stripped of their cytoplasm with the exception of the basophil. Basophils are counted along with the total WBC count and the lobularity index (LI). The LI is a measure of difference between the positions of two cell populations. Basophils are identifiable by their large low-angle scatter (Figure 14).

The reticulocyte reaction chamber measures low-angle and high-angle scatter as well as absorption of each cell counted. The absorption data are used for the classification of reticulocytes or mature red blood cells. Low-angle and high-angle scatter are proportional to cell size and hemoglobin concentration and light absorption is proportional to ribonucleic acid (RNA) contained in the cells (Figure 15). The reticulocyte hemoglobin concentration (CHr) is a parameter that can be used in the early detection of functional iron deficiency and anemia.

The ADVIA 70 hematology system processes a full CBC and five-part differential. The ADVIA 60 is a smaller unit that analyzes 16 different parameters and a three-part differential. The ADVIA S60 is a compact system combines the HEMA-TEK staining system.

Additional Hematology Automation

Automated Reticulocyte Counting

Reticulocyte counting is one of the last manual cell testing procedures. Many analyzers now have onboard automated reticulocyte counting. Automation of the traditional

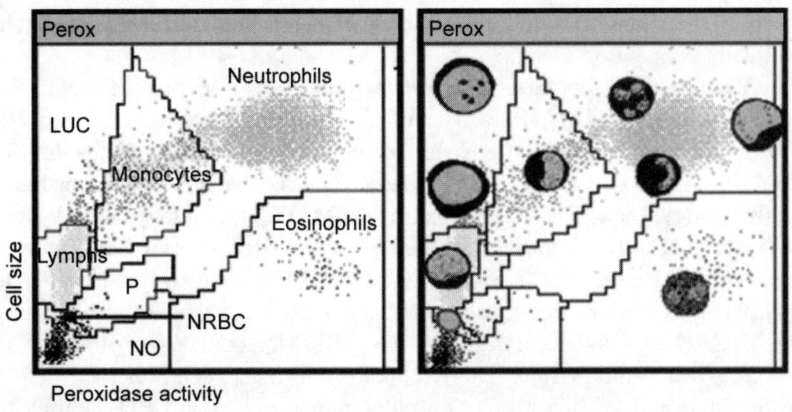

FIGURE 13. Bayer Advia 120 peroxidase scatterplot. (*From Bayer International Atlas of Hematology 1996, Courtesy of Bayer HealthCare, Diagnostics Division*)

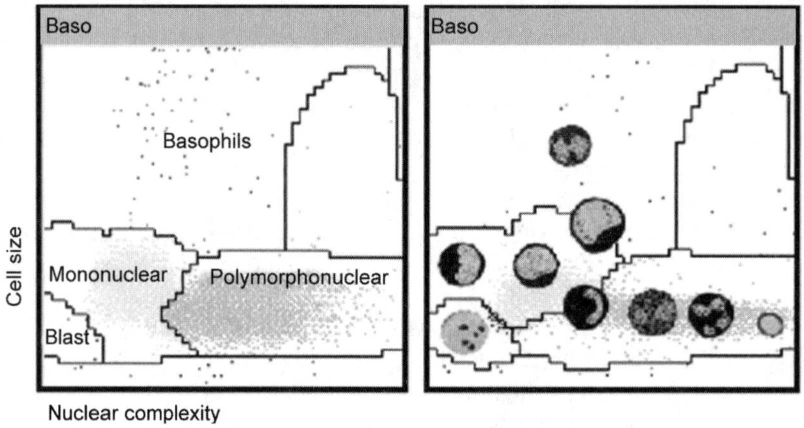

FIGURE 14. Bayer Advia 120 baso/lobularity scatterplot. (*From Bayer International Atlas of Hematology 1996, Courtesy of Bayer HealthCare, Diagnostics Division*)

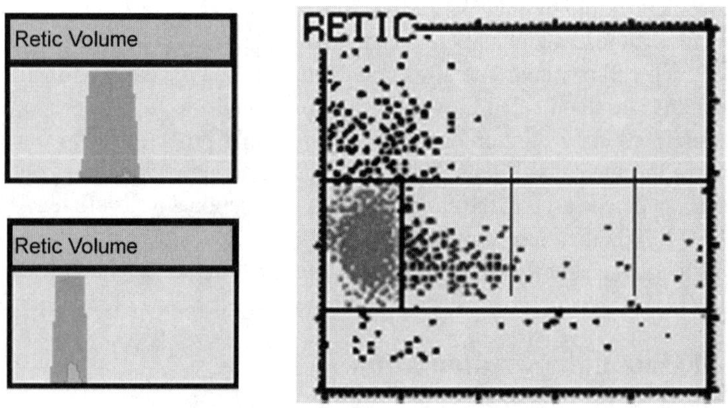

FIGURE 15. Bayer Advia 120 reticulocyte scatterplot. (*From Bayer ADVIA 120 Hematology System 2002, Courtesy of Bayer HealthCare, Diagnostics Division*)

reticulocyte count has allowed for increased precision and accuracy. It has also expanded the analysis of the young RBC, providing new parameters and indices that may help in the diagnosis and treatment of anemia.

The following analyzers have reticulocyte counting as part of their menu: Beckman Coulter GEN-S, STKS, and MAXM which utilizes a new methylene blue stain and VCS technology. The STKS and MAXM systems need some manual preparation. The GEN-S is fully automated. The Abbott CELL-DYN 3500 utilizes a thiazine dye (new methylene blue N) and MAPSS technology. The CELL-DYN 400 also uses MAPSS technology but adds fluorescent detection. It also is fully automated. Sysmex SE series (Roche) uses flow cytometry and auramine O stain. The XE 2100 utilizes a patented fluorescent dye and flow cytometry. ADVIA 120 (Bayer) uses a laser optic flowcell and oxazine 75, a nucleic acid binding dye.

The **MICRO 21** (Cellavision, http://www.cellavision.com) uses a form of artificial intelligence called NeuralVision. This technology locates, identifies, and displays the reticulocyte images on a high-resolution color monitor. The MICRO 21 uses the new methylene blue preparation and a minimum of 1000 RBCs is scanned. The MICRO 21 locates up to 5000 cells, stores the images, and records the number of reticulocytes included in those RBCs scanned. Percent reticulocytes is calculated, and then the images are presented to the reviewer to confirm.

Automated Erythrocyte Sedimentation Rate

The erythrocyte sedimentation rate (ESR) is the rate in millimeters at which the RBCs fall in a given period of time. The two traditional methods performed are the Westergren and Winthrob. Both methods allow red cells to stand at room temperature for 1 hour, and the degree of settling is measured. The test is an indirect measurement of plasma protein changes that occur in many disease processes.

The **StaRRsed** (RR Mechatronics, http://www.mechatronics.nl) is a fully automated ESR analyzer that compares its results to the traditional Westergren in 30 minutes or at 1 hour. The instrument has a citrate dilution system and only requires 1.6 mL of EDTA blood. A carousel holds 120 glass-bore Westergren tubes. The sample is aspirated into the analyzer, and a 4:1 citrate to blood ratio is made. Diluted blood is loaded into the glass Westergren tubes. The ESR can be measured after 30 minutes or the traditional 1 hour. The Westergren tubes are then emptied, washed, dried, and ready for reuse. Measured and temperature-corrected ESR reports are printed out.

Elan Diagnostics (http://www.elandiagnostics.com)

The Ves-Matic™ system determines ESR by the principle of optoelectronic sensing. This methodology is based on the measurement of the change in opacity of a column of blood as the red cells settle. Blood is collected in special Vacu-Tec tubes that contain an anti-coagulant. The tubes are place at an 18° angle to accelerate sedimentation. Results are obtained in 20 minutes.

Streck Laboratories (http://www.streck.com)

The ESR-8 is an automated ESR instrument manufactured by Analys Instrument AB, Stockholm, Sweden. The instrument measures the sedimentation rate of erythrocytes in 2.0-mL vacuum tubes. Results are measured in millimeters per hour (Westergren). Measuring time is 30 minutes.

Hema Technologies (http://www.hematek.com)

The ESR Plus and ESR STAT 180 are direct-read analyzers that provide an ESR from 20 μL of whole blood collected from a fingerstick or venipuncture. The principle of operation is centrifugal/laser optics/kinetics method. ESR results are complete in 3 minutes.

COAGULATION

Testing of blood plasma factors and PLTs depends on seeing the clotting process directly or microscopically. The first whole blood clotting time was done in 1780 by William Hussen who noted that blood taken from healthy people clotted in 7 minutes while blood from persons with some disease states took from 15–20 minutes up to 1.5 hours.

In 1897 Brodie and Russel begin observing the process on a glass slide. A drop of blood was placed on a glass cone in a temperature-controlled glass chamber agitated by an air jet. Blood clotted in 3 minutes and clotting was complete at 8 minutes. In 1905, Golhorm used a wire loop attached to a glass tube. In 1910, Kottman observed an increased viscosity in clotting blood in a Koaguloviskosimeter. Blood was rotated at 20°

12–15 times per minute. In 1936, Baldes and Nygaard added photoelectric tracings called a coagelgram, depicting changes in shape by light transmittance.

BBL introduced the Fibrometer in the 1960s. This instrument provided mechanical registration of clots that allowed more reproducible timing and an expression of the clotting process.

Methods

Electrical Impedance

This method utilizes two probes, one of which is stationary, and one of which moves (Figure 16). The movement allows for detection of a clot, by breaking the current and stopping the timer. This manual method is dependent on having clean probes and good technique. There is no interference with lipemia or hemolysis.

Ball Method (Mechanical Clot Detection)

This method measures increased plasma viscosity with an iron ball in an electromagnetic field. The ball swings in a pendulum motion. Increased viscosity causes the ball to stop and signals the formation of a clot (*see* Figure 16).

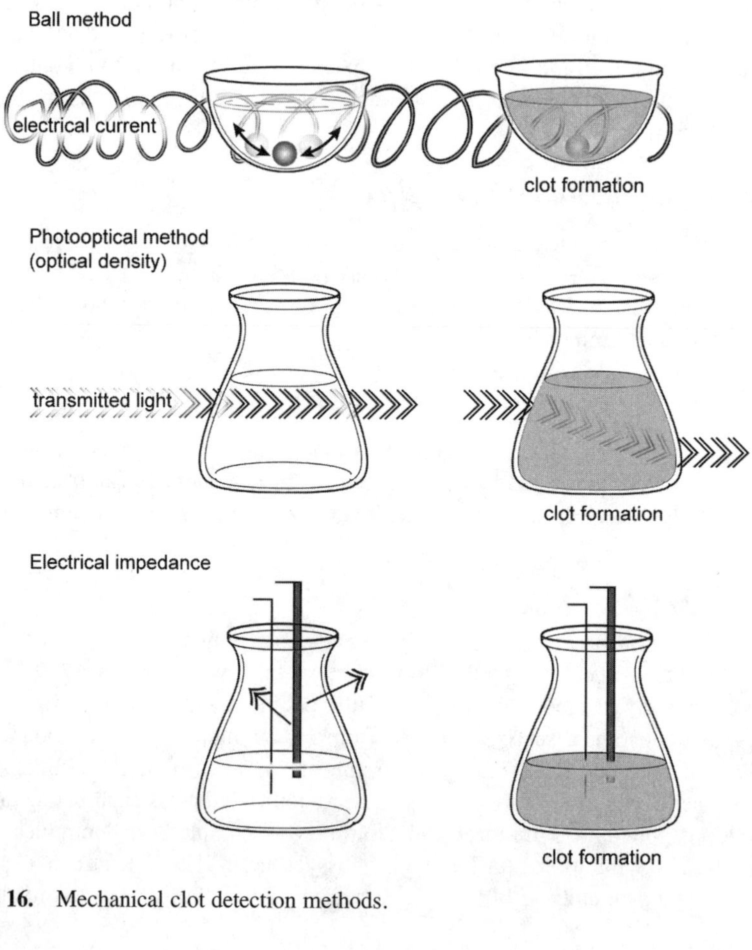

FIGURE 16. Mechanical clot detection methods.

Photooptical

In this method, plasma optical density is measured. Light passes through a sample and the beam is detected by a photodetector that monitors the intensity of the light beam. When the clot forms, light transmittance is decreased, and the endpoint is detected. This can be detected by two methods:

- **Turbidity:** Light is parallel to the photodetector.
- **Nephelometry:** Light is at a 90° angle to the photodetector, and it measures scattered light.

Errors can occur when plasma is viscous, e.g., lipemia or hyperbilirubinemia. This viscosity hampers the ability of the instrument to detect a change in optical density. In addition, a low-fibrinogen level produces a flimsy clot, with the result that the instrument has difficulty reading the clot (*see* Figure 16).

Instrumental Considerations

The most important component in choosing an instrument is knowing what is the best fit for the institution.

- Is an instrument with a variety of testing ability needed, or is it just for routine testing?
- Does it matter if it does 350 tests per hour if the laboratory only does 200 per day?
- Are cap piercer and robotic capabilities necessary?

Remember all the bells and whistles will have to be dealt with if they break.

Definitions

Bidirectional. This interface allows automatic transmission from (download) and to (upload) the local or the host (mainframe) computer.

Random Access. This feature allows the system to perform both turbidimetric and absorbance assays simultaneously. This is accomplished by the ability of the instrument to read at different wavelengths.

Alphanumeric Character Handling. This feature enables the instrument to distinguish between numbers and letters. It has the capability to handle both, without having to convert from one to the other.

Open System. An open system is defined as an instrument that allows different reagents other than the specific manufacturer's reagent.

Positive Patient Identification. This type of identification ensures that the instrument reads the bar code at the testing site in order to identify the patient and minimize mistakes.

Calibrations. The ability of an instrument to be calibrated to other instruments is important; it ensures results that correlate. It is especially helpful when several instruments at different locations are being used.

Features

Continuous Loading. This feature refers to the instrument's capacity for loading samples. Additional samples may be added without interrupting work in progress.

Factor Parallelism. This is a method for identifying factor inhibitors. The patient sample is graphed versus the calibration curve and can be viewed quickly for visual confirmation of an inhibitor.

Robotic. Automated systems help to ensure that high-quality information is generated rapidly and flawlessly. Robotic capabilities include sorting, routing, centrifugating, destopping, aliquotting, cap piercing, and testing. Several companies offer total laboratory automation equipment. It is important to look at workflow, the type of laboratory, size, scope of operation, type of specimens, and range of tests.

Maintenance. An important consideration, maintenance refers to the amount and type of technical time required for daily setup as well as periodic maintenance. This time should be minimal, but not so minimal as to compromise the quality of the specimen and present problems with carry-over. When an instrument breaks down, can a technologist fix it, and how much time will be required?

Cap Piercing. Does the instrument have the ability to access samples without removing the cap? This feature minimizes biohazard exposure. When moving to a system with cap piercing, the results should be compared to the present open-tube system.

Reflexive Testing. When a specimen gives an abnormal result, either high or low, the instrument has the ability to reflex automatically to another dilution, a rerun, or even additional testing.

Consumables. The materials used in testing may include cuvettes, tubes, tubing, and reagents. These are purchased from the instrument manufacturer and can be costly. While consumables may be obtained from another source less expensively, if there is a problem, technical support may not be available from the manufacturer.

Quality Control. It is important to understand the quality control features on the instrument. Such features include the capacity for file storage, calculation of means, and standard deviation. Levy-Jennings charts help to determine shifts and trends. Such features may not be as important if the laboratory information system (LIS) has the capability to automate this function. In addition, it is important to know what type of peer review program and support services the manufacturer will supply.

Chromogenic Substrates. Instruments with this feature have the ability to measure reagents that are linked to the chromophore p-nitroaniline that is cleaved from a substrate. This yellow color is then read at 405 nm.

Carry-Over. Some instruments sample by using probes. If there are not sufficient rinse cycles, there may be carry-over. This factor is important in determining if assays can be run simultaneously or independently. Some reagents may be "sticky" and contaminate other samples. If there is greater than a 10% difference, residual reagents may be contaminating samples.

Choosing Reagents

One of the most important tasks after choosing an instrument is to look at the reagent system. Reagents have the most impact on the quality of the results produced. Precision testing should be included to ensure the reproducibility or the result within the system. Several options should be considered, based on the working of the laboratory.

Prothrombin Time (PT) Reagents

Reagents for PT testing can be either a rabbit brain thromboplastin or a recombinant reagent. A decision also must be made on whether to choose an insensitive reagent with high International Sensitivity Index (ISI) or a low ISI which has greater sensitivity. The recommendation by the College of American Pathologists is to use a reagent with an ISI of <1.7.

Activated Partial Thromboplastin Time (aPTT) Reagents

This reagent is phospholipid based, and the concentration of phospholipid is important to consider. It will be used in determining whether the reagent is sensitive enough to use in screening patients for a lupus anticoagulant. The lower the concentration of phospholipid, the more sensitive the reagent is to picking up an inhibitor.

Sensitivity of Reagents

It is important to know that a normal PT and aPTT reflect factor levels of about 40%. This is accomplished by diluting a known concentration of normal plasma with factor-deficient plasma and performing a PT/aPTT with the reagents chosen. The seconds are graphed against the known percent activity. The upper limit of the normal range should correspond to a factor level of about 40%. This ensures that the reagents will perform well as a screen for abnormalities in the PT and aPTT.

Coagulation Instruments

Diagnostica Stago Inc. (Parsippany, NJ)

The STA series is a viscosity-based system. The ball's motion is activated by two coils working alternatively to maintain a natural oscillation. Reagent is added to a sample and detection begins. As the ball oscillates left and right, the chronometer starts and the amplitude of the ball is measured. The motion remains constant when no clot is present. When a clot appears, amplitude decreases. Therefore, this method is insensitive to colored plasma, hemolysis, lipemia, bilirubin, and turbid reagents. For a summary of these instruments, see Table 1.

Bio/Data Corp. (MCA 310)

The MCA 310 uses a microfiltration technology that has the ability to produce PLT-poor plasma in 20 seconds from a primary whole blood specimen without centrifugation. This instrument is based on fibrin endpoint detection by change in absorbance. It is fully automated with random-access testing capable of performing PT, aPTT, and fibrinogen assays. A signal will detect if plasma is hemolyzed, grossly lipemic, or clotted. The throughput is about 240 results per hour. It also has stat capabilities.

Beckman Coulter Inc./Instrumentation Laboratories (Brea, CA)

These instruments use turbidimetric and absorbance technology. There is a large range of instruments from benchtop to high throughput (*see* Table 2). Features include random access for clotting and chromogenic and immunological assays. Continuous loading eliminates the need for interrupting work in progress. Larger instruments such as the ADVANCE have the capacity to measure fibrin strand formation, to analyze clot curves, to identify bar codes, and to run up to 240 PT tests per hour.

TABLE 1. Diagnostica Stago instruments

Instrument	Tests/methodology	Features
STA Compact	Clot based Chromogenic Immunologic	DM, QC RR, BD LIS, BC
STA Hemostasis	Clot based Chromogenic Immunologic	DM, QC RR, BD LIS, BC
STA-R Hemostasis	Clot based Chromogenic Immunologic	DM, QC, BD RR, RFLX LIS, BC, CAP ROB

Key: DM = data management, QC = onboard charts, LIS = transfer to information system, BC = bar code, RR = rerun, BD = bidirectional, RFLX = reflexive testing, CAP = cap piercer, and ROB = robotic capabilities.

TABLE 2. Beckman Coulter instruments

Instrument	Tests/methodology	Features
Electra 1400/1800C	Clot based Chromogenic	DM, QC, BD RR, RFLX, LIS, BC
ACL 100	Clot based	LIS
ACL 1000	Clot based	QC, LIS, BC
ACL 7000	Clot based Chromogenic Immunologic	DM, QC, BD LIS, BC
ACL 9000	Clot based Chromogenic Immunologic	DM, QC, BD LIS, BC RFLX, RR
ACL Advance	Clot based Chromogenic Immunologic	DM, QC, BD LIS, BC RR

Key: DM = data management, QC = onboard charts, LIS = transfer to information system, BC = bar code, RR = rerun, RFLX = reflexive testing, and BD = bidirectional.

Trinity Biotech USA (St. Louis, MO)

The AMAX series is unique in that these instruments are capable of performing both optical and mechanical methods for determining clot formation. This series also is capable of chromogenic and immunoturbidimetric testing. These instruments are random-access analyzers with fast (<3 minutes) results and a high throughput. Efficient quarter-volume testing for routine assays makes testing very cost efficient. Table 3 provides additional information.

bioMerieux Inc. (Durham, NC)

Photooptical detection with an halogen light source is used in the bioMerieux instruments, which include a wide range from a benchtop for routine assays to special testing. This system has the capability to utilize calibrators; therefore, similar results are obtained regardless of instruments, reagent lots, or location, and similar reference ranges can be maintained year after year. Dyes are also used in routine reagents which enables verification of proper volume delivery of sample and reagents. In addition, a feature on this instrument is the wave-form analysis. This is a set of mathematical parameters. Following activation of the coagulation system, thrombin is formed and converts fibrinogen into a fibrin monomer, further polymerizing it into an insoluble fibrin clot. This process is monitored photooptically (transmittance over time). A sigmoid wave-like pattern appears. A lag phase is observed because a critical fibrin fiber needs to be achieved before a measurable change in transmittance occurs. Rapid polymerization into a larger clot occurs along with a concomitant sharp, almost linear, decrease in transmittance. When the fibrin clot is fully formed, a steady plateau is observed. This wave-form analysis provides more information than clot time alone (Figure 17). These patterns show different forms when looking at patients on heparin, patients with hemophilia, and patients that are factor-deficient, as well as patients with disseminated intravascular coagulation. This analysis can be a valuable adjunct when looking at patients with coagulopathies. Table 4 provides additional details on these instruments.

TABLE 3. The AMAX series

Instrument	Tests/methodology	Features
KC1/ KC4	Clot based	DM, QC, LIS
AMAX 200	Clot based Chromogenic Immunologic	DM, QC RR, BD LIS, BC
AMAX 400	Clot based Chromogenic Immunologic	DM, QC RFLX, RR, BD LIS, BC
AMAX Destiny	Clot based Chromogenic Immunologic	DM, QC RR, LIS, BC

Key: DM = data management, QC = onboard charts, LIS = transfer to information system, BC = bar code, RR = rerun, RFLX = reflexive testing, and BD = bidirectional.

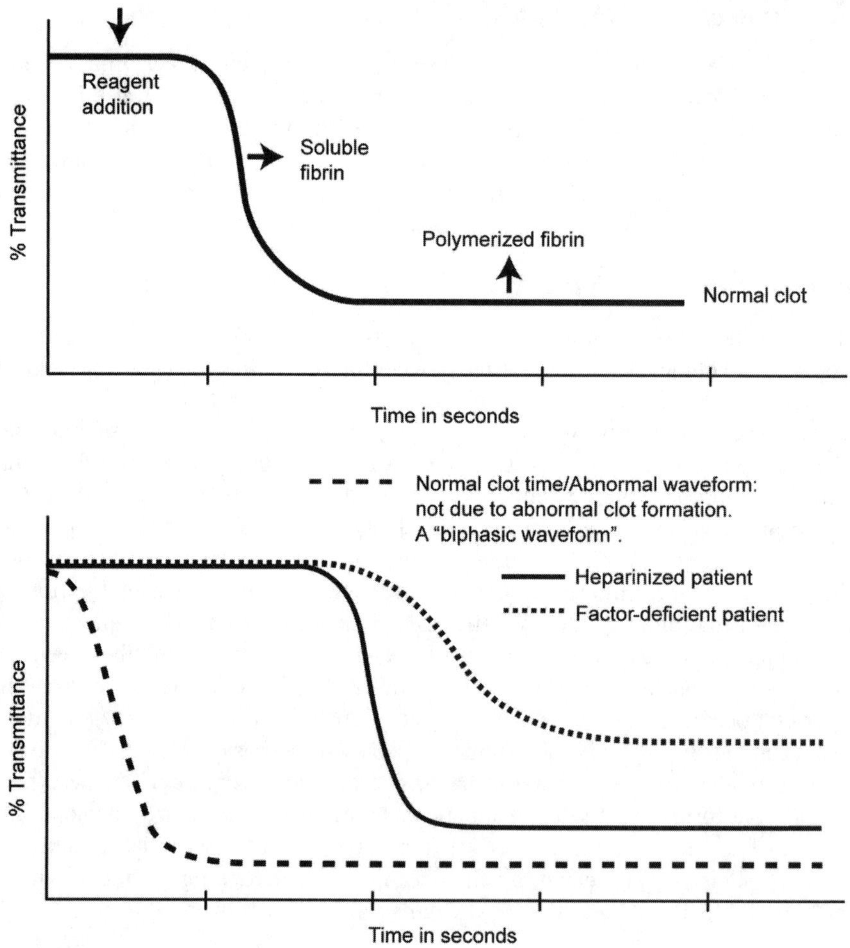

FIGURE 17. Waveform analysis.

TABLE 4. bioMerieux instruments

Instrument	Tests/methodology	Features
MDA II	Clot based Chromogenic Immunologic	DM, QC BD, ROB LIS, BC
Coag-A-Mate XM	Clot based	
Coag-A-Mate MTX-II	Clot based Chromogenic	DM, QC RR, LIS, BC, BD

Key: DM = data management, QC = onboard charts, LIS = transfer to information system, BC = bar code, RR = rerun, BD = bidirectional, and ROB = robotic capabilities.

Dade Behring Inc. (Deerfield, IL)

The Sysmex instruments are based on optical density clot detection. The testing menu includes clot-based, chromogenic, and immunologic methods. The BCS has a feature that enables the operator to autocalibrate the instrument. A modem allows technical service to operate from outside calls. The CA7000 delivers 550 results per hour. This is the fastest throughput of any coagulation analyzer, providing an answer every 7 seconds. In addition, it has 20-parameter random-access capabilities, as well as being able to reflex to another test. See Table 5 for details.

Helena Laboratories (Beaumont, TX)

These instruments (*see* Table 6) utilize photooptical detection sources, regardless of turbidity. Sensitivity is enhanced through direct readout. A green light-emitting diode (LED) eliminated the need for interference filters. This system is a pump system that is capable of reading four samples in a 1/2 volume mode.

D-Dimer Testing: Standalone Instruments

Miniquant™ (Trinity Biotech, St. Louis, MO)

The Miniquant is a two-channel laser automated optical instrument. It is based on latex agglutination and the rate of aggregation. This is compared to a standard curve using known concentrations of D-dimer. The curve can be stored in the instrument. In the presence of D-dimer, latex-coated monoclonal antibodies form aggregates, resulting in increased turbidity. The increase in scattered light is proportional to the amount of D-dimer in the sample.

TABLE 5. Dade Behring instruments

Instrument	Tests/methodology	Features
Sysmex CA500	Clot based Chromogenic	DM, QC BD, LIS, BC
Sysmex CA1500	Clot based Chromogenic Immunologic	DM, QC RR, RFLX, BD LIS, BC, CAP, ROB
BCS	Clot based Chromogenic Immunologic	DM, QC RR, RFLX, BD LIS, BC
Sysmex CA7000	Clot based Chromogenic Immunologic	DM, QC RR, RFLX, BD LIS, BC, CAP ROB

Key: DM = data management, QC = onboard charts, LIS = transfer to information system, BC = bar code, RR = rerun, BD = bidirectional, RFLX = reflexive testing, CAP = cap piercer, and ROB = robotic capabilities.

TABLE 6. Helena Laboratories instruments

Instrument	Tests/methodology	Features
Cascade M-4	Clot based	QC, LIS
Cascade M	Clot based	QC, LIS
Thor	Clot based	QC, CAP RR, RFLX LIS, BC, BD

Key: QC = onboard charts, LIS = transfer to information system, BC = bar code, BD = bidirectional, RR = rerun, RFLX = reflexive testing, and CAP = cap piercer.

There is no interference from bilirubin of 0.2 or hemoglobin up to 6.7 mg/dL; however, lipids can cause decreased results, and lipemic samples can be diluted. The assay range is 75–5000 ng/mL. It has a negative predictive value of 100% for pulmonary embolism. The test is performed in less than 3 minutes.

Vidas D-Dimer (Marcy-l'Etoile, France)

The assay principle combines a two-step enzyme immunoassay sandwich method with a final fluorescent detection (ELFA). A solid phase receptacle (SPR) is coated with anti-FbDP monoclonal mouse antibodies. The antigen to be detected is sandwiched by the labeled antibody. There is a series of dynamic reactions where reagents are aspirated in and out of the SPR several times. The increased kinetics allow for decreased incubation times. The fluorescence is measured at 450 nm. The intensity of the fluorescence is proportional to the concentration of the antigen present in the sample. The results are calculated in relation to two calibration curves that have been stored.

This test takes about 1 hour and is considered the "gold standard" for D-dimer testing, with a sensitivity and negative predictive value of 100%. Factors measured include hemolysis (up to 300 μmol/L), lipemia, bilirubinemia (up to 278 μmol/L), and rheumatoid factor (up to 396 IU/mL). The assay range is 45–10,000 ng/mL.

Platelet Aggregometers

PLT aggregation measures the ability of PLTs to adhere. This test can be performed in whole blood or in PLT-rich plasma. See Table 7 for a listing of instruments.

Whole Blood Aggregation

This test measures impedance change in blood viscosity. This is accomplished by looking at impedance between two electrodes immersed in a sample of whole blood. Whole blood aggregation modulates PLT behavior in vivo due to its interaction with WBCs. Leukocytes release prostacyclin and PLT-activating factor. Erythrocytes are able to bind prostacyclin and release ADP. In addition, when using PLT-rich plasma (PRP), a subpopulation of PLTs may be lost in centrifugation, e.g., large PLTs, hyperactive PLTs.

Optical Aggregation

PLT-rich plasma is prepared with a standard PLT count of 250,000–320,000. The change in turbidity is measured by adding agonists. Infrared light transmission is used to measure

TABLE 7. Platelet aggregometers

Instrument	Type	Principle	Other
Chronolog Chronolog Corp. Haverston, PA	2-channel 4-channel 2-channel	Whole blood Optical density	Hooked up to aggrolink interface. Stores patterns and prints reports. Lumi.
PAP-4 (BioData Corp.)	4-channel	Optical density	Can be hooked up to a computer interface. Stores patterns and prints reports. Windows based.
PACKS-4 Helena Laboratories Beaumont, TX	4-channel	Optical density Chromogenic	Platelet agg ATIII, Protein C Heparin

changes in shape and aggregation. The difference in light transmittance between PRP and PLT-poor plasma is determined. Changes in shape result in a decrease in transmittance, and aggregation results in an increase in light transmission.

Lumi-aggregation

Lumi-aggregation provides a measurement of aggregation and release defects and detects secretion and storage pool deficiency. It provides direct unequivocal measurement and quantification of ATP release. Chronolume (luciferin-luciferase) is added to the sample. Leukocyte generation of superoxides is measured by addition of luminol to the sample.

Other Platelet Instruments

Dade Behring PFA-100®

The PFA-100 simulates primary hemostasis. It is a quantitative measure of PLT function in anticoagulated blood. A cartridge with a biologically active membrane is coated with collagen. This serves as a matrix for PLT deposition and attachment. Whole blood is collected in sodium citrate and is aspirated through a 150-μm capillary aperture into the cartridge. All components are in the cartridge where testing takes place. In addition to the collagen, cartridges contain either adenosine diphosphate (ADP) or epinephrine (EPI). Saline buffer triggers the ADP or EPI to become solubilized. Under high shear rates of 5000–6000 second^{-1} and standardized conditions, PLT attachment, activation, and aggregation are measured in closure time and seconds. The EPI/collagen cartridge is the most sensitive cartridge and will be abnormal in the presence of aspirin for example. Prolongation with the ADP/collagen cartridge would indicate a PLT disorder of high severity. The PFA-100 has been shown to have a 100% negative predictive value when diagnosing von Willebrands disease.

Thrombelastograph® Haemostasis Analyzer (TEG)

TEG analysis is based on two processes. The first process results in a clot. The second process determines how the clot will affect the patient, i.e., will the patient have normal hemostasis, hemorrhage, or develop thrombosis? A clot's physical property is measured by the use of a spiral stationary cylindrical cup. This uses whole blood that is oscillated at an angle of 4° 45″. Each rotation lasts 10 seconds. A pin is suspended in the blood by a tension wire and monitored for motion. The fibrin PLT bonds affect the magnitude of the pin motion; therefore, the motion is directly related to the strength of the clot as it retracts or lyses. Motion will then decrease. This movement is converted to an electrical signal which is then delivered as a profile. These results measure the time for the first fibrin strand to be formed, and the kinetics of clot formation as well as the strength and dissolution of a clot. This method combines the interactive process of cell components that make blood clot. TEG is a global test that helps to determine if a patient is bleeding due to surgery, heparin, or a coagulopathy. It does not identify specific factor deficiencies, inhibitors, or activators that require a coagulation test. This process can aid in the choice of blood products for treatment as well as reduce the amount of required blood components.

Hemodyne Hemostasis System

This instrument simultaneously provides information on PLT function and clot ultrastructure in whole blood. PLT function is determined by measuring the forces developed by PLTs as they undergo cellular contraction. This measurement of PLT contractile force (PCF) has been shown to be a sensitive indicator of global PLT function. Clot structure is determined by measuring the elastic modulus (EM), or rigidity of the network of polymerizing fibrin, PLTs, and erythrocytes. These measurements provide a true global picture of hemostatic balance in a complete physiological test environment. The test uses whole blood and is completed in 15 minutes. The results are directly calculated and presented in standard physical units of force.

Ichor and Plateletworks®

This is a self-contained whole blood PLT aggregation assay that provides a standard CBC with PLT count and PLT aggregation. Ichor uses the laboratory standard of electronic impedance variation generated by the actual passage and counting of each cell type through the instrument's microaperture. Aggregation testing is based on performing a PLT count before and after intentional PLT activation using either collagen or ADP as the agonist. A sample of whole blood is added to a blank tube as well as an agonist tube. Both tubes are run, and results are available within minutes.

Point-of-Care Testing: Coagulation

There are several challenges with point-of-care (POC) testing. Coagulation testing has a diverse selection of assays, with a growing test menu. The activated clotting time (ACT) monitors heparin dosing during cardiac surgery, cardiac catherization, and dialysis. The PT manages long-term warfarin therapy. Some devices also look at aPTT testing. Table 8 summarized some available instruments.

Most errors occur in the preanalytical and postanalytical phases. The National Committee for Clinical Laboratory Standards (NCCLS) suggests that a comprehensive guideline should be developed that enables users, manufacturers, and regulators to identify potential sources of error in test systems and implement processes to manage identified errors using new quality management models. There is a great need for good quality control (QC). The responsibility of QC falls on the laboratory. The purpose of QC in POC testing is to verify the integrity of performance characteristics of the testing device and its

TABLE 8. Point-of-care coagulation instruments

Instrument/manufacturer	Tests	Sample type/ method	Features
IStat Abbott Abbott Park, IL	ACT	Fingerstick/WB Electrogenic	QC, DM, LIS LO, BCS, ID
AvoSure PT PRO Avocet Medical Inc. San Jose, CA	PT	Fingerstick/WB Plasma	QC, DM, ID LO Fluorescent
Rapidpoint Coag Bayer Diagnostics Tarrytown, NY	PT/aPTT ACT HMT	Fingerstick/WB Plasma Fibrin clot impede	QC, LO, DM ID, LIS
Actlyke Helena Beaumont, TX	ACT	WB Electromechanical	QC
GEM PCL Instrumentation Laboratory Lexington, MA	PT/aPTT ACT	Fingerstick/WB Mechanical endpoint Optical detection	QC, DM, LIS
Hemochron International Technidyne Corp, Edison, NJ	PT/aPTT ACT	WB Mechanical clot detection	QC, DM,
ProTime Microcoagulation System, International Technidyne Edison, NJ	PT Optical detection	Fingerstick	QC, LO
ACT II Medtronic Cardiac Surgery Minneapolis, MN	PT/aPTT ACT	Venipuncture Mechanical clot	QC, DM
CoaguChek Pro Roche Diagnostics Indianapolis, IN	PT/aPTT ACT	Fingerstick/WB Laser photometry Iron particles	QC, LO, DM LIS, ID

Key: DM = data management, QC = onboard charts, LIS = transfer to information system, BCS = bar code scanner, LO = lockout, and ID = positive patient identification.

corresponding reagents. Several options are available in coagulation testing. Onboard controls (OBC) are introduced into several units; however, they just state the controls are acceptable, but they really do not evaluate the system. Electronic controls are microchips that are incorporated into testing devices. Having protective devices, e.g., QC lockout, can help to reduce errors due to abnormal QC.

It is important to remember that testing is occurring in whole blood. This contains RBCs, WBCs, and PLTs that all contribute to coagulation. In order to compensate for this, manufacturers have electronically adjusted times to mimic that of plasma samples. It is important to know the therapeutic range for the instrument being used.

One advantage of POC testing is that results are more timely (9 minutes versus 22 minutes–8 hours). Direct costs are higher, but reimbursement is better. Using POC devices can be convenient to patients as well as streamlining workflow.

An important issue in POC testing is connectivity. That is the ability to transmit information from POC instruments to and from the laboratory, and throughout the hospital and healthcare system. Additional questions that should be asked are:

- How accessible is the information?
- Can it be downloaded to an LIS, with patient identification and retrievable data?
- How portable is the unit?
- What is the test volume?
- Is liquid QC available?
- What is the instrument's test menu?

Methods

Various methods are currently used, utilizing various instruments (Table 8). Some of the important aspects of POC testing are discussed in the following sections.

Magnetic Rod. A sample is placed in an instrument and a detector senses the rod. When clotting begins, the rod within the tube is displaced and is no longer sensed by the detector. The clot time is displayed in seconds.

Laser Photodetector. These detectors monitor the interval between the application of the blood sample and cessation of its flow. The clotting time is measured in seconds.

Mechanical Endpoint Clotting Mechanism. Formation of a clot is measured when movement is stopped by the clot.

Optical Clot Detection. This method measures changes in light transmittance due to clot formation.

Iron Particles. Particles mixed with the sample move in magnetic fields. Reflectance photometry detects changes in particle movement with clot formation.

Tests

The Activated Clotting Time. This test is a measure of the time required for a specimen of fresh whole blood to clot upon exposure to a blood coagulation activator. Diatomaceous earth may be used as an activator. Silica may be used; it is unaffected by aprotinin, which is used in conjunction with heparin during cardiopulmonary bypass surgery.

Prothrombin Time. The prothrombin time in POC testing monitors the usage of warfarin therapy. This oral anticoagulant is taken daily and affects the vitamin K-dependent factors (II, VII, IX, X, and proteins C and S) by rendering them nonfunctional, impairing fibrin formation. Warfarin requires frequent monitoring because the drug can be affected by diet.

International Normalized Ratio (INR). This parameter is calculated with the patient's PT. It is important in warfarin therapy, in that it is the number that provides a standard result, i.e., regardless of the instrument/reagent used, this INR will normalize the result. This is accomplished by an equation that uses the reagent's assigned ISI. The ISI is given by the manufacturer as a correction factor to represent the PT that would have been achieved if the most sensitive reagent was used, human brain thromboplastin which has an ISI of 1. The College of American Pathology recommends using an ISI of <1.7.

Activated Partial Thromboplastin Time (aPTT). Testing is used for monitoring heparin therapy. There is no correlation between the aPTT and heparin dosing, so there is no method to standardize the assay. The result must be interpreted using the normal range and the therapeutic range for the assay method used. This test can be difficult to correlate with coagulation instruments, due to the comparison between using whole blood and plasma, the lack of standardization, and preanalytical variables; it should be approached with caution.

Heparin Management Tests (HMT). This test is used to replace the ACT. It is used to measure heparin management. HMT is more accurate for high-dose heparin that is seen in surgery. It is unaffected by shifts in temperature or hemodilution, resulting in reproducible results.

URINALYSIS AUTOMATION

The analysis of urine has been around for many years. Urinalysis provides diagnostic information about the patient's condition from the color, clarity, odor, and chemical constituents of the urine. Modern urinalysis has expanded its scope to include not only the physical properties of urine but the chemical composition and a microscopic examination. The physical portion of urinalysis includes color and clarity. The chemical portion includes glucose, protein, ketones, blood, pH, bilirubin, urobilinogen, nitrite, leukocytes, and specific gravity. The microscopic examination includes the enumeration of RBCs, WBCs, casts, bacteria, and crystals. Urinalysis is still an integral and important part of the examination. For many years, urinalysis was performed manually. As with any other manual test, there was a need for standardization and reproducibility. Reagent strips were developed for the chemical analysis of urine. Other efforts made were to increase the consistency of reagent strip reading and to increase the number of specimens that could be analyzed. Automation has improved color and visual discrimination, improved precision, reproducibility, and increased productivity.

Automated instruments in urinalysis include strip readers, semiautomated analyzers that are operator dependent, fully automated chemistry analyzers, and the complete "walk-away" urinalysis workstation.

Operation

Reflectance Photometry

The reflectance principle uses light reflection or scattered light from the test reagent pads. The reagent pads are impregnated with reagents, which react colorimetrically with various analytes in urine. When light strikes a reagent pad, some light is absorbed and the remaining light is scattered in all directions. A monochromatic light is directed toward the test pads. A filter is placed between the monochromatic light and the test pad. A LED is used to provide a specific wavelength that is needed for each test pad reaction. The light is then reflected to a photodetector and an analog/digital converter, resulting in a linear relationship. As light reflects from the test pad, it decreases in proportion to the intensity of color produced by the concentration of the test substance. The reflectance photometer measures the color change of each reagent pad. The degree of color change in the pad is directly related to the concentration of the particular constituent in urine. A comparison of light reflection from the test pads and known concentrations is then reported.

Flow Cytometry

Flow cytometry is the measurement of the physical characteristics of cells with the use of a laser light source. Each cell can be measured for the intensity of scattered light, which includes cell size, cell density, and cell morphological detail. Hydroplanar positioning is a process that forces all particles in urine to flow in a single plane as they pass in front of the microscope. Laser light, forward light scatter, and fluorescent staining help with the identification of individual characteristics of urine sediment. Images of the analytes are captured using a video camera and strobe illumination to freeze the motion of elements in the flow cell. The computer analyzes multiple freeze-frame images for size and number. The urine flow can be evaluated by using low- and high-power magnification. Formed elements that are identified are RBCs, WBCs, bacteria, casts, and crystals.

Specific Gravity

Specific gravity is defined as the density of a substance as compared with the density of distilled water. The specific gravity of urine is a measure of the density of the dissolved chemicals or particles in urine. The number and molecular size of the solutes affect specific gravity. Specific gravity is an assessment of the concentration and diluting ability of the kidneys. Specific gravity can be measured by reflectance, refractometry, and mass gravity.

Refractometry

Refractometry is based on the refractive index. The refractive index compares the velocity of light in air with the velocity of light in a solution. The velocity is dependent on the concentration of particles present in a given solution. A monochromatic light beam and a prism are used to bend light. As the number of particles increases in a solution, the velocity of light decreases and the angle of light refraction increases. The angle or refractive index is mathematically converted to specific gravity.

Mass Gravity Meter

Specific gravity is determined by harmonic oscillation. Urine is added to a hollow U-shaped tube and sound waves of a fixed frequency are transmitted to one end of the tube by electromagnetic coil. A current is applied to the coil, which vibrates the tube at a frequency causing harmonic oscillation. The timed cycle of the oscillation is proportional to the density of the specimen. The change in frequency as it exits the end of the tube is directly proportional to the specific gravity.

Instrumentation

Several companies offer automated instruments to standardize sample processing, analyze reagent strips, and report results. Additional features now offered are automated microscopic analysis with flow cytometry, software classification and enumeration of formed elements, quantitative and semiquantitative results, flagging of abnormal results, and better data management.

For the chemical portion of routine urinalysis, most instrumentation uses reflectance photometers. Urine is added to a reagent strip and placed into the instrument. The strip moves into the reflectance photometer, an appropriate light source and wavelength are used, the reflectance data are collected and calculated, and results are recorded. In semiautomated and some fully automated analyzers, the physical and microscopic portion is done manually. The new technology using flow cytometry allows the microscopic examination to be done by automation. This technology allows better standardization because of the high variation of personnel identifying urine sediment. As the technology progresses, the analysis of other body fluids is on the horizon.

Bayer Instrumentation (Clinitek® and Clinitet Atlas, http://www.bayerdiag.com)

The Clinitek 100 and 200+ (Bayer Instruments) are semiautomated urine strip readers. All Clinitek analyzers use the Multistix strip reagent for urinalysis. These analyzers use the dry chemistry technology and a reflectometer. Reagent strips are manually dipped into the urine and placed on a platform. A tungsten light source and a filter wheel are used to select the proper wavelength for each reagent pad. Urine color and clarity are manually entered. A bidirectional interface to upload and download patient identification is available with the Clinitek 200+. The Clinitek 500 features an advanced read head design that can determine urine color and nonhemolyzed trace blood automatically. It also contains a bar-code reader for rapid data entry. All microscopic examination is performed manually.

The fully automated Clinitek Atlas performs 12 tests by reflectance colorimetry. Urine is automatically added to the reagent strips. Specific gravity is read by using a fiber optic refractive index method. Light is transmitted through a specially shaped fiber optic. The dry chemistries are contained in a continuous roll to minimize reagent handling. Each reagent roll contains reagent areas for testing glucose, bilirubin, ketone, occult blood, pH, protein, urobilinogen, nitrite, leukocyte esterase, and color. Clarity is measured by the transmission and scattering of light that passes through the specimen. The Clinitek 500 uses a bar code for sample identification. The analyzer also has flagging ability for samples requiring a microscopic examination or confirmatory testing.

Behring Diagnostics Inc. (Rapimat II/T, http://www.behringdiagnostics.com)

The Rapimat II/T (Behring Diagnostics) is a semiautomated urine chemistry analyzer that also uses reflectance photometry. The instrument utilizes 13 separate reflectometers. Each includes a LED and a phototransistor detector. The reflectance reading of each chemical reaction is taken. This analyzer has the capability to correct urine color using a blanking pad, to measure ascorbic acid to correct for possible interference, and to use a thermostatic heating of the leukocyte esterase reagent pad to enhance the enzymatic reaction. Strips are manually dipped into the urine and placed on the conveyer belt. Abnormal results are flagged and manual microscopic examinations are performed.

Roche Diagnostics (Miditron® Junior II, Miditron M, URISYS™ 2400, http://labsystems.roche.com)

The Miditron Junior II and the Miditron M (Roche Diagnostics) are semiautomated urine chemistry analyzers for standardized reflectance photometry. The Miditron M uses six individual reflectometers to read the test reagent pads. It also contains two heads each with three LEDs that use a monochromatic light source and a phototransistor. The reagent strip is manually dipped into the urine and placed on a transport tray that takes the specimen into the analyzer for incubation timing and analyte measurement. A color reference pad on the reagent strip compensates for urine color. Both physical and microscopic characteristics are entered manually. The Miditron M analyzer is designed for online connections to central PC/HOST, sediment terminal, external printer, bar-code reader, and an external SG-meter. Both analyzers use Combur® test strips, which are marketed in Canada as Chemstrip®. (Combur–Test and Chemstrip are trademarks of the Roche group.)

The URISYS 2400 is a fully automated chemical urine strip system. The measuring system uses a reflectance photometer, LEDs for the light source, and three different wavelengths. Urine specimens are loaded into the racks, and the volumes are detected, and then the samples are automatically mixed. The URISYS 2400 system uses cassettes to supply 400 test strips. The analyzer provides the complete test parameters of protein, glucose, ketone, urobilinogen, bilirubin, blood pH, and clarity by turbidimetry and specific gravity by refractometry.

Sysmex (Sysmex UF-100, http://sysmex.com)

The Sysmex UF-100 uses laser flow cytometry, impedance, forward light scatter, and differential fluorescent staining to identify and count urine sediment. Of all previously mentioned analyzers, this is the only one that does not do the chemistry testing; it only does the microscopic evaluation. This analyzer can be combined with the Bayer Clinitek Atlas or any other chemistry strip reader to offer a fully automated urinalysis to include physical, chemical, and microscopic examination.

Uncentrifuged urine is aspirated into the analyzer. Flow cytometric analysis of the urine specimen identifies and counts cells based on their size and fluorescent staining. The sample is stained with two dyes. One dye is phenanthridine, which stains nuclear material. Carbocyanine is the second dye, and it stains cell membranes and mitochondria. The specimen is hydrodynamically focused and is passed through a laser. Particles are measured by the change in impedance, height, and width of fluorescence and light scatter. Data are presented in histograms and scatterplots. Sysmex adaptive cluster analysis translates the data to enumeration and formed element classification. At a rate of 100 samples per hour, the UF-100 identifies and counts the formed elements in urine sediment.

International Remote Imaging Systems (Yellow IRIS, Model 500 Urinalysis Work Station, and Model 939Udx Urine Pathology System, http://www.proirs.com)

The Yellow IRIS and model 500 workstations are capable of performing specific gravity, chemical analysis, and slideless microscopic identification from an uncentrifuged urine specimen. Urine is poured over the chemical strip, and reactions are measured by reflectance at two different wavelengths. Specific gravity is determined by the IRIS mass gravity meter, which analyzes sound wave frequency. A standard amount of urine is placed in a U-shaped tube. Sound waves of fixed frequency are transmitted to one side of the tube. The change in frequency as the sound wave exits the tube is directly related to specific gravity. Flow chamber and planar hydrodynamic positioning perform microscopic analysis. Urine is forced into a moving stream and all particles are in a single plane as they pass the optical path of the microscope. Multiple freeze-frame pictures are taken by a high-intensity strobe light as the particles pass the microscope. Data are generated as to size, shape, density, and number of each particle. Particles are placed into three low-power and five high-power groups and are presented to the operator for final identification.

The 939Udx urine pathology system employs real-time video flow imaging cytometry. This automated analyzer has the capability to automatically perform, classify, and report all parts of urinalysis. The system consists of three components. These components perform automated strip chemical analysis, specific gravity, color, clarity, and microscopic evaluation. A test strip is dipped into the unspun urine and placed into the photometer for chemical analysis. The next step is the urine is sent to the flow microscope where color and clarity are measured. The sample is then delivered to the sample chamber for mixing with stain. The stained sample enters the flow cell where analytes are imaged by a video camera. Low-power and high-power examinations are used. The images are digitized and sent to the view station computer for final processing and classifying. Neural net automation software, a patented software, uses autoclassification, which automatically counts and classifies RBCs, WBCs, bacteria, squamous epithelial cells, hyaline casts, yeast, crystals, sperm, mucus, and amorphous and WBC clumps.

Both the IRIS and Sysmex manufacturers are developing systems to analyze body fluids other than urine. The advantage for doing other body fluids is that preparation is easier and identification can be standardized.

ADDITIONAL READING: HEMATOLOGY

Abbott Laboratories. CELL-DYN 3500 system operator's manual. Abbott Park, IL, 1996.

Abbott Laboratories. CELL-DYN 3500 system operator's manual. Reticulocyte package. Abbott Park, IL, 1999.

Abbott Laboratories. CELL-DYN: the classification of white blood cells by laser light scatter signature. Abbott Park, IL, 1995.

Alpert NL. ADVIA 120 hematology system, clinical instrument systems. Vol 15, No. 6, 1999.

Bayer Corp. ADVIA 120 hematology system. Tarrytown, NY, 2002.

Bayer Corp. ADVIA 120 operation's guide. Tarrytown, NY, 1998.

Beckman Coulter, Inc. Coulter GEN S system: clinical case studies, 1996.

Beckman Coulter, Inc. The Coulter LH 700 series hematology systems, bulletin 9223, 2001.

Beckman Coulter, Inc. The LH reticulocyte count and associated parameters, bulletin 9232, 2001.

Bersch C. Hematology analyzers. MLO Med Lab Obs, February 2003.

Brugnara C, vonKapff CT. Bayer international atlas of hematology. Bayer Diagnostics, 1996.

Coulter Electronics, Inc. Coulter casebook: VCS technology, PN 420628t-2a, Hialeah, FL, 1989.

Coulter Electronics, Inc. Coulter casebook: the Coulter histogram differential with interpretive report. Hialeah, FL, 1989.

Coulter Electronics, Inc. GEN system book of knowledge, user's guide. Miami, FL, 1997.

Coulter Electronics, Inc. STKS hematology system. Hialeah, FL, 1991.

Coulter Electronics, Inc. STKS operation's guide. Hialeah, FL, 1992.

Coulter Electronics, Inc. STKR product reference manual. Hialeah, FL, 1988.

Drew NO. Differential redesigns. Advance for Administrators of the Laboratory, May 2002.

Harmening D. Clinical hematology and fundamentals of hemostasis (chapter 29). In: Principles of automated differential analysis, 4th ed. Philadelphia: FA Davis, 2002.

James E. The future of automation, Advance for Medical Laboratory Professionals, January 2003.

King D. Take advantage of advances. Advance for Medical Laboratory Professionals, May 2002.

Lehmann C. Saunders manual of clinical laboratory science. Philadelphia: WB Saunders, 1998.

McKenzie S. Textbook of hematology (chapter 29). In: Automation in hematology, 2nd ed. Baltimore: Williams and Wilkins, 1996.

Noble S. Hematology analyzers. MLO Med Lab Obs 2002;34(5).

Roche Diagnostics. Sysmex XE-2100, a new class of analyzer, PN 861-4186-1299. Indianapolis, IN, 1999.

Rodak B. Hematology: clinical principles and applications (chapter 40). In: Cell counting instrumentation, 2nd ed. Philadelphia: WB Saunders, 2002.

Statland B, Jetton M, Walters J, Hyder D. Implementation of the automated five part differential. Baxter Diagnostics, 1990.

Stiene-Martin E, Lotspeich-Steininger C, Koepke JA, eds. Clinical hematology principles, procedures, correlations (chapter 42). In: Multiparameter hematology instruments, 2nd ed. Philadelphia: Lippincott, 1998.

Turgeon M. Instrumentation in hematology. In: Clinical hematology theory and procedures, 3rd ed. Philadelphia: Lippincott Williams and Wilkins, 1999.

Ward K, Lehmann C, Leiken A. Automated hematology analyzers. In: Clinical laboratory instrumentation and automation. Philadelphia: WB Saunders, 1994.

ADDITIONAL READING: COAGULATION

Ansell J, Tiarks C, Hirsh J, McGehee W, Adler D, Weibert R. Measurement of activated partial thromboplastin time from a capillary (fingerstick) sample of whole blood. Am J Clin Pathol 1991;95:222–7.

bioMerieux. Instrument literature, waveform analysis technology on the MDA systems.

bioMerieux. VIDAS D-dimer, instrument literature. Durham, NC, 2002.

Biopool Miniquant D-dimer, instrument literature, Ventura, CA.

Chronolog Corp. Chronolog aggregation systems improve platelet function studies, instrument literature. Haverston, PA.

Coagulation analyzers. CAP Today, January 2003;19–33.

Dade Behring hemostasis, instrument literature. Deerfield, IL, 1998.

Dean KJ. Impacts of connectivity on point-of-care anticoagulation testing. Advance for Administrators of the Laboratory, July 2001;64–8.

Diagnostica Stago. Viscosity-based detection system, instrument literature. Parsippany, NJ.

Felder R. Automation planning tools. Advance for Administrators of the Laboratory, January 2003;23–6.

Franks B, Zucker ML. At the bedside. Monitoring, managing POC coagulation. Advance for Administrators of the Laboratory, March 2003;10.

Helena Laboratories. Instrument literature. Beaumont, TX, 2000.

Howdijh W. Analysis of clot waveforms on the MDA system: theory and applications, Organon Teknika, 2000.

Humberston SK, Nicholls PD. Challenges of point-of-care coagulation. Advance for Administrators of the Laboratory, October 2001;58–66.

Instrumentation laboratory. Instrument literature. Lexington, MA, 2001.

Koepke J. Practical laboratory hematology, pp 329–34, chapter 37, pp 626–8.

Kundu SK, Heilmann EJ, Sio R, Garcia C, Davidson RM, Ostgaard RA. Description of an in vitro platelet function analyzer—PFA-100. Semin Thromb Hemost 1995;21(Suppl 2):106–12.

Niles IL, Navickos I, Cohen E. Thrombelastograph haemostasis analyzer, TEG. Haemoscope News, Issue #5, pp 1–8.

Ortel T, James A, Thames EH, Moore KD, Greenberg CS. Assessment of primary hemostasis by the PFA-100: analysis in a tertiary care center. Thromb Haemost 2000;84:93–7.

Owen CA. A history of blood coagulation. Rochester, MN: Mayo Foundation, p 191.

Pontius CA. Finding control in quality control of unit-use prothrombin time tests. MLO Med Lab Obs 2001;33(5):38–42.

Reynolds P. Coagulation analyzers: variety of tests, designs. MLO Med Lab Obs 2002;33(11): 42–4.

Riess H, Braum G, Brehm G, Hiller E. Critical evaluation of platelet aggregation in whole blood human blood. Am J Clin Pathol 1986;85:50–6.

Solomon HM, Mullins RE, Lyden P, Thompson P, Hudoff S. The diagnostic accuracy of bedside and laboratory coagulation: procedures used to monitor the anticoagulation status of patients treated with heparin. Am J Clin Pathol 1998;109:371–8.

Trinity Biotech USA. Instrument literature. St. Louis, MO, 2002.

ADDITIONAL READING: URINALYSIS

Auxter S. Urinalysis—beyond strips and microscopes. Clinical Laboratory News, November 2002.

Bayer Diagnostics. Clinitek Atlas automated urine chemistry analyzer operations manual. April 1999.

Brunzel N. Chemical examination of urine and automation in the urinalysis laboratory (chapter 7). In: Fundamentals of urine and body fluid analysis. Philadelphia: WB Saunders, 1994.

Conrad ME, Jackson JA, Campbell JA. Semi-automated urine chemistry analyzer. American Clinical Laboratory, July 1991.

Graff L. A handbook of routine urinalysis. Philadelphia: Lippincott, 1983.

International Remote Imaging Systems. Yellow Iris operations manual, IRIS, 1992.

McBride L. Instrumentation in the urinalysis and body fluids laboratory. In: Textbook of urinalysis and body fluids. Philadelphia: Lippincott, 1998.

McLane MA. Urinalysis: something old, something borrowed and something blue, Advance for Medical Laboratory Professionals, April 2002, Vol 14, No. 8.

Miles Diagnostic Division. Modern urine chemistry manual. Elkhart, IN, 1991.

Miles Diagnostic Division. TechniTips. Elkhart, IN, October 1992.

Ringsrud K, Linne J. Urinalysis and body fluids: a color text and atlas. St. Louis: Mosby, 1995.

Strasinger S. Urinalysis and body fluids (appendix A, urinalysis automation), 4th ed. Philadelphia: FA Davis, 2001.

Chapter 12

Microbiology Analyzers

Karen C. Carroll and Larry G. Reimer

Automation has played a significant role in clinical microbiology laboratories since its introduction in the 1960s. Early instrumentation focused primarily on urine screening. Since that time, instruments have become more sophisticated and have been well integrated into laboratory workflow, shortening time to detection of common pathogens, improving interpretation, and standardizing work practices. This chapter includes a discussion of nonmolecular testing platforms available to clinical microbiology laboratories in the following broad categories:

- Organism identification
- Susceptibility testing
- Blood culture instrumentation
- Systems for mycobacteria growth, detection, and susceptibility testing
- Urine analyzers

SYSTEMS FOR MICROBIAL IDENTIFICATION

Currently available identification systems utilize one of several principles for identification of microorganisms. Most of these principles are dependent upon organism growth. The most common principle involves detection of changes in pH from utilization of carbohydrates (acidic pH) or protein (alkaline pH). Other growth-dependent systems include carbon source utilization with colorimetric end detection (MicroLog System, Biolog Inc., Hayward, CA) and detection of volatile or nonvolatile acids chromatographically to analyze cell wall cellular fatty acids [Sherlock® Microbial Identification System (MIDI, Inc., Newark, DE)] (1, 2). In addition to growth-dependent substrate reactivity, newer automated instruments have also incorporated detection of preformed enzymes using either chromogen or fluorogen release for enzymatic reaction detection. Such reactions can be detected more quickly (2–4 hours) than methods that are based upon organism growth.

The strength and accuracy of any identification system depend upon the extent of its available **database** and how the database was constructed. Ideally, the database should include a mixture of type strains, clinical strains, including those with unusual or aberrant biochemical reactions, and common environmental isolates. Databases contain hundreds to more than a thousand entries against which unknown organisms are compared. Most manufacturers provide updated versions of their databases every few years. Computer-based algorithms convert biochemical profiles and other substrate information into a probability index to determine the identification of unknown bacteria. Users should familiarize themselves with the limitations of the databases. Laboratorians should validate results and should provide feedback to manufacturers in the event of aberrant results and for a high frequency of misidentified or unidentified isolates. What follows is a brief description of automated identification systems currently available in the United States. Table 1 summarizes the features of these systems. Many of the instruments discussed also have the capability to perform susceptibility testing.

VITEK® and VITEK 2® (bioMerieux, Inc., Durham, NC)

The VITEK system has been available since the early 1980s. The five available models are based upon the number of cards they process: 32, 60, 120, 240, and 480. The test cards themselves are the size of a playing card, and they contain either 30 or 45 microwells containing either substrates for organism identification or antimicrobials in the case of the susceptibility testing cards (*see* Systems for Susceptibility Testing later). Isolates are identified through detection of pH changes based upon growth of organisms in the presence of certain substrates. This system and its various software versions have been extensively reviewed in the literature (3–5).

The VITEK 2 is the newer version of the VITEK system. This is a fully automated system that allows for continuous access. Compared to its predecessor, improvements include the introduction of fluorescent technology with optics designed to read all 64 wells in the work cards every 15 minutes. Identification and susceptibility testing cards are prepared using a standardized inoculum equivalent to 0.5–0.63 McFarland standards. Workflow is standardized through a "Smart Carrier" cassette that allows for specimen tracking from the time the specimen inoculum tube is prepared at the bench to the final report. This is accomplished through a memory chip that contains information for the bar-code-labeled suspensions in that load. Two platforms exist, the VITEK 2 (60-card capacity) and the VITEK 2-XL (120-card capacity) (6). The gram-negative identification cards have 64 wells that contain 41 biochemical tests (21 conventional substrates and 20 preformed enzymes), two negative control wells, and 21 blank wells. In 2004, bioMerieux introduced the 64-well 2GN card, which is entirely colorimetric. The 64-well gram-positive identification card has 22 enzymatic tests, 16 fermentation tests, two carboxylase tests, and tests for urease, pyruvate, optochin, novobiocin, polymyxin B sulfate, and 6.5% NaCl. The yeast identification card consists of 47 biochemical tests including 20 carbohydrate assimilation tests. The VITEK database uses a series of algorithms to classify answers into several confidence levels: excellent, very good, good, and acceptable.

In a study that evaluated 482 enteric strains representing 21 genera and 60 species, the VITEK 2 correctly identified 85.9% at the excellent-to-good confidence level (6). Another 7.1% (34 isolates) were correctly assigned but at a low level of discrimination (6). Of the remaining isolates, 3.9% (N = 19) could not be identified and 3.1% (N = 15) were misidentified at the low level of discrimination (6). Most of the problems occurred with lactose-positive *Salmonella* spp. In the same study, 103 isolates of nonenteric gram-negative bacilli representing 21 genera and 30 species of organisms (glucose fermenting, glucose nonfermenting, oxidase positive, and oxidase negative) were also evaluated (6). Again, 85.4% of strains were correctly assigned with excellent-to-good confidence levels, 9.7% were correctly identified at a low level of probability, three isolates (2.9%) were misidentified, and two strains were not identified (6). The overall accuracy was 93% for enterics and 95.1% for nonenterics (6). Similar results were seen in a larger study of 684

Enterobacteriaceae and 174 non-*Enterobacteriaceae*, where overall accuracy to species level of identification was 95.9% and 92.5%, respectively (7). The current version of the software is 7.01, and it contains 48 genera and 112 species (2).

Several studies have examined the ability of the VITEK 2 to accurately identify gram-positive cocci (7–9). Gavin et al. (7) using challenge strains of *Enterococcus* sp. and viridans streptococci found excellent performance with *Enterococcus faecalis* and *E. faecium* strains but poor performance (72% accuracy) with other enterococci and the viridans streptococci. In a study of 405 clinically significant staphylococci recovered from bloodstream infections, Spanu et al. (8) found an overall accuracy of 95.6% compared to an expanded phenotypic characterization and molecular testing, when necessary. Similar results for staphylococci were reported by Ligozzi et al. (9). In that study, the VITEK 2 system also performed well for *Streptococcus agalactiae* (96.5% accuracy) and *S. pneumoniae* (96.9% accuracy) identification as well (9).

Finally, a published report evaluated the ability of the VITEK 2 to accurately identify 241 clinical isolates representing 21 species of yeasts. It found that correct identification was obtained for 222 of the strains (92.1%) (10).

MicroScan® Microbiology Systems (Dade Behring, Inc., Deerfield, IL)

MicroScan microbiology systems are available in two platforms, the WalkAway® SI System and the autoSCAN®-4 System. The WalkAway system integrates rapid and conventional overnight testing for identification and susceptibility testing on one instrument. It is available in a 40- or 96-panel capacity instrument. The instrument automatically incubates panels, adds reagents, and interprets results. This instrument allows for simultaneous processing. Users may buy identification only (ID), susceptibility testing (AST) only, or combination panels.

The autoSCAN-4 provides automated bacterial ID and AST with traditional, conventional overnight panels. There are more than 150 organisms included in the identification database of these systems.

Table 1 lists the panels that are currently available for identification.

Several studies have evaluated the Rapid Neg ID panel for identification of *Enterobacteriaceae*, other glucose fermenters, and gram-negative nonfermenters (11, 12). For the identification of the most commonly isolated *Enterobacteriaceae* and nonfermenters, the Rapid Neg ID3 panel (software v.22.01) had overall accuracies of 79% at 2.5 hours of incubation and 89% at 24 hours (11). Performance of this same panel (software v.22.28) for the identification of non-*Enterobacteriaceae* gram-negative bacilli was less encouraging with overall accuracy, including additional testing, of 74.6%; 20.2% of the organisms could not be characterized (12). The conventional overnight panels (Neg Combo type 12) demonstrated an overall correct identification of 96% when a large group on nonfermenters was tested on the autoSCAN-W/A along with additional testing recommended by the manufacturer. The performance of the autoSCAN was similar to that of the VITEK GNI+ (accuracy with supplemental testing of 92.3%) (5).

There are fewer papers that examine the accuracy of these systems for identification of a broad range of gram-positive cocci. A study performed in Spain evaluated 99 clinical isolates of staphylococci with the Rapid Pos Combo ID Panels (13). Overall, including eight isolates that required additional testing, the WalkAway identified 94% of the isolates to species level (13). In addition, the Pos Combo Panel type 11 of the WalkAway 96 identified *Enterococcus faecalis* and *E. faecium* quite well (accuracy of 99.6% and 78.3%, respectively), but its performance for identification of other enterococcal species was not reliable (14).

TABLE 1. Automated systems for bacterial identification

System	Manufacturer	Principle	Current test cards; number of species in database	Instrument capacity	References
VITEK Legacy	bioMerieux, Inc. (Durham, NC)	Growth-dependent pH-based reactions from carbohydrate utilization or protein utilization	GNI + V1311[a] (104 organisms) GPI card V1305 (49 organisms) YB card V1303 (36 organisms) ANI card V1309[b] (80 organisms) NHI card V1308 (30 species) UID-3V1102 UID-1V1106	32/120 cards	1–5 www.biomerieux-usa.com
VITEK 2 VITEK 2-XL	bioMerieux, Inc. (Durham, NC)	Fluorescent detection of preformed enzymes	100 gram-negative bacilli; 46 gram-positive cocci; 50 yeast	60 cards (VITEK); 120 cards (VITEK 2-XL)	6–10 www.biomeriuex-usa.com
MicroScan WalkAway SI MicroScan autoSCAN-4 System	Dade Behring, Inc. (Deerfield, IL)	Fluorescent detection of preformed enzymes; conventional growth-dependent substrate utilization	Gram-negative combination panels[a] (44 genera, 125 species of gram-negative bacilli) B1017-119 B1017-135, 136 B1017-300, 301, 302 B1017-138 Urine B1017-303, 304, 305 Urine panels B1017-78 Urine B1017-130 Neg BP combo 11 B1017-131 Neg BP combo 12 B1017-306 Neg BP combo 30 B1017-307 Neg BP combo 31 Gram-positive combination panels B1017-124 B1017-200 B1017-201 B1017-125 BP combo 9 B1017-202 BP combo 20	40/96 cards Unlimited capacity	1, 11–14 www.dadebehring.com

BD Phoenix 100	BD Diagnostic Systems (Sparks, MD)	Fluorescence, chromogen and pH-based technology including detection of preformed enzymes	160 gram-negative organisms 140 gram-positive organisms (see Table 2 for panels)	99 panels	2, 15, 16 www.bd.com/ds/
OmniLog–fully automated MicroLog–semi-automated	Biolog (Hayward, CA)	Carbon source utilization–tetrazolium chemistry	500 gram-negative organisms 318 gram-positive organisms 359 anaerobic bacteria 267 yeast, version 6.01	Unlimited capacity	1, 2, 17, 18 www.biolog.com
Sherlock Microbial Identification System	MIDI Sherlock® library and software (Newark, DE) Agilent Gas Chromatographs, Agilent Technologies (Palo Alto, CA) 6850, 6890 single column, 6890 dual columns	Cell wall fatty acid analysis	480 gram-negative organisms 240 gram-positive organisms 359 anaerobic organisms 300 environmental organisms 50 "fastidious" organisms 194 yeast 28 mycobacteria	Sherlock 4.5 Microbial Identification System 60-card capacity	1, 2, 19, 20 www.midi-inc.com
Sensititre ARIS2X	Trek Diagnostic Systems, Inc. (Westlake, OH)	pH detection of substrate utilization in microtiter plate format	140 gram-negative organisms 39 gram-positive organisms	64 plates	2 www.trekds.com

Key: GNI = gram-negative identification; GPI = gram-positive identification; YB = yeast; ANI = anaerobes; NHI = *Neisseria*, *Haemophilus*, and other fastidious organisms; and UID = identification of urinary pathogens directly.

[a] Listed in product literature as overnight conventional panels that perform combination identification and susceptibility testing.

[b] Direct reading only.

BD Phoenix™ Automated Microbiology System (BD Diagnostic Systems, Sparks, MD)

The Phoenix automated microbiology system is a relatively new, fully automated system that identifies a broad range of gram-positive and gram-negative bacteria. The system includes an instrument, software, disposable panels, broths for identification (ID) and susceptibility testing (AST), and a susceptibility testing indicator. The ID method employs modified conventional, fluorogenic, and chromogenic substrates. The instrument can analyze up to 100 ID and AST combination panels simultaneously. The disposable test panels contain 136 microdilution wells and is available in ID, ID/AST, and AST-only formats. The panels are read every 20 minutes by the instrument. Final results for identification are available in 2–12 hours. Several studies performed in Europe (15, 16) indicate agreements of 97%–100% for gram-positive cocci and 92%–96% for gram-negative bacilli, including *Enterobacteriaceae* and nonfermenters, compared to conventional phenotypic identification methods (15, 16).

Sensititre® Microbiology Systems (TREK Diagnostic Systems, Inc., Westlake, OH)

The Sensititre microbiology system performs both identification and susceptibility testing. The identification portion of the system is designed to identify the most common aerobic gram-negative and gram-positive bacteria. Presumptive identification can be performed in about 5 hours but definitive identification to species level requires overnight incubation. Testing is performed in microtiter plates, and each test plate is designed to identify three separate organisms. The substrate profile (~32 biochemical tests per organism for each panel) is not as extensive as some of the other systems currently available. The plates can be read by the semiautomated Sensititre AutoReader® or the fully automated Sensititre ARIS® system.

MicroLog™ and OmniLog® (Biolog Inc., Hayward, CA)

The Biolog microbial identification and characterization systems allow for identification of more than 1900 species of aerobic and anaerobic organisms including yeast and filamentous fungi (v.6.01). These systems may be of particular interest to reference laboratories that are often asked to characterize environmental pathogens recovered from clinical sources of infection, particularly from immunocompromised patients. The company offers a fully automated system called the OmniLog instrument which incubates, reads, and interprets up to 50 microplates. This instrument has the flexibility of user-defined incubation temperatures (off-line). The software is Windows® based. The semiautomated system called the MicroLog™ MicroStation™ includes instrumentation and software to read the microplates, a turbidimeter for inocula preparation, and an eight-channel repeating electronic pipetter. The user provides the computer. Both systems are based upon the principle of carbon source utilization (95 discrete tests), which uses a novel patented redox chemistry based on reduction of tetrazolium. A standardized inoculum of the organisms to be identified is made in 0.85% saline. Users must use the Biolog media for subculture prior to inoculation. An aliquot is inoculated into each well of a specific 96-microwell plate (e.g., gram-negative, gram-positive, etc.). A metabolic "fingerprint" of the inoculated organism is generated which can be used to create dendrograms and other analyses. These systems have been utilized by ecologists, pharmaceutical companies, and public health laboratories. Few published reports exist regarding the performance of these systems in mainstream clinical laboratories. In the report by Tang et al. (21), 72 unusual gram-negative bacilli were evaluated using the MicroLog system (v.3.50). There was an 87.5% concordance with conventional methods. The system encountered problems with some strains of *Klebsiella*, *Enterobacter*, and *Serratia.* Similar difficulties with species from these same genera were seen in the study by Holmes et al. (v.3.01A) (17). An early study on the performance of the Biolog system for staphylococcal identification reported poor performance (~74% accuracy with repeat testing) (18). At the time of this writing, there are no recently published reports of the current version of the database with respect to gram-positive bacteria and yeast identification. However, of the automated identification systems currently available, this system has one of the most extensive databases.

BIOMIC®-IDTree™ (Giles Scientific, Inc.)

Using nonproprietary methods and materials, this system identifies commonly encountered aerobic and anaerobic bacteria and yeast) based upon the algorithms in the NCCLS M35 document (abbreviated identification of bacteria and yeast) (22). The system consists of a series of flowcharts based upon colony morphology, and various biochemical and enzymatic tests that the user performs. The system is designed to identify 95% of commonly encountered urinary tract pathogens and 80% of those organisms from other nonsterile body sites. The identification component of this system is not automated, but complements the microbiology analyzer susceptibility testing method that the manufacturer also markets (*see* Systems for Susceptibility Testing discussed later). This identification system would not likely suffice as a standalone system for large-volume laboratories, but it may complement existing, more expensive instrumentation by rapidly dispensing with straightforward pathogens from nonsterile sites and urine specimens, thereby reducing costs.

Sherlock® Microbial Identification System (MIDI, Inc., Newark, DE)

The Sherlock microbial identification system uses gas chromatography to identify organisms on the basis of the cell wall fatty acid profiles of bacteria and yeast. The system consists of an Agilent Technologies (Palo Alto, CA) gas chromatograph and ChemStation, the MIDI database, and MIDI fatty acid pattern recognition software loaded onto a Windows 2000 based computer, to identify more than 2000 strains of clinical and environmental, aerobic and anaerobic bacteria and yeast. In addition, in collaboration with the U.S. Army Medical Research Institute of Infectious Diseases, the company has recently created a "bioterrorism library" to identify accurately and rapidly six select bacterial agents and related organisms. There are more than 400 publications in the literature regarding the utility of this methodology. Applications of this technology reach beyond the clinical laboratory and include environmental, food, animal, and applied microbiology, among others.

The technology requires a standardized approach that includes growing organisms under specified culture conditions, saponification of the lipid cell wall components and methylation of the fatty acids, extraction of the methylated fatty acids into organic solvent, and analysis of the extracted fatty acids by gas chromatography (19, 20). Advantages of the MIDI system include the extensive library, automation, and after initial capital expenditure, the low per specimen cost (~$2.50 per sample). It is also as rapid, and in some cases more rapid, than some of the currently available identification systems. Because of its expansive database, this system may be particularly well suited to the reference laboratory setting.

MIDI also offers the Sherlock mycobacteria identification system which is FDA-cleared for identification of the *Mycobacterium tuberculosis* complex (Mtb complex). Particularly helpful is the ability to differentiate *Mycobacterium bovis* BCG from other members of the Mtb complex. The system is based upon analysis of mycolic acids derived from cultures of suspect mycobacteria. In brief, HPLC requires the following steps (23):

1. Disruption/saponification of fatty acids from a pure growth of mycobacteria
2. Extraction of fatty acids
3. Evaporation of the extract
4. Derivatization of fatty acids
5. Clarification of sample
6. HPLC analysis of mycolic acids
7. Pattern recognition

The Sherlock system automates many of these steps, and the pattern recognition software interprets the profiles and allows for mycobacteria identification (24).

SYSTEMS FOR SUSCEPTIBILITY TESTING

BIOMIC Microbiology Analyzer (Giles Scientific)

The BIOMIC microbiology analyzer includes the BIOMIC vision system that is a high-resolution color digital camera that automatically reads and interprets standard disk diffusion plates in less than 1 second. The user sets up the standard disk diffusion Mueller Hinton agar plates, but the zones of inhibition are standardized and interpreted by the instrument. Results may be reported both qualitatively and quantitatively (MIC). The instrument can be interfaced to any laboratory information system. The current version of the BIOMIC vision system interprets standard disk diffusion, fastidious organisms on sheep blood agar, yeast MICs, and E-test results. There are few published studies on this system. One study compared the performance of the BIOMIC to the VITEK system. The overall MIC correlation for close to 3000 organism–drug combinations was 92.6%. For categorical interpretations, the overall agreement was 97.4%. Compared to the VITEK system, the BIOMIC was considerably less expensive—57.4% savings per test (25). In another study, which compared the BIOMIC video-assisted read to manual zone size interpretations, there were four false susceptible results and six minor errors by the video system (26).

MicroScan Systems

As previously discussed, there are two forms of available automation for the MicroScan systems, the fully automated WalkAway-SI and the autoSCAN-4 system. Both systems accommodate panels that are ID only, AST only, or the combination. Available panels for both systems are listed in Table 2. The rapid panels, which are read on the WalkAway system, provide gram-negative AST results in 3.5–7 hours, while the turnaround time for the gram-positive rapid AST panels ranges from 4.5 to 16 hours. The autoSCAN-4 is designed to read only the conventional, growth-dependent overnight panels including an ESBL plus panel and the MICroSTREP Plus™ panel.

In the last 5 years, there have been relatively few published papers that evaluate a large collection of organisms for susceptibility testing using these systems. Most of the available publications focus on problem pathogens such as *Staphylococcus aureus*, enterococcus, *Streptococcus pneumoniae*, and *Pseudomonas aeruginosa* (14, 27, 29, 30). The sensitivity and specificity of the conventional panels and rapid panels for detection of methicillin resistance among *S. aureus* are reported to be 74%, 97% and 100%, 89%, respectively (29). Likewise for detection of high-level aminoglycoside resistance and vancomycin resistance among enterococci, there is excellent agreement of the WalkAway Combo Panel type 11 to conventional methods (96% and 100%, respectively) (14). The MICroSTREP plus frozen panels can be used to perform MIC testing on all streptococci. No very major errors and close to 100% overall correlation with standard reference methods were seen in one study that evaluated the use of these panels for testing a challenge panel of *S. pneumoniae* (30). Unfortunately, such excellent results have not been seen when testing both mucoid and nonmucoid strains of *P. aeruginosa* from cystic fibrosis patients (27). Correlation of the WalkAway system with reference broth microdilution methods was unacceptable. There was a 17% very major error rate for all drugs tested (27).

In terms of information systems, the company has available the LabPro Information Manager and LabPro Alert Software (v.1.51). The latter warns the microbiologist of atypical ID and AST results or results that may be of importance to infection control personnel. The user may incorporate the manufacturer's 75 pre-defined rules or develop customized algorithms/alerts. Examples of some of the features include recognizing isolates that are reportable to public health authorities and alerting the user to microbial resistance patterns that may require infection control measures.

VITEK Systems

Table 2 lists the current test card configurations for the VITEK and VITEK 2 instruments. The VITEK has 45-well standard susceptibility test cards. For gram-negative bacilli, there are 20 available test panels that offer up to 18 different antimicrobial agents. If the user would like to test additional agents, an extension card, GNS-127, is also available and in combination with one of the standard cards, allows for testing 32 antimicrobics. For gram-positive susceptibility testing, three standard test card configurations offering up to 18 agents per card are currently available.

The VITEK 2 cards are designed to detect problem, resistant organisms such as vancomycin-resistant enterococci and extended spectrum β-lactamase producing gram-negative bacilli. Currently, there are two gram-positive susceptibility test cards and six gram-negative test cards.

Both systems have a variety of software applications. These include the VITEK DataTrac™, which gathers data and formats them into many reports such as those used for epidemiology. The VITEK Expert System™ validates organism identification and susceptibility testing combinations and alerts the user to mismatch patterns, unusual resistance trends, etc. The CAR or conditional antimicrobial reporting program allows the user to suppress results of drugs that are toxic, inappropriate, not on an institution's formulary, or too costly for initial use.

BD Phoenix

A description of the capacity of the Phoenix instruments was provided previously in the discussion on ID systems. The Phoenix AST broth requires the addition of one drop of the AST indicator (oxidation–reduction indicator based on resazurin). Then 25 μL of the standardized ID suspension is transferred to the AST broth, resulting in a final inoculum of 5×10^5 colony-forming units (CFU)/mL. The AST broth is then added to the AST side of a Phoenix panel. Since this system is not yet widely available in the United States, there are relatively few publications on its performance. Essential agreement and categorical

TABLE 2. FDA-approved automated instruments for susceptibility testing

System	Manufacturer	Cards/panels	Software programs	References
VITEK	bioMerieux, Inc.	Gram-positive panels: GPS 105, GPS 106, GPS 107, GPS 109, GPS 110, GPS 111 Gram-negative panels with ESBL test: GNS 120, GNS 121 Gram-negative urine isolates: GNS 203, GNS 204, GNS 206 Gram-negative cards: GNS 108, GNS 115, GNS 118, GNS 122–127	VITEK DataTrac™ VITEK Expert System™ bioLiaison® CAR (conditional antimicrobial reporting) Quality Control Bidirectional computer interface (BCI) 7.02	2, 25, 27, 28 www.biomerieux-usa.com
VITEK 2		AST-GP 61 (staph, enterococcus, group B strep) AST GP 62 (*S. pneumo*) AST-GN04–AST-GN11	See above	www.biomerieux-usa.com
autoSCAN-4 WalkAway-SI	Dade Behring Microscan	Conventional overnight panels: Gram-negative B1017-308 MIC 30, B1017-309 MIC +4 Gram-positive conventional panels B1017-203 MIC 20, B1017-109 MICroSTREP™	LabPro Alert System Software (v.1.51)	2, 27, 29–31 www.dadebehring.com
BIOMIC Vision	Giles Scientific Inc.	NA	PC Windows-based bidirectional interface with 2500 expert rules; custom epidemiology reports available	25, 26

Sensititre	TREK Diagnostics	Anaerobic MIC plate Gram-negative MIC plate HPB susceptibility plates[a] ESBL confirmatory MIC plates *Streptococcus pneumoniae* MIC plate YeastOne® with Caspofungin Customized panels are available		32 www.trekds.com
BD Phoenix	BD Diagnostics Systems (Sparks, MD)	NMIC/ID 101, 104, 107, 108 —gram-negative MIC and ID panels NMIC 101, 104, 107, 108 —gram-negative MIC panels (no ID) PMIC/ID, 101—gram-positive MIC and ID PMIC-/00—gram-positive MIC (no ID) SMIC/ID—streptococcal MIC and ID (complete panel scheduled for availability in the United States in July 2005) SMIC—streptococcal MIC (complete panel scheduled for availability in the United States in July 2005)	BDXpert system v.4.01A Phoenix embedded software v.5.02A EpiCenter Data Management software v.5.10A Bidirectional LIS interface	www.bd.com/ds/

Key: ESBL = extended spectrum β-lactamase; ID = identification; and MIC = minimum inhibitory concentration.

[a]Tests both *Haemophilus influenzae* and *Streptococcus pneumoniae.*

agreement with reference broth microdilution testing for staphylococci, enterococci, and streptococci were 93.3% and 97.3%, respectively, in the study by Fahr et al. (16). In one study (15), 100% concordance for categorical results for AST of *Enterobacteriaceae* compared to agar dilution was seen, but the results for gram-negative nonfermenters revealed problems with ciprofloxacin and only an 80% categorical agreement for *Stenotrophomonas maltophilia* and trimethoprim–sulfamethoxazole.

TREK Diagnostics

TREK Diagnostics manufactures a variety of Sensititre® susceptibility testing products for aerobic and anaerobic, fastidious, gram-positive, and gram-negative bacteria as well as yeast. Users may purchase the manufacturer's 96-well microtiter plate panels or, for an additional cost, custom design their own. The plates have vacuum-dried antibiotics only, so that the user may add appropriate broth (which the manufacturer also markets) specific to the organism tested. The shelflife is 18–24 months at room temperature storage. Plates can be read manually or by any one of a number of TREK's semiautomated or automated instruments. The company provides manual viewboxes, electronic pipettes, autoinoculators, semiautomated plate readers (SensiTouch reader and computer database system), and a completely automated system called the Sensititer ARIS® which provides incubation and reading for both the identification and susceptibility testing panels.

Sensititre broth microdilution plates have been available for two decades and have been favorably compared to standardized "gold standard" broth microdilution, agar dilution, disk diffusion methods, and E-test and to a variety of other automated systems such as the VITEK and the WalkAway instruments (28, 31, 33). A recent prospective study performed in the microbiology laboratory of a 250-bed suburban teaching hospital compared the ARIS instrument to the WalkAway system (32). The ARIS demonstrated 93.5% essential agreement for gram-positive organisms and a 95.8% essential agreement for gram-negative organisms compared to the WalkAway system. The very major error rate was 0.4% for both categories of pathogens (32).

BLOOD CULTURE INSTRUMENTS

Overview

The history of blood culture instruments in clinical microbiology laboratories has been well described (34–36). The introduction of automated instruments in clinical microbiology was initiated in the 1970s with the first blood culture monitoring machine. The BACTEC™ 460 (Becton Dickinson Biosciences) was a semiautomated device that required manual loading of blood culture bottles onto a conveyer belt with each bottle sampled one at a time on each run through the machine. A set of sensing needles penetrated the diaphragm at the top of each bottle. Each bottle contained ^{14}C-labeled substrates which, when utilized by microorganisms, released $^{14}CO_2$ into the gas phase of the bottle. This gas phase was sampled from the dead space in the top of the bottle and when $^{14}CO_2$ was present, the bottle was identified as positive. A simple printout showed the radiometric readings for each bottle, and an arbitrary cutoff was used to identify bottles that were positive. Bottles were loaded into the instrument once or twice a day for a reading. Bottles were sampled multiple times over several days of incubation, but there was no attempt to compare readings on the same bottle from one cycle to the next. The BACTEC system initiated the time period when manual gram stains and subcultures from blood culture bottles could be eliminated. Although results were somewhat variable from study to study when this system was compared to manual blood cultures, most supported the capability of this instrument to achieve detection rates of microorganisms similar to manual broth cultures in a time frame similar to or slightly better than those manual systems.

There were disadvantages, however. Most importantly, the detection system utilizing ^{14}C-labeled substrates forced laboratories to deal with state-imposed regulations for appropriate disposal of radioactive material. A second generation of instruments using nonradiometric detection of CO_2 was introduced in the mid-1980s to overcome this problem, but the method of sampling and manual manipulation of bottles remained unchanged. In addition, the needles entering the top of each bottle sometimes transferred organisms from one bottle to another, resulting in false-positive specimens. Multiple case reports appeared in the literature of outbreaks of pseudobacteremia associated with both the first- and second-generation BACTEC instruments.

In the late 1980s, the current generation of monitoring instruments was designed with significant changes in technology. The vast majority of laboratories in the United States have now adopted one of these instruments into routine laboratory practice. These instruments by three different manufacturers have several features in common. They are all self-contained modular units into which bottles are placed in individual slots, coded into a single computer monitoring system, and monitored from this "cell" without further hands-on manipulation. Monitoring occurs on an ongoing basis with repeated cycles of data recording every few minutes, hence bottles are monitored on a continuous basis. This both allows for the potential of earlier detection of positive bottles and the elimination of false-positives with more frequent data points and smoother transitions along data points. These systems are now called **continuous-monitoring blood culture systems, or CMBCSs**. All monitoring occurs from a detection system that makes observations from outside the bottles, eliminating the possibility of cross-contamination. Over time, multiple media have been created to individualize detection approaches by patient group, hospital location, or hospital system. Studies show clear improvement in the overall detection of microorganisms. Equally important, it is now possible to detect the majority of episodes of bacteremia within a few hours with the continuous stream of data analysis coming from each bottle.

Specific Instruments

There are now three commercially available automated blood culture instruments. A comparison of these three systems is shown in Table 3. The **BacT/ALERT®** system (bioMerieux, Inc.) was the first of the CMBCS's introduced. It was upgraded in 1999 to a smaller size and a more advanced system for technologist interaction. All bottles within the system are rocked at 30 cycles per minute. The system detects CO_2 production when

TABLE 3. Comparison of current blood culture instruments

System	Principle of detection	Manufacturer	Comments
BacT/Alert	Colorimetric detection of CO_2 production	bioMerieux, Inc.	The first CMBCS, redesigned 1999
BACTEC 9000 Series	Fluorescent detection of CO_2 production	Becton Dickinson Biosciences	Three different instruments with variable bottle capacities
ESP	Pressure change detection from gas production by organisms	TREK Diagnostic Systems, Inc.	Fewer media formulations for individual patient groups

carbon source substrates are metabolized by organisms. A colorimetric disk at the base of each bottle is able to identify this CO_2 production. The instrument's computer monitors colorimetric readings throughout the incubation of the bottle and plots the colorimetric changes within each bottle over time. Characteristic plots consistent with microorganism growth have been created and are the basis of the detection method. Several formulations of media are available including standard aerobic and anaerobic broths, FAN aerobic and anaerobic media that contain charcoal and Fuller's earth to absorb and inactivate antibiotics, and multiple varieties of lower volume broths for pediatric patients.

The second system introduced was a new generation of instruments **BACTEC™** (Becton Dickinson Biosciences), the 9000 series, with three instruments that vary in the number of bottles that can be entered into the machine. Bottles are all rocked at 34 cycles per minute. Like the BacT/ALERT, a sensing disk is in the base of each bottle and is used to monitor the production of CO_2. Unlike the BacT/ALERT, the mechanism for detection is to determine a fluorescent change instead of a colorimetric one. The computer plots fluorescent changes in each bottle over time, and, like the BacT/ALERT, has a pattern of fluorescent change that identifies the growth of microorganisms. Medium formulations include standard aerobic and anaerobic media, Plus media that contain resin beads to absorb and inactivate antibiotics, an anaerobic lytic medium, a separate resin-containing medium formulated for pediatric patients, and the Myco/F-Lytic medium for detection of mycobacteria and fungi.

The third system, the **ESP** (TREK Diagnostic Systems, Inc.), uses a different mechanism for monitoring. Bottles are placed in the instrument and fitted with an adapter. Aerobic bottles are rotated at 160 rpm while anaerobic bottles are not agitated. As gases are produced during metabolism of substrates by organisms, the adapter is used to monitor pressure changes in the gas phase of the bottle. The computer attached to this system plots the pressure change within each bottle over time and identifies positive bottles based on the increased presence of gas. The many medium formulations available for the other systems are not available for the ESP.

There have been multiple comparisons of these instruments. Summaries of these studies have been published in a number of reviews (34–36). Early studies evaluated the individual instruments with manual systems or against each other. While subtle variations existed, it was generally true that these instruments performed similarly to manual systems and to each other. There have been more recent comparisons of different media formulations which show some variations (36–40). While individual variations exist, the use of any of these instruments results in acceptable recovery of microorganisms in 1–1.5 days.

Whereas CMBCSs have dramatically affected clinical microbiology practice, they are not perfect. The detection of bacteremia or fungemia as accomplished by blood cultures requires hours to days of incubation. More rapid detection of infection should remain an important goal. Whereas these CMBCSs perform well in general, each type of medium, and to some extent each instrument, misses some organisms associated with infection. Some types of microorganisms grow poorly or not at all in conventional blood culture broths. The detection of infection with these organisms requires alternative approaches such as molecular amplification technology or immunological methods. Finally, while CMBCSs do an excellent job of detecting the presence of organisms, they have no intrinsic role in the identification or susceptibility testing of the causative organism. Additional steps using complementary technologies are necessary before a final result is obtained. These additional steps add even more time to a process that already takes longer than would be ideal within the framework of clinical decision-making. The next important advance in technology will be to be able to provide the final identification and approach to management of the patient during the initial few minutes of the evaluation process.

MYCOBACTERIA DETECTION AND SUSCEPTIBILITY TESTING SYSTEMS

The first semiautomated system for detection of mycobacteria in clinical samples, the radiometric BACTEC 460 (Becton Dickinson Biosciences, Inc.) was introduced in the 1980s and clearly was a major advance for its time. It shortened the time to detection of Mtb by 2 weeks, became a useful standard for susceptibility testing, and was semiautomated (41). However, there were some distinct disadvantages such as cross-contamination of culture bottles, the requirement for needles for inoculation, radioactivity, and the fact that the bottles had to be loaded manually (42). This system has been largely replaced by more fully automated instruments that do not require radiolabeled compounds for organism detection.

Three major systems for detection of mycobacteria in clinical samples are currently FDA-cleared in the United States. Two of these systems, the ESP® culture system II (TREK Diagnostics, Inc.) and the Mycobacteria Growth Indicator Tube (MGIT®) (Becton Dickinson Biosciences, Inc.) are approved for both culture and susceptibility testing. The MB/BacT system is approved only for culture. All three systems have been extensively evaluated in the literature. A brief description of each instrument follows and Table 4 contains a synopsis of the performance characteristics based upon several large studies of each system. In general, these systems are as rapid as, or may possibly detect Mtb complex 1–2 days sooner than, the radiometric BACTEC 460 system. None of the systems is sensitive

TABLE 4. Performance characteristics of automated mycobacteria detection systems

System	% Recovery mycobacteria		TTD (days)		% False-positives	% Contamination	Comments	References
	TB	ALL	TB	ALL				
ESP culture system II	74–85	71–79	18.7–19.0	17–18	1.3–2.7	8–19	Isolates more *M. gordonae* than MGIT; unreliable for *M. xenopi* detection	43, 44
MGIT	77–88.9	64–87.4	9.3–14.4	8.7–13.1	0.7–0.95	5.4–17.1	System designed to inhibit growth of *M. gordonae*	44–46
MB/BacT system	84.5–93.6	78.8–91.6	11.5–20	13.9–26	0[a]	4.6–10.2	Problems detecting *M. xenopi*	

Key: TTD = time to detection; TB = *Mycobacterium tuberculosis*; and All = indicates all species of mycobacteria.
[a]Only one paper commented on the false-positive results.

enough to detect all mycobacteria, so the addition of solid media to complement the liquid-based culture systems is still required.

The **ESP culture system II** is a fully automated, continuously monitored broth-based culture system approved for both culture and susceptibility testing of mycobacteria. ESP bottles contain oleic acid–albumin–dextrose–catalase (OADC)-enriched, Middlebrook 7H9 medium, and Myco PVNA (polymyxin B, vancomycin, nalidixic acid, and amphotericin B). The bottles also contain a compressed sponge which provides a platform for growth (43). The medium in the bottle is specifically designed to maximize both consumption and production of gas as a by-product of microbial detection. The instrument detects organism growth by measuring the gas pressure changes within the headspace of a culture bottle. The same instrument that is used for routine blood and sterile body fluid cultures can accommodate the mycobacteria culture and Mtb susceptibility testing, obviating the need for duplicate instruments. Instrument capacities include room for 128, 256, or 384 bottles.

MGIT contains 7 mL of Middlebrook 7H9 broth base to which is added OADC. PANTA (polymyxin B, amphotericin B, nalidixic acid, trimethoprim, and azlocillin) antibiotic mixture is added by the user to reduce contamination by competing normal microbial flora. The bottom of the tube contains silicone which is imbedded with an O_2-sensitive ruthenium metal complex. When organisms grow, the O_2 is depleted, thereby allowing the ruthenium complex to fluorescence and hence signal that a microorganism is present. The MGIT tubes can be read manually, in a small capacity instrument, the BACTEC automated 9000 MB, or in a large capacity instrument, e.g., the 960. The automated instruments are noninvasive and monitor the tubes every 60 minutes.

The **MB/BacT ALERT 3D** system (Organon Teknika, Durham, NC) is an automated, continuously monitored colorimetric CO_2 detection system. The MB/BacT bottles contain 10 mL of modified Middlebrook 7H9 broth enriched with casein, bovine serum albumin, and catalase (47). A proprietary antibiotic supplement, 0.5 mL, containing amphotericin B, azlocillin, nalidixic acid, polymyxin B, trimethoprim, and vancomycin is added by the user.

In terms of susceptibility testing, the MGIT AST SIRE system is FDA-cleared for isoniazid, rifampin, ethambutol, and pyrazinamide. The ESP culture system II is approved for isoniazid, rifampin, and ethambutol. Both systems compare favorably with the agar proportion method and the BACTEC TB 460 for testing the four primary antituberculosis drugs (45–51).

URINE ANALYZERS

There are four major, completely automated urine screening systems available in the United States. Two of these, the Coral UTIscreen™ (Coral Biotechnology, San Diego, CA) and the Cellenium (TREK Diagnostic Systems, Inc., Cleveland, OH), are specifically designed to detect significant bacteriuria. The other two systems, the Sysmex UF-50 and UF-100 (Sysmex Inc., Mundelein, IL) and the IRIS 939 UDx™ urine pathology system (IRIS Diagnostics, Chatsworth, CA) are automated urine analyzers. Only the performance of the latter two systems with respect to their ability to screen for urinary tract infection (UTI) will be addressed in this chapter. Although the Cellenium is discussed below, at the time of this writing, it had been withdrawn from the market (personal communication, Trek Diagnostics).

The **Coral UTIscreen bacterial ATP assay** uses the luciferen-luciferase reaction to assay for adenosine triphosphate (ATP) released from living bacterial cells directly from sterile urine samples (52). First, the urine specimen is treated with a somatic cell release agent (SRA) which destroys ATP from somatic cells. After incubation, an agent is added which suppresses the ATP-destroying enzyme so that bacterial ATP can be measured.

A reduced form of luciferin reacts with bacterial and/or yeast ATP in the presence of the enzyme luciferase to produce the oxidized form of luciferin, adenosine monophosphate, and light, which is measured by a luminometer (WAVE 180 automated luminometer). The light signal is converted to relative light units (RLU) which are proportional to the amount of ATP in the urine sample. The readings are converted to positive or negative results which correlate clinically to colony-forming units (CFU) (52). Up to 180 urines can be screened at one time using this system. In a study performed in a large regional central laboratory in Canada (52), the UTIscreen had a sensitivity of 86%, specificity of 75.5% with positive and negative predictive values of 45% and 95.9%, respectively, compared to conventional bacterial culture (52). Routine use resulted in same day reporting of 65% of all urine culture results because these specimens did not require subsequent culture (52). This system should not be used with visibly bloody urine, because blood falsely elevates the RLU (52).

There are no published peer-reviewed articles to date on the **Cellenium system** (TREK Diagnostic Systems, Inc.). This system is designed to detect, quantify, and classify pathogenic bacteria and yeast as well as detect leukocytes from fresh urine samples within 30 minutes. The principle of operation is as follows. Selective molecular fluorescent staining is combined with computerized video imaging to perform rapid urine screening. An aliquot of urine is robotically dispensed into a cassette to which the molecular stains are added. The cassette is then automatically coupled with a porous membrane. A thin layer of stained microorganisms is deposited on the membrane by vacuum filtration. The membrane is examined by computerized fluorescent microscopy imaging which correlates results to the colony-forming units per milliliter (CFU/mL) of standard cultures. The instrument has a throughput of 70 specimens per hour. The current status of this instrument is uncertain since it has been withdrawn from the market.

Sysmex Inc. has available two fully automated urine cell analyzers, the **Sysmex UF-50** (50 samples per hour) and **UF-100** (100 samples per hour). Each instrument uses a combination of fluorescent technology and scattered light intensity and impedance technologies to detect and quantify 10 formed elements in urine (53). Problematic specimens are flagged for manual microscopic analysis. Depending upon the software version and the instrument, cut-off values for significant bacteriuria include an assessment of the number of leukocytes per milliliter of sample and the bacterial forward-scatter light intensity. In an evaluation of the UF-50 compared to semiquantitative urine culture, Okada et al. (53) found an accuracy of 78.5% and sensitivity and specificity of 83.1% and 76.4%, respectively. In a study of the UF-100, Zaman et al. (54) found the system to be unsuitable in predicting outcome of urine cultures using 10^4 CFU/mL as the diagnostic criterion for UTIs. Differences between the two studies may have included such factors as software version, definition of UTI, and failure to manually screen "flagged" samples that may have contained interfering substances (55).

Finally, the **939UDx urine pathology system** (IRIS Diagnostics, Chatsworth, CA, and Boehringer Mannheim Corp., Indianapolis, IN) incorporates imaging flow cytometry, CHEMSTRIP® reagents, and microcomputer technology into a completely automated walkaway urine analyzer. Workflow begins with loading bar-coded samples into the instrument carousel for the chemical analysis. The instrument reads the bar code, mixes the sample, and aspirates 3 mL of sample. A 10-parameter CHEMSTRIP is wetted robotically and transmits the results to the microcomputer (56). If a microscopic analysis is required, the microscopic analyzer mixes the sample, aspirates it, then stains it to visualize elements, and passes it to the flow microscope where captured photographic images are made and stored. Users can define parameters for autorelease of results and those results which require operator review (57). The system's throughput ranges from 70 to 250 urine samples per hour, depending upon whether full microscopic analysis is requested. One study found a sensitivity of 94.9% for detecting UTI when both the bacterial and white cell counts were combined (57). The specificity was 54.4%; however, the negative predictive value was 98.5% and about 50% of specimens could be reported as negative on the same day. This system appears comparable to other automated methods for detection of UTI.

REFERENCES

1. O'Hara CM, Weinstein MP, Miller JM. Manual and automated systems for detection and identification of microorganisms. In: Murray PM, Baron EJ, Jorgensen JH, Pfaller MA, Yolken RH, eds. Manual of clinical microbiology, 8th ed. Washington, DC: American Society for Microbiology, 2003:191–2.
2. O'Hara CM. Manual and automated instrumentation for identification of *Enterobacteriaceae* and other aerobic gram-negative bacilli. Clin Microbiol Rev 2005;18:147–62.
3. Bourbeau PP, Heiter BJ. Comparison of the Vitek GNI and GNI+ cards for identification of gram-negative bacteria. J Clin Microbiol 1998;36:2775–7.
4. O'Hara CM, Westbrook GL, Miller JM. Evaluation of the Vitek GNI+ and Becton Dickinson Microbiology Systems Crystal E/NF identification systems for identification of members of the family *Enterobacteriaceae* and other gram-negative, glucose-fermenting and non-glucose-fermenting bacilli. J Clin Microbiol 1997;35:3269–73.
5. Sung LL, Yang DI, Hung CC, Ho HT. Evaluation of the autoSCAN-W/A and the Vitek GNI+ AutoMicrobic system for identification of non-glucose-fermenting gram-negative bacilli. J Clin Microbiol 2000;38:1127–30.
6. O'Hara CM, Miller JM. Evaluation of the Vitek 2 ID-GNB assay for identification of members of the family *Enterobacteriaceae* and other nonenteric gram-negative bacilli and comparison with the Vitek GNI+ card. J Clin Microbiol 2003;41:2096–101.
7. Gavin PJ, Warren JR, Obias AA, Collins SM, Peterson LR. Evaluation of the Vitek 2 system for rapid identification of clinical isolates of gram-negative bacilli and members of the family *Streptococcaceae.* Eur J Clin Microbiol Infect Dis 2002;21:869–74.
8. Spanu T, Sanguinetti M, Ciccaglione D, D'Inzeo, Romano L, Leone F, et al. Use of the VITEK 2 system for rapid identification of clinical isolates of Staphylococci from bloodstream infections. J Clin Microbiol 2003;41:4259–63.
9. Ligozzi M, Bernini C, Bonora MG, De Fatima M, Zuliani J, Fontana R. Evaluation of the VITEK 2 system for identification and antimicrobial susceptibility testing of medically relevant gram-positive cocci. J Clin Microbiol 2002;40:1681–6.
10. Graf B, Adam T, Zill E, Gobel UB. Evaluation of the VITEK 2 system for rapid identification of yeast and yeast-like organisms. J Clin Microbiol 2000;38:1782–5.
11. O'Hara CM, Miller JM. Evaluation of the MicroScan rapid neg ID3 panel for identification of *Enterobacteriaceae* and some common gram-negative nonfermenters. J Clin Microbiol 2000;38:3577–80.
12. O'Hara CM, Miller JM. Ability of the MicroScan rapid gram-negative ID type 3 panel to identify nonenteric glucose-fermenting and nonfermenting gram-negative bacilli. J Clin Microbiol 2002;40:3750–2.
13. Saa AI, Vivas J, Tinajas A, Barbeyto L, Rodriguez LA. Evaluation of the MicroScan system for identification of staphylococci. J Basic Microbiol 1999;39:373–6.
14. d'Azevedo PA, Dias CAG, Goncalves ALS, Rowe F, Teixeira LM. Evaluation of an automated system for the identification and antimicrobial susceptibility testing of enterococci. Diagn Microbiol Infect Dis 2001;40:157–61.
15. Stefaniuk E, Baraniak A, Gniadkowski M, Hryniewicz W. Evaluation of the BD Phoenix automated identification and susceptibility testing system in clinical microbiology practice. Eur J Clin Microbiol Infect Dis 2003;22:479–85.

16. Fahr AM, Eigner U, Armburst M, Caganic A, Dettori G, Chezzi C, et al. Two-center collaborative evaluation of the performance of the BD Phoenix automated microbiology system for identification and antimicrobial susceptibility testing of *Enterococcus* spp. and *Staphylococcus* spp. J Clin Microbiol 2003;41:1135–42.
17. Holmes B, Costas M, Ganner M, On SLW, Stevens M. Evaluation of Biolog system for identification of some gram-negative bacteria of clinical importance. J Clin Microbiol 1994;32: 1970–5.
18. Miller JM, Biddle JW, Quenzer VK, McLaughlin JC. Evaluation of the Biolog for identification of members of the family *Micrococcaceae*. J Clin Microbiol 1993;31:3170–3.
19. Vandamme PAR. Taxonomy and classification of bacteria. In: Murray PM, Baron EJ, Jorgensen JH, Pfaller MA, Yolken RH, eds. Manual of clinical microbiology, 8th ed. Washington, DC: American Society for Microbiology, 2003,191–2.
20. Welch DF. Applications of cellular fatty acid analysis. Clin Microbiol Rev 1991;4:422–38.
21. Tang YW, Ellis NM, Hopkins MK, Smith DH, Dodge DE, Persing DH. Comparison of phenotypic and genotypic techniques for identification of unusual aerobic pathogenic gram negative bacilli. J Clin Microbiol 1998;36:3674–9.
22. National committee for clinical laboratory standards: abbreviated identification of bacteria and yeast; approved guideline. NCCLS Document M35A, Wayne, PA: NCCLS, 2002.
23. Butler WR, Guthertz LS. Mycolic acid analysis by high-performance liquid chromatography for identification of *Mycobacterium* species. Clin Microbiol Rev 2001;14:704–26.
24. Kellogg JA, Bankert DA, Withers GS, Sweimler W, Kiehn TE, Pfyffer GE. Application of the Sherlock mycobacteria identification system using high-performance liquid chromatography in a clinical laboratory. J Clin Microbiol 2001;39:964–70.
25. Berke I, Tierno PM Jr. Comparison of efficacy and cost-effectiveness of BIOMIC VIDEO and Vitek antimicrobial susceptibility test systems for use in the clinical microbiology laboratory. J Clin Microbiol 1996;34:1980–4.
26. Korgenski EK, Daly JA. Evaluation of the BIOMIC video reader system for determining interpretive categories of isolates on the basis of disk diffusion susceptibility results. J Clin Microbiol 1998;36:302–4.
27. Burns JL, Saiman L, Whittier S, Krzewinski J, Liu Z, Larone D, et al. Comparison of two commercial systems (Vitek and MicroScan-WalkAway) for antimicrobial susceptibility testing of *Pseudomonas aeruginosa* isolates from cystic fibrosis patients. Diagn Microbiol Infect Dis 2001;39:257–60.
28. Kohner PC, Patel R, Uhl JR, Garin KM, Hopkins MK, Wegner LT, et al. Comparison of agar dilution, broth microdilution, E-test, disk diffusion, and automated Vitek methods for testing susceptibilities of *Enterococcus* spp. to vancomycin. J Clin Microbiol 1997;35:3258–63.
29. Swenson JM, Williams PP, Killgore G, O'Hara CM, Tenover FC. Performance of eight methods, including two new rapid methods, for detection of oxacillin resistance in a challenge set of *Staphylococcus aureus* organisms. J Clin Microbiol 2001;39:3785–8.
30. Jorgensen JH, McElmeel ML, Crawford SA. Evaluation of the Dade MicroScan MICroSTREP antimicrobial susceptibility testing panel with selected *Streptococcus pneumoniae* challenge strains and recent clinical isolates. J Clin Microbiol 1998;36:788–91.
31. Guthrie LL, Banks S, Setiawan W, Waites KB. Comparison of MicroScan, MICroSTREP, PASCO, and Sensititre MIC panels for determining antimicrobial susceptibilities of *Streptococcus pneumoniae*. Diagn Microbiol Infect Dis 1999;33:267–73.
32. Chapin KC, Musgnug MC. Validation of the automated reading and incubation system with Sensititre plates for antimicrobial susceptibility testing. J Clin Microbiol 2003;41:1951–6.
33. Morace G, Amato G, Bistoni F, Fadda G, Marone P, Montagna MT, et al. Multicenter comparative evaluation of six commercial systems and the national committee for clinical laboratory standards M27—a broth microdilution method for fluconazole susceptibility testing of *Candida* sp. J Clin Microbiol 2002;40:2953–8.
34. Dunne WM Jr, Nolte FS, Wilson ML. Cumitech 1B, Blood Cultures III. JA Hindler, coordinating ed. Washington, DC: American Society for Microbiology, 1997.

35. Reimer LG, Wilson ML, Weinstein MP. Update on detection of bacteremia and fungemia. Clin Microbiol Rev 1997;10:444–65.
36. Weinstein MP, Reller LB. Commercial blood culture systems and methods. In: Truant A, ed. Manual of commercial methods in clinical microbiology. Washington, DC: American Society for Microbiology, 2001:12–21.
37. Archibald LK, Dobbie H, Kazembe P, Nwanyanwu O, McKnight C, Byrne T, et al. Utility of paired BACTEC MYCO/F LYTIC blood culture vials for detection of bacteremia, mycobacteremia, and fungemia. J Clin Microbiol 2001;39:1960–2.
38. McDonald LC, Weinstein MP, Fune J, Mirrett S, Reimer LG, Reller LB. Controlled comparison of BacT/ALERT FAN aerobic medium and BACTEC fungal blood culture medium for detection of fungemia. J Clin Microbiol 2001;39:622–4.
39. Mirrett S, Reller LB, Petti CA, Woods CW, Vazirani RS, Weinstein MP. Controlled clinical comparison of BacT/ALERT standard aerobic medium with BACTEC standard aerobic medium for culturing blood. J Clin Microbiol 2003;41:2391–4.
40. Wilson ML, Mirrett S, Meredith FT, Weinstein MP, Scotto V, Reller LB. Controlled clinical comparison of BACTEC Plus Anaerobic/F to standard anaerobic/F as the anaerobic companion bottle to Plus Aerobic/F medium for culturing blood from adults. J Clin Microbiol 2001;39: 983–9.
41. Roberts GD, Goodman NL, Heifets L, Larsh HW, Lindner TH, McClatchy K, et al. Evaluation of the BACTEC radiometric method for recovery of mycobacteria and drug susceptibility testing of *Mycobacterium tuberculosis* from acid-fast smear-positive specimens. J Clin Microbiol 1983;18:689–96.
42. Conville PS, Witebsky FG. Inter-bottle transfer of mycobacteria by the BACTEC 460. Diagn Microbiol Infect Dis 1989;12:401–05.
43. Tortoli E, Cichero P, Chirillo MG, Gismondo MR, Bono L, Gesu G, et al. Multicenter comparison of ESP culture system II with BACTEC 460TB and with Lowenstein-Jensen medium for recovery of mycobacteria from different clinical specimens, including blood. J Clin Microbiol 1998;36:1378–81.
44. Williams-Bouyer N, Yorke R, Lee HI, Woods GL. Comparison of the BACTEC MGIT 960 and ESP culture system II for growth and detection of mycobacteria. J Clin Microbiol 2000;38:4167–70.
45. Hanna BA, Ebrahimzadeh A, Elliott LB, Morgan MA, Novak SM, Rusch-Gerdes S, et al. Multicenter evaluation of the BACTEC MGIT 960 system for recovery of mycobacteria. J Clin Microbiol 1999;37:748–52.
46. Yan JJ, Huang AH, Tsai SH, Ko WC, Jin YT, Wu JJ. Comparison of the MB/BacT and BACTEC MGIT 960 system for recovery of mycobacteria from clinical specimens. Diagn Microbiol Infect Dis 2000;37:25–30.
47. Piersimoni C, Scarparo C, Callegaro A, Tosi CP, Nista D, Bornigia S, et al. Comparison of MB/BacT ALERT 3D system with radiometric BACTEC system and Lowenstein-Jensen medium for recovery and identification of mycobacteria from clinical specimens: a multicenter study. J Clin Microbiol 2001;39:651–7.
48. Bergmann JS, Woods GL. Evaluation of the ESP culture system II for testing susceptibilities of *Mycobacterium tuberculosis* isolates to four primary antituberculous drugs. J Clin Microbiol 1998;36:2940–3.
49. Ruiz P, Zerolo FJ, Casal MJ. Comparison of susceptibility testing of *Mycobacterium tuberculosis* using the ESP culture system II with that using the BACTEC method. J Clin Microbiol 2000;38:4663–4.
50. Bemer P, Palicova F, Rusch-Gerdes S, Drugeon HB, Pfyffer GE. Multicenter evaluation of fully automated BACTEC Mycobacteria Growth Indicator Tube 960 System for susceptibility testing of *Mycobacterium tuberculosis*. J Clin Microbiol 2002;40:150–4.
51. Tortoli E, Benedetti M, Fontanelli A, Simonetti MT. Evaluation of automated BACTEC MGIT 960 system for testing susceptibility of *Mycobacterium tuberculosis* to four major antituberculosis drugs: comparison with the radiometric BACTEC 460TB method and the agar plate method of proportion. J Clin Microbiol 2002;40:607–10.

52. Semeniuk H, Noonan J, Gill H, Church D. Evaluation of the Coral UTI Screen^{TM} system for rapid automated screening of significant bacteriuria in a regional centralized laboratory. Diagn Microbiol Infect Dis 2002;44:7–10.
53. Okada H, Sakai Y, Miyazaki S, Arakawa S, Hamaguchi Y, Kamidono S. Detection of significant bacteriuria by automated urinalysis using flow cytometry. J Clin Microbiol 2000;38:2870–2.
54. Zaman Z, Roggeman S, Verhaegen J. Unsatisfactory performance of flow cytometer UF-100 and urine strips in predicting outcome of urine cultures. J Clin Microbiol 2001;39:4169–71.
55. Delanghe JR, Langlois MR, Wuyts B, DeBuyzere ML. Performance of urinary flow cytometry in predicting outcome of urine cultures. J Clin Microbiol 2002;40:2314–5.
56. Koontz AE. Automation of laboratory urinalysis. *www.irisdiagnostics.com/education/reference/labua.shtml.*
57. Hughes C, Roebuck MJ. Evaluation of the IRIS 939 UDx flow microscope as a screening system for urinary tract infection. J Clin Pathol 2003;56:844–9.

Chapter 13

Immunohematology Analyzers

Elizabeth Cascone and Deborah Firestone

The implementation of managed care in the 1980s and the subsequent emphasis on cost containment has placed the operating expenses of the hospital-based laboratory under intense scrutiny. The revenue recouped no longer balances the cost of staffing and supplying and operating the transfusion medicine service and the other departments in the clinical laboratory.

Blood banks in particular are under increased regulatory scrutiny with the implementation of and requirement to comply with the Food and Drug Administration's current good manufacturing practices (cGMP) regulations. These factors have made the process of acquiring blood and blood products, and testing and delivering these products to patients in need, considerably more demanding and expensive. Perhaps the most troubling sign of times to come is the fact that the U.S. Bureau of Labor Statistics projects the need for 5300 new medical technologists (MT) and medical laboratory technicians (MLT) annually through 2008; however, there will not be a sufficient number of qualified personnel to fill these positions. The three major contributing factors to the problem are:

- More than 50% of the current laboratory workforce is over the age of 47
- A decline in the number of people choosing the laboratory professions as a career
- A decrease in the number of NAACLS (National Accrediting Agency for Clinical Laboratory Sciences) training programs for MTs and MLTs

The decrease in the number of available and qualified graduates from MT and MLT programs to fill these positions, coupled with the projection that "baby boomers" will begin retiring from their laboratory positions within the next 5–10 years is likely to increase significantly the laboratory staffing challenge that currently exists.

Blood banks are presently under pressure to find alternate strategies for performing safe, cost-effective testing in an environment operating under the mandates of cGMP. Some laboratories have responded to this challenge by utilizing personnel with minimal technical experience and expertise, creating an environment in which there is the potential for serious errors; most have undertaken "cross-training" programs in which all laboratory technical staff are trained and expected to perform in any laboratory section that requires additional personnel on any given day. While this may resolve the critical issue of providing "bodies" to perform necessary tasks, it does not provide the technical personnel an opportunity to become intensively trained and adept in any one clinical laboratory discipline.

The market within which healthcare is practiced, and laboratory services are delivered, is certainly no longer simple. It is into this environment that automation and semi-automation using gel and solid-phase technology are being introduced, validated, and adopted. These technologies build on and modify the simple, reliable, and versatile tube agglutination testing that has been the standard method for ABO grouping, Rho(D) typing, antibody detection, antibody identification, and compatibility testing since the early 1900s.

In the hospital/transfusion service, instruments are generally chosen for their:

- Simplicity of use
- Adaptability to cGMP
- Suitability for the laboratory workload and available workspace
- Reliability, precision, and accuracy
- Initial cost
- Purchase or lease pricing
- Cost of operation

Instruments selected for use in a blood center are generally chosen for all of these reasons as well as their ability to test large numbers of samples (high volume) and provide results rapidly.

The intent of this chapter is not to advocate one technology over the other but rather to present information that the reader can use as a guide when making decisions about the feasibility of adopting a particular technology. Some additional information can be found under *Suggested Reading*.

SOLID-PHASE TECHNOLOGY

Capture Technology

Capture Technology (Figure 1) by Immucor Inc. is an example of semiautomated solid-phase technology. Capture-R® Ready-Screen and Capture-R® Ready-ID are modified solid-phase antibody detection systems using predispensed reagent red cells. The membranes of red cells are bound to, then dried onto, the surfaces of polystyrene microtitration strip wells. Membrane antigens are used to capture red cell-specific IgG antibodies from serum or plasma. These systems employ a low ionic potentiator, positive and negative control sera, and an indicator reagent consisting of anti-IgG-coated intact red cells. See Figure 2.

In the first step of Capture-R® Ready-Screen or Ready-ID procedures, two drops of a low ionic potentiator and one drop of test serum or plasma are added to each test well. Serum or plasma is incubated in the wells for at least 15 minutes at 37 °C. During this incubation period, red cell antibodies, if present, bind to the surfaces of antigen-positive reagent red cell membranes.

Step two prepares the test wells for the addition of the indicator by rinsing the wells with phosphate-buffered saline. The indicator system, a type of antiglobulin reagent, consists of red cells coated with anti-IgG. The indicator red cells attach through their anti-IgG component to IgG antibodies that have bound to immobilized reagent red cell membranes. The anti-IgG component of the indicator red cells also binds readily to unbound (or free) IgG molecules in the test serum. Thus, the wash step must be taken to ensure that unbound IgG antibodies capable of neutralizing the antiglobulin component of the indicator red cells are removed from the wells.

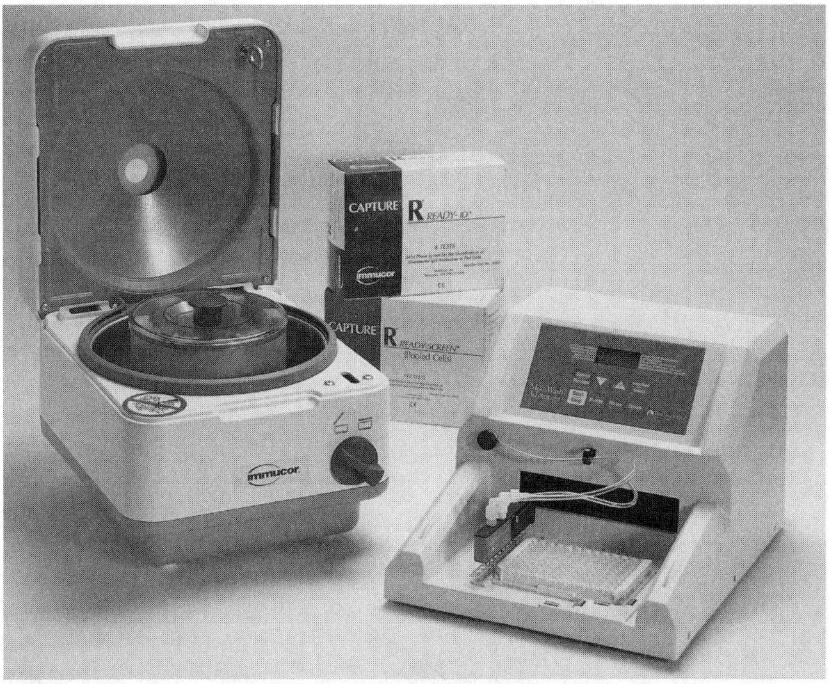

FIGURE 1. The Capture system. (*Courtesy of Immucor*)

Then one drop of indicator red cells is added to each of the washed wells. Centrifugation applied to the system places the indicator red cells in contact with the antibodies bound to the immobilized membranes. In the case of a negative test, there will be no antibodies bound to the reagent membranes to impede the settling of the indicator red cells during centrifugation. As a consequence, they migrate to the bottom of the wells where they form tight cell buttons in the middle. In the case of positive tests, the migration of the anti-IgG-coated indicator red cells is impeded by anti-red cell antibodies bound to the immobilized reagent red cell membranes. As a consequence of bridges formed between the red-cell-directed antibodies and anti-IgG, the indicator cells bind to part, or all, of the monolayer surface.

ABS 2000

The ABS2000 (Figure 3) by Immucor Inc. is a fully automated blood bank instrument that utilizes hemagglutination and patented solid-phase technologies.

Blood may be tested to determine:

- The red blood cell (RBC) ABO and Rh group: red cells from the intended RBC recipient are tested with ABO Blood Grouping reagents to determine the ABO group.
- Cell grouping results are confirmed with tests performed with the patient plasma and ABO Serum Grouping Reagent Red Cells. Red cells are typed with two reagents containing different IgM monoclonal Anti-D to determine their D antigen status.
- The presence of unexpected serum or plasma IgG alloantibodies to RBC antigens that could cause diminished survival or accelerated destruction of transfused donor red cells. Patient plasma is tested with antibody screening reagents to detect unexpected IgG RBC antibodies.

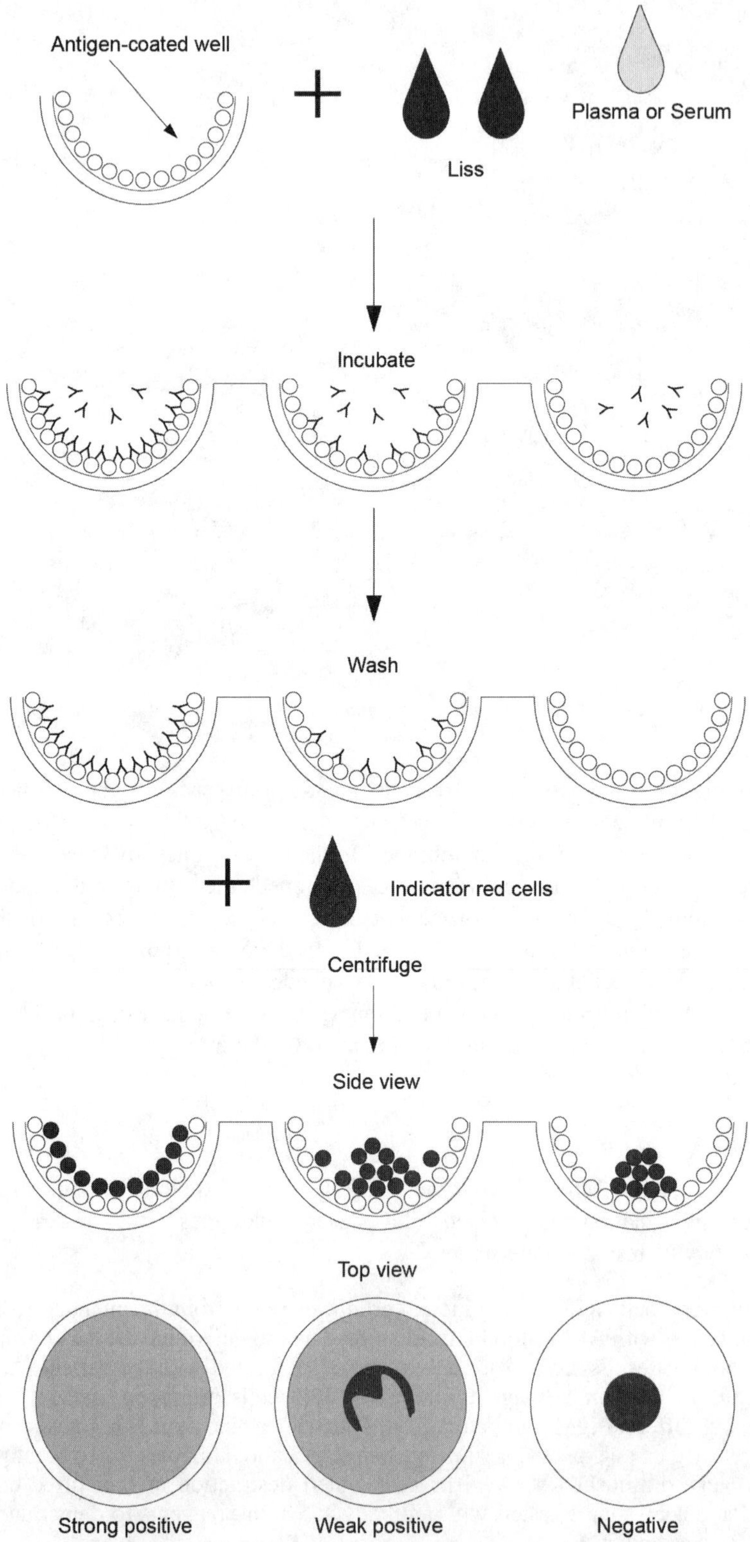

FIGURE 2. Capture test procedure. (*Courtesy of Immucor*)

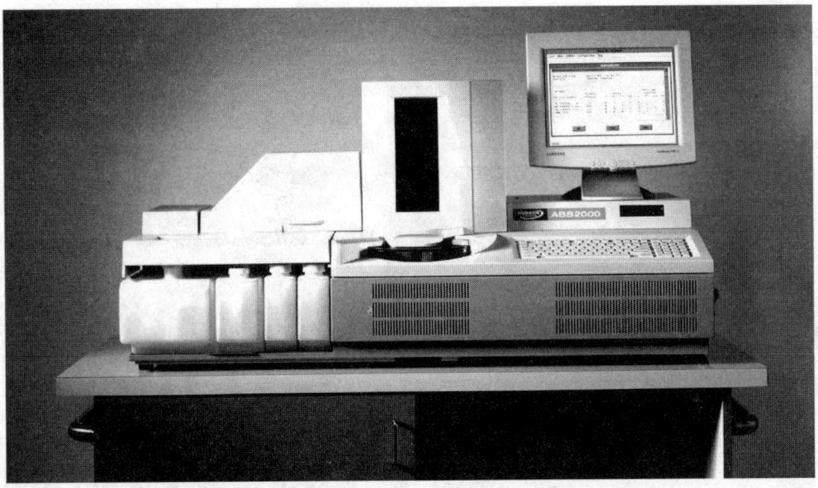

FIGURE 3. The ABS2000. (*Courtesy of Immucor*)

The ABS2000 has been designed to maximize testing efficiency. Operation of the instrument is simplified because all test programs are operated in the same manner. Operator involvement with test programs entails:

1. Selecting the test protocol from the menu bar
2. Checking and filling or emptying waste bottles and reservoirs
3. Unloading used test strips and samples that have completed batch processing
4. Loading new reagents, test strips, and samples
5. Selecting the assay and initiating the run sequence

Before the instrument starts testing, it will automatically:

1. Perform self-diagnostics.
2. Prime and wash the probe with deionized water.
3. Prime the washer manifold.
4. Empty the contents of the intermediate waste collection vessel into the primary waste container.
5. Mix reagent red cells.
6. Check the reader and filter to ensure proper performance capabilities.

The ABS2000 scans the sectors and carriers of the carousel and scans the track to identify reagents, strips, and samples. It prompts the operator to enter manually, via the keyboard, any sector, reagent, strip, or specimen identifications that were not readable by the bar-code scanner or absorbance reader. The instrument checks for the presence of all required reagents strips and cleaning supplies (on the carousel) and for the volume in each reagent vial. It displays a list of those that are missing or deficient and also determines if strips are dirty and unsuitable for testing.

Once the instrument has verified that the appropriate samples and supplies are present, it schedules all steps of the desired test and executes each at the appropriate time. The expected completion time of the test batch then is displayed on the screen. If an insufficient volume of sample is encountered during a test, the instrument records the sample as a failure and continues processing the remaining samples in the batch.

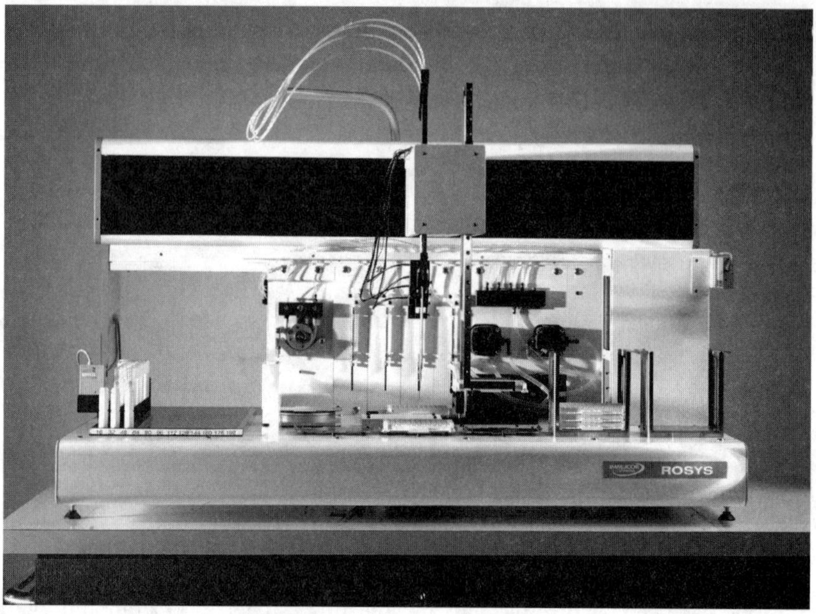

FIGURE 4. The ROSYS Plato. (*Courtesy of Immucor*)

Once a test batch is completed the instrument cleans various components. It also analyzes the data obtained from the reader and interprets the results for each test. The results are stored by test batch on the hard disk. Batch results can be viewed on the ABS2000 screen by the operator using the batch results utility or by printing the results via the optional printer. Test results can be transferred to a floppy disk or downloaded to the laboratory's data management system.

ROSYS Plato

The ROSYS Plato by Immucor Inc. is a walkaway system for automating microplate assays. See Figure 4.

This system offers the following instrument features:

- **Positive sample identification:** Bar codes on sample tubes are automatically read from any position in the microplate.
- **Sample capacity:** Automatically processes up to 96 samples in tubes of different sizes.
- **Sample integrity:** Liquid level sensor allows processing samples of variable volumes.
- **Precision pipetting:** High-precision fluidic system provides volumetric accuracy of reagent and sample with negligible carryover.
- **Efficiency of process:** Microplates are presented to the pipette probes on the most efficient orientation for fluid transfer (Figure 5).
- **User friendliness:** Windows®-based software allows the flexibility to handle large and small test batches.
- **Objectivity of results:** The hemagglutination and solid-phase assay reader that utilizes an optical system provides an electronic interpretation of the assay results which are electronically downloaded.
- **Broad menu:** Open system profile provides the ability to process microplate assays that utilize either hemagglutination or solid-phase testing.

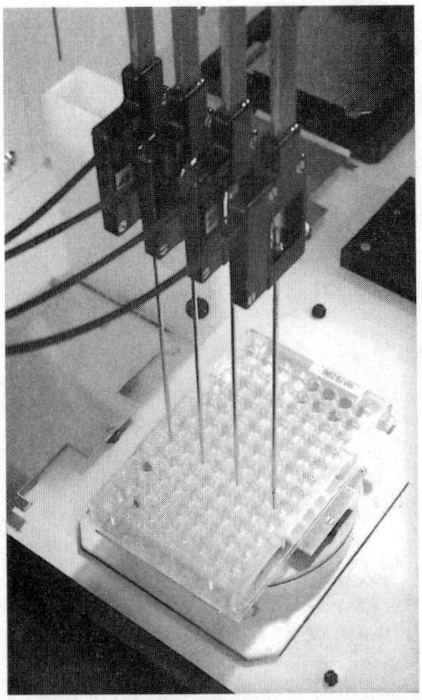

FIGURE 5. ROSYS pipetting. (*Courtesy of Immucor*)

- **Complete system:** With a reagent and sample loading device, an incubator, and a washer, this system allows walkaway processing.
- **Consolidated and compact workstation**
- **Improves cGMP:** Standardized automated assay steps, reduced technological attended time, reader accommodates manufacturer-prepared hemagglutination strips and precoated solid-phase strip well plates.
- **Increases productivity**

DIAS PLUS System

The DIAS PLUS System by Immucor Inc. is designed for 24-hour-a-day operation and high throughput with minimal scheduled maintenance. It offers the following features:

- Positive sample identification for microplate, primary sample tubes, and reagents
- Proven reliability
- 12-Tip configuration for rapid sample and reagent delivery
- Positive displacement pipetting for sample integrity
- Processes more than 300 tests per hour
- Continuous access processing
- Bar-coded sample processing throughout the entire process
- Automated transport of sample plates to and from each module
- Scheduling software to ensure that each step is performed at the correct time, to display workload information, and to display timelines in a graphic format for easy interpretation
- Event log created and saved to a computer file during processing to provide process tracking

- Biohazardous materials captured in a sealed container "closed system" during plate washing
- Temperature of each plate constantly monitored in a holding area to increase process capacity
- Digital settings for accurate centrifugation speeds
- Four-plate capacity
- Calibrated for both hemagglutination (ABO and Rh typing) and for solid-phase (antiglobulin) testing
- Microwells scanned by optical system
- Reactions interpreted electronically
- Integrated bar-code reader for sample identification

GEL TECHNOLOGY

ID-MTS Gel Technology (Ortho-Clinical Diagnostics) (Figure 6)

Lapierre and colleagues first described the gel test for detecting interactions between red blood cell antigens and antibodies in 1990. Gel technology operates on the principle that an inert matrix can be used to separate agglutinated red blood cells from those that are not

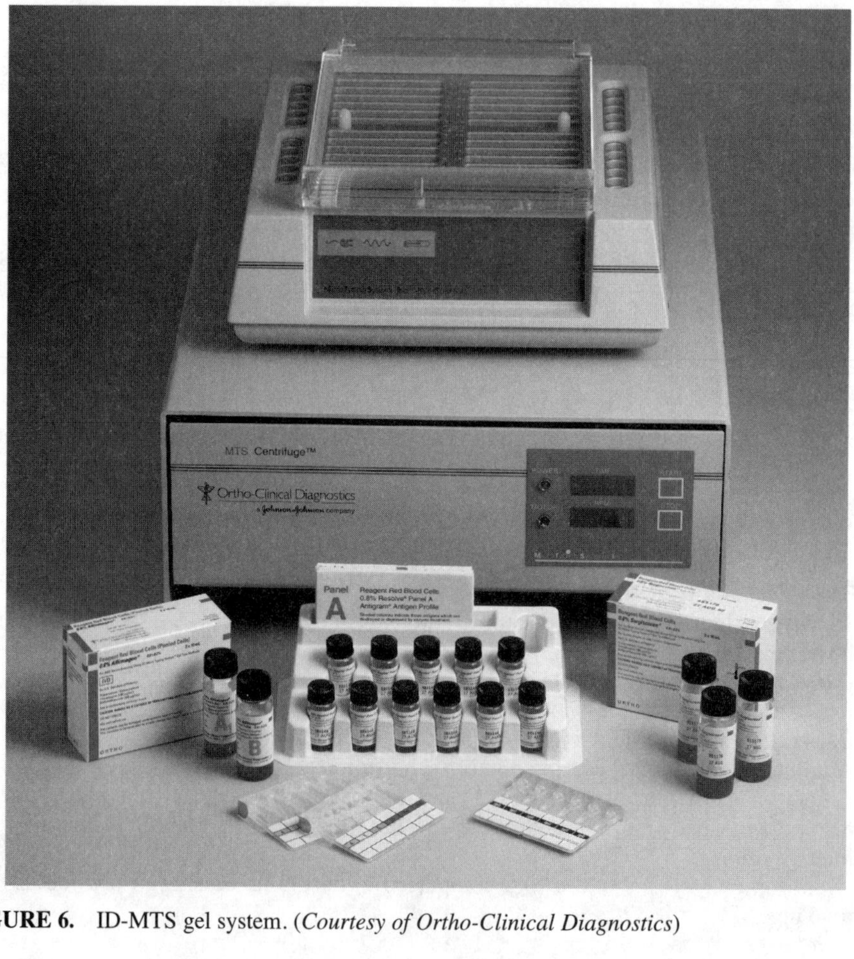

FIGURE 6. ID-MTS gel system. (*Courtesy of Ortho-Clinical Diagnostics*)

agglutinated. ABO forward and reverse typing, Rh typing, RBC phenotyping, antibody detection and identification, direct antiglobulin testing, and compatibility testing can all be performed using this technology.

Six microtubes, also known as microcolumns, filled with gel are packaged into a cassette or card for easy handling. Each microtube consists of an upper reaction or incubation chamber that is situated on top of the gel-filled microtube.

Test sample (serum/plasma and/or cells) is added to the reaction chamber at the top of the microtube. An air bubble serves as a barrier to prevent the reactants from entering the gel during the reaction phase. The cards are incubated, if necessary, followed by centrifugation.

Agglutinated RBCs are trapped in the gel and the strength of agglutination is based on the position of the red blood cells in the gel column (*see* Figure 7).

Tests differ by the sample added to the reaction chamber, the specificity of the antisera in the gel, and the incubation time and temperature and centrifugation of the reactants. Table 1 illustrates the distinguishing characteristics of each test.

There is some inherent subjectivity in the interpretation of results based on a number of factors including the position of agglutinated cells within the gel, centrifugation time and speed, and the potential for "false" agglutination. The vertical (upper and lower) position, not horizontal (right to left) position, of cells within the gel is important to consider when interpreting 2+ reactions. Fibrin or other forms of debris associated with certain samples (cord blood, frozen samples, serum) may trap unagglutinated red blood cells on top of the gel. Insufficient centrifugation may result in a more positive result by preventing unagglutinated red blood cells from traveling to the bottom of the tube. Conversely, excessive centrifugation may produce a more weakly positive result due to the fact that excess pressure is being placed on weak agglutinates, causing them to pull apart and migrate to the bottom of the microtube.

Automation using gel technology can be implemented at the facility's own pace. One option is the Manual ID-MTS workstation, which consists of the following components: pipettor, incubator, and centrifuge. The technology can be semiautomated by adding the MTS-Reader M to the Manual ID-MTS workstation to read the cards electronically, and the MTS-Reader SA to centrifuge and read cards. Lastly, the combination of the TECAN Megaflex-ID™, which is an automated liquid-handling device that can dispense reagents and samples to the ID-MTS gel cards, and MTS-Reader M allow the technology to be automated from initial scan to test result (*see* Figure 8).

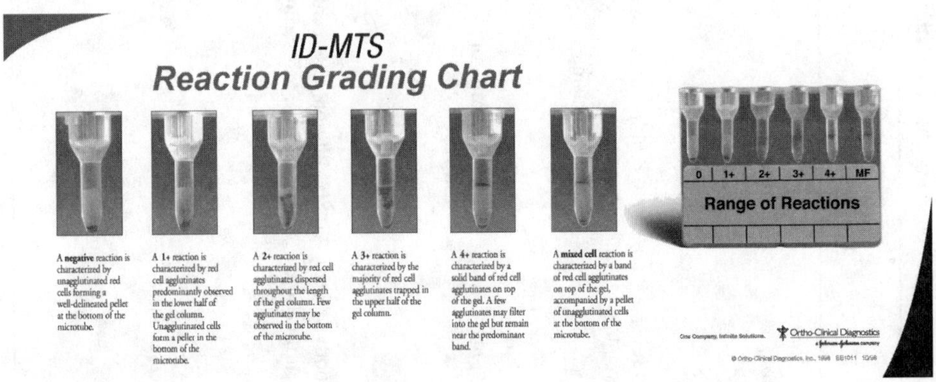

FIGURE 7. ID-MTS range of reactions. (*Courtesy of Ortho-Clinical Diagnostics*)

TABLE 1. Distinguishing characteristics of gel technology tests

Test	Sample added to reaction chamber	Reagent in gel	Antibody–antigen reaction	Incubation	Centrifugation
ABO forward grouping	4% (±1) dilution of test RBCs	Anti-A Anti-B	Antigen on RBC (if present) reacts with corresponding antibody in gel.	No incubation required	• Agglutinated RBCs become trapped in gel. • Unagglutinated RBCs form a pellet on the bottom of the microtube.
ABO reverse grouping	0.8% dilution of A_1 and B cells; test serum/plasma	No reagent added	Antibody in test sample (if present) reacts with corresponding antigen on reagent RBC.	No incubation required	• Agglutinated RBCs become trapped in gel. • Unagglutinated RBCs form a pellet on the bottom of the microtube.
Rh typing	4% (±1) dilution of test RBCs	Anti-D No reagent in control card	Antigen on RBC (if present) reacts with anti-D in microtube. No reaction takes place in the reaction chamber of the control microtube.	No incubation required	• Agglutinated RBCs become trapped in gel. • Unagglutinated RBCs form a pellet on the bottom of the microtube.
Antibody screen/ identification	0.8% dilution of screening/ panel cells; test serum/ plasma	Anti-IgG	Antibody in test sample (if present) reacts with corresponding antigen on screening/panel cells.	Microtube is incubated at 37 °C	• Reagent RBCs that become sensitized with antibody from the test sample during the incubation process are agglutinated by the anti-IgG antiglobulin reagent in the gel. Agglutinated RBCs become trapped in gel. • Unagglutinated RBCs form a pellet on the bottom of the microtube.

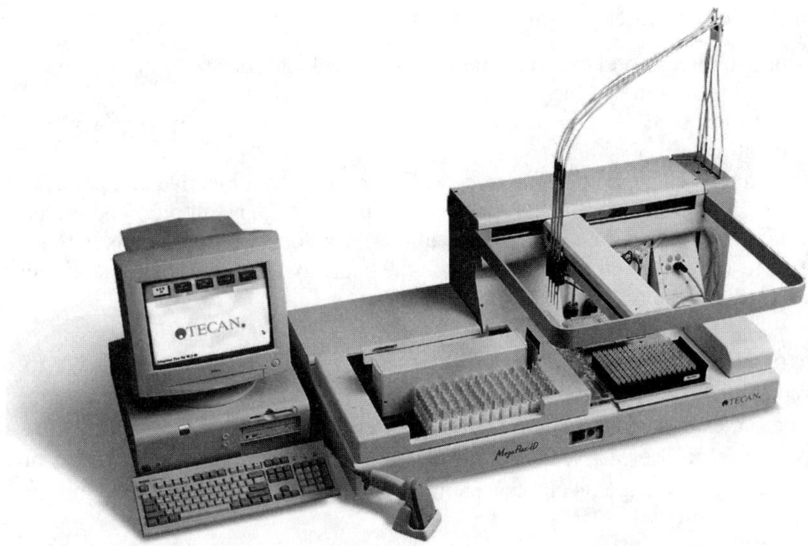

FIGURE 8. Tecan MegaFlex-ID. (*Courtesy of Ortho-Clinical Diagnostics*)

TECAN Mega Flex-ID and MTS Reader M (Ortho-Clinical Diagnostics)

The operating features of this technology include the following:

- Wide-angle scanner to scan patient identification
- Positive identification bar-code capabilities to track patient sample from initial scan to test results
- Automated sample processing
- Efficient, high-throughput with the capacity to process 256 sample tubes and 64 gel cards per run at a speed of 150 sample tubes in 15 minutes
- Electronic reporting to host computer systems
- Continuous and batch modes
- Stat interrupt capability
- Automatic gel card reading
- High-resolution image analysis
- Links with a laboratory information system to ensure safe data transfer
- Image and result storage capability for future review

When a laboratory chooses to implement a new technology, it is expected that the benefits will outweigh the disadvantages. The benefits reported in the literature for gel technology are:

Fewer manipulative procedures: Requires transfer of a gel card (which holds six microtubes) from a rack, to an incubator, to a centrifuge, no addition of antiglobulin reagent (it is embedded in the gel), and no required validation of negative reactions at the antiglobulin phase.

Stable end points: The card can be read as many times as necessary and reactions in gel cards are said to be stable for two to three days after the test is performed, providing an opportunity for the card to be read by as many people as necessary (on the same or different shift) in order to provide confirmatory review of reactions.

Less subjectivity in interpreting results

- Agglutinated red blood cells are trapped in the gel and the strength of agglutination is based on the location of the red blood cells within the gel.
- Reactions are read as soon as cards are removed from the centrifuge with no further manipulation.
- Although red cell separation provides a clearer and more objective end point, subjectivity is not completely eliminated based on the fact that the result recorded is based on an individual technologist's visual examination of the location of red cells within the gel.
- The inclusion of an automatic reader has the capacity to virtually eliminate subjectivity when reading results.

Standardization of sample/reagents added: The use of a calibrated pipette to deliver measured amounts of reagent red blood cells and test sample to the reaction chamber of the microtube serves to standardize the antibody/antigen ratio and reproducibility of results.
Increased safety: Use of plastic microtubes eliminates exposure to glass test tubes and smaller quantities of reagents and test sample reduces exposure to biohazardous materials.

The following are factors to consider when introducing automation into a hospital transfusion service and evaluating instrumentation in the workplace:

Costs and savings of operation

- Comparison of costs of reagents and supplies to costs of ALL supplies and reagents for current methodology
- Potential savings in labor (hands-on testing time reduced, allowing personnel to perform other tasks)
- Potential maintenance, repair, and replacement savings from retirement of some equipment (centrifuges, cell-washers, microscopes, timers, waterbaths)
- Potential savings in costs associated with quality control and validation of retired equipment (reagents, supplies, staff time)
- Potential savings in costs associated with the disposal of biohazardous waste
- Potential savings from reduced number of "false positive" tests or detection of clinically unimportant antibodies that must be investigated

Vendor reliability

- Evaluate current and past experiences with vendors as reagent suppliers
- Network with current users to assess their experiences—positive and negative—regarding the effects of validation, implementation, use, and operational costs of the new technology

Test volume and workflow

- Test volume: number of samples tested on a daily basis
    - Assess current and projected workload
    - Assess current and projected staffing requirements
- Workflow
    - Some testing (e.g., next day surgery, prenatal work ups) can be "batched"; other testing is unscheduled or requires immediate processing (stat). Determine if proposed transition is adaptable to the demands of the laboratory customers.
    - Review functions performed by MTs and MLTs and assess the potential to transition to implementation of new technology.

- Develop and validate a workflow process to accommodate requirements of the new technology.

Available space

- Determine requirements of new equipment—single large space (automated plate technology) or multiple smaller spaces (gel technology).
- Determine which instruments can be removed to free space.
- Consider rearranging equipment and benches if possible to accommodate and expedite work with new technology.

Adaptability of staff

- Resistance to change
- Ability to learn new techniques and processes
- Willingness to adapt to new processes
- Ability to include part-time employees in training and updates

Availability of and ability to create and execute follow-up and back-up procedures

- Develop a reliable and cost-effective process to deal with positive and inconclusive tests and testing failures.
- Clearly delineate the process to interpret unclear or equivocal test results and the methods to be used for any additional investigation required.
- Train all personnel in the use, interpretation, and follow-up testing of the new technology selected

> Potential cost reductions can be reduced significantly when staff members are not trained and prepared to deal confidently with the sensitivity of these testing procedures—both manual and automated.

Accuracy of test results/patient safety (validation)

Perform parallel studies, involving a referee if necessary, to assess and resolve discrepancies between new and current methodologies. This may provide useful information to determine if the predicted benefits of cost and staff reduction of the new technology may be reasonably expected in the environment in which it will be used.

SUGGESTED READING

Hannah DM. Transfusion service automation. ADVANCE for Administrators of the Laboratory 2001;10 (http://www.advanceforal.com/editorial/al/10-1-2001/)

http://www.immucor.com/

http://www.orthoclinical.com/

Judd WJ. 'New' blood bank technologies. Clin Lab Sci 1998;11:106–13.

Mybeck JF. Bringing blood bank automation into the 21st century. ADVANCE for Administrators of the Laboratory 2000; 9/10. (http://www.advanceforal.com/editorial/al/10-1-2000).

Smith T. On the brink of crisis. ADVANCE for Administrators of the Laboratory. June 10, 2002 (http://www.advanceforal.com/pastarticles/jun10_02feature3.html)

Walker PS. New technologies in transfusion medicine. Lab Med. 1997;28:259–62.

Chapter 14

Flow Cytometry Instrumentation and Clinical Applications

Candace Golightly and Marc Golightly

In the clinical diagnostic field, flow cytometry has long been regarded as an esoteric, eccentric, and an expensive methodology for arriving at an answer that usually could be obtained by more traditional and less expensive methods. The exceptions to this have always been in the diagnosing and staging of leukemias/lymphomas and other cancers and in the monitoring of HIV patients. In these areas, flow cytometry has proved to be an invaluable unique clinical laboratory diagnostic tool, often arriving at the diagnosis where other methods have failed. Recently, as flow cytometry has advanced by the application of new methodology and monoclonal antibodies, it has replaced and become the method of choice for several long-time established clinical tests [NBT test for chronic granulomatous disease, acidified serum test and sucrose hemolysis test for paroxysmal nocturnal hemoglobinuria (PNH), and the Kleihauer-Betke test for fetal hemoglobin]. In these cases, flow cytometry is so superior in performance in terms of accuracy and sensitivity over the traditional methods that meaningful validation against the traditional methods is often difficult. In addition, bead array technology has now been applied to flow cytometry for the quantitation of specific antibodies and various soluble proteins down to picogram amounts, which will open endless applications of flow cytometry in clinical diagnostics. The other area in which flow cytometry has been invaluable has been clinical and basic research. Here, flow cytometry is capable of purification and analysis that is often just not possible or practical by any other means.

This chapter is devoted to the recent developments in instrumentation and diagnostic testing. The field is rapidly changing with ever-increasing flexibility and features to consider in instrumentation and testing. With regard to instrumentation, emphasis will be put on user-selectable features and options including sensitivity issues between instruments, software/analysis platforms, machine processing platforms (digital versus analog), laser type/capability/maintenance issues, and expandability/upgrade ability issues. The discussion of the diagnostic testing will concentrate on those areas in which flow cytometry has demonstrated unique ability, superior performance, or future potential over currently available diagnostic testing.

INSTRUMENTATION

Analyzers and Sorters

Flow cytometers are of two types: analyzers and sorters. The most common instrument in the clinical diagnostic laboratory is the analyzer. This just reflects the fact that sorters, which not only analyze but also can physically separate or sort different cell populations, are much more expensive and presently there are very few requirements to sort cells on a clinical basis. Furthermore, since sorters are primarily research instruments, some clinical software analysis packages have not even been written for these instruments, which further limit their clinical usefulness.

Anatomy of Instrumentation

The flow cytometry analyzers and sorters can be broken down into three component systems (*see* Figure 1):

- **Fluidics:** the plumbing and hydraulics for the specimen handling includes sampling, injection into flow cell, and finally collection (for sorters) or waste.

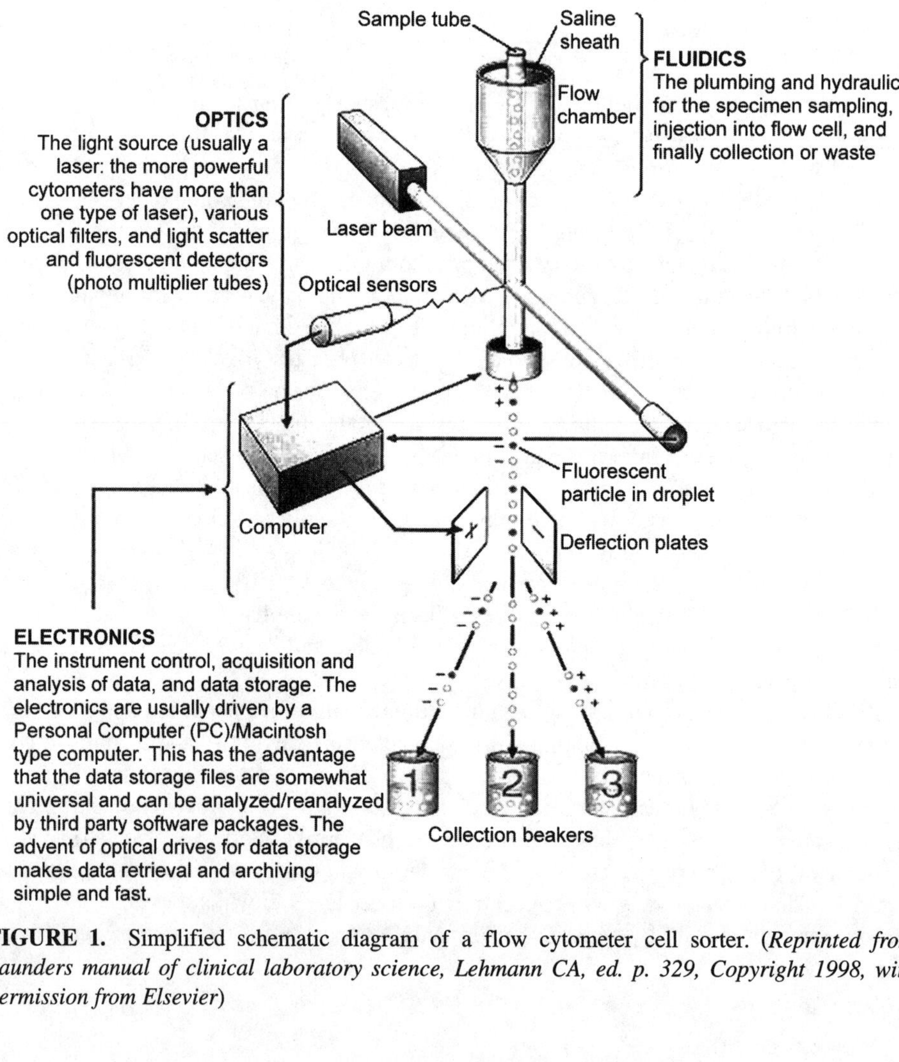

FIGURE 1. Simplified schematic diagram of a flow cytometer cell sorter. (*Reprinted from Saunders manual of clinical laboratory science, Lehmann CA, ed. p. 329, Copyright 1998, with permission from Elsevier*)

- **Optics:** included here are the light source (usually a laser, most cytometers come standard with two different lasers and some of the more powerful cytometers have three or four lasers), various optical filters, and light scatter and fluorescent detectors (photomultiplier tubes).
- **Electronics:** this involves the instrument control, acquisition and analysis of data, and data storage.

Fluidics. One cell at a time, flow cytometers interrogate and collect the resulting data at a very high rate of speed. The cytometer's flow cell is responsible for preparing the sample so that it can be presented to the laser light source in a single-cell fluid stream. The sample, in an isotonic fluid, is forced through the flow cell surrounded by another isotonic fluid (referred to as sheath fluid) to produce a laminar flow. It is this sample stream within a stream that creates an optimal differential pressure for cells to enter the conical nozzle assembly and exit the orifice of the nozzle for intersection by the laser light source. After intersection with the laser, the sample is either collected as waste or, in the case of sorters, the stream is vibrated and broken up into droplets. If done properly, most droplets will contain one cell, which can be given an electrical charge. As the charged droplet falls (the cytometer keeps track of where any particular droplet will be at any given time), it passes charged electric plates which then can deflect the charged droplet left, right, or not at all, depending on the instrument settings, thus sorting the individual cells.

Optics. Most cytometers come standard with two different lasers and some powerful cytometers have three or more lasers. The light source is necessary for quantitating intrinsic cellular parameters as well as extrinsic cell properties obtained by excitation and differential emission of added fluorochromes. Laser light sources are different from other light sources in that they are monochromatic or of a single wavelength with parallel waves of light. Many different types of laser have been used and include gas ion lasers (argon, krypton, helium–neon), diode lasers, and dye lasers. Diode lasers are the newest lasers to be used in cytometers and, in the beginning, had been plagued by some stability and shortened life problems. At the time of this printing, these issues seem to have been resolved. The information encoded in the scatter of the laser light and emission of the fluorescent light is then separated and directed into individual photomultiplier tubes (PMT) through a series of complex beam splitters, dichroic mirror, and wavelength selective filters (*see* Figure 2). With the addition of new fluorescent dyes, four-color analysis is easily performed with two lasers. Again, the more complex machines with three and four lasers are mainly the sorters and research grade analyzers.

Electronics. Light signals collected by the cytometer's PMT detectors are converted to digital signals by the instrument's computer. The instrument electronics are usually controlled and driven by standard personal computer (PC)/Macintosh type computers, which are very easily upgraded for speed, performance, and new data storage capabilities. The advent of CD and DVD-R, RW drives for data storage makes data retrieval and archiving simple and fast. Since the data storage files are somewhat universal, there are also third-party software packages available by which the data can be analyzed/reanalyzed. However, to date, the manufacturer's software is adequate for most clinical analysis required and, in fact, is often preferable. The advantage of the third-party software is in the research applications where it is often more flexible and less expensive. Researchers can take their data with them and reanalyze/print from their own computers.

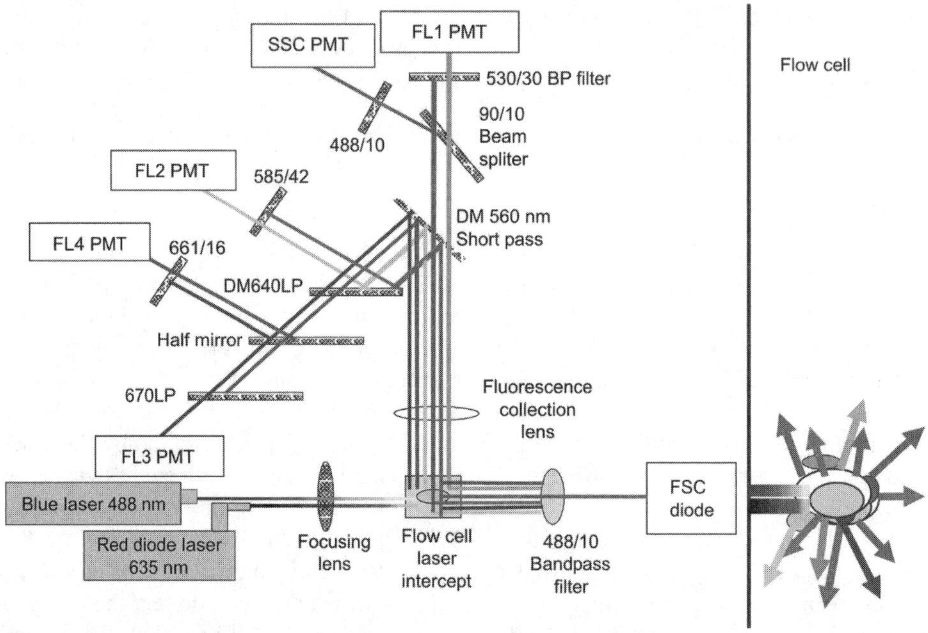

FIGURE 2. PMT, filter, lens, and mirror configuration in a dual laser cytometer.

Theory of Operation

The specimen types that can be analyzed by flow cytometry include those that can be manipulated into a single cell suspension. These include but are not limited to ascites fluid, bone cores and bone marrow, cerebrospinal fluid, lymph nodes, fine needle aspirates, peripheral blood, products of conception, pleural fluid, spleen, solid tumors, and paraffin-imbedded tissue. The single cell suspension can then be labeled with an appropriate panel of fluorescent monoclonal antibodies assembled in groups of up to four colors per aliquot specifically designed for the diagnosis being considered. The actual labeling procedure is simple and similar to any direct fluorescent antibody test procedure. To further simplify things, there are procedures to label the whole blood without any purification or separation procedures.

Flow cytometry has gained a great deal of popularity among clinicians since it has several advantages over histology and immunohistology. One is that the results are quantitative (both in absolute numbers and fluorescent intensity/antigen density), although there is a trend away from numbers and just to designate level of positivity. The other advantage is the cytometer's shear statistical brute force capability. Most instruments are capable of analyzing up to 10,000 events per second. It is easy to see that very rare cells can be analyzed with high statistical significance not possible by other methods. As with most high technology, there is a down side. The main disadvantage of the cytometer is that it is still an expensive technology (although coming down in price) and requires highly trained individuals to operate and interpret the results. Another possible pitfall is that the architecture of the tissue is lost during specimen preparation. It is often important to examine the cells in the context of the surrounding tissue. Finally, there is the very real potential to lose highly fragile cells during preparation and analysis (large cell lymphomas are particularly troublesome in this regard). For these reasons, flow cytometry is not a replacement to standard histological and immunohistologic procedures but an added secondary procedure, which ideally should be used when the diagnosis by traditional, less expensive means is difficult.

Analysis/Software

Data from the cytometer initially are analyzed to determine the light-scattering properties of the cells; this defines the cell population to be examined further. When the laser beam hits the cell, light is scattered in all directions but is collected in the 90° direction (90LS) and low forward angle direction (*see* Figure 2). The 90LS scatter gives an indication of the internal cellular complexity (related to the density of the cell), the more 90LS, the higher the density of the cell. Forward angle light scatter (FALS) is related to the size of the cell, the higher the FALS, the larger the cell. Plotting both of these light-scattering parameters along two axis results in a very characteristic pattern for the different cell types. Mature lymphocytes, monocytes, and granulocytes can be identified easily based on light scatter alone. Abnormal size and/or dense cells can often be identified and distinguished from normal populations on this basis alone. At this point, the population(s) of interest can be identified for fluorescent analysis and further characterization. Another popular method for the initial identification of the cell to be further examined is to use only the 90LS and plot it against CD45 fluorescence. CD45 stains almost all leukocytes and with characteristic fluorescent intensities. This method has the distinct disadvantage that CD45 must be included in every tube, which significantly increases the cost of testing. Besides that, both methods have advantages and disadvantages, but the authors have never found a case where one method was clearly superior or outright missed an abnormal population.

Once the population(s) to be examined is identified by the initial analysis, the analysis of the fluorescent properties (via fluorescent-labeled monoclonal antibody markers) of the gated cells in question can be examined. This means that only fluorescent data are reported on the cells having the light-scattering properties that the operator identified in the initial analysis and excludes all others. In most clinical cytometry laboratories, up to four markers (antigens) can be examined on a single cell at the same time. This is done using four different monoclonal antibodies labeled with four different fluorochromes. While performing multiple color analysis can represent a savings in labor/reagent costs, the main advantages of this type of analysis is in the clinical diagnostic arena. The advantages are twofold. First, the number of cells required for meaningful analysis is greatly reduced. This has allowed analysis of specimens not previously able to be analyzed due to low cell yield, e.g., fine needle aspirates, bone cores, cerebrospinal fluid specimens. Second, the presence of several specific markers on the same cell is extremely important and often critical to the diagnosis. For example, CD5 (marker for T cells and a small subpopulation of B cells), CD19 (marker for B cells), CD23 (B cell subpopulation), and CD10 (Calla) when all run together in four colors are a combination fairly specific for chronic lymphocytic leukemia (CLL). CLL cells are almost always B cells at the stage of maturity that marks with CD5, CD19, and CD23 but are CD10 negative. When a large number of these cells are present, the diagnosis of CLL can be made, excluding many other leukemias.

The fluorescent data should be examined for both the absolute/percent of cells that are positive and the fluorescent intensity, which as previously stated is related to antigen density of the marker being investigated. The fluorescent intensity (antigen density) is important to further defining the maturational stages and phenotype of the cells in question and is playing an ever-expanding role in defining certain diagnostic and prognostic criteria.

Features

The instruments are changing and improving at a rapid rate. In addition, the number of companies making these instruments has increased, giving the potential buyer more choices than the "Big Two." Competition between the companies is fierce. For the major players, it is also competition for the monoclonal antibodies reagents which, for large university medical centers, amounts to a sizable sustained revenue for the companies if they can secure the reagent contract. This being said, there are bargains to be had for the informed consumer when one knows the strengths and weaknesses of each instrument and a decision is based on this information.

Sensitivity

Not all cytometers are the same in sensitivity. They have different light paths, optics, and electronics, all of which affect the sensitivity to detecting low-level fluorescence. This is an area that is becoming even more important as low-level fluorescence and shifts in fluorescence are very meaningful in certain clinical situations. When purchasing a second cytometer or trading in a cytometer, it is imperative to examine the two different instruments side by side on the same samples. Pay careful attention not only to percentages, but also, more importantly to the fluorescent levels (mean peak channel fluorescence). Differences are usually apparent on samples expressing dim fluorescence. The authors' experience has been that these differences are usually manufacturer specific. For first-time buyers, it will be difficult to get both manufacturers in at the same time for side-by-side comparison since the field/sales reps will for the most part be running their machines. In this case, running the same samples at the same time may be difficult. There are preserved flow cytometry cellular controls, which are available, and these could be used which would eliminate donor variability over time. Standardized fluorescent beads are also commercially available.

Capability and Reliability

The choice of analyzer/sorter should be matched for the anticipated usage. Bigger and more expensive is not always better. The authors have seen a case where money was allocated for a new cancer center which included flow cytometry. In this case, the administrator contacted the instrument manufacturer and placed an order for the biggest and best cytometer, assuming it would meet the center's needs. Unfortunately, the large research grade sorters are not oriented to clinical usage and, in fact, some clinical testing cannot even be performed on these instruments because the clinical software has not been written for these machines. Another issue to consider is service record of the company. Most companies promise good service and turnaround; however, the reality may be somewhat different. Check with other institutions in the area regarding their experience with the company's service. This is critical to clinical and one-cytometer sites.

Other Issues

Other issues to consider are the instrument platform and the computer platform. Instruments are available in analog and digital platforms. Some flexibility and convenience is lost on the analog platforms; however, these instruments perform extremely well and by no means should be discounted on this basis. Eventually, most manufacturers will be completely digital. The controlling computers come in PC and MAC formats. This is pretty much an individual choice and some manufacturers are even considering giving the buyer the option of either one. In practicality, either one is fine since the operating systems are converging and the software is similar. Finally, a consideration toward the laboratories' future needs should be addressed. Can the instrument be upgraded with the desired options at a future date and where is the company going with the instrument that is being considered (i.e., phasing out or continuing development)?

CLINICAL APPLICATIONS

Functional Leukocyte Testing

Chronic Granulomatous Disease (CGD)

CGD is characterized by defective killing of intracellular microorganisms due to mutations in one of the four known components of the NADPH oxidase system. This system is responsible for the generation of superoxide and related antimicrobial oxidants. Diagnosis of CGD requires the demonstration of an abnormal oxidase system in the polymorphonuclear cells of affected patients. In the past this has been performed using a dye reduction test (nitroblue tetrazolium or NBT test) where leukocytes are stimulated to reduce the dye that turns blue/purple and are scored qualitatively by eye. There is a slide methodology based on the same dye test that is semiquantitative; however, both methods are very subjective and accuracy is not high. The flow cytometry procedure (CGD test by flow cytometry) directly labels and stimulates cells in whole blood enabling the diagnosis of patients with CGD or X-linked carriers. The cells are labeled with dihydrorhodamine 123, which is oxidized when the cells are stimulated to undergo the oxidative burst with phorbol myristate acetate. The oxidized form of dihydrorhodamine 123 is fluorescent. The results are quantitative, objective, and extremely sensitive which easily allows detection of carrier states. This technique is particularly useful for the diagnosis of CGD in very young infants due to the small volume of blood required.

The results are expressed as a ratio of the mean peak channel fluorescence of the stimulated granulocytes over the mean peak channel fluorescence of unstimulated granulocytes (neutrophil oxidative index or NOI). A NOI ratio greater than 100 is considered responsive but usually it is much higher than that. For example, in the healthy control patient in Figure 3, this ratio is 1614 (fluorescence on the x-axis is extremely intense and shifted to the right when the granulocytes are stimulated). In the two twin patients (20 months old)

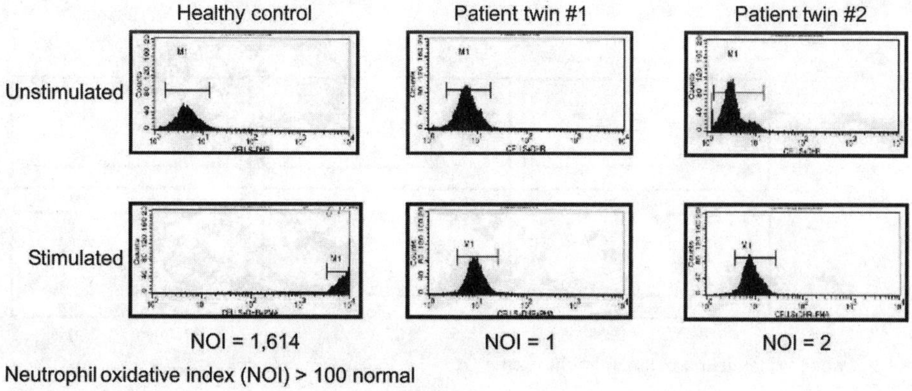

FIGURE 3. Neutrophil oxidative burst test for a patient with CGD.

with CGD who presented in the hospital at the exact same time, there is very little shift or expression of fluorescence after the granulocytes are stimulated (as demonstrated in Figure 3 with NOIs of 1 and 2, respectively).

The detection of carriers is by the detection of a bimodal peak, one peak expressing normal stimulation and one peak expressing the deficient characteristic. This is due to two populations of granulocytes in the carrier (i.e., normal and abnormal). Figure 4 demonstrates the results for the mother and older sibling of the twins presented in Figure 3. The older sibling also had CGD, however this was unknown at the time of diagnosis of the twins. The sibling had a more than normal number of infections as an infant but these infections were managed by antibiotics and never worked up. The mother demonstrated the bimodal peak characteristic of a carrier. The flow cytometry method for detection of CGD is now the method of choice due to its accuracy, objectivity, and sensitivity. The NBT test should no longer be ordered.

Leukocyte Adhesion Deficiency (LAD)

LAD is a rare inherited immunodeficiency disorder characterized by an absence or reduced expression of a group of cell surface leukocyte adhesion molecules which results in the inability of polymorphonuclear cells to adhere to the vascular endothelium and to opsonized microorganisms. The clinical hallmarks of this disease are recurrent infections, nonpurulent necrotic soft tissue lesions, delayed wound healing, persistent granulocytosis, gingivitis, and/or periodontitis. Typically, the adhesion molecules examined are CDIIb and CDIIc (expressed on monocytes, granulocytes, and natural killer cells) and CD18 (expressed on lymphoid and myeloid cells). This procedure involves the direct stimulation of these molecules with phorbol 12-myristate 13-acetate and examines the absolute expression of these molecules and the functional up regulation of the molecules as indicated by increases in fluorescent intensity of expression. The advantage of this procedure is that it is a functional assay which can be performed on very little blood (heel/fingerstick), thus allowing the diagnosis of LAD on very young infants.

Paroxysmal Nocturnal Hemoglobinuria (PNH)

PNH is a rare acquired chronic hemolytic anemia that arises from a somatic mutation in a hematopoietic stem cell. Most hematopoietic cell lines may be affected by the intrinsic membrane defect. This defect renders the red cells highly susceptible to complement-mediated lysis, resulting in the characteristic hemolysis. This is the basis of the two

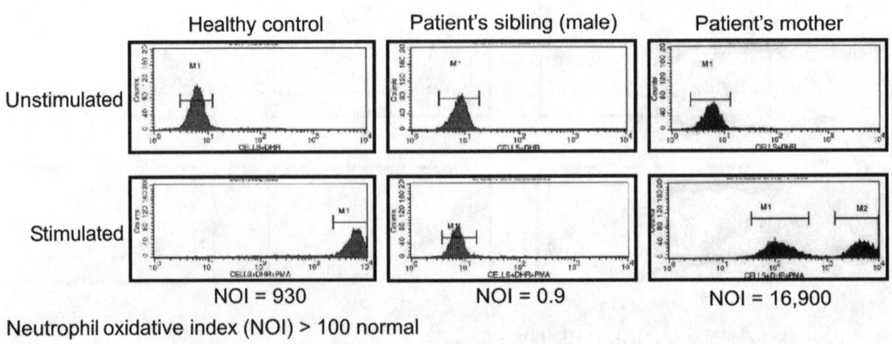

FIGURE 4. Neutrophil oxidative burst test for the family of a CGD patient.

standard tests for this disease: acidified serum test (Ham test) and the sucrose hemolysis test. Both of these tests are still in use today; however, in 1996 a flow cytometry test was put forth as the method of choice since it is more sensitive, specific, and less labor intensive. The flow cytometry test looks for the expression of glycosylphosphatidylinositol (GPI) anchored proteins. In PNH this glycolipid anchor is missing or defective and therefore all surface proteins, which are held to the membrane by this glycolipid, are also missing or reduced. There are many different proteins that are anchored in this fashion on lymphocytes, monocytes, granulocytes, and erythrocytes. Patients with PNH vary considerably in their severity since the defect arises from a somatic mutation of a hematopoietic stem cell. The extent of this clone and their progeny as well as the type of mutation (over 100 different mutations have been described) determine the severity. Generally, PNH patients fall into four classes of GPI-linked antigen expression:

- Patients whose expression of antigen is completely lacking and the fluorescent intensity is similar to the negative (isotype) control. These are designated as having Type III cells.
- Patients have a population of cells with totally deficient expression (Type III) and a population of cells with normal expression (designated Type I cells).
- Patients have a population of cells with partial (lower fluorescence than normal) antigen expression (designated as Type II cells) and a population of normal Type I cells.
- Patients have a combination of Types I, II, and III.

The most commonly examined GPI-linked proteins are CD55 (decay-accelerating factor which disassembles C3/C5 convertase) and CD59 (protectin which binds C8, C9 and prevents assembly of membrane attack complex or MAC) on granulocytes and CD14 (monocyte LPS receptor) on monocytes. In a normal person, CD55 and CD59 are expressed on all granulocytes (Figure 5). The PNH patient in Figure 5 demonstrates Type I (normal expression) and Type II (partially deficient) cells present. In this example, the granulocyte expression of GPI-linked proteins reveals the classic bimodal peaks. Two-color contour plots can also present these data (not shown). In this case, the quadrant markers and mean channel fluorescence are used to quantitate the populations. Of note, both the acidified serum test and the sucrose hemolysis test were negative for this patient and flow cytometry easily detected the PNH cells.

Fetal Cells in Maternal Circulation

The presence of fetal cells in the maternal circulation, resulting from fetal–maternal hemorrhage, may be attributed to a variety of causes including fetal and/or placental trauma and various obstetrical emergencies. In addition to these emergency situations, hemorrhage of Rh+ fetal blood into Rh– maternal blood may result in the formation of Rh-reactive antibodies in the mother, causing an adverse effect on the current pregnancy and even more devastating effects on subsequent pregnancies (hemolytic disease of the newborn). This Rh immunization may be prevented by the administration to the mother of anti-Rh immunoglobulin after delivery.

Fetal hemoglobin tests have been used to indicate fetal–maternal trauma as well as a guide in determining the amount of RhIg to administer clinically. This is done by using the percentage of fetal hemoglobin-containing red cells to calculate the partial volume of fetal blood in the maternal circulation. The Kleihauer-Betke (KB) test has been used since 1957 to detect fetal–maternal hemorrhage and to approximate the volume of fetal red blood cells (RBCs) in the maternal circulation. However, despite widespread use, the KB

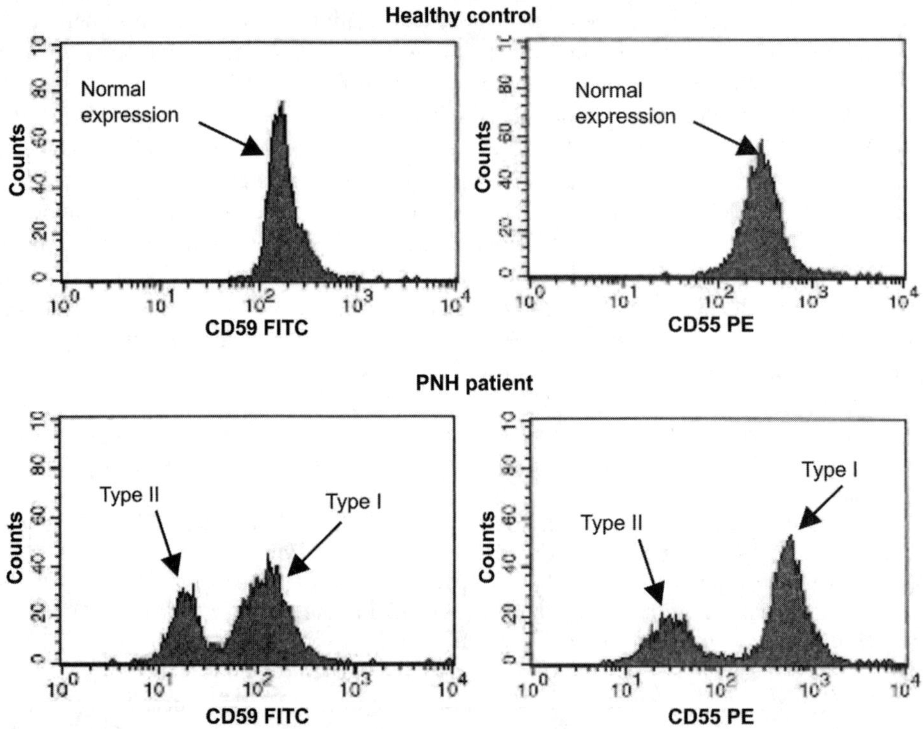

FIGURE 5. Type I and Type II cells in PNH patient.

acid elution test is limited to a detection sensitivity of about 0.5% of fetal cells and has been questioned regarding its accuracy in the context of acute trauma. In addition, errors frequently arise due to interobserver subjectivity, as well as the need to manually count substantial numbers of maternal and fetal erythrocytes to determine the percentage of fetal cells present.

Recently, flow cytometric methods have been employed to enumerate fetal cells in the maternal circulation. This test is based on a monoclonal antibody directed to fetal hemoglobin (hemoglobin F). The presence and amount of fetal hemoglobin in the erythrocytes identifies the fetal red cells. Erythrocytes containing fetal hemoglobin may be found in individuals of any age, but with lower amounts of fetal hemoglobin compared to fetal red cells. These cells have been termed F cells (not to be confused with fetal cells). Clinical conditions that involve significant anemia may result in elevated levels of F cells. Included in this list are hereditary anemic diseases such as sickle cell anemia and thalassemia major. High levels of F cells may also exist in adults with a group of genetic disorders referred to as hereditary persistence of fetal hemoglobin. The flow cytometric test can easily distinguish between F cells and fetal red cells (F cells have a much lower fluorescence than fetal red cells which are bright).

The histogram shown in Figure 6 identifies the fetal RBCs by the small peak labeled M1. This is reported as a percentage of all RBCs. Of interest is the fact that flow cytometry has been reported to be able to detect 1 fetal RBC per 100,000 maternal RBCs. The sensitivity needed for routine clinical use is approximately 1 fetal RBC per 200 maternal RBCs. The sensitivity, ease of performance, accuracy, and reproducibility make flow cytometry the method of choice for fetal RBC determinations.

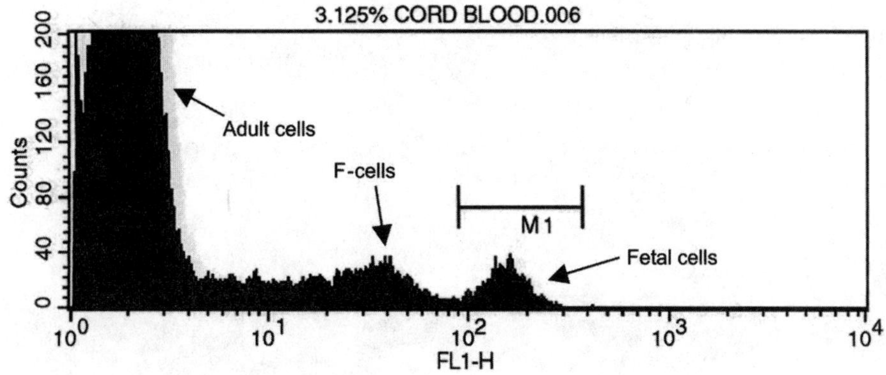

Histogram Statistics

Sample ID: 3.125% CORD BLOOD Acquisition Date: 10-Jan-01
Gate: G3 Gated Events: 47734
Total Events: 50000

Marker	% Gated	% Total	Mean	Geo Mean	CV	Median	Peak Ch
All	100.00	95.47	9.05	2.75	312.19	2.04	1
M1	3.12	2.97	155.03	151.44	21.74	152.61	158

FIGURE 6. Fetal hemoglobin test by flow cytometry.

Cytometric Bead Array Technology

Cytometric bead arrays or multiplexed solid phase particle-based immunoassays are a new technology that uses different fluorescent beads to measure multiple soluble analytes simultaneously by flow cytometry. Currently there are three areas using this technology (autoimmune, cytokine quantitations, and transplantation), some of these are advanced enough to have FDA clearance for clinical testing. It is anticipated that this technology may well revolutionize the ability to do multiple testing on a single specimen. However, ultimate development of this for clinical purposes may be hampered somewhat by regulations prohibiting unnecessary testing and does raise some serious compliance/informed consent issues even if the unwanted tests are suppressed. One area where this ability is superbly fitted to the clinical need is in transplant HLA typing and panel reactive antibodies (PRA) determinations where multiple determinations are indeed required.

This technology uses beads that have been infused with a fluorescent dye (usually a red dye) at different concentrations and therefore are distinguishable from each other on the level of fluorescence observed. To detect autoantibodies, the specific beads would be coated with individually purified autoantigens. Each bead with a different level of fluorescent dye would be coated with a different autoantigen. After incubation of the patient's serum and subsequent binding of any autoantibodies present to their respective beads, the beads are incubated with a fluorescein (green) labeled anti-Ig. Any beads with autoantibodies on them will now be both red and green, which can be read easily and distinguished on the flow cytometer (Figure 7). Currently, one manufacturer has put the determination of nine specific autoantibodies in a format using a dedicated flow cytometer in semiautomated software driven format. The FDA has cleared this test for in vitro diagnostic use. This is such a radical departure from the firmly entrenched standard autoimmune testing

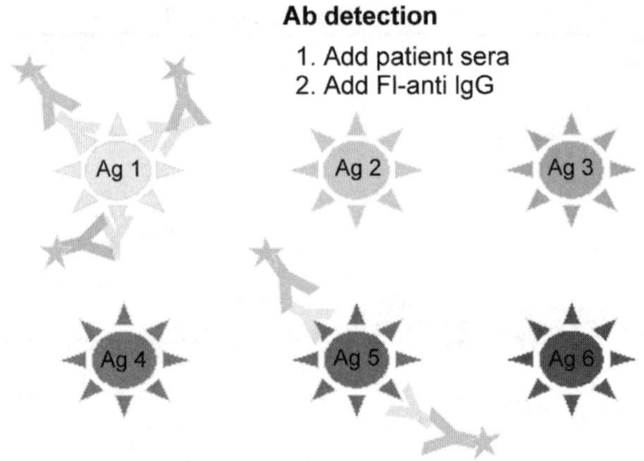

FIGURE 7. Cytometric bead array schematic for antibody detection.

(ANA pattern recognition and ELISA testing) that correlation studies (while always important) are especially pertinent to this new technology and to clinician understanding of the new testing protocols. In addition, all tests are performed whether they were ordered or not and the information is available (albeit suppressed). This does raise some possible regulatory issues, which should be addressed by the appropriate regulatory agencies. Another example of this type of bead array assay is the determination of PRA in potential renal transplant recipients. This test is currently FDA- and ASHI-cleared. However, it has not yet been cleared to replace the standard complement-dependent cytotoxic techniques and is listed as supplementary testing. It is anticipated that in the near future it will be cleared to replace the old technology, much like flow cytometry cross-matching is currently cleared to replace the microlymphocytotoxicity test for renal transplantation. The interested reader is referred to the Additional Reading section at the end of this chapter for further information about these tests.

Another configuration of the bead array technology is the detection of soluble proteins (other than autoantibodies). This uses an alteration of the technique already discussed. In this case, an antigen capture technique is used. Specific antibodies to the desired analytes are coated on the different beads (Figure 8). The unknown specimen is then incubated with the beads, followed by development with fluorescein (green) labeled specific anti-analyte antibodies. Figure 9 gives an example of the negative control where none of the different beads fluoresces green. The different levels of red fluorescence distinguish the specific beads. Figure 10 demonstrates three beads that are positive and three that are negative. When specific standards are run, a standard curve can be generated and the amount of each analyte present can be quantitated based on the green fluorescent intensity. These assays are extremely sensitive and are accurate down to the 2-pg/mL range.

Leukemia/Lymphoma Phenotyping Advances

The theory in the diagnosis of leukemias and lymphomas by flow cytometry has changed very little over the years and there are books devoted to the subject. The interested reader is referred to the Additional Reading section at the end of this chapter for detailed information regarding this subject. The following summarizes what is new to phenotyping in regard to instrumentation and reagents. What has changed is knowledge of cell surface antigens that are expressed on various cells and the vast availability of different monoclonal antibody reagents to these antigens. The other technical improvement has been the

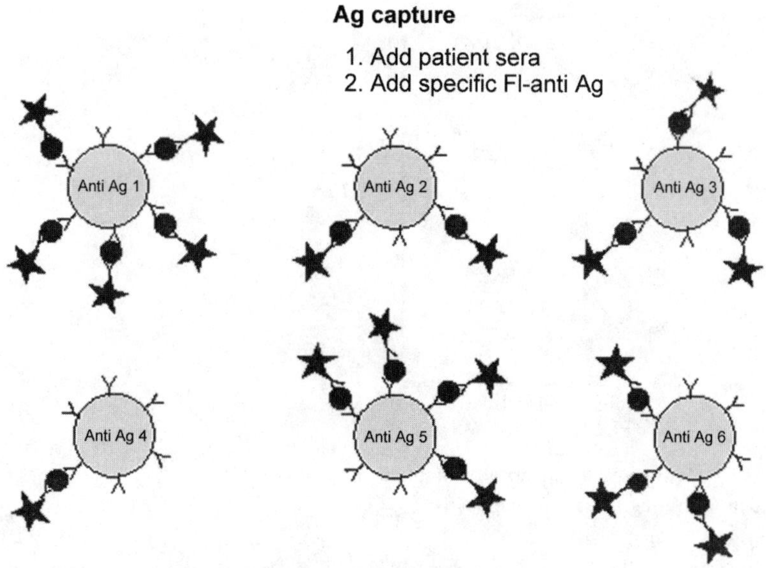

FIGURE 8. Cytometric bead array schematic for antigen detection.

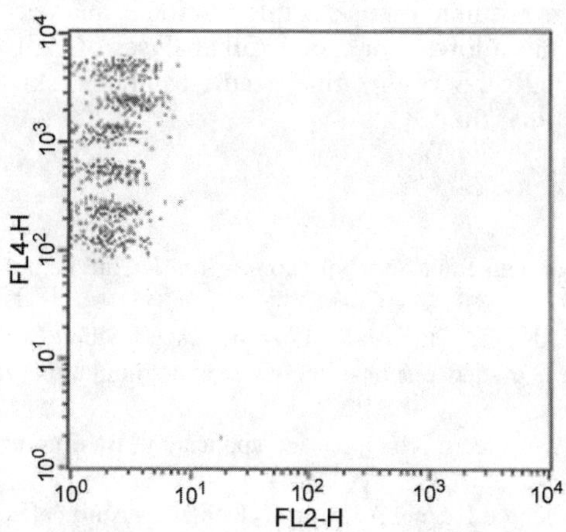

FIGURE 9. Cytometric bead array: dot plots of negative specimen demonstrating the six negative beads.

routine use of four-color analysis on the two laser analyzers in the clinical setting. This has two advantages over the more traditional two-color techniques:

- The ability to examine four antigens at the same time on a single cell, in many cases, allows the user to classify and subclassify the cell populations in much greater detail. This is very important when one is trying to look for residual disease after treatment where there is a requirement to detect very small populations of malignant cells in a virtual sea of other normal cells. Using four-color techniques, these residue populations can be identified much easier by putting an antibody panel together which may uniquely identify the leukemic cells from other similar but normal regenerating cells. This is done by examining and discriminating subtle fluorescent intensity differences and differences within the 16 different antigen combinations possible with four-color

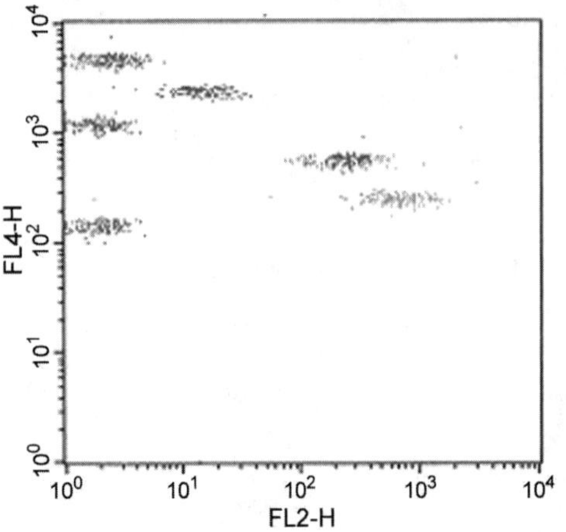

FIGURE 10. Cytometric bead array: dot plots of positive specimen demonstrating three positive beads.

analysis. This is in contrast to the four possible combinations with two-color analysis. Therefore, it is much easier to find that unique profile for the malignant population and therefore identify them at very low levels.

- The second advantage is that the sample size required for useful information is markedly reduced using four-color analysis. This has allowed for successful analyses of samples in which the cell yields are traditionally poor, e.g., fine needle aspirates, skin biopsies, bone core samples, and cerebrospinal fluid.

ADDITIONAL READING

Bagg A, Kallakury BVS. Molecular pathology of leukemia and lymphoma. Am J Clin Pathol 1999;112(Suppl 1):S76–92.

Bass DA, Parce JW, DeChatelet LR, Szejda P, Seeds MC, Thomas M. Flow cytometric studies of oxidative product formation by neutrophils: a graded response to membrane stimulation. J Immunol 1983;130:1910–7.

Bauer KD, Duque RE, Shankey TV. Clinical flow cytometry, principles and application. Baltimore: Williams & Wilkins, 1993.

Bene MC, Kolopp Sarda MN, El Kaissouni J, De March Kennel A, Mole C, Kohler C. Automated cell count in flow cytometry: a valuable tool to assess CD4 absolute levels in peripheral blood. Am J Clin Pathol 1998;110:321–6.

Borowitz MJ, Rubnitz J, Nash M, Pullen DJ, Camitta B. Surface antigen phenotype can predict TEL-AML1 rearrangement in childhood B-precursor ALL: a Pediatric Oncology Group study. Leukemia 1998;12:1764–70.

Breen C, Golightly M. Lymphoproliferative diseases. In: Lehmann C, ed. Saunders manual of clinical laboratory science: Philadelphia: Saunders, 1998:325–38.

Bronson RA, Peresleni T, Golightly M. Progesterone promotes the acrosome reaction in capacitated human spermatozoa as judged by flow cytometry and CD46 staining. Mol Hum Reprod 1999;5(6):507–12.

Campana D. Monitoring minimal residual disease in acute leukemia: expectations, possibilities and initial clinical results. Int J Clin Lab Res 1994;24:132–8.

Darzyniewicz Z, Crissman JA. Flow cytometry: methods in cell biology. Vol 33. San Diego: Academic Press, 1990.

Freedman AS. Cell surface antigens in leukemias and lymphomas. Cancer Invest 1996;14(3): 252–76.

Garratty G, Arndt PA. Applications of flow cytofluorometry to red blood cell immunology. Cytometry 1999;38:259–67.

Golightly MG, Moss RB. Natural killer cells and lymphokine activated killer cells: their reactivity with monoclonal antibody. In: Cheremisinoff P, ed. Biotechnology, current progress. Lancaster, PA: Technomic Publishing Co., 1991,1:103–18.

Henderson LO, Marti GE, Gaigalas A, Hannon WH, Vogt RF Jr. Terminology and nomenclature for standardization in quantitative fluorescence cytometry. Cytometry 1998;33:97–105.

Keren DF, Hedstrom DL. Contemporary approaches to anti-nuclear antibody serology. J Clin Ligand Assay 1999;22:50–5.

Keren DF, McCoy JP, Carey JL. Flow cytometry in clinical diagnosis, 3rd ed. Chicago: DSCP, 2001.

Knapp W, Strobl H, Majdic O. Flow cytometric analysis of cell-surface and intracellular antigens in leukemia diagnosis. Cytometry 1994;18:187–98.

Loken MR, Parks DR, Herzenberg LA. Two-color immunofluorescence using a fluorescence-activated cell sorter. J Histochem Cytochem 1997;25:899–907.

O'Gorman M, Corrochano V. Rapid whole-blood flow cytometry assay for diagnosis of chronic granulomatous disease. Clin Diagn Lab Immunol 1995;2:227–32.

Oshimi K. Lymphoproliferative disorders of natural killer cells. Int J Hematol 1996;63(4):279–90.

Paietta E, Andersen J, Wiernik PH. A new approach to analyzing the utility of immunophenotyping for predicting clinical outcome in acute leukemia. Eastern Cooperative Oncology Group. Leukemia 1996;10(1):1–4.

Qwens MA, Loken MR. Flow cytometry principles for clinical laboratory practice: quality assurance for quantitative immunophenotyping. New York: Wiley-Liss, 1995.

Radbruch A. Flow cytometry and cell sorting, 2nd ed. New York: Springer-Verlag, 1999.

Rosse WF. Paroxysmal nocturnal hemoglobinuria. In: Hoffman R, Benz EJ, Furie B, Shattil SJ, Cohen HJ, eds. Hematology: basic principles and practice, 2nd ed. New York: Churchill Livingstone, 1995:370–81.

Schwartz A, Marti GE, Poon R, Gratama JW, Fernandez-Repollet E. Standardizing flow cytometry: a classification system of fluorescence standards used for flow cytometry. Cytometry 1998;33:106–14.

Shapiro H. Practical flow cytometry, 3rd ed. New York: Wiley-Liss, 1995.

Stelzer GT, Shults KE, Loken MR. CD45 gating for routine flow cytometric analysis of human bone marrow specimens. Ann NY Acad Sci 1993;677:265–80.

Sutherland DR, Anderson L, Keeney M, et al. Toward a worldwide standard for CD34+ enumeration? J Hematother 1997;6:85–9.

Tabbara IA: Allogeneic bone marrow transplantation: acute and late complications. Anticancer Res 1996;16(2):1019–26.

Thor AD, Moore DH II. Prognostic and predictive markers in breast cancer. In: Winchester DJ, Winchester DP, eds. Breast cancer: atlas of clinical oncology. Hamilton, Ontario: Decker, 2000:113–30.

Van Dilla MA, Dean PN, Laerum OD, Melamed MR. Flow cytometry: instrumentation and data analysis. Orlando: Academic Press, 1985.

Warzynski MJ, Rosen MH, Golightly MG, Steingart RH, Otto RN, Rezuke WN, et al. An acute form of T gamma lymphoproliferative disease presenting with massive splenomegaly—importance of immunophenotyping for diagnosis. Clin Immunol Immunopathol 1993;67:100–8.

Weir EG, Cowan K, LeBeau P, Borowitz MJ. A limited antibody panel can distinguish B-precursor acute lymphoblastic leukemia from normal B precursors with four color flow cytometry: implications for residual disease detection. Leukemia 1999;13:558–67.

Williams NN, Daly JM. Flow cytometry and prognostic implications in patients with solid tumors. Surg Gynecol Obstet 1990;171:257–66.

Chapter 15

Molecular Diagnostics Technology

Carl T. Wittwer and Noriko Kusukawa

What is "molecular diagnostics?" In its broadest sense, molecular diagnostics includes all aspects of clinical testing. However, as commonly used today, molecular diagnostics specifically implies analysis of nucleic acids, i.e., ribonucleic acid (RNA) and deoxyribonucleic acid (DNA). The double helical structure of DNA was correctly proposed in 1953. Fifty years later, the ordering of more than 92% of the 3 billion adenine (A), cytosine (C), guanine (G), and thymine (T) bases of the human genome was established through the Human Genome Project (1).

This chapter covers technologies for the analysis of nucleic acids that are particularly relevant for the clinical laboratory. Cytogenetics, proteomics, and techniques commonly used by anatomic pathologists (in situ hybridization, FISH) are not covered. Various genomes and the spectrum of genetic changes that are of interest in humans, bacteria, and viruses are considered. This is followed by a general discussion of methods to detect and characterize nucleic acids. Often, nucleic acid amplification is necessary to observe the sequence alterations of interest, so amplification techniques are discussed next, followed by specific descriptions of genotyping methods. Finally, real-time techniques that allow amplification, detection, quantification, and genotyping in a closed-tube system are described.

GENOMES AND THEIR SEQUENCE VARIATION

Each cell in the human body contains two copies of a 3.2 billion sequence code comprising double-stranded DNA. Although this DNA is packaged into 46 chromosomes, if stretched end-to-end, the total length of the DNA double helix in each cell would be more than 2 meters. Table 1 lists important aspects of the **human genome**, including variations important in clinical diagnostics.

Three-quarters of human DNA is **intragenic** or between genes and is not directly involved in coding for proteins through the processes of transcription into mRNA and translation into protein. Intragenic DNA contains most of the simple sequence repeats (SSRs) present in the genome. These repeats are known as microsatellites or short tandem repeats (STRs) when the repeat unit is 1–13 bases, and minisatellites or variable number of tandem repeats (VNTRs) when the repeat unit is 14–500 bases. SSRs are critical markers in genetic linkage studies and forensic identity testing. The most common SSRs are dinucleotide repeats such as AC and AT. On average, approximately one SSR occurs every 2000 bases.

TABLE 1. The Human Genome and its sequence variation

The Human Genome (1)

- 3.2 Billion base pairs
  - 23 Chromosomes (47–245 million base pair each)
  - 75% Intragenic
    - 45% Parasitic (transposon-derived repeats)
    - 5% Segmental duplications
    - 3% Simple sequence repeats (SSRs, STRs)
    - 22% Other
  - 25% Genes
    - Number of genes: 30,000
    - Average values for a gene:
      - Base pairs: 27,000
      - Number of exons: 9
      - Coding sequence: 1340
      - Number of amino acids: 447
    - 24% Intronic
    - 1.1%–1.4% Exonic

Sequence Alterations[a]

- 99.9% Equality (one difference every 1250 bases between random haploid genomes)
  - Single nucleotide polymorphisms (SNPs) identified every 100–300 bases
    - 97% Noncoding
    - 3% Within exons
  - Mutations
    - 70% SNPs
      - 49% Missense (amino acid substitution)
      - 11% Nonsense (termination)
      - 9% Splicing
      - <1% Regulatory
    - 23% Small indels
    - 7% Gross lesions (large indels, repeats, rearrangements, complex)

Epigenetic Alterations

- Variable initiation
- Alternative splicing
- Methylation

[a]Data compiled from reference 1 and the human mutation database (http://archive.uwcm.ac.uk/uwcm/mg/hgmd0.html)

One-quarter of the human genome consists of genes. There are about 30,000 genes in the human genome. The average gene covers 27,000 bases, but only about 1300 of these bases code for amino acid sequence. These coding areas are interspersed throughout the gene and are known as **exons.** On average, there are about nine exons per gene. The non-coding areas between exons are known as **introns.** Within a gene, 95% of the sequence is covered by introns, while only 5% consists of coding sequence within exons. When both intragenic sequence and genes are considered, coding sequence comprises only 1.1%–1.4% of the genome.

Sequence Variation Within the Human Genome

There is approximately 99.9% sequence identity between random copies of the genome. That is, within or between individuals, two copies of the genome show, on average, one difference every 1250 bases. Depending on the viewer's perspective, this degree of variation may seem staggeringly high or conveniently low. For example, with more than 3 billion bases in the genome, even a variation of <0.1% results in more than 2 million sequence variations. From another perspective, if less than 1 in a 1000 bases are different between genomes, more than 99.9% of the work to sequence any copy of the human genome has already been accomplished. To describe the differences between genomes, the relatively rare changes in sequence need to be cataloged. Techniques that identify sequence differences, rather than perform de novo sequencing, are known as **resequencing** methods. Instead of identifying the specific sequence, or **genotype**, only the differences between two genomes are identified. Since most of the sequence between genomes is identical, these screening or "scanning" techniques can be very useful.

The most common sequence variations are single-base changes, also known as **single nucleotide polymorphisms** or **SNPs**. Millions of SNPs have been described, and many new SNPs will be reported. Some SNPs are common in the population with allele frequencies of from 0.1 to 0.5, while others are very rare. Although an SNP has been identified about every 100–300 bases, many of these are not common in the population. The vast majority of SNPs (97%) occur in noncoding regions; only 3% of SNPs are associated with exons.

Sequence Variations that Cause Human Disease

Many sequence variations in the genome do not affect human health. For example, most of the intragenic sequence variations, e.g., SNPs and SSRs, are not associated with disease. Similarly, most of the SNPs in introns, except for splicing and regulatory mutations, are not known to affect gene function. In addition, some of the SNPs within exons are silent alterations that do not code for a change in amino acid sequence because of the redundancy of the genetic code. Still other SNPs in exons code for amino acid changes that do not affect protein function.

When only sequence alterations that are known to cause disease, or "mutations" are considered, most are SNPs, followed by insertions/deletions and gross lesions (Table 1). Approximately 70% of disease-causing mutations are SNPs. Most of these result in an amino acid change and are known as **missense mutations**. Approximately 11% of disease-causing mutations are **nonsense** mutations that change an amino acid coding triplet to a termination codon, resulting in premature polypeptide chain termination. Approximately 9% of disease-causing mutations alter the splicing sites located just outside of an exon, resulting in altered concatenation of coding sequences. Finally, less than 1% of disease-causing mutations are regulatory mutations that affect the efficiency of transcription by altering promoter/enhancer regions in introns.

After SNPs, small insertions/deletions are the next most common class of mutations, accounting for about 23% of human sequence alterations that cause disease. An insertion refers to the presence of extra bases while deletion implies the absence of certain bases in comparison to a reference sequence. Because choice of the reference sequence is at times arbitrary, both insertions and deletions are often considered together as one class of sequence variant called **indels**.

After SNPs and small indels, the remaining mutations are mostly larger lesions and comprise only 7% of human mutations. These include whole gene duplications and deletions, SSR expansions (e.g., trinucleotide repeat expansions), gene rearrangements (e.g., B- and T-cell gene rearrangements), and complex polymorphic loci related to health and disease (e.g., HLA).

Often, sequence variants are inherited together in a contiguous block, or **haplotype**. Disease associations may depend not on any particular mutation, but on the overall effect of several linked alleles that define the haplotype. When the haplotype linkage is strong, genotype determination at a single locus may identify the haplotype and disease association. However, if the haplotype linkage is weak, or when the disease association and/or haplotype linkage is first being established, methods for determining the cis/trans phase of alleles at distant loci are necessary.

Most human genetic material is present in two copies, with the exception of the sex chromosomes in males and mitochondrial DNA. The presence of only a single copy of genes on the X and Y chromosome in males leads to well-known sex-linked disorders. In contrast, the 16,500 bp mitochondrial genome is present in more than 1000 copies per cell, constituting about 0.3% of human DNA. Allele fractions may vary over a wide range when all mitochondria in a cell are considered. That is, mutations in mitochondrial DNA are **heteroplasmic**, meaning the ratio of wild type to mutant alleles can vary almost continuously, sometimes resulting in a wide range of symptoms when only one mutation is involved.

Human Epigenetic Alterations

In addition to the sequence alterations just considered, epigenetic alterations, including alternative splicing and methylation affect gene expression. Even though the number of genes may be limited to 30,000, variable transcription initiation and exon splicing may produce up to three times as many mRNA transcripts and protein products.

Methylation of cytosine to form 5-methylcytosine occurs frequently; about 70% of CpG dinucleotides in the human genome are methylated (2). Although not inherited, interest in this "5th base" has increased recently as correlations to cancer have been reported. CpG islands are about 1000 bases in length and are often found near the 5′-end of genes. These regions consist of clusters of CpG dinucleotides that are usually not methylated in normal cells. However, CpG methylation correlates with condensed chromatin structure and promoter inactivation of tumor suppressor genes.

Bacterial Genomes and Sequence Alterations

Bacterial genomes are considerably less complex than human or other eucaryotic genomes. Common bacteria have only one chromosome, usually a circular DNA double helix of 4–5 million base pairs long, about 1000 times less than the amount of DNA in a human cell. About 90% of the DNA in bacteria codes for protein. Intragenic regions are small, there are no introns, and few repeated DNA segments. In the common bacteria, *Escherichia coli*, there are about 4300 genes.

In addition to the large circular chromosome that carries essential genes, bacteria also carry accessory genes in smaller circles of double-stranded DNA known as **plasmids**. Plasmids range in size from 1000 to more than 1,000,000 base pairs. Plasmids are important in molecular diagnostics; pathogenic factors and antibiotic resistance are often encoded by plasmids.

The bacterial repertoire of DNA can be altered by:

- Gain or loss of plasmids
- Single-base changes and small indels as in eucaryotic genomes
- Larger segmental rearrangements, including inversions, deletions, and duplications

Some genes such as those for ribosomal RNA are present in many copies and can be used to identify different species of bacteria.

Viral Genomes and Sequence Alterations

Viral genomes are considerable less complex than bacterial genomes. Common viruses that infect humans vary in size from about 5000 to 250,000 bases, or 20–1000 times less than the amount of nucleic acid in *E. coli*. Because viruses utilize the host's cellular machinery, they do not need as many genes; small viruses may only encode several genes while the larger viruses can encode hundreds. The viral genome consists of either DNA or RNA, and the nucleic acid may be single stranded or double stranded, linear or circular with one or multiple fragments and/or copies. Similar to bacteria, there are no introns. In fact, in some viruses the exons overlap, with different reading frames coding different products from the same nucleic acid sequence. Noncoding regions are usually present at the terminal ends of linear genomes. Repeat segments are often found as terminal or internal repeats and may be inverted.

Sequence alterations in viruses are common. Areas of high sequence variation may be interspersed between conserved domains. Higher rates of variation may allow escape from antibody recognition. Common mutations in viruses include point mutations and indels. Sequence diversity within a viral species may be so great that consensus sequences for molecular typing may be difficult to find.

NUCLEIC ACID DETECTION AND CHARACTERIZATION METHODS

Direct Detection Methods

UV Absorbance

Although colorless, nucleic acids absorb in the ultraviolet (UV). If a double-stranded nucleic acid preparation is pure, a 50-μg/mL solution has an absorbance of 1.0 at 260 nm. Single-stranded nucleic acids have a stronger absorbance, so only about 30 μg/mL gives an absorbance of 1.0. More precise estimates for oligonucleotides are based on dinucleotide contributions (3). The change in absorbance of DNA that occurs with the transition from single strand to double strand is known as the **hypochromatic shift**. When DNA is heated, it melts at a characteristic temperature, depending on the fraction of Gs and Cs, length, and sequence of the double-stranded portion (4), a process that can be measured by UV absorbance.

Staining of Nucleic Acids with Fluorescent Dyes

Although absorbance measurements are simple and precise, they are not sensitive. In contrast, fluorescent dyes that stain nucleic acid are 1000 to 10,000 times more sensitive than absorbance measurements. The most familiar example of a nucleic acid dye is ethidium bromide, an intercalating dye used to visualize bands of nucleic acid separated by size after gel electrophoresis. Cyanine dyes, such as SYBR Green I, have recently become very popular stains for nucleic acids in gels or solution. With the right optics, single molecules of DNA can be visualized with nucleic acid stains (5). Nucleic acid dyes can also be used to monitor amplification in real-time, and fluorescent melting curve analysis is now commonly used in molecular diagnostics (6).

Complementary Labeled Probes

In general, absorbance and generic fluorescence measurements do not discriminate between different nucleic acid sequences, i.e., they are not sequence specific. Specificity in nucleic acid assays almost always comes from the hybridization of two complementary nucleic acid strands. The complement to the target sequence is labeled with a radioactive, fluorescent, or electronic label and becomes a probe that specifically binds to the target. Historically, clones in plasmids were the source of probe sequence and were jealously guarded by laboratories and used as currency for collaborations. Today, probes are usually either synthesized directly as oligonucleotides or created by PCR (7). Molecular diagnostics has truly become "democratized," with equal availability of information and basic tools to all researchers.

Use of complementary probes requires hybridization to the target. This happens rapidly if the concentration of the probe and target are high (e.g., after amplification), but it may require hours or days if the concentrations are low (8, 9).

Radioactive Probes

Radioactive labeling can produce very hot probes with high sensitivity. Most common is ^{32}P-labeling through the alpha phosphate of a nucleotide that is incorporated into a probe by nick translation or random hexamer priming of a template. Also popular is **kinasing**, labeling the 5′-end of a DNA strand with ^{32}P or labeling the 3′-end with terminal deoxyribonucleotidyl transferase (TDT). Radioactive probes are becoming less popular with the availability of more convenient fluorescent and chemiluminescent probes.

Fluorescent Probes

Automated oligonucleotide synthesis has made fluorescent nucleic acid probes widely available. Assay designs with hybridization probes conventionally required a separation step. However, more recent homogeneous fluorescent techniques that do not require removal of excess free probe include fluorescent polarization, fluorescent resonance energy transfer (FRET), and fluorescent quenching. Fluorescent polarization can be used to distinguish free from bound label if the molecular rotation of the probe changes upon binding (10). Molecular rotation primarily depends upon the size of the molecule, so binding of a small probe onto a large target results in a polarization increase that can be measured. FRET techniques depend on the distance between two spectrally distinct fluorescent labels. The two labels are either brought closer together through hybridization, or end up farther apart, often through hydrolytic cleavage of a dual-labeled probe (11). Finally, fluorescent quenching or augmentation can occur with hybridization of a fluorescent oligonucleotide to its target. The effect depends on the specific fluorescent dye and the inherent quenching from G residues in the target and/or probe (12, 13). Alternately, quenching moieties can be purposely incorporated into the probe (14, 15).

Electronic Probes

Electronic detection of nucleic acid hybridization is an area of active research. Several designs attach a capture probe to an electrode surface. If the complementary target is present, it binds to the capture probe. The target, in turn binds to an electroactive, signaling probe that incorporates ferrocenyl derivatives that can be detected by AC voltammetry (16). Another design also uses capture, target, and signaling probes, although the signaling probes are attached to metal nanoparticles that change the conductivity between electrodes (17). Although labeled probes are usually used, detection with unlabeled probes has also been demonstrated. An unlabeled probe anchored to a field-effect sensor can detect hybridization to target by an increase in the local charge (18). It is difficult to make electronic methods sensitive and specific enough so that amplification is not required.

Indirect Detection Methods

Well-known indirect methods of detection can be used for nucleic acid detection, especially when the nucleic acid targets have been amplified. These methods usually require derivatized probes, multiple separation and washing steps, and often employ bifunctional conjugates for detection. For example, if a 5′-biotin-labeled probe and an adjacent 3′-digoxigenin-labeled probe are mixed with amplified target in the presence of a DNA ligase, the probes are joined together with biotin on one end and digoxigenin on the other. The probe can be immobilized on a strepavidin-coated plate, and color developed through an anti-digoxigenin antibody, alkaline phosphatase conjugate, and appropriate substrates (19).

Nucleic acids can also be linked to indicator molecules that emit light spontaneously under certain conditions. Chemiluminescence occurs when organic compounds are exposed to certain chemicals and the resulting reaction produces light. For example, when acridinium esters are exposed to hydrogen peroxide at high pH, light is emitted (20). Bioluminescence occurs when biomolecules produce light through catalysis of certain substrates. Alkaline phosphatase and peroxidase are examples of enzymes that can act on luminescent substrates to emit light. Luciferase is another example of a bioluminescent molecule. Luciferase has been used as an indicator of ATP generation in pyrosequencing (21). Electrochemiluminescence is initiated at an electrode surface in the presence of certain chelates of ruthenium (II). Once activated by charge transfer, chemiluminescence occurs (22).

Characterization/Multiplexing Methods

In addition to nucleic acid detection, characterization is usually required. Even if sequence-specific probes are used for detection, additional parameters that allow multiplex detection of more than one target are very useful. What are the characteristics of nucleic acids that can be used for differentiation and multiplexing?

Molecular Weight

The molecular weight of a single- or double-stranded nucleic acid is one of the most convenient and powerful ways to characterize different fragments. Size-separation of nucleic acids is usually achieved by electrophoresis through a matrix and the mobility is correlated to the length of the nucleic acid. For example, agarose gel electrophoresis is often used to size RNA or DNA fragments between 50 and 10,000 bases. Another example is the characterization of sequencing reaction products that require single-base resolution. Denaturing polyacrylamide gel electrophoresis (PAGE) in slab gels and capillary electrophoresis (CE) through linear polymers are both used for sequencing (23). PAGE, thin-layer chromatography, and high-pressure liquid chromatography (HPLC) are all common methods for separating and purifying oligonucleotides based on size.

Mass spectroscopy can be used for nucleic acid mass determination. Gentle methods of ionization, specifically matrix-assisted, laser desorption, time-of-flight mass spectroscopy (MALDI-TOF), allow typing of single-base extension products (24). Mass spectroscopy is most useful in characterizing small single-stranded fragments and can be used in the quality control of oligonucleotide synthesis.

Conformation

In addition to length, nucleic acid shape or conformation affects mobility through a matrix. For example, single-stranded DNA usually migrates differently from double-stranded

DNA of the same length. Furthermore, when different single-stranded nucleic acids of the same length fold, they form different shapes, depending on the sequence. When electrophoresis is used to measure differences in the shape of single strands, the technique is known as single-stranded conformation polymorphism analysis or SSCP (25).

When two strands of nucleic acid anneal together, the shape of the duplex depends on how well the sequences complement each other. If the sequences are perfectly matched, the duplex is referred to as a **homoduplex**. If the sequences are not completely complementary, **heteroduplexes** are present. Base mismatches result in bubbles and indels cause loops. Any variation from the regular double helix retards migration during electrophoresis. When electrophoretic migration is used to identify heteroduplexes, the technique is known as heteroduplex analysis (26). Instead of using electrophoresis, HPLC methods can also be used for heteroduplex analysis. The column is run at an elevated temperature to partly denature the heteroduplex products, a technique known as denaturing high-performance liquid chromatography or dHPLC (27).

Denaturing gradients can be applied during separation so that the conformation of the nucleic acid changes during electrophoresis. When the denaturant is a concentration gradient of a chemical, the method is known as **denaturing gradient gel electrophoresis (DGGE)** (28). When the denaturing gradient is temperature, the analogous method is **temperature gradient gel electrophoresis (TGGE)** (29, 30).

Fluorescence

Different fluorescent labels can be distinguished by their excitation and/or emission wavelength (color) and by fluorescent lifetime. Even though the wavelengths of different fluorescent labels often overlap, mathematical compensation algorithms are well developed, routinely applied, and highly accurate, particularly when the effect of temperature is considered (3). Examples include four-color sequencing and multicolor probe techniques. Time-resolved fluorometry can be used to distinguish labels that differ in fluorescent lifetime in addition to color. Different lanthanide labels, typically europium, terbium, and samarium, are attached to probes and distinguished based on their rate of decay after a flash of light (31).

Melting Curve Analysis

The melting curve of a duplex under defined conditions of buffer, ionic strength, and concentration is a characteristic property of the duplex. Conventional melting curve analysis using absorbance requires high concentrations of purified duplex. In contrast, fluorescent analysis can easily follow the melting transition of amplified products without any purification or manipulation. Fluorescent dyes can be used to characterize different DNA fragments (6) and melting analysis of labeled probes can genotype polymorphisms such as SNPs (11, 32).

High-resolution amplicon melting analysis is a new development with promise for discriminating different genotypes over an entire amplified fragment. Fluorescent-labeled primers (33), or certain double-stranded DNA (dsDNA) dyes can be used (34). The melting curves of different homozygotes are distinguished by melting temperature (Tm), and different heterozygotes are discriminated by the melting curve shape (Figure 1).

Spatial Separation

One way to keep track of different analyses that use the same detection method is to separate them in space. Multiplexing on a surface by spatial separation is generally known as

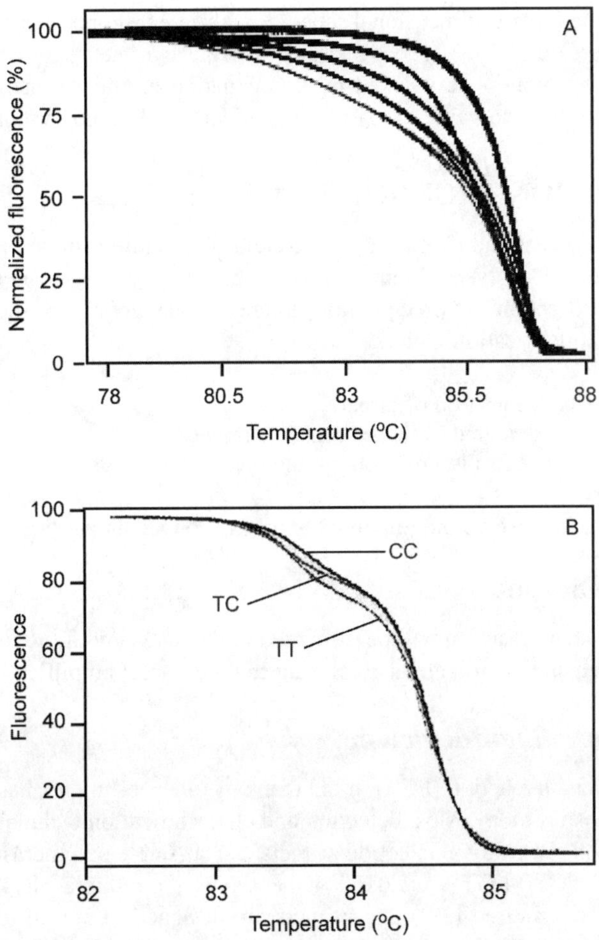

FIGURE 1. High-resolution melting analysis of PCR products in a closed-tube system. A: high-resolution melting curves for a 113 bp β-globin amplicon using a labeled primer. Wild type (AA) is at the top right. Curves for the heterozygous beta-globin SNP variants (AE, AS, AC, and SC) are shown in order progressing to bottom left. Two different samples for each genotype were amplified and are displayed. All heterozygotes were distinguishable from each other and the wild-type sequence. Rapid cycle PCR and melting analysis required, in total, less than 30 minutes (reprinted with permission from reference 33). B: high-resolution melting curves for a 544 bp amplicon of the gene HTR2A using the dsDNA dye, LCGreen I, including one common SNP locus. Duplicate samples of each genotype (CC, TC, and TT) were amplified by PCR. The melting curves showed two apparent melting domains. All genotypes were similar in the higher melting temperature domain, but differed in the lower melting domain where the SNP was located. (*Reprinted with permission from reference 34*).

array technology. Dot blots, line probes, 96-well microtiter plates, and high-density microarrays are familiar examples. Nucleic acid probes are arrayed on a matrix and every spot, well, or pixel is treated identically through the hybridization and detection process. Nucleic acid probes can be synthesized directly on the arrays, physically spotted, or addressed electronically (35). Arrays can be interrogated by any detection method, although fluorescence is most common.

Instead of one- or two-dimensional separation, different probes can be attached to different microspheres, and fluorescence measured by flow cytometry or through a fiber optic (36). The different probes are indexed by impregnating the microspheres with different amounts of spectrally resolvable dyes (37) or semiconductor nanocrystals (38).

AMPLIFICATION TECHNOLOGIES

Most methods to detect and characterize nucleic acids require sample preparation and/or amplification before analysis. Methods of sample preparation prior to amplification include organic extraction and precipitation, and reversible binding to silica or other matrices. Methods of amplification include:

- Increasing the concentration of target
- Amplifying specific signal in the presence of target
- Increasing the concentration of probe in the presence of target

Some of the more interesting and important amplification techniques are shown in Table 2.

Target Amplification

The polymerase chain reaction will be discussed in detail. Many of the topics covered for the polymerase chain reaction are also relevant to other target amplification techniques.

The Polymerase Chain Reaction

The polymerase chain reaction (PCR), more than any other technique, has enabled routine molecular diagnostics today. Most detection and characterization techniques require prior PCR amplification. Two oligonucleotide primers, a heat-stable polymerase, nucleotides of each base (dATP, dCTP, dGTP, and dTTP, collectively referred to as dNTPs), and the target in question are required (39). The primers are designed to anneal to opposite target strands so that the polymerase extends each primer toward the other. The samples are temperature-cycled between three temperatures, a high temperature sufficient to denature the target, a low temperature that allows annealing of the primers to the target, and a third temperature optimal for polymerase extension.

The primers are placed close enough together so that the polymerase extends each strand through the other priming site. If the efficiency of each cycle is optimal, the number of targets for priming and extension doubles each cycle (efficiency = 2.0). This means that under ideal conditions, the amount of target increases over 1000-fold after 10 cycles, 1,000,000-fold after 20 cycles, and one billion-fold after 30 cycles. At some point however, the efficiency of amplification falls and the amount of product plateaus, either from exhaustion of components or competition between primer and product annealing (11).

Rapid Cycle PCR. Automated instruments that cycle between temperatures using familiar conical tubes and metal heating blocks focus on accurate temperature control of the heating block at equilibrium, not on dynamic control of the sample temperature. As a result, temperature control at the sample is not well defined and long cycle times have become standard to ensure that the samples reach target temperatures. Reproducibility between instruments and manufacturers is poor and PCR often takes 2–4 hours to complete a typical 30-cycle amplification. The temperature cycling needs of PCR are surprisingly different from the usual engineering solution.

TABLE 2. Amplification technologies

	Abbreviations	Template	Oligos	Enzymes	Temperature	Reference
Target amplification						
Polymerase chain reaction	PCR	DNA	2	1	Cycling	39
Ligase chain reaction	LCR	DNA	4	1	Cycling	40
Transcription-based amplification	NASBA SSSR/3SR TMA	RNA/DNA	2	3	Isothermal[a]	41
Strand displacement amplification	SDA	DNA	4	2	Denature + Isothermal	42
Loop-mediated amplification	LAMP	DNA	4[b]	1	Denature + Isothermal	43
Linked-linear amplification	LLA	DNA	10–20	1	Cycling	44
Signal amplification						
Branched DNA	bDNA	RNA/DNA	Many	1	Multiple Incubations	45
Serial-invasive amplification	SISAR	DNA	3	1	Denature + Isothermal	46
Probe amplification						
Q-beta replicase		DNA/RNA	1[c]	1	Isothermal	47
Rolling-circle amplification	RCA	DNA	2–4	2	Denature + Isothermal	48
Isothermal oligo amplification		RNA/DNA	2	2	Isothermal[1]	49

[a]Initial denaturation is required for double-stranded DNA targets; [b]The four primers include six target recognition sequences; [c]The target sequence is embedded within the sequence of a replicatable RNA.

Denaturation, annealing, and extension are very rapid reactions as shown by experiments in capillaries (50). The actual time required for PCR depends on the size of the product, but when less than 500 bp in size, a 30-cycle amplification can easily be completed in 15 minutes. Furthermore, rapid amplification improves specificity. Product specificity is optimal when annealing times are less than 1 second. Denaturation is complete with a denaturation time of less than 1 second. However, the extension time needs to be adjusted for the length of the PCR product to ensure acceptable yield. Conventional temperature cycling compromises quality and time-to-result for convenience under the guise of high throughput.

Hot Start Techniques. When primers anneal to other primers or to undesired template regions, primer "dimers" and other unexpected products may be extended and amplified. This process is initiated during PCR preparation when the primers, template, and polymerase are all together at temperatures well below the annealing temperature of PCR. At these low temperatures the polymerase has decreased, but measurable activity, and some complexes may be extended to create undesired PCR templates. There are several ways in which the formation of these products can be minimized.

Hot start techniques limit polymerase activity until the temperature is raised. The enzyme can be manually added to the reaction after the samples reach a high temperature. Alternately, a physical barrier of wax can separate the essential components in the reaction. When the wax melts at high temperature, the components are mixed by convection. Another method uses an antibody or aptamer to bind and inactivate the polymerase at room temperature. At high temperature, the binding agent is released, activating the polymerase. Finally, the polymerase itself can be modified so that it is activated by heat, usually requiring an extended initial denaturation period.

Low-Copy Limitations. When PCR is performed under optimal conditions, a single copy of target can be detected. However, the statistical probability of getting that single copy into the reaction tube needs to be considered. If a PCR reaction is spiked with a dilute solution of template with an average of one target copy, some tubes will have no target (in fact, this will happen about 40%–45% of the time), while others will have one or more copies as determined by the Poisson distribution. If there is an average of two copies per tube, approximately 10% of the tubes will have no template and will provide a false-negative result. About five copies on average are necessary for 99% of the tubes to include at least one copy. Of course, this limitation of low-copy analysis is true for any amplification technique.

Preventing False-Positive Results—Contamination Control Measures. Because PCR can detect a single target molecule, the risk of contamination is similar to that of a microbiology laboratory. Sources of contamination include cross-contamination between samples within a run and contamination between runs with the amplification product. Contamination with PCR product can be a serious problem when gels are used for detection and characterization, particularly with open horizontal slab gels. Over a billion copies of product per reaction end up in the gel buffer and can easily turn the lab into a Dr. Seuss fiasco (51). The best way to prevent product contamination is to not let the product out of the tube. Methods that perform amplification, detection, and characterization in the same tube are called **closed-tube methods** and greatly reduce the risk of product contamination. If closed-tube analysis is not possible, PCR products can be modified chemically to prevent further amplification (52). Even with these precautions, a negative control or blank (all reactants except the target) remains an important control for PCR.

Preventing False-Negative Results—Inhibition Control Measures. PCR is surprisingly resilient and does not require highly purified nucleic acid. However, clinical samples can contain impurities that remain after sample preparation and inhibit polymerase activity. The potential for inhibitors suggests that if a product is not amplified, a control reaction is necessary to prove that the mixture supports amplification. Failure to amplify the control template indicates that the sample needs to be purified further to remove PCR inhibitors. In practice, with most sample types and well-defined preparation methods, inhibition rarely occurs.

Ligase Chain Reaction

In the ligase chain reaction (40), four oligonucleotides and a DNA ligase are used. Two of the oligonucleotides anneal directly adjacent to each other on the target. When they are joined (ligated), they form a target for the remaining two oligonucleotides (and vice versa). Just like PCR, temperature cycling is used and the target is ideally doubled each cycle.

Transcription-Based Amplification

This class of amplification reactions is partly based on retroviral replication (41). Isothermal target amplification, using the collective activities of reverse transcriptase, RNase H, and RNA polymerase are common to these methods. Usually a single-stranded RNA is the beginning template. A reverse transcriptase is used to synthesize a cDNA strand from the template RNA with a primer that has an RNA polymerase promoter as a 5′-tail. The RNA strand of the RNA/DNA duplex is then digested with RNAse H, followed by synthesis of dsDNA with an opposing primer. The promoter sequence on the dsDNA then promotes transcription of multiple copies of single-stranded RNA by the RNA polymerase, completing the cycle. Like PCR, all reagents can be included in one mixture and amplification is exponential with completion in less than an hour. Unlike PCR, temperature cycling is not required (except for an initial heat denaturation, especially if a DNA template is used). The method is particularly advantageous when the target is RNA (e.g., HIV and HCV in blood bank nucleic acid testing) and is used in several commercial assays, including nucleic acid sequence base amplification (53), self-sustained sequence replication (41), and transcription-mediated amplification (54).

Strand Displacement Amplification

Another isothermal amplification technique is strand displacement amplification (42). After heat denaturation of DNA in the presence of four primers, dCTP, dGTP, dUTP, and the modified deoxynucleotide, dATPαS, two enzymes are added, an exonuclease-deficient polymerase and a restriction enzyme. The two flanking primers that enter into exponential amplification have a restriction site added to their 5′-end, and get nicked by the restriction enzyme, allowing displacement of strands that can in turn be primed, extended, and nicked. Deoxy-ATPαS is needed so that the restriction sites include a hemiphosphorothioate linkage resulting in single-strand nicking instead of double-strand cutting.

Loop-Mediated Amplification

The target amplification methods presented so far produce a defined length of RNA or DNA according to the placement of the primers. In loop-mediated isothermal amplification (LAMP), multiple populations of repeated stem-loops produce concatenated structures of variable length and branching (43). After DNA denaturation, the process is isothermal, requiring four primers and a polymerase. Two of the primers each recognize two distinct sequences on the target DNA, resulting in loops forming at the end of extension products. Repeated strand displacement DNA synthesis results in the final mixture of products.

Linked-Linear Amplification

If two PCR primers include elements that cannot be replicated, an exponential expansion is reduced to arithmetic accumulation. However, if multiple nested sets of internal primers (also nonreplicable) are included, product accumulation (at least in theory) can approach that of PCR. This process is known as linked-linear amplification (44). It requires a polymerase, several sets of nested primer pairs, and thermal cycling similar to PCR.

Signal Amplification Techniques

Instead of increasing the concentration of target, signal amplification techniques use nucleic acids to magnify the detection signal. Two methods are in common use.

Branched DNA (bDNA)

The bDNA approach hybridizes the target nucleic acid to multiple capture probes affixed to a microtiter well. This is followed by hybridization to a series of extender, preamplifier, and amplifier probes. The final, highly branched amplifier probe includes multiple copies of an enzyme that act on a chemiluminescent substrate to produce light (45). The nucleotide analogs isoC and isoG can be used to increase specificity of the signaling cascade.

Serial-Invasive Amplification

When two probes overlap on one target, an **invasive cleavage reaction** can be catalyzed by certain structure-specific nucleases. The cleaved fragment, in turn, can cause invasive cleavage of a secondary hairpin probe. The hairpin probe can be designed as a fluorogenic indicator by using a reporter/quencher pair of dyes that are separated by cleavage. This serial sequence of events, primary invasion and cleavage, followed by secondary invasion and cleavage of an indicator probe, is known as the serial-invasive signal amplification reaction, or SISAR (46). After DNA denaturation, cooling, and the addition of enzyme, the reaction is run at a temperature that results in recycling of both the primary and secondary reactions.

Probe Amplification

In this class of amplification techniques, the concentration of probe increases if the target is present. Similar to target amplification, a large amount of nucleic acid makes detection relatively easy.

Q-beta Replicase

A replicatable RNA probe is amplified exponentially in the presence of the RNA-directed RNA polymerase, Q-beta replicase (47). The probe is a recombinant RNA hybrid that includes sequence complementary to the target embedded in a naturally occurring template for the enzyme. Separation of bound from unbound hybrid is necessary before detection with Q-beta replicase.

Rolling-Circle Amplification

If a primer is annealed to a closed circle of DNA in the presence of a processive, displacing polymerase, the complement of the circle will be synthesized over and over again with displacement of the tandem repeats (48). If two primers are used in opposite orientation, progressively more complex branches will be formed in an exponential reaction. Rolling-circle amplification can be triggered by ligation of the two ends of a linear probe on template DNA. Ligation may happen directly, after polymerization through a gap, or after annealing of an additional, allele-specific oligonucleotide.

Isothermal Oligo Amplification

Short oligonucleotides, 8–16 bases in length can be linearly produced at a constant temperature in the presence of a polymerase and a nicking enzyme (49). The replication can be exponential if the amplification template is in excess and contains two complementary copies of the signal oligonucleotide. The signal oligonucleotide, or trigger, is originally produced by hybridization of a **trigger template** to the target, generating the oligonucleotide trigger by extension and nicking.

GENOTYPING METHODS

There are many genotyping methods. The best choice depends on several factors, including the types of sequence alterations present, for example:

- Highly variable loci are efficiently typed by sequencing.
- Simple sequence repeats are best sized by electrophoresis after PCR.
- SNPs can be rapidly typed in closed tubes by melting curve analysis.

Turnaround time and throughput requirements are also considerations. The needs of high-volume genomic research are different from a clinical reference laboratory, a medical clinic, or the stat laboratories of the future. A recent compilation of articles on molecular diagnostics is one source for further reading (55). Most of the following methods use PCR for amplification before genotyping.

Sequencing

DNA sequencing (23) is now a technique routinely performed in the clinical laboratory. The actual nucleic acid sequence of a DNA fragment can be determined and compared to a reference sequence with an accuracy around 99.9% (one misidentified base in 1000). Often the sequence is analyzed on both strands (sense and antisense), providing even greater accuracy. Any deviation from the reference sequence is identified using computer programs matching the sequences. Base changes resulting in a stop codon, altered amino acid code, or frame shift (deletions or insertions) are identified.

The most common sequencing strategy uses PCR in the first step to amplify the region of interest, followed by a variation of the chain-termination reaction developed by Sanger in the late 1970s (56). This technique generates fragments terminated at various lengths by incorporation of one of four dideoxynucleotide base analogs during extension from the sequencing primer. Dideoxynucleotides lack the 3′-hydroxyl group (OH) as well as the 2′-OH on the pentose ring, and because DNA chain growth requires the addition of deoxynucleotides to the 3′-OH group, incorporation of this base analog terminates chain growth. The most common method for generating these terminated fragments is **cycle sequencing**, which consists of thermally cycling to repeat the Sanger reaction by use of a thermostable DNA polymerase, ensuring efficient utilization of the primers. The fragments generated by the Sanger reaction are tagged with a fluorescent dye (either by use of labeled primers or labeled terminator dideoxynucleotides), then separated by denaturing polyacrylamide gel or capillary electrophoresis, and detected by automated fluorescent detection as the fragments travel past the detector. When fluorescent-labeled primers are used, the termination reaction for each of the four bases needs to be performed in separate tubes, and then combined prior to electrophoresis. The use of four terminators each having a different color label has made it possible to significantly streamline the process requiring only one tube for the reaction. About 600 bases are routinely resolved by a 2.5-hour run on capillary electrophoresis instruments.

DNA sequencing is most commonly used in infectious disease testing, such as genotyping of HCV and analysis of HIV for drug resistance assessment. Whole gene sequencing for the detection of disease-causing mutations is still an expensive proposition, whether it is for population screening (in which the majority of samples will not have a mutation) or even for patients affected with the disease. Therefore, in genetic testing, DNA sequencing is often performed only after an initial **mutation scanning assay** has identified samples that contain sequence alterations.

Pyrosequencing

Pyrosequencing (21) is a method to determine the nucleic acid sequence of short segments without the use of electrophoresis. A sequencing primer is hybridized to the template (usually generated by PCR), and incubated in the presence of four enzymes, DNA polymerase, ATP sulfurylase, luciferase, and apyrase. The instrument adds one of the four dNTPs to the reaction, and if it is complementary to the template strand at the next position, DNA polymerase extends the primer. Each incorporation event is accompanied by release of pyrophosphate (PPi) in quantities equimolar to the amount of incorporated nucleotide. The release of PPi is monitored by conversion of PPi into ATP, and ATP in the presence of luciferase generates light. The light intensity is proportional to the number of nucleotides incorporated. Apyrase, which is a nucleotide-degrading enzyme, continuously degrades ATP and any unincorporated dNTPs. As the process is repeated by adding one dNTP at a time, the complementary DNA strand is built and the nucleotide sequence is determined. The nucleotide dATPαS is used instead of dATP because it is a substrate for the polymerase, but not the luciferase. This automated technique is useful when the sequence of a large number of short segments needs to be determined.

Oligonucleotide Extension

Minisequencing, also known as single-base primer extension or single nucleotide extension (SNE), requires annealing of an primer to a single-stranded PCR product immediately adjacent to, but not including, the SNP site. This is followed by enzymatic extension of the primer in the presence of a polymerase and dideoxynucleotide terminators. Each of the four terminators is labeled with a unique label so that the incorporated base can be identified. The most common label is fluorescent, so that electrophoresis can be performed on an automated DNA sequencing instrument. This allows multiplexing by using primers of varying lengths so that several SNPs can be resolved in an electrophoresis run.

Oligonucleotide extension assays can also be analyzed by matrix-assisted laser desorption ionization time-of-flight (MALDI-TOF) mass spectrometry (24). With mass spectroscopy, no label is necessary because all four nucleotides differ in mass. However, salt and excess dNTPs interfere, requiring several purification steps through PCR, single-strand isolation, primer extension, and mixing the sample with the desorption matrix. Despite its complexity, the process can be automated.

Allele-specific PCR is a simple genotyping method that is based on a preference by the polymerase to extend perfectly matched primers. If the 3′-end of a primer complements the allele, extension (and amplification) will occur. If there is a mismatch, amplification will be less efficient or not occur at all. This strategy can be used for distinguishing a gene from its pseudogenes and for genotyping of SNPs. By monitoring for products each cycle (real-time analysis), it is easy to observe differences in efficiency, genotype, and even calculate allele frequencies in pools of DNA for population studies (57).

Fragment Size

Many conventional molecular techniques rely heavily on identification of fragment size by gel electrophoresis. For example, if cellular RNA is isolated, run out on a denaturing gel, blotted, and exposed to a specific probe, mRNAs that hybridize to the probe will be identified as bands, a process known as **Northern blotting**. If DNA is digested with a restriction enzyme, the DNA will be cut at specific sequences and a wide range of DNA fragment sizes will result. If the digested DNA is run out on a gel, blotted, and probed, the process is known as **Southern blotting**. Southern blot analysis provides information on structural alterations such as large deletions, duplications, insertions, rearrangements, and the number of repeats within probed fragments. Polymorphisms detected by this technique are known as **restriction fragment length polymorphisms (RFLPs)**. Southern and Northern analysis is labor intensive and, when possible, has been replaced by amplification methods.

When PCR is followed by restriction enzyme digestion, the PCR product is cut into fragments. If the restriction enzyme is chosen so that the sequence recognized is present in one allele but not another, different alleles show different banding patterns after gel electrophoresis and staining. This method, known as PCR/RFLP is a very common method of genotyping that any laboratory can perform.

Instead of allele-specific digestion, allele-specific ligation can also be used for genotyping. For example, if a PCR-generated target is hybridized to adjacent probes in the presence of a DNA ligase, the two probes will be joined if and only if the probes are homologous to the target at the point of ligation. In one format, a fluorescent-labeled probe is common to both alleles, and two other allele-specific probes compete for ligation and differ in electrophoretic mobility. Many loci can be analyzed at once on automated sequencing instruments by controlling the mobility of the allele-specific probes (58). Ligation can also be used to join two ends of a long, single "padlock" probe when both ends perfectly anneal to adjacent sites on the target. The resulting circle can be amplified by rolling-circle amplification (48).

Hybridization Techniques

All hybridization assays are based on the ability of single-stranded nucleic acids to form double-stranded hybrids. The process requires that probe and target nucleic acid are mixed under conditions that allow hybridization, and a method to detect any resulting double-stranded hybrids. The probe is a nucleic acid whose identity is known, and the target or sample is a nucleic acid whose concentration or identity is not known. The hybridization may be tethered to a surface or free in solution. Both solid phase and liquid phase assays are used in the clinical laboratory.

Surface Hybridization

Nucleic acids bound on a solid matrix can still bind complementary nucleic acids. Solid phase assays are useful because multiple samples can be processed together, facilitating control, washing, and separation procedures. However, hybridization on a solid support is less efficient than solution hybridization and the kinetics are slower and more difficult to predict.

Dot Blots and Line Probes. Conventional hybridization assays on membranes are known as dot blots or line probes, depending on the geometry of the individual spots. After the nucleic acids are immobilized, the membrane is incubated with complementary nucleic acid at a constant temperature, followed by one or more washes to discriminate matched from mismatched nucleic acid. The method allows multiple probe–target hybridizations to be carried out simultaneously under identical conditions.

Usually, amplified fragments of target DNA are used. Multiple samples may be attached to the membrane and interrogated with solution phase probes (similar to a Southern blot). Alternately, if multiple probes are bound to the membrane in a **reverse dot blot**, the amplified DNA from one sample can be interrogated at multiple loci. Usually, the nucleic acid in solution is labeled with radioactivity or fluorescence. Interpretation of hybridization assays is usually qualitative. As the level of multiplexing increases, it becomes challenging to find a hybridization condition that provides adequate discrimination for all probe–target combinations.

Arrays. Microarrays further extend the concept of increasing the density of individual hybridization assays. Microarrays, also called DNA arrays or DNA chips, were developed in the 1990s (59, 60). In microarrays, the spot size is typically less than 200 μm in diameter so that one array can contain thousands of spots. Microarrays are fabricated on solid surfaces (usually glass, but also gel pads and gold). The probes may be synthesized on the array, addressed electronically, or spotted with the aid of robotics. To synthesize probes in situ, the entire chip is exposed to one of the base precursors (A, C, G, or T) and light is used to extend only the desired elements with that base. The process is repeated until the probes are the desired length. Another approach is to use a matrix of electrodes covered with individual gel pads. Each probe (or sample) is addressed electronically to the desired elements by electrophoresis and immobilized in the gel with biotin–streptavidin capture. Both of these methods, as well as mechanical spotting with "arrayers" require a lot of work to produce the chips. Even so, because of their massively parallel capacity, microarrays have attracted great interest in applications where thousands of analyses are useful. Examples include discovery experiments using expression arrays for mRNAs and the correlation of SNPs to disease. Medium-density arrays cover the middle ground between high-density microarrays and classical dot blots or line probes (35, 37, 61).

Solution Hybridization

Hybridization in solution is faster and more precise than hybridization on a surface. Classical methods of solution hybridization required separation of the bound and free label by exclusion chromatography, electrophoresis, or capture of the probe–target hybrid by hydroxyapatite, magnetic beads, or other affinity capture agent. For example, if an RNA–DNA hybrid is formed, an immobilized antibody against RNA–DNA complexes can be used in a **hybrid capture assay**.

Recently, solution hybridization has been combined with amplification, detection, and quantification all in the same tube. These homogeneous, nonseparation or real-time assays, do not require any additions, washing steps, or separation steps.

Quantitative Real-Time PCR. Amplification methods are only quantitative under certain conditions. Variations in sample preparation, the presence of enzyme inhibitors, and the eventual plateau of amplification are major concerns. Amplification reactions that require temperature cycling have a quantitative advantage over isothermal reactions because the reaction rate is limited (paced) by the thermal cycling. Real-time PCR offers a convenient and systematic approach to quantification by monitoring the amount of product each cycle (62). In contrast to endpoint analysis where multiple reactions were necessary to ensure accurate quantification, real-time PCR monitors the progress of the reaction with cycle number and uses the position of the curve to calculate the initial target concentration. Quantitative PCR is usually carried out with reference standards of known amounts. The standards can be PCR products, plasmids, or RNA packaged into synthetic virus particles to mimic real viruses. For accurate quantification by endpoint analysis, the need for internal controls that compete for the same primers is generally accepted (competitive PCR). In contrast, real-time PCR usually employs external quantification standards that are in different tubes. The number of standards needed and types of controls necessary continues to be actively discussed.

One of the advantages of real-time PCR is its large dynamic range. Figure 2A shows an extended range of external standards in a typical real-time PCR. As the initial template concentration increases, the curves shift to earlier cycles. The cycle where fluorescence first rises correlates inversely to the log of the initial template concentration (Figure 2B). This cycle is actually a virtual cycle that includes a fractional component determined by interpolation that can be calculated by several methods. The most common methods include using a horizontal threshold after baseline adjustment and using the second derivative maximum of each curve. The second derivative method appears to be more precise (62).

Viral Load Methods. Perhaps the most common clinical use of real-time PCR is in the assessment of viral load, particularly for HIV and HCV. The clinical need for quantification is well established and real-time methods can give rapid and precise answers. However, other amplification systems, particularly transcription-based and branched DNA methods are also available in this highly competitive field.

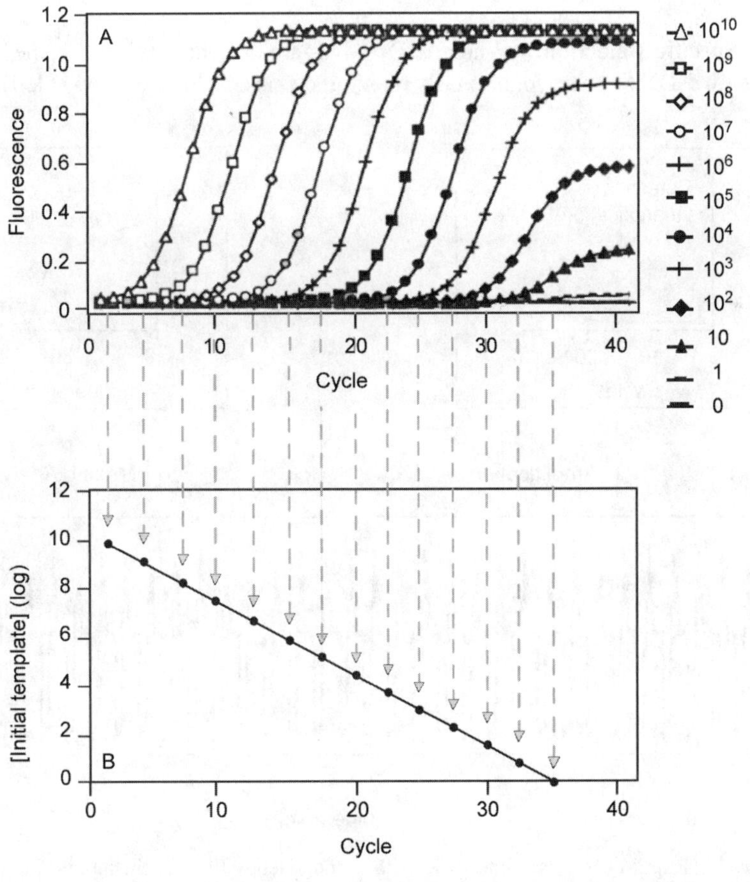

FIGURE 2. Idealized standard curves for quantitative real-time PCR over a 10^{10}-fold range of initial template concentration. A: the logistic equation was used to generate titration curves with an efficiency of 2.0. The carrying capacity was progressively decreased at 10^4 copies and below. Actual standard curves will vary from this ideal, depending on the fluorescent indicator used (11). B: the second derivative maximum of each curve is plotted as a fractional cycle number against the log of the initial template concentration. (*Reprinted with permission from reference 62*)

Melting Curve Analysis. Not only can amplification, detection, and quantification be performed by solution hybridization, but detailed genotyping information can also be obtained. Genotyping is best performed in the same tube by monitoring the melting of hybridized duplexes during controlled heating, producing a melting curve signature for the duplex. Such a signature monitors duplex binding over a range of temperatures, compared to the single temperature analysis of conventional hybridization techniques such as dot blots or microarrays. The advantages of a complete melting curve also holds when only homogeneous techniques are compared. For example, methods that rely on hydrolysis for signal generation and/or those that acquire data at only one temperature generally result in more genotyping errors (63). Amplification and melting analysis are a powerful combination that only requires temperature control and sampling of fluorescence. Most of the other genotyping techniques discussed require complex separation and/or detection equipment after PCR. Real-time PCR with melting curve analysis allows detection, quantification, and genotyping in less than 30 minutes (Figure 3) without ancillary processing or additional equipment. A book series on methods and application of rapid-cycle, real-time PCR has been published (64–66).

Primer-Specific Detection. When dsDNA dyes are present during PCR, the conversion of single- to dsDNA can be continuously monitored (11) (*see* Figure 4, lower left). Although

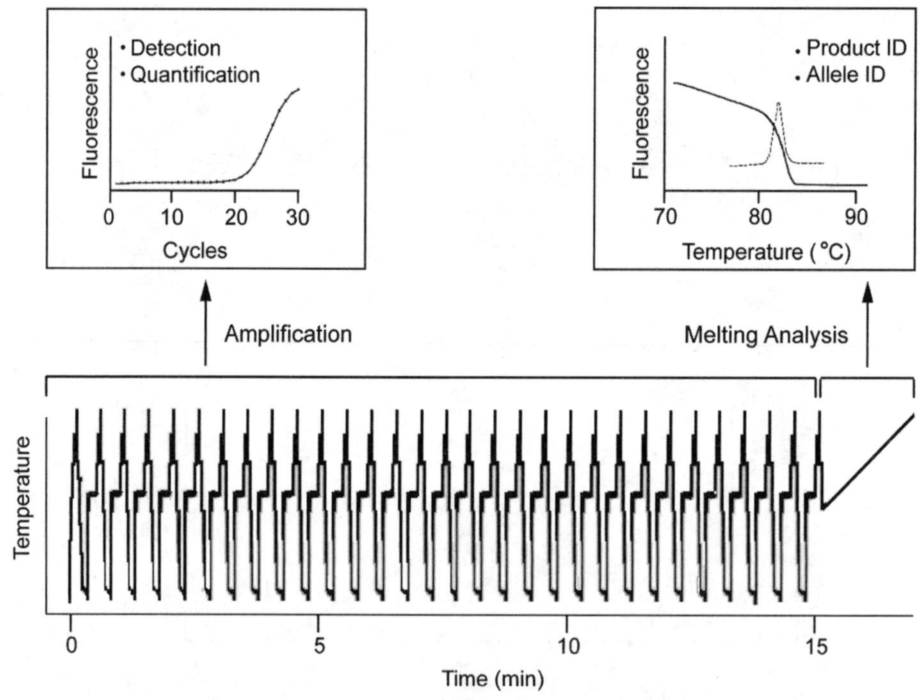

FIGURE 3. Rapid cycle, real-time PCR with homogeneous fluorescent monitoring. With rapid cycle PCR, 30-second cycles are typical, requiring about 15 minutes for 30 cycles. During cycling, data for detection and quantification are obtained by monitoring fluorescence once each cycle at the end of extension. Amplification is immediately followed by continuous acquisition of a melting curve during relatively slow heating (0.1–0.4 °C/second). The melting curve plot can be optionally converted to a derivative plot. Melting curves are used to identify PCR products (6, 33, 34) and sequence alterations (32). (*Reprinted with permission from reference 62*)

ethidium bromide was the first dye used in real-time PCR (67), SYBR Green I is more commonly used today. Introduced to real-time PCR in 1997 (11), SYBR Green I has fluorescent properties similar to fluorescein, allowing the same optics to be used for both. During PCR, SYBR Green I also distinguishes double- from single-stranded DNA better than ethidium bromide (62). SYBR Green I is commonly used for real-time quantification when the expense and specificity of a probe is not needed. Specificity can be improved by acquiring fluorescence just under the melting temperature of the desired product (68). High-resolution melting curve analysis (34) can even genotype SNPs from PCR product melting curves (Figure 1). SYBR Green I can be used to monitor PCR once each cycle or to continuously monitor hybridization throughout amplification at all temperatures (Figure 4, left).

Fluorescent-labeled primers can also be used to monitor PCR. In one system, a primer labeled with a fluorophore and a quencher in a hairpin conformation straightens out during PCR, resulting in an increase in fluorescence (69). If the sequence of the primer is carefully considered, the quencher moiety is not necessary (13). Labeled primers can be used for amplicon genotyping by melting analysis because of fluorescent changes observed with hybridization (33).

In another primer-specific design, isoC and isoG are incorporated into a nonhomologous 5′-tail of an allele specific primer (70). The tail is not replicated during PCR and hybridizes to quenched dual-labeled probes that form a **double flap gap**. This structure is a substrate for polymerase 5′-exonuclease activity and the probe is hydrolyzed, separating the quencher and thereby increasing reporter fluorescence.

One advantage of fluorescent-labeled primers over dsDNA dyes is that multiplexing is possible. However, with both dsDNA dyes and labeled primers, reaction specificity depends on the specificity of the primers. Any double-stranded product that is formed is at risk of detection, including primer dimers. Therefore, hot start techniques, temperature

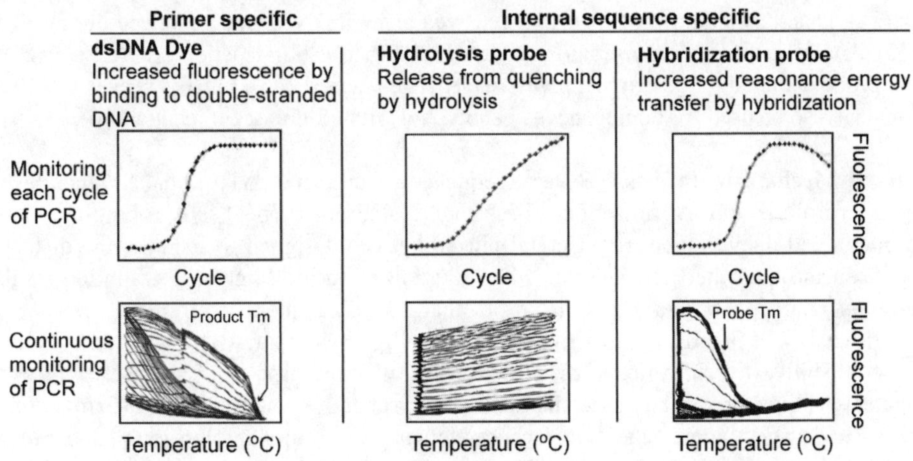

FIGURE 4. Typical real-time PCR amplification monitored with SYBR Green I, hydrolysis probes or hybridization probes. Reactions monitored once each cycle are displayed on fluorescence versus cycle number plots (top). Continuously monitored reactions are shown on fluorescence versus temperature plots (bottom). Note the reversible hybridization information inherent in the reactions monitored with SYBR Green I and hybridization probes. Product melting temperature (Tm) can be determined with SYBR Green I, and probe Tm is apparent when hybridization probes are used. For both hybridization and hydrolysis probes, fluorescence is not proportional to product amount, most obviously seen at higher cycle numbers. (*Reprinted with permission from reference 62*)

discrimination by collecting real-time data at a high temperature, and melting curve analysis to confirm the desired product are useful.

Fluorescent probes that hybridize to PCR products during amplification change fluorescence by two possible mechanisms:

- A covalent bond between two dyes is broken by hydrolysis or made through ligation.
- The fluorescent change follows reversible hybridization of the probe to the target.

Following this distinction, when an irreversible covalent bond is involved, the probes are called **hydrolysis probes**. When a probe reversibly changes fluorescence on duplex formation, they are called **hybridization probes** (71). One major difference between the two probe types is that melting analysis is possible with hybridization, but not hydrolysis, probes. The cycle-by-cycle and continuous amplification plots of the two probe types, along with a dsDNA dye for comparison, are shown in Figure 4.

Reversible Hybridization. Hybridization probes change fluorescence upon hybridization, usually by fluorescent energy transfer. One fluorophore can be placed on a primer and the other on a probe (32), or the interacting fluorophores may be placed on adjacent probes (72). The 3′-ends of the probes are blocked to prevent extension. If the deoxyguanosine content of the probe and target is considered, only a single probe with one fluorophore can be used (12). Single probe, single fluorophore assays using fluorescent enhancement of thiazole orange have also been reported (73).

Irreversible Hydrolysis. If a probe labeled with a fluorophore and a quencher is hydrolyzed during PCR and the labels are separated, fluorescence will increase. The most common technique uses the 5′-exonuclease activity of the PCR polymerase to hydrolyze the probe and dissociate the labels (14). A minor groove binder can be used to increase specificity (74). Dual-labeled probes can also be cleaved using a DNAzyme generated during PCR (75). Another example is the serial-invasive signal amplification reaction, where cleavage of the probe is linked to the original invasive cleavage reaction (46). Finally, irreversible ligation can also be used for homogeneous genotyping with a fluorescent readout (76).

Mixed Mechanism Probes. Several sequence-specific methods probably function by both hydrolysis and hybridization. These include hairpin probes, self-probing amplicon primers, and displacement probes. Hairpin probes are designed to increase the distance between the quencher and reporter when hybridized to the target (15). Similarly, self-probing amplicon primers have a hairpin that separates quencher from reporter when hybridized (77). Finally, competitive displacement probes separate quencher and reporter by competitive hybridization (78). However, in all three cases, polymerases with exonuclease activity are usually used and the labeled probes are potential substrates for exonuclease cleavage. Indeed, the fluorescence versus cycle number plots often look more similar to irreversible hydrolysis than reversible hybridization (Figure 4). Conversely, many exonuclease probes, especially probes labeled on each end (79) show significant reversible hybridization signals.

Comparison of Closed-Tube SNP Genotyping Methods. Methods for homogeneous SNP analysis in a closed-tube system differ greatly in their level of complexity (Table 3). All these methods use fluorescence and solution hybridization, and the number of oligonucleotides required varies from 2 to 8. The simpler techniques do not

TABLE 3. Closed-tube methods for SNP typing[a]

Method	Number of Oligos	Mods[b]	Mods/Oligo[c]	Alleles	Technique[d]	Reference
Amplicon melting	2	0	0	2 or more	PCR/melting	34, 80
Unlabeled probe melting	3	0	0	2 or more	PCR/melting	81
Real-time allele-specific PCR	3	0	0	2	Real-time PCR	57
Allele-specific PCR with a GC clamp	3	1 GC tail	1	2	PCR/melting	82
Single probe melting	3	1	1	2 or more	PCR/melting	32
Two probe melting	4	2	1	2 or more	PCR/melting	72
Ligase-mediated FRET	5	3	1	2	Endpoint	76
5′-Exonuclease	4	4	2	2	Endpoint	14, 79
Dual-labeled hairpin	4	4	2	2	Endpoint	15
Self-probing amplicon	3–4	6	3	2	Endpoint	77
3′-Minor groove binder 5′-exonuclease	4	6	3	2	Endpoint	74
Serial invasive signal amplification	5	4	2	2	Endpoint	46
Allele-specific PCR double flap gap	5	8	2	2	Endpoint	70
Ligation with rolling-circle amplification	8	4	2	2	Endpoint	48

[a]Listed in order of approximate complexity; [b]Number of total oligonucleotide modifications (usually fluorophore or quencher additions); [c]Maximum number of modifications per oligonucleotide; [d]Endpoint assays can be monitored in real time, but real time instrumentation is not necessary.

require probes at all, while some of the more complex require up to three labels or modifications on each probe. Some of the methods that use melting analysis will detect more than two alleles if present, while those based on allele-specific amplification or endpoint analysis are limited to two. Figure 5 illustrates three different methods of SNP genotyping that utilize melting analysis differing in the number of labeled oligonucleotides that are required.

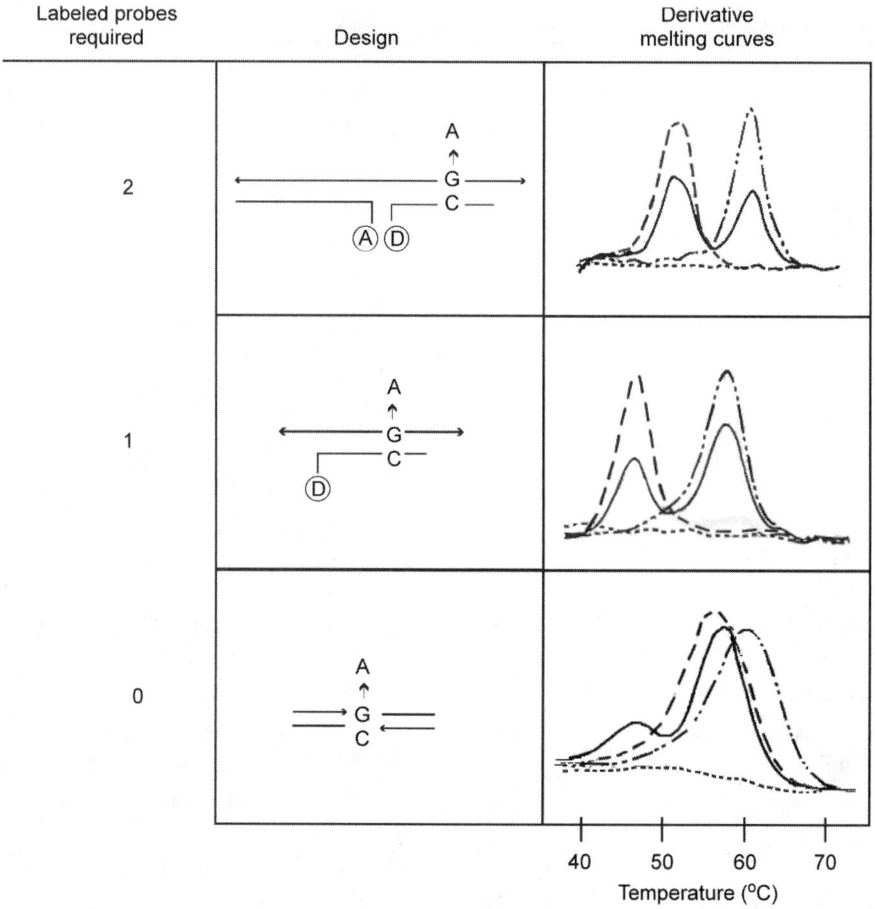

FIGURE 5. Homogeneous, closed-tube SNP genotyping by melting analysis. Three different fluorescent methods that require different numbers of labeled probes are shown. Conventional melting curve analysis for genotyping requires two probes (top), one labeled with a donor fluorophore (D) and the other labeled with an acceptor fluorophore (A). One of the probes anneals to a consensus sequence and is more stable than the other probe placed over the polymorphic site. As the temperature is raised, the less stable probe melts off, revealing the genotypes by their stability difference. Derivative melting curves are shown with a negative template control (dots), homozygous mutant (dash), heterozygous (solid), and homozygous wild type (dash-dot-dot) genotypes displayed. In the middle design, only one probe is used. The change in fluorescence results directly from quenching or enhancement of a donor fluorophore upon hybridization (D). Finally, SNP genotyping without any probes is possible in the presence of the dye LCGreen I (34, 80). A small product flanking the polymorphism is amplified in the presence of the dye. Different homozygotes have different melting temperatures, and heterozygotes show a heteroduplex peak. Melting acquisition requires only 1–2 minutes.

Haplotyping

Allele-specific PCR is the most common method used for haplotyping (83). Another method uses single molecule dilution of genomic DNA to separate alleles physically, followed by amplification and analysis (84).

TABLE 4. Commercial suppliers of molecular diagnostics systems

Company	Technology	http://www
Roche Diagnostics	PCR	roche-diagnostics.com
Abbott	LCR	abbottdiagnostics.com
Gen-Probe	TMA	gen-probe.com
B-D Biosystems	SDA	bd.com
Digene	Hybrid capture	digene.com
Affymetrix	Arrays	affymetrix.com

Methylation Status

To detect CpG methylation, DNA is first treated chemically with bisulfite, which changes any 5-methylcytosines (but not unmethylated cytosines) to uracils. This is usually followed by an allele-specific PCR that discriminates between cytosines and uracils at the PCR primer sites. The amplification is best done in real-time to obtain quantitative information. An interesting alternative is to detect the cytosine-to-uracil changes within a PCR product by melting curve analysis (85). Each methylated base results in conversion of a C::G base pair to an A::T base pair within the PCR product, lowering the melting temperature of the resultant PCR products as detected by SYBR Green I.

COMMERCIAL SUPPLIERS

In this chapter, the authors made an effort not to refer to commercial suppliers or to make comparative judgments between commercial instruments and systems. However, Table 4 includes web links to several manufacturers of clinical molecular diagnostics instrumentation.

FINAL NOTE

Conventional molecular analysis often requires many steps, including sample preparation, amplification, and analysis. As a result, automated methods have been successfully developed. However, simple techniques that do not require automation are always better than equivalent, more complex methods. Techniques that require separation and washing steps are being replaced with nonseparation methods that are rapid and homogeneous with data available in real-time.

REFERENCES

1. Lander ES, Linton LM, Birren B, Nusbaum C, Zody MC, Baldwin J, et al. Initial sequencing and analysis of the human genome. Nature 2001;409:860–921.
2. Laird PW. The power and the promise of DNA methylation markers. Nat Rev Cancer 2003;3:253–66.
3. Wittwer CT, Herrmann MG, Gundry CN, Elenitoba-Johnson KS. Real-time multiplex PCR assays. Methods 2001;25:430–42.
4. von Ahsen N, Wittwer CT, Schutz E. Oligonucleotide melting temperatures under PCR conditions: nearest-neighbor corrections for Mg(2+), deoxynucleotide triphosphate, and dimethyl sulfoxide concentrations with comparison to alternative empirical formulas. Clin Chem 2001;47:1956–61.

5. Gurrieri S, Wells KS, Johnson ID, Bustamante C. Direct visualization of individual DNA molecules by fluorescence microscopy: characterization of the factors affecting signal/background and optimization of imaging conditions using YOYO. Anal Biochem 1997;249: 44–53.
6. Ririe KM, Rasmussen RP, Wittwer CT. Product differentiation by analysis of DNA melting curves during the polymerase chain reaction. Anal Biochem 1997;245:154–60.
7. Hopfenbeck JA, Holden JA, Wittwer CT, Kjeldsberg CR. Digoxigenin-labeled probes amplified from genomic DNA detect T-cell gene rearrangements. Am J Clin Pathol 1992;97:638–44.
8. Wetmur JG. DNA probes: applications of the principles of nucleic acid hybridization. Crit Rev Biochem Mol Biol 1991;26:227–59.
9. Wittwer CT, Herrmann MG. Rapid thermal cycling and PCR kinetics. In: Innis M, Gelfand D, Sninsky J, eds. PCR methods manual. San Diego: Academic Press, 1999:211–29.
10. Kwok PY. SNP genotyping with fluorescence polarization detection. Hum Mutat 2002;19: 315–23.
11. Wittwer CT, Herrmann MG, Moss AA, Rasmussen RP. Continuous fluorescence monitoring of rapid cycle DNA amplification. Biotechniques 1997;22:130–1, 134–8.
12. Crockett AO, Wittwer CT. Fluorescein-labeled oligonucleotides for real-time PCR: using the inherent quenching of deoxyguanosine nucleotides. Anal Biochem 2001;290:89–97.
13. Nazarenko I, Pires R, Lowe B, Obaidy M, Rashtchian A. Effect of primary and secondary structure of oligodeoxyribonucleotides on the fluorescent properties of conjugated dyes. Nucleic Acids Res 2002;30:2089–195.
14. Lee LG, Connell CR, Bloch W. Allelic discrimination by nick-translation PCR with fluorogenic probes. Nucleic Acids Res 1993;21:3761–6.
15. Tyagi S, Bratu DP, Kramer FR. Multicolor molecular beacons for allele discrimination. Nat Biotechnol 1998;16:49–53.
16. Yu CJ, Wan Y, Yowanto H, Li J, Tao C, James MD, et al. Electronic detection of single-base mismatches in DNA with ferrocene-modified probes. J Am Chem Soc 2001;123:11155–61.
17. Park SJ, Taton TA, Mirkin CA. Array-based electrical detection of DNA with nanoparticle probes. Science 2002;295:1503–6.
18. Fritz J, Cooper EB, Gaudet S, Sorger PK, Manalis SR. Electronic detection of DNA by its intrinsic molecular charge. Proc Natl Acad Sci USA 2002;99:14142–6.
19. Nickerson DA, Kaiser R, Lappin S, Stewart J, Hood L, Landegren U. Automated DNA diagnostics using an ELISA-based oligonucleotide ligation assay. Proc Natl Acad Sci USA 1990;87: 8923–7.
20. Nelson NC, Cheikh AB, Matsuda E, Becker MM. Simultaneous detection of multiple nucleic acid targets in a homogeneous format. Biochemistry 1996;35:8429–38.
21. Ronaghi M, Uhlen M, Nyren P. A sequencing method based on real-time pyrophosphate. Science 1998;281:363, 365.
22. Blackburn GF, Shah HP, Kenten JH, Leland J, Kamin RA, Link J, et al. Electrochemiluminescence detection for development of immunoassays and DNA probe assays for clinical diagnostics. Clin Chem 1991;37:1534–9.
23. Franca LT, Carrilho E, Kist TB. A review of DNA sequencing techniques. Q Rev Biophys 2002;35:169–200.
24. Pusch W, Wurmbach JH, Thiele H, Kostrzewa M. MALDI-TOF mass spectrometry-based SNP genotyping. Pharmacogenomics 2002;3:537–48.
25. Orita M, Iwahana H, Kanazawa H, Hayashi K, Sekiya T. Detection of polymorphisms of human DNA by gel electrophoresis as single-strand conformation polymorphisms. Proc Natl Acad Sci USA 1989;86:2766–70.
26. Highsmith WE Jr, Jin Q, Nataraj AJ, O'Connor JM, Burland VD, Baubonis WR, et al. Use of a DNA toolbox for the characterization of mutation scanning methods. I: construction of the toolbox and evaluation of heteroduplex analysis. Electrophoresis 1999;20:1186–94.
27. Xiao W, Oefner PJ. Denaturing high-performance liquid chromatography: A review. Hum Mutat 2001;17:439–74.

28. Abrams ES, Murdaugh SE, Lerman LS. Comprehensive detection of single base changes in human genomic DNA using denaturing gradient gel electrophoresis and a GC clamp. Genomics 1990;7:463–75.
29. Wartell RM, Hosseini S, Powell S, Zhu J. Detecting single base substitutions, mismatches and bulges in DNA by temperature gradient gel electrophoresis and related methods. J Chromatogr A 1998;806:169–85.
30. Gao Q, Yeung ES. High-throughput detection of unknown mutations by using multiplexed capillary electrophoresis with poly(vinylpyrrolidone) solution. Anal Chem 2000;72:2499–506.
31. Halminen M, Sjoroos M, Makela MJ, Waris M, Terho E, Lovgren T, et al. Simultaneous detection of IFN-gamma and IL-4 mRNAs using RT-PCR and time-resolved fluorometry. Cytokine 1999;11:87–93.
32. Lay MJ, Wittwer CT. Real-time fluorescence genotyping of factor V Leiden during rapid-cycle PCR. Clin Chem 1997;43:2262–7.
33. Gundry CN, Vandersteen JG, Reed GH, Pryor RJ, Chen J, Wittwer CT. Amplicon melting analysis with labeled primers: a closed-tube method for differentiating homozygotes and heterozygotes. Clin Chem 2003;49:396–406.
34. Wittwer CT, Reed GH, Gundry CN, Vandersteen JG, Pryor RJ. High-resolution genotyping by amplicon melting analysis using LCgreen. Clin Chem 2003;49:853–60.
35. Heller MJ. DNA microarray technology: devices, systems, and applications. Annu Rev Biomed Eng 2002;4:129–53.
36. Oliphant A, Barker DL, Stuelpnagel JR, Chee MS. BeadArray technology: enabling an accurate, cost-effective approach to high-throughput genotyping. Biotechniques 2002 Jun;Suppl:56–8, 60–1.
37. Kellar KL, Iannone MA. Multiplexed microsphere-based flow cytometric assays. Exp Hematol 2002;30:1227–37.
38. Xu H, Sha MY, Wong EY, Uphoff J, Xu Y, Treadway JA, et al. Multiplexed SNP genotyping using the Qbead system: a quantum dot-encoded microsphere-based assay. Nucleic Acids Res 2003;31:E43.
39. Saiki RK, Gelfand DH, Stoffel S, Scharf SJ, Higuchi R, Horn GT, et al. Primer-directed enzymatic amplification of DNA with a thermostable DNA polymerase. Science 1988;239:487–91.
40. Wiedmann M, Wilson WJ, Czajka J, Luo J, Barany F, Batt CA. Ligase chain reaction (LCR)—overview and applications. PCR Methods Appl 1994;3:S51–64.
41. Guatelli JC, Whitfield KM, Kwoh DY, Barringer KJ, Richman DD, Gingeras TR. Isothermal, in vitro amplification of nucleic acids by a multienzyme reaction modeled after retroviral replication. Proc Natl Acad Sci USA 1990;87:1874–8.
42. Walker GT, Linn CP, Nadeau JG. DNA detection by strand displacement amplification and fluorescence polarization with signal enhancement using a DNA binding protein. Nucleic Acids Res 1996;24:348–53.
43. Notomi T, Okayama H, Masubuchi H, Yonekawa T, Watanabe K, Amino N, et al. Loop-mediated isothermal amplification of DNA. Nucleic Acids Res 2000;28:E63.
44. Reyes AA, Ugozzoli LA, Lowery JD, Breneman JW 3rd, Hixson CS, Press RD, et al. Linked linear amplification: a new method for the amplification of DNA. Clin Chem 2001;47:31–40.
45. Collins ML, Irvine B, Tyner D, Fine E, Zayati C, Chang C, et al. A branched DNA signal amplification assay for quantification of nucleic acid targets below 100 molecules/ml. Nucleic Acids Res 1997;25:2979–84.
46. Hall JG, Eis PS, Law SM, Reynaldo LP, Prudent JR, Marshall DJ, et al. Sensitive detection of DNA polymorphisms by the serial invasive signal amplification reaction. Proc Natl Acad Sci USA 2000;97:8272–7.
47. Lomeli H, Tyagi S, Pritchard CG, Lizardi PM, Kramer FR. Quantitative assays based on the use of replicatable hybridization probes. Clin Chem 1989;35:1826–31.
48. Lizardi PM, Huang X, Zhu Z, Bray-Ward P, Thomas DC, Ward DC. Mutation detection and single-molecule counting using isothermal rolling-circle amplification. Nat Genet 1998;19:225–32.
49. Van Ness J, Van Ness LK, Galas DJ. Isothermal reactions for the amplification of oligonucleotides. Proc Natl Acad Sci USA 2003;100:4504–9.

50. Wittwer CT, Garling DJ. Rapid cycle DNA amplification: time and temperature optimization. Biotechniques 1991;10:76–83.
51. Seuss D. The cat in the hat comes back! New York: Random House, 1958.
52. Espy MJ, Smith TF, Persing DH. Dependence of polymerase chain reaction product inactivation protocols on amplicon length and sequence composition. J Clin Microbiol 1993;31:2361–5.
53. Compton J. Nucleic acid sequence-based amplification. Nature 1991;350:91–2.
54. Giachetti C, Linnen JM, Kolk DP, Dockter J, Gillotte-Taylor K, Park M, et al. Highly sensitive multiplex assay for detection of human immunodeficiency virus type 1 and hepatitis C virus RNA. J Clin Microbiol 2002;40:2408–19.
55. Bruns D, Lo YMD, Wittwer CT. Molecular testing in laboratory medicine: selections from clinical chemistry. Washington, DC: AACC Press, 2002.
56. Sanger F, Nicklen S, Coulson AR. DNA sequencing with chain-terminating inhibitors. Proc Natl Acad Sci USA 1977;74:5463–7.
57. Germer S, Holland MJ, Higuchi R. High-throughput SNP allele-frequency determination in pooled DNA samples by kinetic PCR. Genome Res 2000;10:258–66.
58. Brinson EC, Adriano T, Bloch W, Brown CL, Chang CC, Chen J, et al. Introduction to PCR/OLA/SCS, a multiplex DNA test, and its application to cystic fibrosis. Genet Test 1997;1:61–8.
59. Schena M, Shalon D, Davis RW, Brown PO. Quantitative monitoring of gene expression patterns with a complementary DNA microarray. Science 1995;270:467–70.
60. Lipshutz RJ, Fodor SP, Gingeras TR, Lockhart DJ. High density synthetic oligonucleotide arrays. Nat Genet 1999;21:20–4.
61. Holloway AJ, van Laar RK, Tothill RW, Bowtell DD. Options available—from start to finish—for obtaining data from DNA microarrays II. Nat Genet 2002;32(Suppl):481–9.
62. Wittwer CT, Kusukawa N. Real-time PCR. In: Persing DH, Tenover F, Relman D, White T, Tang Y, Versalovic J, et al., eds. Molecular microbiology: diagnostic principles and practices. Washington, DC: ASM Press, 2003.
63. Teupser D, Rupprecht W, Lohse P, Thiery J. Fluorescence-based detection of the CETP TaqIB polymorphism: false positives with the TaqMan-based exonuclease assay attributable to a previously unknown gene variant. Clin Chem 2001;47:852–7.
64. Meuer S, Wittwer CT, Nakagawara K. Rapid cycle real-time PCR—methods and applications. Berlin: Springer, 2001.
65. Reischl U, Wittwer CT, Cockerill F. Rapid cycle real-time PCR—methods and applications: microbiology and food analysis. Berlin: Springer, 2002.
66. Dietmaier C, Wittwer CT, Sivasubramanian N. Rapid cycle real-time PCR—methods and applications: genetics and oncology. Berlin: Springer, 2002.
67. Higuchi R, Fockler C, Dollinger G, Watson R. Kinetic PCR analysis: real-time monitoring of DNA amplification reactions. Biotechnology (NY) 1993;11:1026–30.
68. Morrison TB, Weis JJ, Wittwer CT. Quantification of low-copy transcripts by continuous SYBR Green I monitoring during amplification. Biotechniques 1998;24:954–8, 960, 962.
69. Nazarenko IA, Bhatnagar SK, Hohman RJ. A closed tube format for amplification and detection of DNA based on energy transfer. Nucleic Acids Res 1997;25:2516–21.
70. Moser MJ, Marshall DJ, Grenier JK, Kieffer CD, Killeen AA, Ptacin JL, et al. Exploiting the enzymatic recognition of an unnatural base pair to develop a universal genetic analysis system. Clin Chem 2003;49:407–14.
71. Wittwer CT, Ririe KM, Rasmussen RP. Fluorescence monitoring of rapid cycle PCR for quantification. In: Ferre F, ed. Gene quantification. New York: Birkhauser, 1998:129–44.
72. Bernard PS, Ajioka RS, Kushner JP, Wittwer CT. Homogeneous multiplex genotyping of hemochromatosis mutations with fluorescent hybridization probes. Am J Pathol 1998; 153:1055–61.
73. Svanvik N, Westman G, Wang D, Kubista M. Light-up probes: thiazole orange-conjugated peptide nucleic acid for detection of target nucleic acid in homogeneous solution. Anal Biochem 2000;281:26–35.

74. de Kok JB, Wiegerinck ET, Giesendorf BA, Swinkels DW. Rapid genotyping of single nucleotide polymorphisms using novel minor groove binding DNA oligonucleotides (MGB probes). Hum Mutat 2002;19:554–9.
75. Todd AV, Fuery CJ, Impey HL, Applegate TL, Haughton MA. DzyNA-PCR: use of DNAzymes to detect and quantify nucleic acid sequences in a real-time fluorescent format. Clin Chem 2000;46:625–30.
76. Chen X, Livak KJ, Kwok PY. A homogeneous, ligase-mediated DNA diagnostic test. Genome Res 1998;8:549–56.
77. Whitcombe D, Theaker J, Guy SP, Brown T, Little S. Detection of PCR products using self-probing amplicons and fluorescence. Nat Biotechnol 1999;17:804–7.
78. Li Q, Luan G, Guo Q, Liang J. A new class of homogeneous nucleic acid probes based on specific displacement hybridization. Nucleic Acids Res 2002;30:E5.
79. Livak KJ, Flood SJ, Marmaro J, Giusti W, Deetz K. Oligonucleotides with fluorescent dyes at opposite ends provide a quenched probe system useful for detecting PCR product and nucleic acid hybridization. PCR Methods Appl 1995;4:357–62.
80. Liew M, Pryor R, Palais R, Meadows C, Erali M, Lyon E, et al. Genotyping of single-nucleotide polymorphisms by high-resolution melting of small amplicons. Clin Chem 2004;50:1156–64.
81. Zhou L, Myers AN, Vandersteen JG, Wang L, Wittwer CT. Closed-tube genotyping with unlabeled oligonucleotide probes and a saturating DNA dye. Clin Chem 2004;50:1328–35.
82. Germer S, Higuchi R. Single-tube genotyping without oligonucleotide probes. Genome Res 1999;9:72–8.
83. Michalatos-Beloin S, Tishkoff SA, Bentley KL, Kidd KK, Ruano G. Molecular haplotyping of genetic markers 10 kb apart by allele-specific long-range PCR. Nucleic Acids Res 1996; 24:4841–3.
84. Ding C, Cantor CR. Direct molecular haplotyping of long-range genomic DNA with M1-PCR. Proc Natl Acad Sci USA 2003;100:7449–53.
85. Worm J, Aggerholm A, Guldberg P. In-tube DNA methylation profiling by fluorescence melting curve analysis. Clin Chem 2001;47:1183–9.

Chapter 16

Selection of Laboratory Automation Technology: Instruments, Workcells, and Systems

Rodney S. Markin and Mary C. Newcomb

Clinical laboratory automation technology has been in operation since the late 1980s. Early adopters in Japan (1980s) (1–4) and in North America (1990s) (5–10) implemented large, full-scale automation systems at significant expense. As with many technologies in the early stage of technological evolution, these systems supported a variety of functional requirements, most of which applied to larger clinical laboratory operations and reference or commercial laboratories.

Over the last 10 years, the implementation of clinical laboratory automation technology has been optimized for the following instrument categories: chemistry, immunoassay/serology, hematology, coagulation, and urinalysis. These instrument/discipline categories represent 70%–80% of the test volume in most typical clinical laboratories (11). As a result of these volume considerations, instrument manufacturers have invested in onboard instrument software and instrument hardware modifications that support a connection to clinical laboratory automation technology. Investment in automation technology to support blood bank operations has been in process for several years. Based upon the complex interpretive issues in blood banking operations, most automation systems applications have not incorporated blood-banking technology into the automation platform.

Visionaries and early adopters such as Dr. David Beckwith and Beth Rokus at Health Network Laboratories (Allentown, PA) and David Thiel and Dr. Scott Whalen (10) at Aultman Hospital (Canton, OH) implemented automation systems for several reasons, including their individual and their respective institutions' understanding of information systems and the value of information as a driver of medical practice and patient care. Visionaries and pioneers outside Japan and the United States, such as Dr. Dina Noff at the Macabbi Healthcare Services in Tel Aviv, Israel, have implemented systems in high-volume outpatient clinical laboratories.

Implementation of the automation system in the laboratory at Aultman Hospital provided an opportunity to evaluate the predicted operational effects of a clinical laboratory automation system. Before and after automation implementation, measurements were taken that showed the results in Table 1.

TABLE 1. Predicted and observed clinical laboratory automation operating characteristics

Category	Predicted[a,b]	Observed[c]
Labor savings	30%	30%
Turnaround time (loaded)	40% decrease	30% decrease
Instrument capacity	48% increase	45% increase
Reagent/supplies savings	Not predicted	10%

[a]Markin RS. University of Nebraska Medical Center Robotics Project 1990, unpublished work; [b]Markin RS. Clinical laboratory automation systems: concepts, designs and future directions. Am Path Rev Winter 1994/95; [c]Markin RS, Whalen S. Laboratory automation: trajectory, technology, and tactics. Clin Chem 2000;45:764–71.

As the level of interest in clinical laboratory automation increased, a group of people interested in clinical laboratory automation petitioned NCCLS to support the development of standards for clinical laboratory automation technology (12). In 1996, the area committee for laboratory automation was officially formed and by December 2000, five documents that describe the basic standards for interconnection of clinical laboratory instruments and information systems to automation systems were published (www.nccls.org) (*see* Volume 1, Chapter 7). The implementation of these standards has significantly decreased the costs of clinical laboratory automation technology and allowed the laboratorians a choice of instruments independent of automation vendor.

Clinical laboratory automation technology has been implemented in more than 300 laboratories in the world in various forms and with a variety of functional capabilities. Clinical laboratory automation technology will likely follow the same growth curve as the laboratory information system (LIS) after 1980 and by 2010, 90% of clinical laboratories in North America will have some level of clinical laboratory automation technology.

Automation technology in molecular diagnostics and microbiology appears to be converging, both using molecular methods for detection and identification. As specimen-processing methodologies that support automation platforms are developed and the detection systems evolve, these assays will be incorporated into automation frameworks. Laboratory automation has become a valuable laboratory management tool!

CLINICAL LABORATORY AUTOMATION THEORY

Clinical laboratory automation theory is simple and contextually parallel to automation implementations in other production environments (13–17). Automation technology is incorporated into the laboratory to:

- Decrease production cost per test
- Increase specimen volume/capacity without a proportional (proportional to preautomation manual methods) increase in labor resources
- Decrease and stabilize turnaround times
- Minimize biohazard exposures
- Enhance patient safety
- Reduce patient length of stay (LOS)

Automation will optimize the overall laboratory operation including the automated and nonautomated sections of the clinical laboratory (Table 2). Investigations into the design and construction of laboratory automation technology were founded upon clinical insight

TABLE 2. Reasons to automate a clinical laboratory

- Decrease production cost per test—**make administrators happy!**
- Increase specimen volume/capacity without a proportional (proportional to preautomation manual methods) increase in labor resources—**medical technologists are a scarce resource.**
- Decrease and stabilize turnaround times—**make your physicians, nurses, and other customers happy and efficient.**
- Minimize biohazard exposures—**protect employees.**
- Optimize the overall laboratory operation including the automated and nonautomated sections of the clinical laboratory—**provide better patient care service.**

TABLE 3. Clinical laboratory automation design guidelines

- Patient care issues supercede engineering principles (using multiple specimen collection container sizes as compared to standardization on one size to make the design simple).
- Automation is an information systems problem, not a hardware problem.
- The overarching process and information system structure should be developed first, then work down to the hardware components.
- Platforms shall be scalable across the range of volumes encountered in clinical laboratories.
- Patients will be cared for in hospitals and health systems and these organizations will have laboratories for the foreseeable future; therefore, design and build a system that will work in hospital-based clinical laboratories.
- Each specimen represents the patient.
- Each specimen is a unique "lot number" or represents a unique set of data in time from the patient (the biological organism).
- Each specimen may have a relationship to another specimen based upon time, tests ordered, the patient's disease, business issues (contractual issues), or ordering physician, for example.

and experience working in the clinical laboratory, a basic understanding of engineering methodology, and supported by the use of simulation modeling and other tools to help predict the system's behavior and evaluate productivity outcomes (Table 3).

The authors' work at the University of Nebraska Medical Center established a base theory, simply stated: laboratory automation should work as a combination of specimen-handling and specimen-processing devices and instruments, connected by a transportation system (a transportation network), under software control, analogous to a computer-integrated manufacturing (CIM) process control software package. The approach was to create a model of the most plausible automation scenario which included preanalytical specimen processing (specimen centrifugation, decapping, aliquotting, sorting), specimen analysis (direct-track sampling by instruments, routing between and among instruments, reflex and repeat testing), and postanalytical specimen handling (specimen recapping, sorting, specimen storage, retrieval for add-on and reflex testing, automated disposal). The original simulation models produced in 1989 through 1991 for a typical hospital laboratory (18–20) showed the following results:

- Labor costs would decrease by up to 30%.
- Specimen volume/system capacity would increase up to 48%.
- Turnaround times could stabilize at approximately 30 minutes from receipt in the laboratory to result reporting after the system is at steady state (dependent upon volumes).
- Reflex and repeat testing could occur in the automated system without additional labor costs in the absence of additional specimen collection needs.
- Aliquotting is not necessary if primary specimens are sampled serially on the automation system prior to using the specimen for manual testing.

During the investigation phase, several important and fundamental concepts were found to differentiate laboratory automation system development (*see* Table 3). In addition, the capital costs of a system should be preserved. During 13 years of development experience, these concepts were followed to develop automation technology that supports the care of the patient in a format designed especially for the hospital laboratories that facilitate acute care environments (21).

The approach, clearly stated at a high level in 1990, is that "clinical laboratory automation is a software problem (16), not a hardware problem." This has proven true over time. This approach to clinical laboratory automation was patterned after a method introduced decades ago in manufacturing environments: CIM, which is based upon the use of an information system (hardware and software) to direct the production of a component or a product through two or more interrelated steps. In early investigations into CIM and the application of industrial CIM software to a laboratory setting, the authors' discovered a distinct difference. In the production environment, one lot number of material may be used to produce many of the same identical products until that lot number is exhausted. In the clinical laboratory, each specimen is a different lot number; in other words, each specimen varies because it is derived from a biological organism at a particular point of time. Since this level of granularity is not available in commercial CIM applications, specific software that supports process control at the level of the instruments, processing devices, and the patient specimens was required (Table 4). To that end, a process control system was designed using an Oracle® database that considers that each specimen represents a patient, is a unique "lot number," and may have a relationship to another specimen (e.g., time drawn) (Table 3).

Clinical laboratory automation process control software must be scalable and flexible. The software should operate on a small framework of automation technology or preanalytical processing station and may be scaled up to operate with transportation systems and a myriad of specimen-handling and specimen-processing devices, instruments, and processes (22). The software approach provides HL7 and ASTM communications to laboratory information and hospital information systems and supports the NCCLS clinical laboratory automation standards (AUTO3-A).

Another important concept is the single terminal control of the system. The single operator in the laboratory can view all of the instruments, their status, and the entire specimen-processing and specimen-handling devices attached to the transportation line,

TABLE 4. Key features of process control software

- Automatic load balancing between similar instruments and the same modules
- Instrument priority assignments based on client-defined rules
- Shared tube processing between multiple instruments to minimize sample volume and primary tube integrity
- Simple or complex aliquotting algorithms
- Automatic repeat, reflex, and delta testing based on user-defined rules that can be instrument specific
- Sample routing decision logic based on instrument onboard reagents combinations
- Continuous sample monitoring and notification if client-defined time on the LAS system has been exceeded before all routes are satisfied
- Immediate operator notification of system conditions displayed on a central PC workstation
- Real-time specimen tracking and reporting options
- Automatic storage and disposal criteria
- Onboard reagent, consumable, and disposable inventory monitoring and control—if provided by the instrument

from a single console; likewise, the laboratory manager should be able to review the workings of an automated laboratory from the office, home, or elsewhere. The software should also have the functionality to allow the vendor to troubleshoot a system remotely and provide online and remote diagnosis and repair of software problems and reporting of hardware problems.

INSTRUMENT CONTROL AND OPERATION IN THE AUTOMATED LABORATORY

One of the most significant components of the CIM approach to laboratory automation is the instrument automation interface: the interface between the instrument and the laboratory automation system (LAS). This interface control allows a level of results processing that previously occurred at the level of the medical technologist; with a CIM command and control approach, errors and simple reflex responses may be handled by the automation system software. Errors and other troubleshooting issues not defined in a low level of rules execution will be routed to an operator for intervention and evaluation.

Process control software should reside on its own IT hardware and manage the entire automation system independent of instrument vendor, instrument type, or capabilities of the LIS. Many suppliers of clinical laboratory automation embed software control features and process control applications within the data manager or instrument manager associated with their particular instrument, thereby rendering the transportation system and other specimen-handling devices "dumb" in the absence of their proprietary instrumentation. From a laboratorian's standpoint, this is a significant problem since the user will then be tied to one vendor for instrumentation and automation solutions. The user should be able to interchange instruments and other specimen-processing devices as long as both the automation vendor and the independent instrument manufacturers adhere to the standards published for these applications (NCCLS AUTO1-A through AUTO 5-A).

> **Key concept:** Process control software that is not independent of the instruments on the system or not independent of the instrument's data manager will inhibit the swapping of instruments in the laboratory. These software-constrained systems are not true "open automation systems," but in fact are marketing mechanisms to bind the laboratory to a vendor, with significant penalties (the cost of the automation system) if their instruments are deselected.

COMPONENTS OF CLINICAL LABORATORY AUTOMATION SYSTEMS

The process control software functions as the "brain" behind the "brawn" of the automation hardware, enabling the LAS functionality that works to enhance laboratory operation. Specimens move throughout the automation system from preanalytical processing, to completion of analytical results, and on to archive or disposal when processing concludes. Scheduling functions determine the most efficient routing for each specimen and manage how the clinical analyzers attached to the automation system are used.

The process control software allows the operator to simultaneously monitor the status of all of the hardware, software, and workcell modules from one PC workstation. The operator can start and stop the transport system, reset the processes for each intelligent device, shut down portions of the system to enable alternate routing, and control the sampling process at the analyzer workcells. Analyzer operational status, error notification, and reagent inventory information (dependent on the capability of the particular analyzer) can be provided to the operator directly.

The process control software is usually a library of programs and a relational database strategy that controls the scheduling, routing, and tracking of specimen carriers on the transport system and their intersection with the instruments and specimen-handling and specimen-processing devices. Process control rules can be designed to direct an entire suite of automation components and laboratory instruments. Automating most of the routine actions in the laboratory—from specimen receipt to specimen storage and retrieval—optimizes maximum efficiency, which benefits laboratory operation. Figure 1 compares the high level IT architecture of an automation system without and with true process control.

LAS software technology can help reduce error rates, improve turnaround times, increase staff productivity and capacity without adding staff, lower labor costs, and standardize operations. The most advanced software technology available in the industry today operates on top of the LAS, monitoring the progress of each specimen, choreographing the quick and efficient production of results, and directing the flow of specimen traffic to optimize throughput and results production. Other major software and interface subcomponents of an LAS include:

- System status monitoring from a single PC workstation
- Real-time interface to LIS
- Scaleable process management
- Reflex and repeat testing capabilities
- Real-time specimen routing and scheduling
- Balanced workload between similar instruments
- Rules-based laboratory operations

A real-time interface to the LIS provides the data that drive the specimen through the random-access process of clinical analysis. Patient demographics, episode of care information, orders, and verified results are sent from the LIS to the LAS. The LAS transmits unverified results from clinical analyzers to the LIS.

Automated interfaces for clinical instrumentation mimic the processes performed by the medical technologist. Presentation of the specimens to the instruments is most efficiently handled by direct-track sampling (DTS) ready instrumentation (NCCLS AUTO-5A). The development of this type of interface was pioneered at the University of Nebraska Medical Center with the clinical diagnostics division of Eastman Kodak (now Ortho-Clinical Diagnostics, a Johnson and Johnson Company).

Analyzers that do not support DTS may be retrofitted with an automation interface that facilitates the loading and unloading of the specimens. Automation vendors have developed many of these types of interfaces, preserving the throughput integrity of the analyzer and supporting "walk-up" operation, if necessary. Instruments work in standalone mode, as well as in conjunction with other instruments as part of a system.

LIS–LAS Interfaces

When communicating with an LIS, the LIS–LAS interface may support either a HL7 protocol (v.2.3 or greater) for the electronic exchange or transfer of data in the healthcare environment (*see* NCCLS AUTO-5A) or the ASTM protocol for HIS and the instrument communication (ASTM 1394). The interface between the hospital/healthcare system LIS receives patient identification, specimen identification, and analytical method request data and

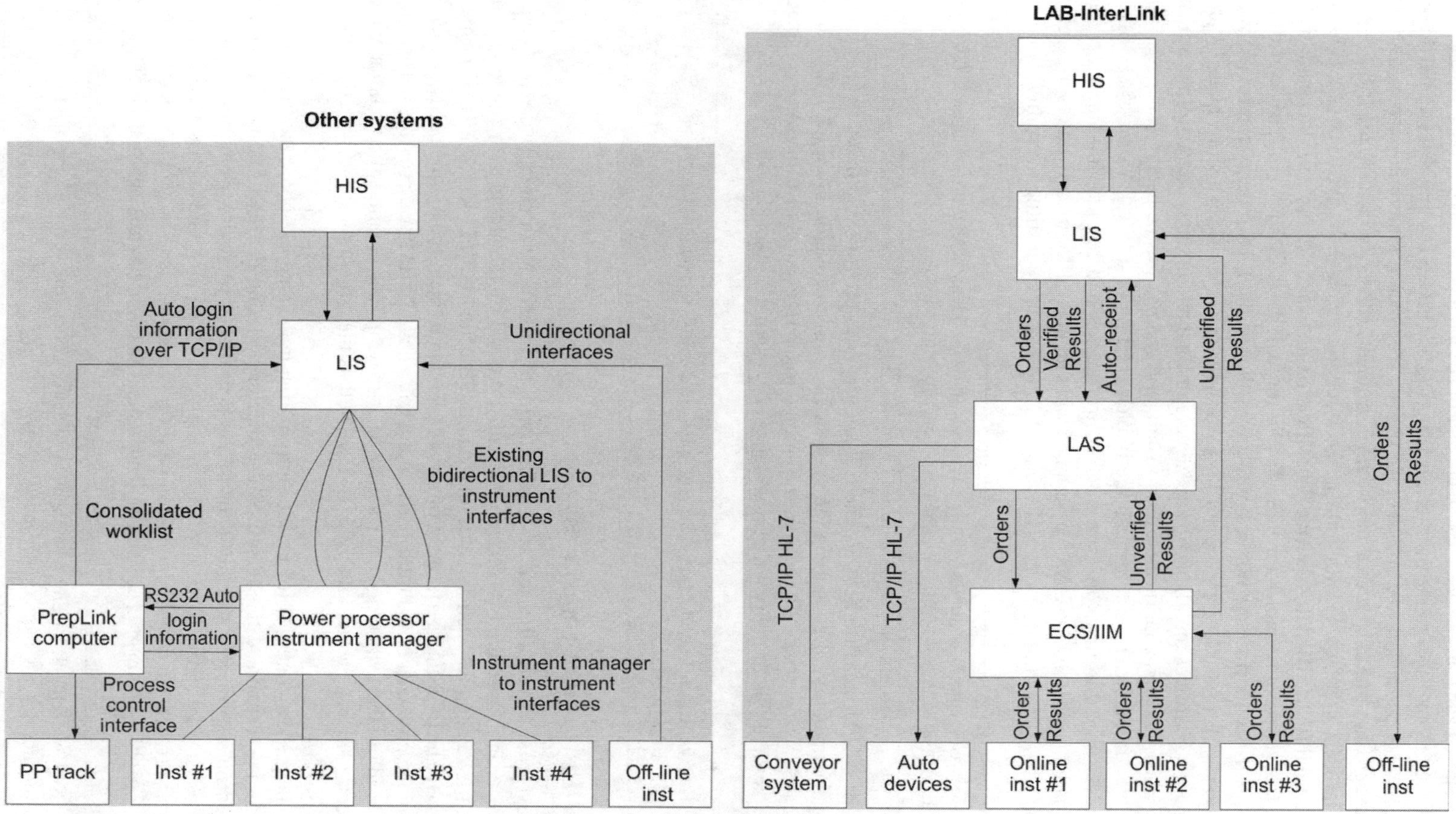

FIGURE 1. Comparison of automation system information technology infrastructure with and without process control software.

creates subsequent transactions through another or second interface to the LAS. Transactions maybe sent by the LAS to the instruments using a standard ASTM protocol (ASTM 1394). These transactions include the upload of the patient, specimen, and test information to specific analyzers. In some LAS architectures, the instruments connect directly to the LIS.

The HL7 interface specification is the standard endorsed by NCCLS (AUTO3-A), JCCLS, and IFCC. The HL7 interface specification allows the transfer of information elements that support the implementation of rules through the LAS software. The costs of the HL7 LIS–LAS interface are not insignificant. Although the LAS process control software usually includes an HL7 protocol LIS–LAS interface, the LIS vendors have created automation interfaces that they consider developmental and at times charge inflated prices for this interface and significant hourly installation charges for their services.

The information passed through the implementation of a LIS–LAS interface will be dependent upon the fields that are selected to transmit and receive. In some cases, the information needed by the LAS may not be available in the LIS, usually due to the lack of the data being transmitted by the HIS to the LIS at a specific institution/facility.

> **Key concept:** You cannot write a rule against a data element that is not in the LAS database. This will be an implementation and operational issue.

The ASTM interface between the LIS and the LAS provides rudimentary functionality for the operation of an automation system. The implementation of the ASTM protocol LIS–LAS interface basically defines the automation system as an instrument as compared to the "system functionality" of current laboratory automation technology.

> **Key concept:** You do not have true process control if you implement an ASTM LIS–LAS interface.

LAS–Instrument Interfaces

The **external communication system/instrument interface manager (ECS/IIM)** component is an off-the-shelf (OTS) product either created by the automation vendor or purchased by a supplier such as Data Innovations (Burlington, VT) which is used in many systems. The ECS/IIM performs protocol conversion to meet the unique needs of each of the unique protocols of the third-party analyzers. The ECS/IIM also provides a user interface to allow the technologist the ability to start, stop, and monitor the communication between each analyzer and the ECS/IIM, as well as the communications with the LIS and ECS/IIM.

The process control software uses information in the database about the transportation system, the location of the analyzers, the specimen(s), and the tests that need to be performed on a specimen, and the status of the instruments to devise a plan for routing the specimen and its carrier to the appropriate analyzer. Using this scheduled plan, the process control software directs the automation hardware components to move the specimen carriers to specific specimen-processing and specimen-handling devices and instruments (23).

> **Key concept:** Replacing the medical technologist at the level of the instrument requires that you replace their functionality.

When the carrier arrives at a workcell (specific specimen-processing and specimen-handling devices and instruments), the process control software passes order information to the instrument controller that instructs the third-party analyzer as to what tests are to be performed on the specimens. Once the specimens have been analyzed, unverified results are transmitted from the third-party analyzer to the ECS/IIM, which then transmits the results to the LIS. When the unverified results arrive in the LIS, the results are available for verification, approval, or rejection by the technologist. As soon as the unverified result is entered into the process control software database, it is forwarded to a rules engine for examination.

Rules Engine

A rules engine is a process control software component designed to use client-specified rules to implement decisions on the automation system when results, analyzer error codes, warnings, flags, or other operational conditions satisfy a condition specified by the rule. If the benefits of laboratory automation and the ability to choose instruments based upon clinical needs are requirements, an "open system" LAS with a rules engine should be selected.

The user may define simple or sophisticated rule sets to reflect the laboratory's operational practices and goals. Specimen containers are routed on the automation system based on these rules, which should be designed to optimize result turnaround time. The created rules are set into motion regardless of which instruments are online with the LAS; system capabilities are not compromised by a lack of compatibility or a lack of process control functionality with the LIS (Table 5).

Rules can be easily subdivided into three broad categories: clinical rules, business rules, and operational rules. **Clinical rules** are defined as rules that affect the patient or the patient's specimen based upon patient attributes. Examples of clinical rule concepts include:

- Order of priority of patient specimen processing is based upon location (i.e., patient location where OR>ER>ICU>5 WEST>outpatient clinics.
- Test reflex ordering or cancellation is based upon diagnosis or ordering physician.

Business rules are defined as rules that affect the business of the laboratory, hospital, or health system based upon business attributes. Examples of business rule concepts include:

- Test reflex ordering or cancellation is based upon contractual obligation (i.e., rules for test allowed per specific contract).
- Prioritization of discounted outside testing is based upon price charged or discount allowed.

Operational rules are defined as rules that affect the operation of the laboratory, hospital, or health system based upon operational attributes. Examples of operational rule concepts include:

- Delivery of specimens to specific instruments is based upon reagent status.

TABLE 5. Benefits of laboratory-specific rules for each patient type, analyte, or body fluid

- Standardize laboratory operational practices
- Enhance productivity and quality
- Equalize staff skill sets and experience
- Produce consistent routing decisions and quality outcomes
- Optimize turnaround time through unique specimen ID support
- Minimize operational delays by issuing immediate status alerts if operator intervention is necessary

- Delivery or routing of specimens to specific instruments is based upon shift (i.e., all instruments of the same configuration or type receive specimens on the day shift, instrument use in the evening shift or night shift is scaled based upon use and reagent availability).

A rules engine can use the client-supplied rules to dilute specimens, repeat analyses, conduct reflexive testing, alert the technologist, or just about any conditional response based upon the data available to the LAS. Regardless of the action taken, all test results are transmitted to the LIS for review by the medical technologist. The process control software components do not alter, delete, compute, calculate, or modify any result derived from a patient's specimen.

Instrument data, such as analytical results, instrument flags, or warnings and errors in conjunction with patient demographic and episodic data, may be used to formulate a rule. The rules engine should actually update the processing rules in real-time as information is added or changed. Most rules engines apply rules to specimens according to the dynamic inputs/variables until all outcomes are satisfied according to the laboratory-defined criteria. Examples of some rules from operational automated installations are shown in Table 6:

> **Key concept:** Independent of which instruments are online with the LAS, system capabilities are not compromised by a lack of compatibility with the LIS.

Reporting Engine

One of the most critical areas of clinical laboratory management is the monitoring and management of clinical, business, and operational processes to ensure the quality of the results produced. On occasion, the healthcare provider or even the patient may question a laboratory result. When this happens, it is customary for the technical staff responsible for quality assurance (QA) in the laboratory to research the validity of the result. This is not an easy task.

TABLE 6. Examples of rules engine applications

Rules set example: The site's procedure requires it to repeat a critical low result from a baby on another equivalent analyzer.

This critical low result < or = 40 mg/dL.
Condition = AQA_critical_limit_low and: age < 30 days
Action = :REPDIFFLAG (repeat to a different analyzer)
Log Message = Above critical low limit

Rules set example: The site's procedure is to repeat a patient sample when the analyzer error codes 'ME' and 'PF' are seen.

If the error codes 'ME' and 'PF' are seen on the repeat, the site will perform a visual inspection on the tube and check the analyzer errors.
Condition = in_error_fields ('ME') AND in_error_fields ('PF') and :Counter =1
Action = REPEQUFLAG
Log Message = ME = Mechanical error and PF = invalid slide response or no slide response
Condition = in_error_fields ('ME') AND in_error_fields ('PF') and :Counter >=2
Action = ALERTFLAG
Log Message = ME = Mechanical error and PF = invalid slide response or no slide response

Raw data that were provided to the LIS for results reporting may not be readily available either from the LIS or the instrument. Results buffer size on the instrument may be limited to a finite number of results or to a specific time frame. A report generator that either cannot access the raw data transactions or is too difficult for laboratory staff to use may search the LIS database. In the case of the latter, requests for data usually go through an experienced LIS system administrator.

A strong data management system (a CIM-like process controller) should provide the data management tools to facilitate this process. These data management functions can be facilitated easily when the raw data are stored in a relational database. LAS systems using the relational databases such as Oracle® provide ad hoc report generation using SQL language support through a user-friendly interface. Correlation studies routinely used to validate results data, i.e., within-run patient correlation, correlation of results data across equivalent analyzers, review of raw results data for instrument errors and flags, and review of quality control (QC) data can be performed using the data extracted from the LAS.

Key concept: The raw transaction data from the instruments, the specimen-processing and specimen-handling devices and the LIS interface are stored in the database and available for examination and correlation. This level of data has never before been available to the clinical laboratory.

One of the features of a true process control system is the ability to collect information from instruments connected to the LAS. The data may be extracted from the LAS table containing unverified results. This table holds data that are directly received from the instrument prior to any manipulation by the technologist or the LIS. Exactly which analyzer reported the results in question and at what time and in which sequence can be ascertained. The data allow determination of what error flags were reported with the results. The result data can indicate that there were some significant errors in the sample management such as sample metering on one of the instruments. Instrument event messaging logs stored in the LAS database can be accessed remotely by field service technicians for pre-emptive instrument maintenance.

The most significant value in this demonstration is the ability to correlate result values across two instruments from one database through a defined time period. Another advantage of this type of data management is the ability to store the raw data electronically for a long period either on the system (by increasing disk capacity locally), or by exporting tables to a long-term electronic storage media (digital tape or compact disk).

CLINICAL LABORATORY AUTOMATION HARDWARE COMPONENTS

Depending on the approach taken in developing automation, either software based or hardware based, several well-defined automation hardware components can be easily translated into functionality (Table 7). These functions are defined in the NCCLS automation standards (AUTO 1-A through AUTO 5-A) as well as being identified in the annual CAP Today survey published in May of each year.

Transportation

In each automation system available and presumably in future automation system designs, a transportation mechanism will be included. The transportation mechanism can be

TABLE 7. Major components of clinical laboratory automation systems

Software	Hardware
Process controller	Transportation
LIS–LAS interface	Loading station
LAS–instrument interfaces	Centrifuge
Rules engine	Decapper
Reporting engine	Specimen integrity monitor
	Instrument interfaces
	Aliquotter
	Recapper
	Sorter
	Storage/retrieval/disposal

conveyor track, which may be integrated into automation components as a separate component, an automated guided vehicle system, or a combination of both. All of the automation systems currently on the market include a transportation mechanism of some sort. In the automation systems that may be characterized as instruments such as the Tecan FE500, a small segment of conveyor mechanism is present within the instrument. In workcells such as the Dade StreamLab® or the Bayer LabCell®, a separate transportation mechanism is present that connects instruments and other components. In the large automation systems including LAB-InterLink® and Beckman Coulter®, transportation systems are designed to connect a variety of system components and instruments. Examples of automation transportation mechanisms are present in Figures 2 through 8.

Loading Station

In many automation systems, some type of loading mechanism is used. A linking station that links the specimens with the specimen carriers or enters the specimen container to the LAS or LIS electronically and identifies it within the automation system database usually accompanies a loading station, which allows individual specimens to be introduced into the system. Loading stations may be incorporated into the other devices such as an automated centrifuge, an automated aliquotter, or an automated storage retrieval and disposal system, depending upon the functionality of each device and the intent of the manufacturer. In the future, loading station-type devices may take on different characteristics. When specimens are identified by a unique container ID, the LAS can provide a receipt transaction to the LIS, which replaces a manual processing step.

Centrifuge

Many automation systems, some automation workcells, and some automation instruments include an automated centrifuge. The automated centrifuge performs separation using the usual centrifugal sedimentation methodologies, the standard rotor and bucket centrifuge under the control of the automation system, or the local automated centrifuge device. In many automated centrifuge components, the software may control the centrifuge speed, time, and temperature during centrifugation. The centrifuge functionality may be incorporated into devices such as the Tecan FE500 or may be a subcomponent of a system such as the LAB-InterLink or Beckman Coulter automation system offerings.

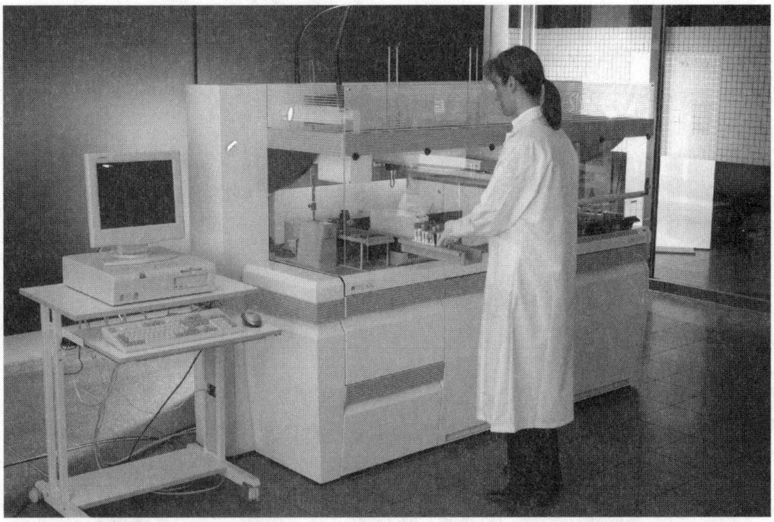

FIGURE 2. Tecan FE-500. (*Courtesy of Tecan U.S., Inc.*)

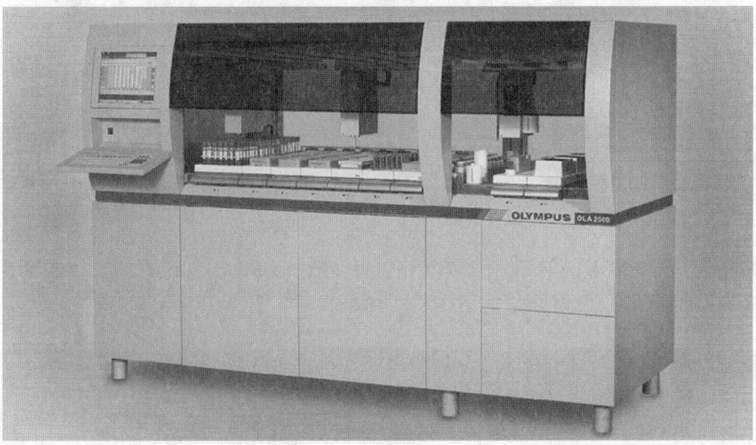

FIGURE 3. Olympus OLA 2500. (*Courtesy of Olympus America, Inc.*)

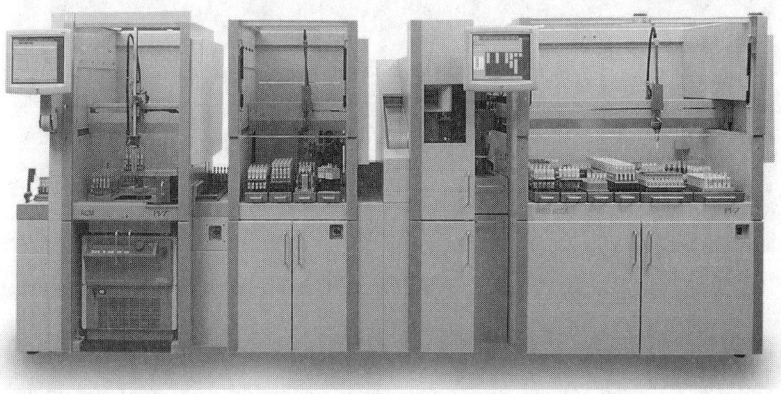

FIGURE 4. PVT specimen processing equipment. (*Courtesy of PVT Lab Systems, LLC*)

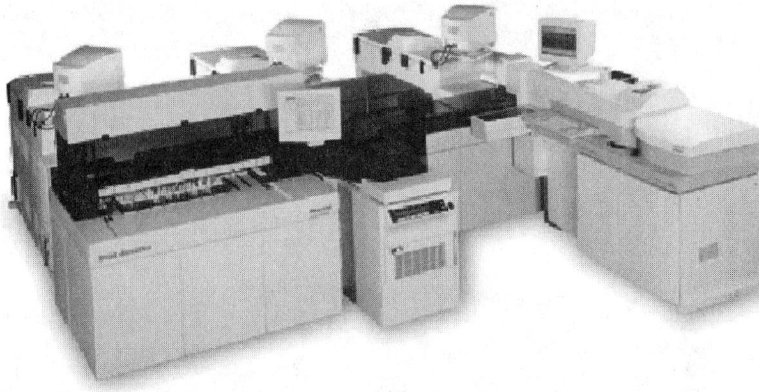

FIGURE 5. Dade Behring StreamLab. (*Courtesy of Dade Behring Inc.*)

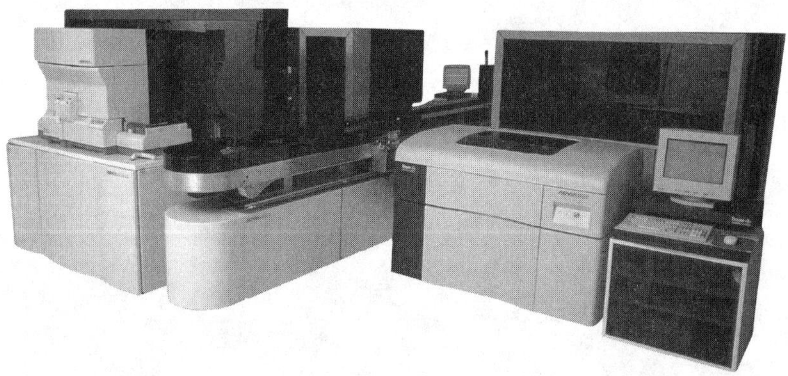

FIGURE 6. Bayer ADVIA LabCell. (©2002. Bayer Healthcare LLC, Diagnostics Division, Tarrytown, NY. ADVIA® and LabCell® are registered trademarks of Bayer HealthCare LLC)

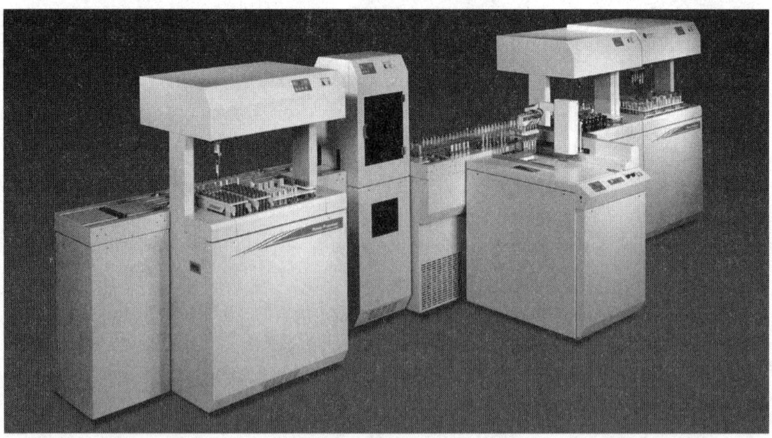

FIGURE 7. Beckman Coulter IDS Power Processor. (*Courtesy of Beckman Coulter, Inc.*)

Decapper

The decapper is required for closure/cap removal so that an uncapped specimen may be presented to devices such as a specimen integrity monitor, an instrument/analyzer, and an aliquotter. The decapper may remove the closures from many different types and brands

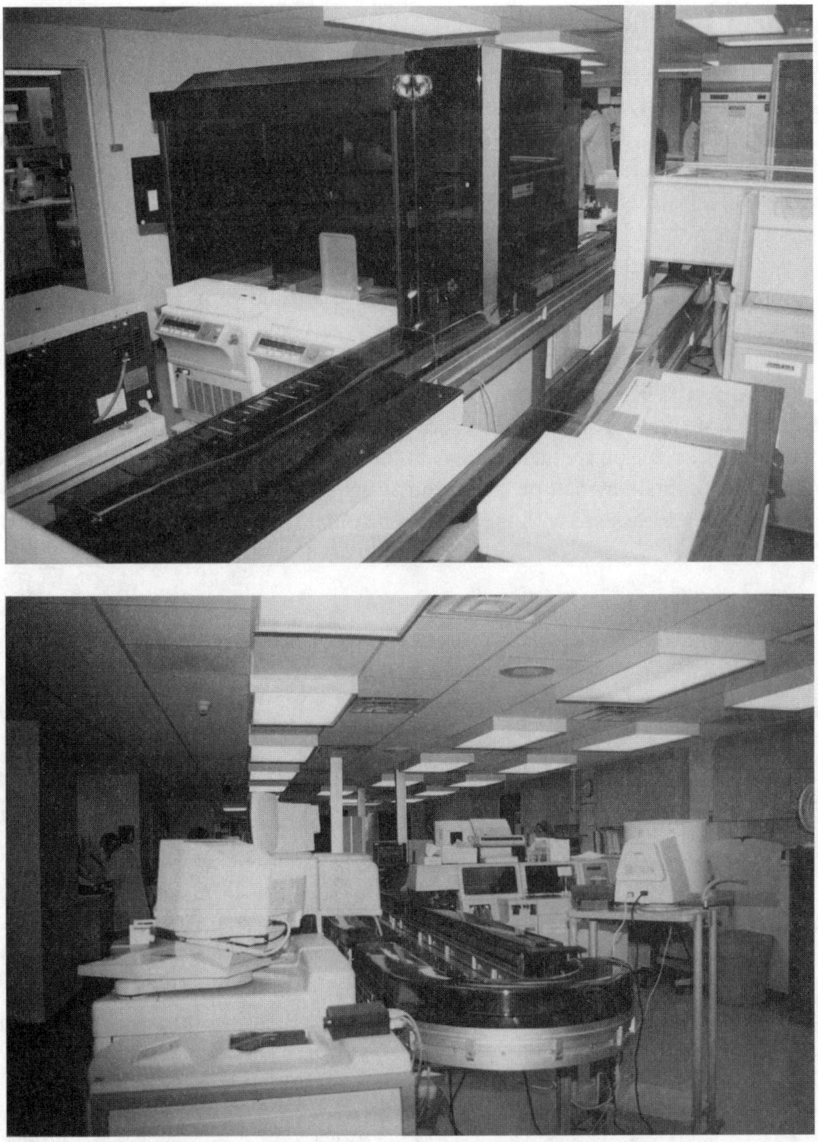

FIGURE 8. LAB-InterLink LAB-Frame automation system. (*Courtesy of the University of Nebraska Medical Center*)

of specimen containers and in some instances has the functionality to remove both depression closures as well as screw-top closures.

Specimen Integrity Monitor

The specimen integrity monitor is a device that allows the determination of hemolysis, icterus, and lipemia prior to the delivery determination of a specimen into an instrument/analyzer (*see* NCCLS AUTO 4-A). The specimen integrity monitor may be a device that is integrated into the automation system independent of instruments. In some implementations, the specimen integrity monitor is implemented through an instrument or many instruments and not a standalone device. The advantage of standalone devices is that prior to the analytical process, the specimen may be identified as one with hemolysis, icterus, or lipemia.

Instrument Interfaces

There are two major types of instrument interfaces: direct-track sampling (DTS) interfaces (23) and robotic analyzer interfaces (RAI). DTS interfaces are those interfaces that are defined within the NCCLS AUTO 5-A standard. The NCCLS AUTO 5-A standard defines a point in space as a reference that allows instrument manufacturers and automation manufacturers the physical measurements and relationships to transportation systems and instruments. In addition, AUTO 3-A defines the communications protocols, connectivity, and messaging required to interface an automated analyzer with a DTS interface to the automation systems. Examples of the DTS interface are shown in Figure 9.

The robotic automation interfaces are specialized devices constructed to link instruments without the AUTO 5-A specified point in space DTS interface and automation systems. Typically, the RAI uses one or many articulated robotic devices to remove a specimen from a transportation system and load in the carrier or specimen rack on the automation interface or on the instrument. In the case that a specimen container is loaded into a specimen container rack on the automation interface, a second movement will be required to move the cassette with the specimen containers onto and off of the instrument.

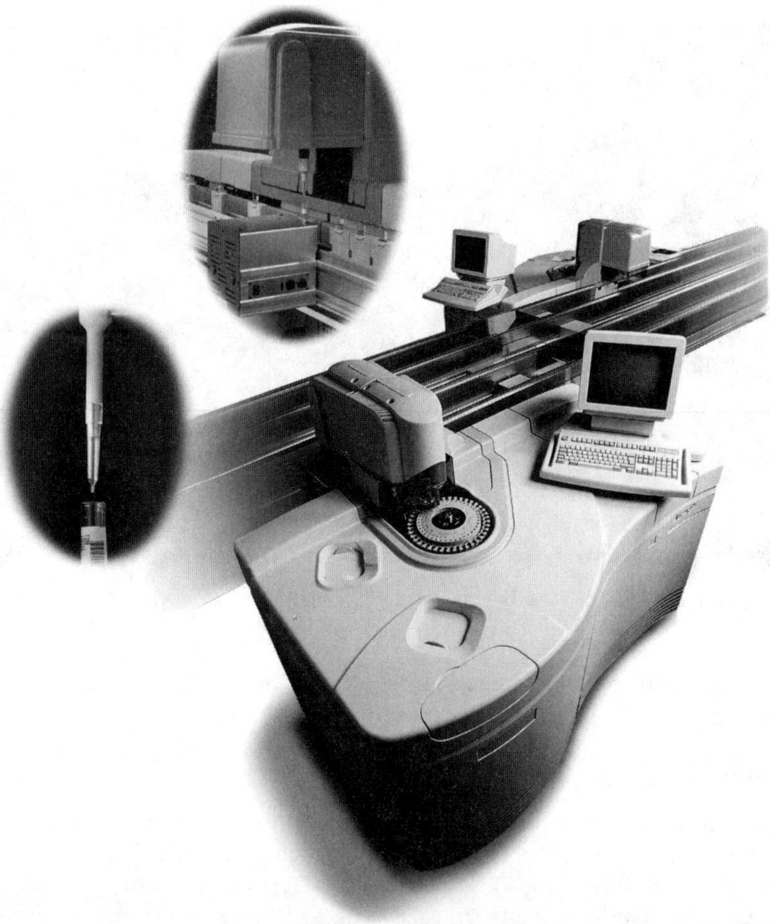

FIGURE 9. Direct-track sampling mechanism incorporated into an Ortho Clinical Diagnostics VITROS 950. (*Courtesy of Ortho-Clinical Diagnostics, A Johnson and Johnson Company*)

When the processing of the specimen is completed on the instrument, the specimen container and/or the rack holding specimen containers will be removed and the specimen container placed back on the transportation system (Figure 10).

Aliquotter

Many automation offerings include aliquotting capability. An aliquotter may be used at many points in the automation process. In a substantial or large automation system, aliquotting would most likely occur near the end of the process for specimens that are used at manual stations or lower volume testing stations to send out to reference laboratories.

Recapper

A recapping device as expected performs the opposite process of a decapper: places a closure back on the specimen container. A recapper may use a pressure-fit closure or a screw-cap closure or in some cases both.

Sorter

A sorter may be used to provide output so specimen containers may be sorted to multiple different formats. Specimens may be sorted to the individual "personality" racks for instrument/analyzers. A sorter may also output specimen containers to a bench specific rack for transportation within an individual laboratory or may put specimens into specialized containers for delivery to a reference laboratory. A sorter may also be used to output specimen containers for short-term and long-term storage.

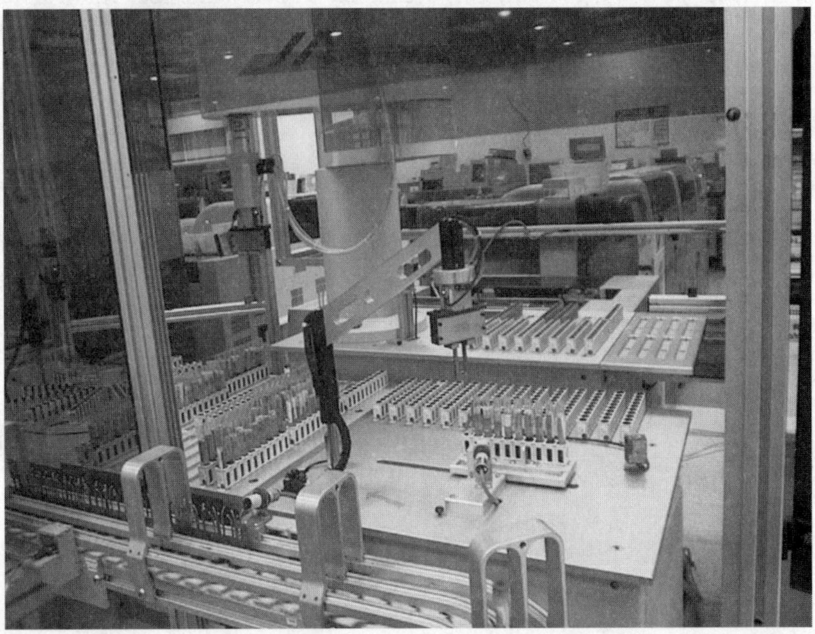

FIGURE 10. Robotic automation instrument interface for Olympus AU series chemistry instrument. (*Courtesy of Maccabi Healthcare Services, Maccabi Megalab, Rehovot, Israel*)

Storage/Retrieval/Disposal

Storage, retrieval, and disposal systems may collect specimen containers from the automation system and provide short-term or long-term storage. A storage/retrieval/disposal system may or may not be refrigerated, depending upon the specimen volume of the laboratory and the duration of specimen storage. Most storage and retrieval systems also allow for disposal of specimen containers through their defined time-out (i.e., 24 hours and 1 minute for a whole blood specimen). Storage and retrieval units may also be used to prepare specimens for long-term storage such as a serum bank or to collect specimens for prospective testing by test code and test result (i.e., the preparation of a collection of serum specimens for future comparison of methodologies for a specific analyte).

INSTRUMENTS, WORKCELLS, AND SYSTEMS

Laboratory automation technology can be categorized into three distinct groups: instruments, workcells, and systems. This categorization is outlined in Table 8.

Automation Instruments

Automation instruments are defined as devices that perform one or many specimen-processing or specimen-handling functions, usually in a standalone mode. Typically, these instruments combine one or many of the following functions: inputting, decapping, centrifuging, liquid level sensing, aliquotting, recapping, and sorting to output racks. The functional combinations are usually dependent upon the marketing requirements of the company selling the technology. Technology marketed by specific in vitro diagnostics vendors usually accentuate the functionality of their specific instrument offerings.

Specimen container output racks are usually specific for a particular instrument. In the case of the Tecan FE500, this instrument can sort to many different configurations of instrument racks. Instruments such as the Olympus OLA series are typically configured to sort to Olympus-specific output racks, with the option to sort to other manufacturers racks. The instruments manufactured by PVT are based upon the technology that supports the

TABLE 8. Sorting the technology

Systems	Workcells	Instruments
Open architecture:	ADVIA Workcell	Tecan FE500
LAB-InterLink	Bayer	
Ortho Clinical	(chem., ia, heme, etc.)	Olympus OLA 1/2/3500
Olympus	Closed system	
Dade Behring		Sysmex Hematology
Roche	StreamLab Workcell	
Bayer	Dade Behring	PVT Specimen Processing
Abbott	(chem.)	
DPC	Closed system	Roche MODULAR
Stago		
Sysmex		
Tosoh		
Beckman Coulter		
Closed architecture:		
Beckman Coulter		

Roche instrument lines. The Roche MODULAR® system is a unique combination of instrument-based automation technology and front-end automation functionality combined into an instrument.

The software capability of these systems is also similar to that of an instrument. The functionality is most useful with unique specimen identification numbers or accession numbers. The interface between the LIS and the automation instrument is typically an ASTM protocol with limited segment content.

The automation instruments do not directly connect to other technologies such as other automation instruments or instruments. The lack of connectivity is potentially a long-term issue for many laboratories, since the capital investment is not conserved when the laboratory or institution requires an upgrade to a workcell or a system. At this time, the only automation technologies that provide an entry-level automation solution that conserves capital investment and provides an upgrade pathway is the front-end processor from LAB-InterLink, Inc., and the Beckman Coulter IDS Power Processor.

Workcells

Automation workcells are typically composed of some automation technology components, such as an input/loading station, centrifugation, decapping, and instruments connectivity. The two workcells currently on the market are the Bayer LabCell® workcell and the Dade StreamLab® workcell.

The Bayer LabCell workcell incorporates hematology, chemistry, immunoassay, and urinalysis instruments. The combination of instruments may handle the bulk of the testing in an average clinical laboratory. The LabCell also uses a more sophisticated software suite as compared to the automation instruments, allowing for routing and balancing of specimen workload across instruments.

The Bayer LabCell is a closed system, simply stated, a system that connects to Bayer equipment, for the purpose of marketing Bayer instruments and reagents. At this writing, the system does not comply with the NCCLS standards and therefore does not accept the addition or substitution of non-Bayer analytical equipment. The interface between the LabCell and the LIS may be at the level of an HL7 or ASTM, and depending upon the segment content, may perform different levels of sorting and prioritization.

The Dade StreamLab workcell incorporates one or many Dade RxL instruments in combination with a transportation system and an input/sorting device. The StreamLab also uses a more sophisticated software package as compared to the automation instruments. Similar to the LabCell, the StreamLab is also a closed system that does not comply with the NCCLS standards. The absence of connectivity and expandability, similar to the automation instruments, limits the use of limited capital resources into the future, and binds the hospital or laboratory to the instrument vendor: a good marketing strategy for the vendor and a less than optimal situation for the laboratory or hospital.

Systems

There are two system vendors currently on the market: the Beckman Coulter IDS Power Processor system and the LAB-InterLink LAB-Frame automation system. Automation systems are characterized as systems composed of components that can be assembled to create the functionality defined by the laboratory. Table 7 and the section on automation components in this chapter define each automation component.

The Beckman Coulter IDS Power Processor is composed of modules that contain track segments with or without automation; specimen-handling functionality including centrifugation, decapping, aliquotting, instrument interfaces, recapping, and sorting to output racks including instrument-specific racks; and storage and retrieval. It can be configured to function as a front-end processing station or a small system configuration, all the way up to and through a large full function automation system. Examples of small front-end systems through larger full function systems are present in many organizations in North America. The Beckman Coulter IDS Power Processor has the capability to connect to many different analyzers and instruments; however, the system is configured to optimize the connections to the Beckman Coulter instruments, specifically the LX-20.

The LAB-InterLink LAB-Frame system is composed of a transportation system that connects to specimen-processing and specimen-handling devices similar to those listed in Table 7. The system is designed to comply with the NCCLS standards for clinical laboratory automation, allowing the use of any NCCLS compliant third-party automation products. The LAB-InterLink LAB-Frame system allows the use of one or many of the automation components in any configuration to create systems that support the turnaround time needs of a laboratory or hospital. The LAB-InterLink LAB-Frame system is constructed to take advantage of the LAB-InterLink process control software, a computer integrated manufacturing approach to laboratory operations. The process control software allows the system to optimize turnaround time on a specimen container and test level to support the needs of the mission of the clinical laboratory and the operations of a hospital. At this writing, this is the most sophisticated automation process control software package on the market.

LABORATORY LAYOUT

Defining the layout of a clinical automation system is a significant task. There are two important caveats when defining the laboratory layout:

- If possible, the trajectory of the clinical laboratory in terms of volume, physical space, remodeling, or other physical and operational changes should be identified and mapped out prior to determining a physical implementation for an automation system.
- Points of reference with respect to the laboratory physical layout should be identified upfront (i.e., utilities for instruments, location of pneumatic tube system stations, significant physical support structures, etc.).

Many automation systems vendors have an automation system layout tool, which is either a software tool, hardware tool, or a combination of both. The software or hardware tool eventually will provide information that will be translated into a computer-assisted design (CAD) software system. Many LAS companies will request CAD drawings of the laboratory layout before and after any physical changes so that the physical implementation of a clinical laboratory system may be laid out. The CAD drawing will be the basis for the physical implementation of the automation system and will be the translation tool used for construction, information system, and electrical workers. Significant caveats to be discussed include the need for securing the automation and the incorporated instrumentation to the floor for earthquake proofing such as is required in the state of California.

Construction Rules

With most automation systems, there are construction rules whether it is the configuration of automation subcomponents (i.e., input station, centrifuge, decapper, analyzers) or physical relationship of the system to other site parameters such as tube systems and electrical services. Most vendors of automation systems suggest the following steps for determining the layout of an automation system.

Step 1

Select the functional areas of the clinical laboratory to automate:

- Preanalytical specimen processing (specimen centrifugation, specimen decapping, specimen aliquotting)
- Specimen analysis (DTS by instruments, routing between and among instruments, reflex and repeat testing)
- Postanalytical specimen handling (specimen recapping, sorting, specimen storage, retrieval for add-on and reflex testing, automated disposal)

Step 2

Choose the preanalytical specimen-processing devices to operate the clinical laboratory. These may include a manual input station, an automated centrifuge, or other input device. Determine the number of modules or options on those modules required for laboratory preprocessing.

Step 3

Arrange the instruments/analyzers in the preferred order around the automation system. Choices will be determined based upon volume, instrument turnaround time, or the type of automation system acquired. Analyzers not currently interfaced with an NCCLS standard DTS interface may require the use of a RAI. The RAI may require development prior to the implementation of the LAS. In order to create an RAI, significant and sustained cooperation is required between the instrument vendor and the automation system vendor. In the absence of cooperation by either vendor, another instrument/analyzer will usually be required to be chosen by the laboratorian.

Step 4

Determine which postanalytical specimen-handling devices are needed for the system, i.e., a recapper, a sorter, and a storage and retrieval unit with or without refrigeration.

Step 5

Arrange all modules in sequential order based upon processing workflow and distribution of specimens and instruments/analyzer throughput. The LAS vendor will have the expertise in-house to help create this priority order.

Step 6

Determine what automation system shape options are available by coordinated discussions with vendors and with input from the automation technology group, the institutional architects, and members of the laboratory automation acquisition team, and then determine the appropriate configuration for the laboratory.

Step 7

Determine a timeline that includes contracting through implementation and testing and begin the process.

Establishing a Proforma for the Automated Laboratory

Hospitals, healthcare organizations, and many other business entities require their officers, directors, and managers to provide financial justification of capital purchases, capital leases, and operational leases. Policy and procedure varies significantly from organization to organization. The policies and procedures for justification of categories of equipment purchase also vary significantly from organization to organization. In some institutions, large capital purchases are made for the benefit of the organization without substantial financial evaluation. Examples of these types of purchases include hospital information systems, LISs, radiology information systems, and financial information systems (24–26). Every hospital has these information systems in the year 2002, and the administrators and employees could not imagine working without these tools.

The evaluation of capital purchases for the clinical laboratory is usually based on per test cost evaluation including **all** associated expenses and labor. The decreasing numbers of medical technologists and medical technology training programs will increase the associated labor costs, just as the shortage in nurses has increased nursing salaries and limited admissions in many hospitals across North America. The decrease in the number of medical technologists will support the demand for automation technology in the coming years (27).

Most organizations require a formal proposal that defines the rationale for purchasing the selected technology, background information, a future look at the operation of the laboratory, and forecast of the future condition of the laboratory's financial statement after the implementation of the technology. Many methods exist to summarize and rank investment opportunities for the acquisition of capital equipment including:

- Payback period
- Accounting rate of return or return on investment (ROI)
- Net present value (NPV)
- Internal rate of return (IRR)
- Discounted payback period
- Profitability index (PI)

The **payback period** is defined as the number of years required to recover the investment costs from the cash flows associated with the project. Payback period analysis use should be secondary to other methodologies since it does not take into account discounting, inflation, risk, or organizational cash flow.

The **accounting rate of return**, more commonly known as the return on investment, is a simple measure of return, usually calculated on a year-to-year basis, and expressed as a percentage. The ROI method may include depreciation and usually does not depend upon cash flows.

The **net present value** is the difference between the present value of the net cash flow generated and the present value of the investment. A net present value of zero means that the cost of capital equals the internal rate of return. A net present value greater than zero is preferable to the internal rate of return as ranking criteria and makes a more realistic assumption that funds can be reinvested at the cost of capital rather than the internal rate of return.

The **internal rate of return** is the discount that equates cash inflows with cash outflows. The internal rate of return is usually solved using a trial-and-error methodology, with many results based upon the year-to-year cash flows. Basically, the internal rate of return is the rate at which funds are presumed to be reinvested.

The **discounted payback period** is the number of years required to recover the equipment expense based upon the present value of the annual discounted cash flows. The discounted payback period is used to determine the breakeven point for the investment versus the useful life of the equipment.

The **profitability index** is the ratio of the present value of cash flows generated by the project and the present value of the investment. This ratio scales a project to the net present value per dollar of investment.

The most commonly used evaluation formula is the accounting **rate of return** or the ROI. The ROI is simple to comprehend, however, it is highly dependent upon cash from year to year. Many people in the organization and many vendors speak to the issue of ROI, however, it is not clear if they really comprehend the cash dependence of the future years. Consulting the chief financial officer is an important step in the evaluation process. Vendors' ROI calculations are rarely reliable, since the vendors do not "run" the operation.

The **discounted payback period** relates to cash flow and may be a more useful discriminator, depending on the organization. The discounted payback period and the other discriminators listed are similar in value for the purpose of an investment. Choose the discriminator or the cluster of discriminators that the organization is comfortable with. The relevant equations are presented in Table 9.

Measuring Operational Change

Measuring the operational change in a laboratory after implementing a clinical laboratory automation system is paramount (28). It is difficult, if not almost impossible, to segregate operational change from the reorganization resulting from implementing automation systems and the direct effect of the automation system itself. A purist would want to measure the effects of both; however, to a pragmatic laboratorian facing significant financial

TABLE 9. Financial Equations

Payback Period

$$PP = \frac{\text{Investment}}{\text{Yearly Return}}$$

Accounting Rate of Return (ROI)

$$ROI = \frac{\text{Investment}}{\Sigma\text{Returns}} - 1$$

Net Present Value (NPV)

$$NPV = \Sigma PV - C$$

$$\Sigma PV = PV_1 + PV_2 + PV_3 + \ldots..$$

$$C = \text{Investment}$$

Internal Rate of Return (IRR)

Discount rate where NPV = zero
(Solve for discount rate in PV calculation.)

Discounted Payback Period

$$PP = \frac{\text{Investment + Cost of Capital}}{\text{Yearly Return}}$$

Profitability Index (PI)

$$PI = \frac{\Sigma\text{PVCashFlows}}{\Sigma\text{PVInvestment}}$$

operating constraints within the hospital or a healthcare system, it is clear that there is a job to do and it must be accomplished.

Every laboratory scientist (whether technologist, chemist, or physician) is trained to perform against a benchmark or standard. In the clinical laboratory automation environment, new benchmarks will be set based upon the operational changes enacted by implementing automation. Only after the reimplementation of laboratory automation in a previously automated laboratory will changes directly attributed to the automation system be able to be justified.

In order to determine the effects of automation, first determine which elements of the clinical laboratory operation to measure both before implementation of automation and after implementation (29). Table 10 provides some suggestions for measuring operational changes affected by the LAS that should be evaluated before and many times after the implementation of a clinical laboratory automation system. (*See* NCCLS AUTO4-A, Vol 21, No. 4 for additional information.)

Caveats and Important Concepts

- Automation technology is complex, more complex than most purchasers suspect.
- Automation technology breaks and/or fails like every other "machine" it requires maintenance, support, and repair.
- Automation theory is complex and as more variables are added, the complexity grows exponentially.
- Not all technology is the same. Pneumatic devices, used in many applications today will aerosolize specimens, i.e., serum and plasma and may result in cross-contamination.
- If automation technology is purchased that does not conform to the NCCLS standards, the products will not fit in an open-system environment.

TABLE 10. Measuring operational changes before and after automation

Measurement	Before	After
Number of full-time equivalents (FTE) in the automated laboratory		
Test volume in the automated laboratory		
Turnaround time for the 20 highest volume tests		
Cost per test		
Cost per requisition		
Number of errors in specimen handling		
Number of errors in test reporting		
Tests per hour		
Tests per FTE-hour		
Number of aliquots generated		
Number of aliquots per specimen		
Specimen retrieval time		
Worker's compensation claims in dollars		
Reagent use–billable tests/test performed		
Supply budget		
Volume per FTE-hour/operating hour		
Errors per FTE-hour		

- Choose a software driven automation solution. Nonsoftware-based or driven automation solutions are usually add-ons to the instruments sold by a vendor and not a system unto themselves.
- Automation technology without a defined upgrade pathway may result in a dead-end technology. Evaluate the upgrade pathway for automation; if the automation system is composed of components, then an upgrade pathway is likely. However, if the purchased technology is a fixed unit, it is usually replaceable, not upgradeable.

LABORATORY AUTOMATION QUESTIONS AND ANSWERS

Is this Laboratory Large Enough to Justify an Automation Investment?

A commonly quoted **rule-of-thumb** is that a laboratory should run 1.0 to 1.3 million tests annually to obtain an acceptable ROI. This rule can be very misleading. Laboratory-to-laboratory variables alter the ROI conditions, not the least of which is the automation system itself (is it preanalytic only, analytic only, what functionality modules are attached, which and how many instruments are online, etc.).

The validity of this estimation is dependent on the cost of the automation technology. Costs have decreased over the years. Options such as intelligent process control software improve the financial return over hardware-based systems. Important qualitative benefits such as improved turnaround time, error reduction, or market positioning can override a marginal difference in the financial determination of value.

What Target Benefits are Used to Help Justify an Investment in Automation?

Financial ROI relies primarily on **space**, **labor**, and **capacity** gains. The economic benefit usually derives from productivity gains and the resulting reduced labor costs.

- **Space**: automation saves costly floor space by consolidating operations. New laboratory construction costs range between $200 and $400 per square foot. Transfer unused space to other high-value or revenue-generating services.
- **Labor**: automation expands laboratories capacity to perform more work without increasing labor hours. Laboratories forecasting significant growth have the added cost-avoidance payback in future months or years as they take advantage of the built-in capacity of an automated laboratory.
- **Capacity**: for example, the laboratory can aggressively grow outreach revenues while improving net margins. This is possible because the cost of technical labor remains static as new clients are added.

What Qualitative, Nonfinancial Benefits can be Expected?

Automation clients point to these quality or general business management benefits. Many of these factors provide considerable indirect financial return.

- **Service quality**: improves turnaround time of results, and reduces the rate of laboratory errors
- **Safety issues**: lowers risk of job-related injury, and lowers risk of biohazard exposure
- **Labor management**: helps solve labor shortage problems, and helps with employee turnover problems
- **Business management**: enhances competitive position, and enables cultural change in the laboratory

Is Front-end Preanalytic Automation Right for this Laboratory?

- **Standalone preanalytic system**: typically this includes centrifugation, decapping, and sorting of specimens. It may also include aliquotting to secondary containers. The labor, capacity, and safety benefits of these systems are limited solely to the central processing department. In the recent past, preanalytic systems were cost-justifiable only in very large laboratories with a high proportion of routine (non-stat) chemistry work.
- **Phased implementation**: the greatest financial payback from automation is derived with a tightly integrated, software optimized, comprehensive system that includes preanalytic, analytic, and postanalytic modules. An option is progressive implementation of functionality/modules over a phased implementation period.
- **Plan 3–5 years ahead**: envision the potential future laboratory, perhaps 3–5 years beyond the first-stage venture into automation. Planning ahead may prevent making a good short-term decision that later proves to be a poor long-term decision.
- **Easily expandable system**: it is advisable to avoid any initial investment in an automation module that is not designed to be easily expanded either for higher capacity or for additional components of automation. It is best to develop a sound strategic plan for automation that considers possible business and capacity scenarios in future years.

What Routine Laboratory Tasks can be Automated?

Automating routine laboratory tasks depends on the comprehensiveness of the vendor's system and how it is configured. An automation system should support the following laboratory tasks:

- In-lab receipt notification (normally performed through the LIS)
- Specimen triage decisions
- Centrifugation
- Uncapping of specimen containers
- Primary container aliquotting to secondary containers, labeling, and distribution of secondary containers
- Specimens delivered to analytic instrument workstations
- Specimens submitted directly to the analyzers for testing
- Unverified results from analyzers reviewed for acceptability (rules-based)
- Instrument error, status, and reagent inventory messages reviewed
- Rules-based rerouting of specimens to analyzers for repeat testing
- Container management and sorting for both automated and manual workstations
- Continuous specimen tracking and retrieval
- Specimen integrity monitoring
- Recapping of containers
- Container storage management

Does it Make Sense to Consider an LAS that Does not Include Front-end Automation?

Successful systems have been installed without preanalytic automation other than a loading station. Centrifuging, decapping, and aliquotting are performed manually, and a fully processed sample is loaded onto the automation track that unites a number of instruments.

- **Island of automation**: these analytic systems focus on consolidating instruments into an island of automation, a form of modular automation technology. Preanalytic modules for analytic islands include (at a minimum) a loading station, decapper, and triage/sorting unit.

- **Process control software**: such software is essential to optimize analytic automation because of the added value of being able to automate repeat testing, dilutions, reflex orders, and automatically adjudicate instrument errors.
- **Closed versus open solutions**: analytic systems are either **closed** or **open** solutions.

The Laboratory Runs a High Number of Stat Orders. Does Automation Help or Hinder Turn-around Time (TAT)?

Stat and routine tests are not the same. When a mixed volume of both stat and routine testing is high, some automated laboratories have found it necessary to retain manual processing of stats to ensure priority handling. This is because most automation systems treat stat and routine specimens the same. Intelligent software makes the difference. The currently available systems and technologies greatly differ. Most preanalytic systems are fairly unintelligent; they are not designed to use process control logic to expedite stat samples. Process control software intelligently alters the routing and handling of specimens based on data such as order status, specimen origin (ER, OR, etc.), ordering physician, etc. Determine whether the automation vendor capabilities built into the software uniquely address stat specimen handling. By making the right changes, most laboratories can expect significant improvements in service quality and reliability. The **right changes** include adjustments to processes, space planning, and implementation of the appropriate configuration.

What is Process Control as Applied to Laboratory Automation?

Process control software technology integrated with robotic hardware modules, analyzers, and an automation transportation system that unites them physically makes an impact on the laboratory. An experienced medical technologist relies on various clinical, quality assurance, instrument, and demographic parameters to qualify a patient result as acceptable for reporting, or takes actions to validate the quality of a result. Yet, it is estimated that roughly 85% of all laboratories results could be automatically verified against an operational rule set. Using automation and process control technology, **standards of practice** are employed to take action to augment the human effort. These rules control the decisions and actions for 80%–90% of all results released from the laboratory. This system consistently and objectively reacts to input parameters (results, QA data, instrument messages, etc.) to produce the same results regardless of the expertise of the technologist or changes in personnel across shifts and departments.

The job of the laboratory staff is to produce quality results in a timely fashion. The vast majority of clinical specimens and results are within normal range. Consequently, the laboratory's technical staff spends a considerable time performing routine and even mundane tasks that require minimal technical skill. The technologist's time and attention is thereby diffused. Automation and process control technology effectively "flips" their attention off the routine and the mundane tasks and onto patient specimens with exceptional or variant results.

Process control **automates routine tasks**. Without automation technology, 70%–80% of an average technologist's time is spent on nontechnical tasks. The automation "system" takes over the routine tasks. It also handles many technical decisions and actions that can be defined through standard rule sets. This process alters the attention ratio of the laboratory staff, 70%–80% of their time is now spent on the most important technical work. Greater attention is given to variant results when there is no time lost on the "normals." Quality is gained and time is saved.

What Distinguishes Open versus Closed Systems?

An open design philosophy creates the opportunity to consolidate "best-of-class" analyzers from multiple vendors into an integrated system. Open system technology is a low-risk investment because it avoids the possibility of losing the automation system if a switch is made to a new instrument vendor at a future date. Open system technology offers the flexibility of swapping one instrument for another with minimal disruption. Instrument vendors typically sell closed systems. Closed systems are purposely designed to integrate (favor) only the instruments of that vendor. Purchase agreements from closed system vendors commonly bundle the automation system with the instruments as a single purchase.

What Other Features Should be Evaluated?

Two fundamental design characteristics that significantly impact how automation systems operate are continuous loop versus one-way track and the use of single specimen container carriers versus rack-style carriers. **Continuous loop and single specimen container carrier** are features best suited for hospital-based laboratories that run a higher rate of stat requests and/or abnormal patient samples. One-way and rack-style systems are optimized for commercial laboratories that run a high percentage of routine or batch testing.

Continuous-loop transport technology offers the flexibility to return specimens to instruments or modules on the automation line. Some systems employ one-way track design with no ability to return specimens to an instrument or an automated module. This limitation is often unacceptable because it forces continued dependency on manual processes. For example, a continuous loop eliminates interrupting a technologist to locate and transport a specimen for repeat or add-on testing or for dilutions. In contrast, a one-way system requires manual retrieval and reloading of specimens to the beginning of the track. It forces manual processing off-line from the automation system.

Specimen carriers are either single specimen containers or multispecimen containers (rack-style). Use of multicontainer racks effectively sacrifices the flexibility required for processing a single sample as unique from the batch (i.e., mixing stat versus routine samples). Other important characteristics include:

- Support of direct container sampling
- Handling of multiple container sizes/types
- Ability to minimize aliquots
- Protection of routine instrument accessibility

Specimen tracking and quick retrieval is a major laboratory challenge poorly addressed by manual systems. Process control software easily solves this problem by knowing where each specimen is at all times and retrieving the specimen either automatically or on-demand by user request, depending on the situation. The continuous-loop track enables the container to be re-routed directly to the appropriate analyzer for testing.

Laboratories at teaching institutions and academic medical centers and/or those with large outreach operations can experience as many as 2000 or more add-on orders each month. The search for some specimens can consume the time of two or three medical technologists and can take 30 minutes or more. Other specimens are never found or are not found quickly enough. In these cases, the ordering physician must be contacted and a new specimen obtained from the patient. If the average time to find a specimen and resubmit it for analysis is 5 minutes, then the labor cost of this effort can range from $50,000 to $80,000 annually.

We Deal with a Mix of Laboratory Errors that Negatively Impact our Productivity or the Quality of our Service. How can Automation Help?

Not all automation systems are equal, but **all** have resulted a reduction in laboratory errors. The use of process management software, a continuous-loop track, and an integrated suite of robotic modules and analyzers are the most important attributes to lower errors.

- Repeat testing that is not performed per protocol for abnormal patient results such as failing delta check, panic results, linearity failure, etc.
- Repeat testing that is not performed per protocol in response to instrument errors such as humidity or temperature problems, short sample, etc.
- Tests not performed because an order for testing is overlooked for some reason
- Required dilution not performed
- Add-on testing not able to be performed because a specimen cannot be located or not located quickly enough
- Unacceptable delays in turnaround time because the specimen cannot be located or not located quickly enough
- Wrong test performed
- Unnecessary patient re-collects because a specimen is dropped and broken or spilled
- Unnecessary patient re-collects because a specimen is lost or cannot be quickly located
- Misplaced or forgotten specimens
- Exposure to infectious disease from improper handling of specimens
- Repetitive task injuries or injuries from broken glass, etc.

SUMMARY AND CONCLUSIONS

During the past 20 years clinical laboratory automation has evolved from several concepts and approaches to a continuum of products ranging from instruments through workcells and system-level implementations. The approaches to solving clinical laboratory operational issues, similar to many other industries, has moved in a direction using software to model, drive, control, and operate many of the technologies that now are used daily if not hourly. The incorporation of clinical laboratory automation technology into the hospital and regional clinical laboratories is as inevitable as the implementation of the laboratory information systems of the 1980s. It is not a matter of "if," but simply a matter of "when" a laboratory incorporates clinical laboratory automation technology and in what form (30–32).

The implementation of the prospective clinical laboratory automation standards published by NCCLS has resulted in a significant change in the clinical laboratory instrument manufacturers approach to vendor–vendor cooperation. The adoption and implementation of these standards has also resulted in a significant reduction and potential savings to the patient and third-party payers through the "re-use" of interface designs that would have been designed as proprietary devices to technologies if left up to the manufacturers' marketing departments. Prospective buyers have learned both what steps to take and which steps to avoid from the information systems market of the 1980s.

The selection of technology during this phase of the lifecycle of automation technology may be viewed as a significant risk by laboratorians and their administrative counterparts. This appears to be a "darned" if you do and "darned" if you do not purchase and implement automation technology in the clinical laboratory. Practically speaking if automation technology, that is compliant with the NCCLS standards is purchased, the buyer is less likely to loose his/her capital investment going forward in the future. The difference is simply risk, purchasing technology that is standard compliant compared with "risky," a result of purchasing non-NCCLS compliant automation technology.

REFERENCES

1. Sasaki M, Hashimoto E. Systematization of clinical laboratory—some problems caused from specimen transport through laboratory reports. Rinsho Byori 1991;39(10):1022–7. (Japanese)
2. Sasaki M, Kageoka T, Ogura K, Kataoka H, Ueta T, Sugihara S. Total laboratory automation in Japan. Past, present, and the future. Clin Chim Acta 1998;278(2):217–27.
3. Sasaki M. An innovative conveyor belt system for a clinical laboratory. J Int Fed Clin Chem 1991;3(1):31–3.
4. Sasaki M. The robotic system of the clinical laboratories. Rinsho Byori 1987;35(10):1072–8. (Japanese)
5. Bauer S, Teplitz C. Laboratory automation, part 1. Total laboratory automation: a view of the 21st century. MLO Med Lab Obs 1995;27(7):22–5.
6. Bauer S, Teplitz C. Laboratory automation, part 2. Total lab automation: system design. MLO Med Lab Obs 1995;27(9):44–50.
7. Boyd JC, Felder RA, Savory J. Robotics and the changing face of the clinical laboratory. Clin Chem 1996;42(12):1901–10.
8. Dadoun R. Impact on human resources: core laboratory versus laboratory information system versus modular robotics. Clin Lab Manage Rev 1998;12(4):248–55.
9. Dadoun R. Case study: automation's impact on productivity and turnaround time. MLO Med Lab Obs 2002;34:36–8.
10. Markin RS, Whalen SA. Laboratory automation: trajectory, technology, and tactics. Clin Chem 2000;46(5):764–71.
11. Markin RS. Clinical laboratory automation: concepts and directions, chapter 7. In Bozzo P, ed. Cost-effective laboratory management. Philadelpia: Lippincott-Raven, 1998:145–62.
12. Hawker CD, Schlank MR. Development of standards for laboratory automation. Clin Chem 2000;46(5):746–50.
13. Markin RS, Sasaki M. A laboratory automation platform: the next robotic step. MLO Med Lab Obs 1992;24(10):24–9.
14. Markin RS. Clinical laboratory automation, chapter 4. In: Clinical diagnosis and management by laboratory methods, 20th ed. Henry JB, ed. Philadelpia: WB Saunders in press, 2001.
15. Markin RS. Clinical laboratory automation systems: concepts, designs and future directions. Am Pathol Rev Winter 1994/5.
16. Markin RS. Implementing automation in a modern clinical laboratory. Chemometrics and intelligent laboratory systems. Lab Inform Manage 1993;21(2,3):169–79.
17. Markin RS. Laboratory automation platform. In: Handbook of clinical automation, robotics, and optimization. Kost GJ, ed. New York: Wiley, 1996:217–34.
18. Markin RS. Challenging the future. Clinical laboratory automation: a paradigm shift. Clin Lab Manage Rev 1993 May–Jun;7(3):243–51.
19. Markin RS. Laboratory automation systems. An introduction to concepts and terminology. Am J Clin Pathol 1992;98(4 Suppl 1):S3–10.
20. Markin RS. Clinical laboratory automation: concepts and designs. Semin Diagn Pathol 1994 Nov;11(4):274–81.
21. Markin RS. Recent trends in clinical laboratory automation. Clin Lab Manage Rev 1998 May–Jun;12(3):176–80.
22. Markin RS. Historical perspectives and critical issues. In: Handbook of clinical automation, robotics, and optimization. Kost GJ, ed. New York: Wiley, 1996:30–42.
23. McPherson RA. Robotics, automation, and the new role of process control. Clin Lab Manage Rev 1998 Sep–Oct;12(5):339–46.

24. Markin RS. Robotics, interfaces, and the docking device. In: Handbook of clinical automation, robotics, and optimization. Kost GJ, ed. New York: Wiley, 1996:235–51.
25. Krempel G. Financial benefits of integrating robotics into an academic medical center core laboratory. Am Clin Lab 2000;19(2):22.
26. Kost GJ, Felder RA. Automation, part 2. Modular stepwise automation and the future of diagnostic testing. MLO Med Lab Obs 1998;30(6):46, 48, 56.
27. Pawlick GF, Smith C, Smith C. A task-targeted automation system: a case study. Clin Lab Manage Rev 1999 Nov–Dec;13(6):351–6.
28. Serrano L. Laboratory automation: a case study. MLO Med Lab Obs 2001;33(7):30.
29. Middleton SR. Developing an automation concept that is right for your laboratory. Clin Chem 2000;46(5):757–63.
30. Young DS. Laboratory automation: smart strategies and practical applications. Clin Chem 2000;46(5):740–5.
31. Gochman N, Quint J. The new millennium in laboratory automation. Ann Clin Lab Sci 1999 Apr–Jun;29(2):104–5.
32. Felder RA, Kost GJ. Automation, part 1. Modular stepwise automation and the future of diagnostic testing. MLO Med Lab Obs 1998;30(4):22–4, 26–7.

Chapter 17

Point-of-Care Testing

Christopher P. Price, Andrew St John, and Jocelyn M. Hicks

The development of point-of-care testing (POCT) over the last two decades marks the completion of a cycle that began with the performance of simple urine tests at the patient's bedside (1). When these tests, such as measurement of glucose in urine, moved away from the patient into separate rooms attached to the ward or the clinic, it heralded what was effectively the formation of a laboratory. Parallel developments led to patients visiting a physician either at a health center (primary care) or at an outpatient clinic attached to a hospital (secondary care), rather than the reverse situation, and this change led to a lengthening of the time taken to making clinical decisions. This delay is not always acceptable for clinicians or patients and so a significant portion of testing has now moved back closer to the patient. POCT is now carried out in a wide range of environments, some of which are set out in Table 1.

POCT can be defined as "any test that is performed in close proximity to the patient which enables a very rapid result to be obtained and action taken immediately." Some of the other names given to this form of testing have included bedside, near patient, physician's office, extralaboratory, decentralized, off-site, ancillary, and alternative site testing (2).

Figure 1 describes the process from patient consultation to implementation of the intervention and the many activities associated with producing a test result. It becomes immediately clear that, from an operational standpoint, there are several benefits from the use of POCT including:

- Reduction in the administrative work associated with test requesting
- Minimization of delays occurring during sample collection, as well as sample requirement
- Lack of delays associated with the need to transport the sample to a testing site; registering receipt of the sample; and the entry of a sample into a complex testing facility
- The use of whole blood samples rather than serum or plasma

Since the introduction of POCT, much has been written about the problems associated with this form of testing. These concerns essentially relate to four areas:

- Patient samples used for POCT may not be appropriate.
- Operators may not be sufficiently well trained to perform the procedure correctly.

- The analytical performance of POCT technology may be inferior to that of the central laboratory.
- Results may not reach the requester, be interpreted correctly, or reach the patient record.

Experience with the technology has resulted in several guidelines for POCT that can minimize these problems (3–6). Today the most challenging issue with POCT is to ensure that POCT is accompanied by changes in clinical practice that allow the best use of the rapidity with which the result can be delivered.

TABLE 1. Locations where point-of-care testing can be employed

Primary Care
Home
Community pharmacy
Health center (general practice, primary care)
Workplace clinic
Physician's office and community clinic
Diagnostic and treatment center
Paramedical support vehicle (ambulance, helicopter, aircraft)
Secondary and Tertiary Care
Emergency room
Admissions unit
Ambulatory diagnostic and treatment center
Operating room
Intensive care unit
Ward (patient floor)
Outpatient clinic

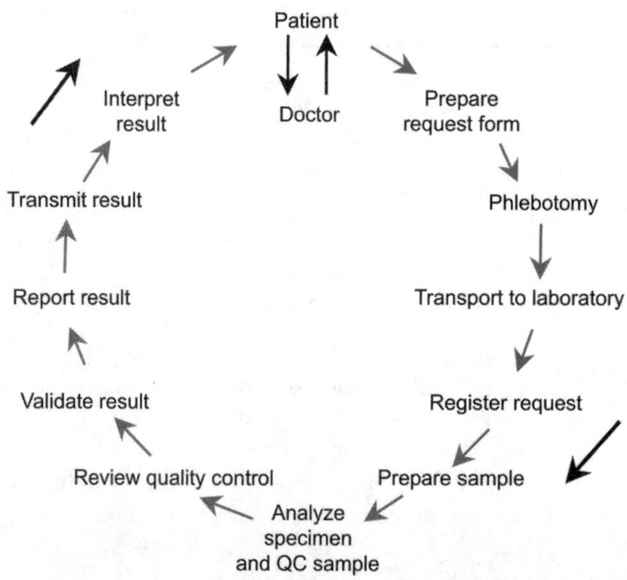

FIGURE 1. Process from patient consultation through to implementation of the intervention.

POCT TECHNOLOGY

A wide range of devices are now used at the point of care, ranging from the relatively simple urine dipstick to the more complex benchtop analyzer that measures up to 20 critical care or routine chemistry analytes. An increasing number of devices are based on a single-use strip or cartridge that is used in conjunction with a reader-type device for quantitation. One classification of the various types of POCT technology is shown in Table 2.

The development, manufacture, and application of instruments to be used at the point-of-care is based on five major requirements or demands. The first is that no sample treatment such as centrifugation is required prior to analysis. Second, since the instrument is likely to be used by nonlaboratory or relatively untrained personnel, it must be robust, reliable, and simple to operate. Third, the time taken to produce a result must be within the normal consultation period between clinician and patient. Fourth, the POCT device must produce results that are concordant with those produced by the central laboratory. A fifth, and more recent demand, is that the device can be easily linked or interfaced to information systems.

Design of POCT Devices

Much of the literature on POCT has concentrated on the advances in **sensor design** that have enabled a growing number of analytes to be measured directly on whole blood and other fluids. A sensor is a device that transforms chemical information directly via a transducer to a measurable signal (7) and for the purposes used here it will include reversible and nonreversible sensors. Figure 2 shows various different sensor designs. The

TABLE 2. Types of point-of-care instruments

Type of technology	Analytical principle	Analytes
Single-use, qualitative or semiquantitative cartridge/strip tests	Reflectance	Urine and blood chemistry
	Lateral-flow or flow-through immunoassays	Infectious disease agents, cardiac markers, HCG
Single-use quantitative cartridge/strip tests with a reader device	Reflectance	Glucose
	Electrochemistry	Glucose
	Reflectance	Blood chemistry
	Light scattering/optical motion	Coagulation
	Lateral-flow, flow-through or solid-phase immunoassays	Cardiac markers, drugs, CRP, allergy & fertility tests
	Immunoturbidimetry	HbA1c, Urine albumin
	Spectrophotometry	Blood chemistry
	Electrochemistry	pH, blood gases, electrolytes, metabolites
Multiple-use quantitative cartridge/benchtop devices	Electrochemistry	pH, blood gases, electrolytes, metabolites
	Fluorescence	pH, blood gases, electrolytes, metabolites
	Multiwavelength spectrophotometry	Hemoglobin species, bilirubin
	Time-resolved fluorescence	Cardiac markers, drugs, CRP
	Electrical impedance	Complete blood count

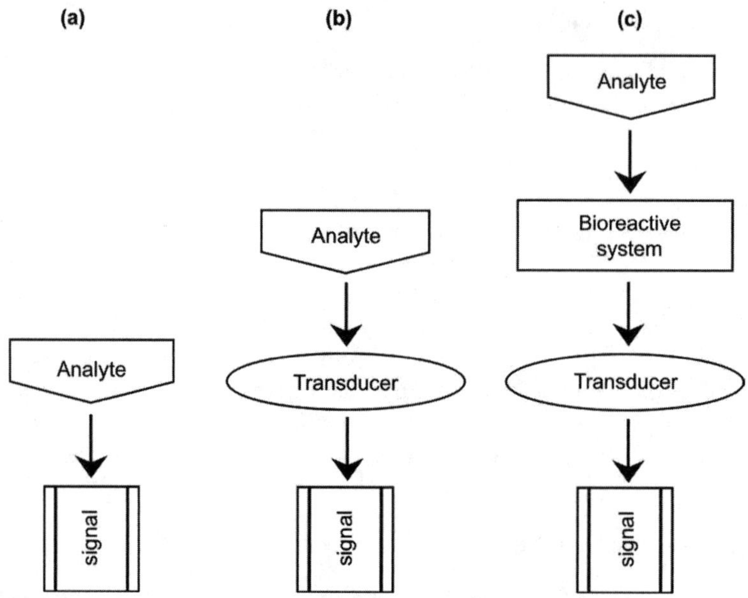

FIGURE 2. Types of sensors used in POCT devices.

chemosensor shown in Figure 2 (a) is an example of where the analyte has an intrinsic property such as fluorescence which enables it to be detected without a recognition element. The chemosensor shown in Figure 2 (b) is a much more common design and is used in many POCT devices. The transducing element might be a chemical indicator or binding molecule that recognizes the analyte to be measured and produces a signal which is usually electrical or optical. A biosensor is shown in Figure 2 (c) and is distinguished from a chemosensor by having a biological or biochemical component as the recognition element. Enzymes are the most common biological element used followed by antibodies and transduction can be via an optical or electrical signal.

The design of the location in the POCT device where the sensing process takes place can be very simple such as a porous pad, a cell, or a surface within a chamber. However, a major design goal in all POCT devices is to simplify the user interface, and, to achieve this, it is often necessary to design complexity into the reaction chamber. This complexity can be achieved through advances in microfluidics and techniques such as moulding, micromachining, photolithography, and screen printing, all of which have played a major role in the development of POCT devices (8).

The **analytical cell** is just one of several design features that are important for producing a successful POCT device. Interaction of the user with the device needs to be easy, demand as few steps as possible, and tolerate minor operator errors. Ideally, following addition of the sample, results should be produced without further intervention. Key interactions may include application of the sample to the device followed by delivery of the sample to the actual sensing component of the strip, cassette, or cartridge; in some cases, sample removal may also require user intervention. In devices other than single strips, all of these steps can be facilitated through the use of LCD screens, touch screens, keypads, bar-code readers, and printers as part of the user interface. User interactions should include identifying the operator and the patient as well as the test to be measured. This will ensure that there is traceability of the person who performed the test and that the results are linked to the correct patient.

In devices that have a reader or quantitative measurement process, **control systems** are required to coordinate all the other subsystems and ensure that processes take place in the correct sequence. These processes include insertion or removal of the strip, cartridge, or cassette into the instrument; temperature control; sample injection or aspiration; sample detection; mixing; timing of reaction and detection process, e.g., absorbance measurement; and waste removal. While the larger devices have pumps and even centrifugation processes to achieve fluid movement, many small microfabricated devices rely upon surface tension to achieve fluid transfer (9).

In recent years, there has been an increasing focus on the **informatics** associated with POCT devices (10). Thus, many devices have facilities for data storage and in some cases data management; the need for these grows in proportion to the size and complexity of the device and testing menu. Data storage will include calibration curve data and quality control limits as well as patient results. In some systems, data transfer and management take place when the meter or reader is linked to a small benchtop device called a docking station. These and other devices will include standard communication protocols that allow data to be transferred to other data management systems (11).

With the exception of critical care or blood gas analyzers and larger benchtop chemistry and hematology analyzers, most POCT measurements are performed on single-use devices. A key requirement of all single-use devices is that they can be manufactured reproducibly so that consistent performance extends across a large number of devices. Furthermore, they have to be stable during storage over a stated period of time which must be in terms of months if not years.

It is impossible to review the wide range of POCT technologies within this chapter. Thus, it will focus on the **principles** of the more common devices and in particular it will highlight those features that contribute toward obtaining a reliable result from the device. Readers requiring detailed information are referred to more comprehensive texts (12, 13) or to the vendors of POCT devices. Examples of POCT devices will be considered in the following categories:

- Single-use qualitative strip tests
- Single-use quantitative cartridge/strip tests with a reader device
- Multiple-use cartridge and benchtop systems

Single-Use Qualitative Strip Tests

This category of POCT device includes qualitative or semiquantitative urine tests or **dipsticks**, probably the most common POCT after glucose measurements. The strips are relatively simple in construction, comprising a pad composed of porous material such as cellulose which is impregnated with reagent and dried (14). More complex pads are composed of several layers, the uppermost of which is a semipermeable membrane that can prevent red cells from entering the matrix. Urine dipsticks can be read visually by comparing the color of the pad to a color chart but increasingly dipsticks, particularly multipad strips, are read photometrically in a small benchtop analyzer.

Despite their overt simplicity, highly sophisticated techniques of mass production are used to produce the urine sticks such as screen printing and inkjet technologies. Reproducible manufacturing of all strip-like devices relies upon the ability to apply precise quantities of reagents onto surfaces, be it a pad, cell, or cartridge surface. There are also critical operator factors including the need to cover the whole pad with the sample and, because the reactions often do not proceed to completion, it is necessary to time the period between placing the sample on the pad and comparing the resulting color to a color chart. In addition, for blood tests it may be necessary to remove all the blood before placing the sample in the reading device meter.

Many urine dipsticks are used in a multipad format where pH, specific gravity, blood, glucose, protein, ketones, leukocytes, urobilinogen, and bilirubin can all be measured on a single strip using reflectance technology. Other developments include two pads for measurement of different concentrations of the same analyte such as hemoglobin, and measurement of both albumin and creatinine to provide an albumin–creatinine ratio. Table 3 shows some of the parameters measured by single or multipad dipsticks.

In the last decade, many different immunosensors have become commercial products and are used for point-of-care measurements of a growing number of parameters including cardiac markers, pregnancy and fertility tests, and infectious disease markers. Immunosensors rely upon an antibody as the recognition agent with detection of the binding event or signal transduction usually via either reflectance or fluorescence spectrophotometry. Many immunosensors employ immunochromatography on various solid phase type materials to achieve separation of the analyte to be detected (15).

A typical immunoassay format in a flow-through device has an antibody covalently coupled to a defined area of the porous matrix. When the patient sample is added, it flows through the matrix and the analyte of interest binds to this antibody. A second labeled antibody which is impregnated in the sample addition area (but not covalently bound) flows with the sample and binds to the analyte, forming a sandwich and trapping the label at the position of the first antibody. If the label is gold sol particles or colored latex, the label can be directly visualized or quantitated by reflectance spectrophotometry using a separate reader device. Another important feature of this type of technology is the incorporation of a built-in quality control that indicates positive if all the reagents have been stored and the device operated correctly.

Several lateral-flow immunosensors exist for the detection of cardiac markers. In one device, plasma is separated from blood by a glass fleece and two monoclonal anti-human

TABLE 3. Analytes measured by single or multipad stick tests

Test	Sample	Chemistry
Glucose	Whole blood	Glucose oxidase
Cholesterol	Whole blood	Cholesterol oxidase
Acetaminophen	Whole blood	Acyl aminohydrolase
Lactate	Whole blood	Lactate dehydrogenase
Uric acid	Whole blood	Uricase
Alanine aminotransferase	Whole blood	Alanine/glutamate
Hemoglobin	Urine	Peroxidase activity
Protein	Urine	Protein error of indicators
Bilirubin	Urine	2,4-dichloroaniline
Urobilinogen	Urine	Ehrlich reaction
Leukocyte esterase	Urine	Pyrrole amino ester hydrolysis
Nitrite	Urine	p-Arsanilic acid reaction
pH	Urine	Double indicator principle
Specific gravity	Urine	Polyacid pH change
Ketones	Urine	Sodium nitroprusside reaction
Alcohol	Urine	Alcohol dehydrogenase
Drugs of abuse	Urine	Homogeneous immunoassay

cTnT antibodies, one conjugated to biotin and one labeled with gold particles, bind to the troponin T in the sample. The antibody–troponin complex then flows in a lateral direction along the cellulose nitrate test strip until it reaches the capture zone where the biotin binds to the streptavidin and immobilizes the complex that is visualized as a purple band by the gold particles attached to one of the antibodies. Unreacted gold-labeled antibody can move further down the strip where it is captured by a zone containing a synthetic peptide consisting of the epitope of human cardiac troponin T and is visualized as a separate but similar colored band. The presence of this second band serves as an important quality control because it indicates that the sample has flowed along the test strip and the device has worked correctly (16).

Several different infectious disease antigens and antibodies can now be rapidly detected with POCT including chlamydia, group A streptococci, *Helicobacter pylori*, infectious mononucleosis, and human immunodeficiency virus. Most commonly these tests use a lateral flow format in conjunction with analytical techniques such as enzyme immunoassay and immunochromatography with urine, serum, plasma, or whole blood samples. An alternative approach uses light reflection and thin-film amplification in what are termed optical immunoassays. The presence of an infectious disease antigen such as Strep A is detected through binding to an antibody coated on a test surface. Light reflected through the antibody film alone produces a gold background that changes to purple when the thickness of the film is increased due to the presence of an antigen (17).

Single-Use Quantitative Cartridge/Strip Tests with a Reader Device

A major development in POCT in the last decade has been development of small reader devices based on reflectance, spectrophotometry, or electrochemistry which has enabled a shift from qualitative to quantitative measurements. This trend commenced with the glucose test strip, which is by far the most common test performed outside of the laboratory due to the high and increasing prevalence of diabetes. Glucose test strips are biosensors that use one of three enzymes as the recognition agent: glucose oxidase (GO), hexokinase (HK), or glucose dehydrogenase (GLDH). Originally detection was by photometry or reflectance but now electrochemical detection is the most common (18). The reactions in one example of an electrochemical glucose strip are shown in Figure 3.

A glucose strip is a film composed of several layers that have specific functions. For photometric systems, erythrocytes must be excluded so the strip includes a separating layer that contains various components including glass fibers, fleeces, membranes, and special latex formulations which retain the cells allowing water and glucose to pass into the analytical layer. In photometric systems, a spreading layer is important for the fast homogeneous distribution of the sample whereas electrochemical strips use capillary fill systems. All of the above layers are supported by a thin plastic material that, in the case of reflectance-based strips, may also have reflective properties through the inclusion of substances such as titanium oxide, barium sulfate, and zinc oxide.

Since their introduction, innovations associated with glucose measurement technology have focused on ease-of-use and on reducing the impact of various factors which can interfere with the measurement. The introduction of electrochemical sensors facilitated the production of smaller, more convenient meters and, perhaps more significantly, made it possible to develop strips that did not require the operator to time the reaction and then wipe the strip. These latter steps can contribute to major operator-to-operator variances.

There are two major **chemical interferences in glucose measurement**. The first group are substances that can be easily oxidized such as ascorbic acid which compete with

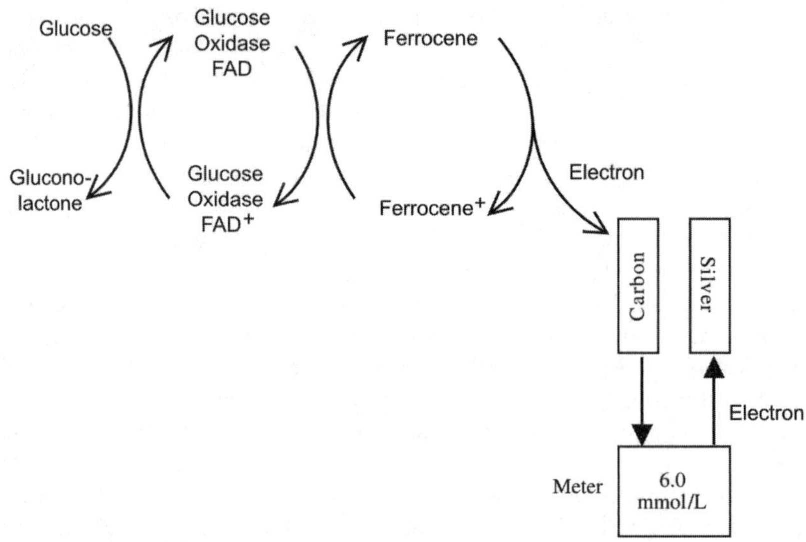

FIGURE 3. The reactions taking place in an electrochemical glucose strip.

hydrogen peroxide for the dyes used in reflectance-based systems and produce inaccurate values. Such substances can also interfere in electrochemical systems but this problem is overcome by using a mediator to cycle glucose oxidase rather than oxygen. However, electrochemical strips using glucose oxidase and mediators can be subject to interference from abnormal oxygen tensions and this has led to manufacturers using glucose dehydrogenase which is only subject to minor interference from oxygen. Inaccuracies resulting from extremes of hematocrit have proved a more difficult problem to resolve and can be a particular problem with neonatal samples in which the hematocrit may be very high. Different strips cope with this problem to varying degrees, depending on the degree to which the strip separates plasma from whole blood.

Like urine strips, reproducible manufacturing techniques over extended periods of time are fundamental to maintaining the quality of glucose measurements. Strips are produced in large batches and after extensive quality assurance procedures each batch is given a code which describes the performance of the batch including the relationship between the photometric or electrochemical signal and the concentration of glucose.

Reflectance technology is also used for measurement of parameters other than glucose in whole blood such as cholesterol, glucose, and urea in the Reflotron® system. Although whole blood is applied, separation of serum or plasma is still required and is achieved through a glass filter that traps red blood cells after which the plasma flows into a glass fiber reservoir. Initiation of the reaction takes place when the strip is inserted into a photometer that presses the reagent layers into contact with the plasma in the reservoir. A magnetic band on the back of the reagent strip is used to store lot-specific calibration data and the test identity, information which is then transferred into the photometer when the strip is inserted (19).

Several immunosensor technologies that are available as visually read, qualitative measurements can also provide a quantitative measurement through a compact reader device. Once again these developments have come about through advances in modern electronics and miniaturization such as the use of charged couple devices, so-called CCD cameras. These are multichannel light detectors, similar to a photomultiplier tube in a spectrophotometer, but with a higher signal-to-noise ratios so that they can detect much lower signal changes at low levels of light. This technology has been incorporated in devices capable of measuring a panel of analytes such as cardiac markers, allergy tests, and fertility tests. In these devices, a mixture of labeled antibodies is impregnated at the origin (sample addition point) and complementary antibodies for the various analytes are immobilized at varying positions along the porous strip.

Single-use, quantitative measurements are also available for critical care analytes such as blood gases and electrolytes. The i-STAT® handheld analyzer is an example of thin-film technology where the sensors or electrodes are wafer structures constructed with thin metal oxide films using microfabrication techniques directly comparable to those used in the computer industry. The results are small single-use cartridges containing an array of electrochemical sensors which operate in conjunction with a handheld analyzer that can be used directly at the bedside (20). Because the sensor layer is very thin, blood can permeate this layer quickly and the sensor cartridge can be used immediately after it is unwrapped from its packing. This is an advantage over some thick-film sensors, which require an equilibration or wet-up time before they can be used to measure blood samples. Optical detection can also be used for blood gas and electrolyte measurements with the advantage that optical sensors do not need to be regularly recalibrated to correct for electrode drift and therefore the sensors can be calibrated once at the time of manufacture (21).

Other analytes that can be measured at point-of-care by single-use, quantitative devices using cassette-type technology include hemoglobin, glucose, cholesterol, or triglycerides by absorbance; glycated hemoglobin by light-scattering immunoassay; and coagulation parameters by various different methodologies, including the use of magnetic particles and changes in sample flow.

Multiple-Use Cartridge and Benchtop Systems

By far the majority of critical care tests such as blood gases are performed outside of the laboratory using relatively large, benchtop, multiple-use analyzers. These instruments were first introduced more than 30 years ago and in many countries, they have been located outside of the central laboratory since their introduction. Since then several major trends have taken place in their development which have facilitated their use at the point-of-care including:

- Extension of the test menu beyond pH and blood gases
- Miniaturization of electrodes or sensors requiring no maintenance
- Cartridge technology with combined sensor and reagent packs
- In-built and automated quality control (QC) functions
- Informatic applications including remote monitoring and maintenance

The larger critical care test menu that can now be measured on what was once called a blood gas analyzer has come about partly through technological advances. However, it also reflects the desire of clinicians to have the ability to measure parameters beyond the traditional pH and blood gas parameters on less than 100 μL of whole blood. The advantage for neonatal and pediatric patients is obvious but there is also increasing concern about iatrogenic anemia in adult patients undergoing intensive therapy for long periods.

While the ability to measure up to 20 or more parameters has undoubtedly added a degree of complexity to the modern critical care analyzer, the overall maintenance requirements of these devices is much less due to modern microelectrodes which have many user-friendly features such as extended no maintenance lifetimes. This trend will continue with the extension of thick-film technology from existing metabolite (glucose and lactate) sensors to pH and blood gas measurements. The advantage of such sensors is that they can be incorporated with reagents and calibrators into a single cartridge that is placed in a small to medium-sized, portable critical care analyzer (22). Each pack has a limited lifetime or will analyze a fixed number of samples, whichever comes first. When the pack has expired, the pack is replaced, a process that, with appropriate training, can be carried out by nonlaboratory staff. This type of cartridge technology has been available for more than a decade but it is now more affordable and has improved features; for these reasons it is likely to grow in popularity.

Other trends that have facilitated the use of critical care analyzers by nonlaboratory staff include the replacement of gas bottles by liquid calibration systems that use a combination of aqueous base solutions and conductance measurements to calibrate the pH, and PCO_2 electrodes while oxygen is calibrated using an oxygen-free solution and room air. The challenge of ensuring that nursing and other paramedical staff analyze quality control samples at regular intervals has been largely solved by incorporating automated QC packages into instruments. Bottles or packs of QC material are sampled at predetermined intervals and onboard software interprets the results and generates alerts if necessary.

The introduction of networking technology throughout medical facilities together with software supplied by analyzer vendors has allowed laboratory scientists to remotely monitor, maintain, and review data from analyzers which may be some distance from the central laboratory (23). Formerly remote instruments required daily visits from laboratory staff with obvious and significant costs but these can be significantly reduced through the implementation of remote management software.

It is likely that the trends in miniaturization alluded to earlier will lead to the development of multiuse-type analyzers measuring parameters other than those traditionally regarded as critical. These include hematological parameters and certain endocrine tests. Single-use devices already exist for these tests but small, compact multiple-use devices are likely to be developed in the future.

Analytical Performance of POCT Technology

One of the major controversies that has existed with POCT is that the rapidity of result is often achieved at the expense of analytical performance. This may be related to poorer precision, interferences, or user errors. For example, while the performance of glucose meters has improved over the years, most meters still do not meet the precision goals of the American Diabetes Association. Recently international consensus was reached on a global strategy to set analytical quality specifications and it has been advocated that this approach should be used to set defined goals for accuracy and precision for all types of testing including POCT (24). Along these lines, several studies have been published that examine these strategies in relation to several POCT tests such as cholesterol and HbA1c (25). In the case of HbA1c it was possible to demonstrate a relationship between the risk of cardiovascular disease and glycated hemoglobin (e.g., as shown in the United Kingdom Prospective Diabetes Study), and thereby identify the potential effect of analytical bias on clinical outcome.

Most current quality specifications are based on published state of the art performance. The problem of this approach for POCT data is that much of the data used to derive the specifications comes from evaluations carried out by well-trained staff. When the test is used in practice, it is likely that those carrying out the test do not reach the same standard of performance. While this problem may by diminished by future improvements in technology, it will remain important for all POCT devices to be used by adequately trained operators.

ORGANIZATION AND MANAGEMENT OF POCT

Successful implementation of POCT depends on having a robust case for the use of POCT, putting in place all of the processes to ensure that the service is properly organized, ensuring that quality is maintained, and fully integrating the POCT service into clinical care with the involvement of all healthcare professionals involved in the patient's care.

Is POCT Required?

The need for POCT is primarily based on the following issues:

- The test and turnaround time required
- Current access to the test
- The decision and action taken upon receipt of the test result
- Whether a faster process is likely to lead to benefit for the patient
- Whether a faster process will improve efficiency within the organization
- Whether there will be cost savings within the organization

The case for a POCT service can be based on responses to a series of questions, which are summarized in Table 4. Clearly, this will identify the test itself but should also explain why the current service is not meeting the needs of the patient or the clinician. Specifically, the case should identify what benefits are likely to accrue to the patient and/or the healthcare provider by introducing a more rapid service. The case will contain an economic assessment of the costs of delivering the current service and the costs associated with the POCT service. The benefits will need to be identified and accounted for in a similar way although this will be more complex as it will involve identifying the cost of other elements of the health service, which may not always be amenable to a simple accounting approach. However, it is important in such an exercise to ensure that the costs associated with the benefits are recognized in terms of those that will free-up resources, as against those that

TABLE 4. Questions to determine the need for a POCT service

- Which tests are required?
- What is the turnround time required?
- What clinical question is being asked when requesting this test?
- What clinical decision is likely to be made upon receipt of the result?
- What action is likely to be taken upon receipt of the result?
- What outcome should be expected from the action taken?
- Why can the laboratory not deliver the required service?
- Will point-of-care testing provide the required accuracy and precision of result?
- Are there staff available to perform the test?
- Are there adequate facilities to perform the test, store the equipment and reagents?
- Will you abide by the organization's point-of-care testing policy?
- Are there operational benefits to this point-of-care testing strategy?
- Are there economic benefits to this point-of-care testing strategy?
- Will a change in practice be required to deliver these benefits?
- Can you deliver the changes in practice that might be required?

may be more associated with an improved quality of care, and ultimately quality of life. Some costs in the latter cannot be readily leveraged, and therefore resources are required to fund the POCT service. This part of the exercise is extremely useful as it often identifies the changes in practice that are required to release the resources in order to fund the new service, as well as the potential difficulties associated with achieving such a change!

In parallel with this needs assessment there should be a risk assessment. The needs assessment primarily looks at the diagnostic service from the perspectives of the patient, clinician, and healthcare organization, whereas the risk assessment concentrates primarily on the procedures and processes that are necessary for ensuring the maintenance of a high-quality service. The issues that should be considered include:

- Quality of performance of the device
- Whether, and how, performance can be compromised by the operator
- Limitations of the device, e.g., in terms of sample type, stability of device, etc.
- Competence of the operator of the device
- Process for result transmission to the caregiver, and transmission into the patient record
- Process for ensuring correct interpretation of results
- Procedures for staff training, continuing education, and assessment of competence
- Adherence to regulatory requirements at local, regional, and national levels
- Changes in practice required to deliver the benefit, and how this will be achieved.

All of these goals can be achieved with the establishment of a number of key policies which are adopted in an organizationwide POCT policy and overseen by a multidisciplinary POCT coordinating committee.

POCT Coordinating Committee

POCT is a very multidisciplinary activity, as indeed is laboratory medicine, and it is important to take an holistic approach to the setting up, organization, and management of a POCT service. Indeed it provides an opportunity for the laboratorian to get out of the laboratory and closer to the patient and the clinician. In order to achieve this, it is necessary to consult with all of the parties involved in delivering such a service. This is best achieved through the setting up of a POCT coordinating committee. Such a committee can be charged with managing the whole process of delivering a high-quality POCT service. Membership of a POCT coordinating committee should comprise representatives of healthcare professionals using the service, those involved in delivering the service, together with a representative of the organizations' management team. The users will include doctors and nurses but may also include a patient. The providers will include at least one representative from the laboratory as well as those involved in the use of other diagnostic and therapy equipment close to the patient, e.g., respiratory physiologists, nurses. Invariably a laboratory professional will chair such a committee as it is the laboratory that provides the necessary backup if there is a POCT service failure. The laboratory professional has the best training and expertise with the analytical issues that are likely to arise. The committee should report to the individual within the organization responsible for the quality of the clinical service, e.g., the medical director (*see* Section on Accountability). The committee should appoint members who will take the responsibility for overseeing the training and accreditation of all POCT operators, and also for QC and quality assurance (QA); in a larger institution this may be a full-time appointment. The work of the committee should be governed by the organization's policy on POCT.

POCT Policy

Most organizations delivering healthcare will operate with a core of policies that guide decision making and which form the cornerstone of ensuring the highest quality of service is maintained. A POCT policy should be within this set of core policies. The POCT policy will specify the responsibility and accountability of all staff associated with POCT. This policy is likely to be part of the organization's total quality management system (26), part of the clinical governance policy (27), as well as being required for accreditation purposes (28). The details of the POCT policy should be drawn up by the POCT coordinating committee and then agreed to by the organization's policy guidance committee and clinical governance committees or their equivalents. The elements of a POCT policy are set out in Table 5.

The policies should include protocols for:

- Equipment procurement
- Introduction of POCT equipment or devices
- Training and certification
- QC and QA

TABLE 5. Elements of point-of-care testing policy

Introduction
- background
- definition
- accreditation of services
- audit of services
Laboratory services in the organization
- location
- logistics
- policy on diagnostic testing
Management of point-of-care testing
- committee and accountability
- officers
- committee members
- terms of reference
- responsibilities
- meetings
Equipment and consumable procurement
- criteria for procurement
- process of procurement
Standard operating procedures
Training and certification of staff
- training
- certification
- recertification
Quality control and quality assurance
- procedures
- documentation and review
Health and safety procedures
Bibliography
Review process

- Audit of utilization
- Maintenance and inventory control
- Documentation
- Accreditation and regulation of POCT

Equipment Procurement

Procuring equipment requires identification of the tests required, the analytical performance (accuracy and precision), and the expectations for the turnaround time for the delivery of the result. It is assumed that a previous audit has determined that the laboratory is unable to provide the level of service required, even with additional investment in logistical support. In addition operational requirements have been identified including the stability of the analyte in the sample and the required consumables, calibration, and QC materials. The operator-dependent steps in the use of the POCT system will need to be either identified in terms of the staffing implications or defined in terms of the staffing resource that has already been identified. A judgment has to be made at some point as to the staffing expertise required to use the device and this may be gleaned from discussions with other users of the system and from evaluation reports.

Evaluation reports are an important resource for providing an independent evaluation of whether the device actually meets the performance claims of the manufacturer. This information can be obtained from the company selling the device, from reports in the peer-reviewed literature, and from published evaluations performed by agencies such as the Medicines and Health Regulatory Agency in the United Kingdom. Performance data will typically include information on the precision and accuracy of measurement, and in relation to the former, should include some assessment of interoperator performance. An important feature of the accuracy of a POCT device will be the concordance between the results produced by the device and by the routine laboratory method. Patients are invariably managed using both analytical systems. The precision (and possibly accuracy of the POCT system) may also be influenced by the frequency of calibration of the system as well as changes in reagent batches.

Several features of analytical devices, including POCT systems, are sometimes difficult to assess in a systematic fashion but can have a major impact on the quality of the final result produced. Some of these factors are due to the device being used by less technically qualified personnel and the fact that devices used outside of the laboratory are not subject to the whole range of QA procedures. These factors may include:

- The effect of potential interferents
- Collection of the appropriate specimen
- The stability of calibrators and reagents
- The potential for operator error, e.g., including delayed sample addition
- Use of incorrect sample volume etc.
- Incorrect reporting of the result, e.g., units of measurement

The likelihood of any of these errors occurring is very difficult to assess; it may be necessary to seek endorsements from current users of the systems as well as possibly conducting some form of internal trial. Clearly the risk of occurrence is best reduced by having a good training and education program in place, which is supported by regular QC and QA. The basic evaluation of analytical performance has been addressed in a number of protocols, including the CLSI (NCCLS) protocol (29).

Although probably seldom performed, it is important to undertake some form of economic assessment of the equipment including the cost of consumables and servicing. It will comprise a comparative exercise between the various point-of-care systems under consideration, and a comparison of costs with the laboratory service. However, it should be kept in mind that any comparison of costs between laboratory and POCT services is likely to show that the cost of the reagents for POCT is higher. This is not unexpected as the laboratory is able to take advantage of the economies of scale to be gained from high-volume testing. However, it is helpful at this point to have a good assessment of the relative staff costs associated with different systems as these are likely to be key features in the decision-making process. It is likely that the chosen system will be operated by staff already performing a wide range of duties involving the care of patients, and therefore the amount of time required to operate the device may be critical. It is important to stress again that the benefits of POCT are going to be seen beyond the boundaries of the laboratory medicine budget and so any economic assessment should attempt to take into account the wider benefits to be achieved with the implementation of POCT.

Introduction of a POCT System

It is always helpful if a laboratory professional takes the responsibility for equipment procurement and then performs a short evaluation of the equipment in order to gain familiarization with the system. Together with any information gained from evaluation reports and conversation with existing users, this experience can form the basis of a trouble-shooting guide for future use by operators. This type of evaluation can also determine the content of the training program that is developed, highlighting any local issues that may arise. This evaluation should also be used to establish the concordance between the results generated with the device and those provided by the laboratory. This information should then be recorded in a introduction manual associated with the equipment. It is likely that the organization will also wish to undertake some form of safety check (e.g., electrical safety), as well as giving the device some form of local code that is entered into the local equipment register.

Training, Certification of Operators, and Maintenance of Competence

The quality of the results produced depends on the robustness of the instrument and the competence of the operator. Those healthcare professionals involved in POCT will generally have received limited training in the use of analytical devices as part of their core professional development. However, they are often involved in the operation of complex pieces of equipment. As POCT systems become simpler in their operation, and possibly as the operator interface shows greater commonality with other monitoring instruments, e.g., in the critical care setting, then the concern about the competence of operators may diminish. However, the importance of a comprehensive training program cannot be underestimated, both for the patient as well as for the operator.

The main features of a training program for any POCT device should include:

- The pathophysiological context of the test
- Clinical requirement for the test
- The action taken upon receipt of the result including critical values
- Patient preparation required
- Sample requirement and collection procedure
- Preparation of the device required
- Test procedure
- QC procedures including interpretation of QC results
- Documentation of result and QC
- Interpretation of patient result and urgency of report required
- Report of patient result to correct person
- Disposal of sample and test device
- Additional health and safety issues

There are a number of approaches to the delivery of the training program that can be tailored to suit the needs of the individual and the organization. These may include formal presentation to groups or on a one-to-one basis, self-directed learning using agreed documentation, or computer-aided learning. Several current models of blood gas and electrolyte analyzers and other types of benchtop analyzers have onboard computer-aided training modules. Satisfactory completion of the training should be documented in a central register as this is the first step to recognizing that the individual is competent. Assessment of competence at the end of training should be undertaken with a combination of questions concerned with understanding and a practical demonstration of the skills gained. Performance of tests on a series of QC materials and repeat testing of samples that have recently been analyzed (parallel testing) can provide a very practical means of assessing the competence of the operator at the conclusion of a training program. The operator can also be shadowed through the whole procedure involved in the POCT, on a minimum of three occasions. Such a training program may also be integrated with those of other pieces of equipment being used in the same environment, e.g., the critical care unit.

A certificate of competence should be issued by a recognized trainer, with a copy given to the successful operator as well as a second copy lodged in a central register of POCT operators for the respective device. The certificate should be dated and an indication given when recertification is expected. The operator may be given a badge to indicate that he/she is a certified operator, as this may help to build the relationship between patient and operator at the time of testing.

Maintenance of competence is achieved through regular practice of skills and continuing education, and these features should all be incorporated into the education and training program. Regular review of performance in QC and QA programs will provide a means of overseeing the competence of operators. This may be a difficult discipline to maintain, particularly when operators are employed on irregular shifts or may not be called upon to perform POCT regularly. It may be necessary to make specific arrangements for individuals to undertake tests on QC material at specified intervals, e.g., once per shift when POCT is undertaken. The error log may also highlight when problems are arising.

However, it is an awareness of the strengths and limitations of the POCT device and the relevance of the test in the clinical situation that will provide the best QA tools. It is also most important to encourage an open approach to the assessment of competence such that operators can themselves seek help if they feel that problems are occurring. An open approach can then be supported with audit and performance review meetings where problems can be aired and developments discussed. The regular assessment of competence should be built into a formal program for recertification that will be a requirement of most accreditation programs.

QC and QA

The internal QC program generally compares the current QC performance with the QC results from previous analyses. External QA takes a longer term view and also addresses other issues relating to the quality of the result. External QA programs provide information on the testing performance of different sites and/or different pieces of equipment or methods including concordance of results. Despite these tools, the foundation for ensuring a good quality service remains a successful training and certification scheme.

Internal QC involves the analysis of a sample for which the analyte concentration is known, either because the material has been analyzed on many occasions and the distribution of results documented, or it has been analyzed independently and the mean and range of results quoted for the method used. Establishing the range of results that are acceptable when analyzing the QC material is a key feature when using such QC materials. The current analytical result is then compared with the range of results deemed to be acceptable (typically the mean ± two standard deviations). The result obtained must then be documented; this may be undertaken using a computer database or using a logbook. Usually it is undertaken using graphical presentation, as this shows the conformity of results and any trends in results that may be occurring. The key feature of the documentation should be that it ensures that comparative performance can be assessed.

There are several issues surrounding **internal QC in POCT**. The first is the frequency of testing. The options for testing include when each sample is run, when each new operator uses the system, when new reagents are set up, and/or when the system is recalibrated. While there appears to be no consistent agreement on the correct approach, it is probably acknowledged that there needs to be a QC check performed when a new batch of reagents is commenced and when the system is recalibrated. Otherwise, guidance on frequency of testing should be based on the reproducibility and overall analytical performance of the system and the number and competence of the operators. The frequency with which the POCT system is used can also be used as a guide; in the hands of an experienced operator the patients' results will provide valuable QC information. In the case of a bench-top analyzer, at least one QC sample should probably be run a minimum of once per shift for a reliable machine, i.e., three times a day. Some critical care analyzers can be programmed to perform a QC check at intervals set by those responsible for the device; in some cases it is set by the manufacturer. In the case of single-use, disposable devices, this strategy cannot completely quality control the test system (30). A similar criticism could be made of early approaches to the QC of reflectance meters, using a reflectance standard strip, namely, that the whole process is not being assessed. In addition, when conventional QC material is run on a unit-use or single-test system, only that testing unit is checked. In this case, there is a greater dependence on the manufacturing reproducibility of the devices to ensure a good quality service. A recent CLSI (NCCLS) guideline documents quality management procedures for unit-use testing, both from a manufacturer's and a user's perspective (31).

External QA or proficiency testing involves analyzing samples sent from a scheme organizer. In this case, the operator has no knowledge of the analyte concentration and therefore it is closer to the real testing situation. The results are sent back to the scheme organizer and a performance report is then sent out a few days later. The report will identify the range of results obtained for the complete cohort of participants and then may be broken down according to the different methods used by participants in the scheme. The scheme may encompass both laboratory and POCT users, which gives an opportunity to compare results with laboratory-based methods. This type of scheme is more concerned with long-term performance, with concordance of results with the laboratory as well as other POCT systems (in other words, a wider consensus view), as well as providing an external proficiency testing system.

There are a number of external QA schemes dedicated to, or including, POCT systems schemes which are run on a national or international basis and there are also some web-based schemes (32–34). External QA schemes can also be run within a hospital or throughout a community of healthcare providers. While the materials for such schemes can be purchased commercially, the schemes are sometimes run by qualified laboratory personnel but commercially organized schemes are also available. The involvement of laboratory personnel provides the opportunity to compare the results being reported by both the laboratory and other POCT sites within the same organization, as well as having the expertise of the laboratorian available to give advice when needed. The overview of performance across a site or community can be important when patients are managed in several departments or when machines break down and samples are taken to other sites for testing.

Poor performance in QC and QA schemes should be properly documented, together with information on the solution to the perceived problem. As part of this exercise it may be necessary to go back and review some of the patients' notes to ensure that incorrect results have not been reported and inappropriate clinical actions taken. There should then be a regular review of all QC and QA data together with the error log to ensure that all of the problems have been identified and the correct action has been taken.

Audit

Audit is another tool used to maintain quality in the POCT setting and it is sometimes easier to conduct in the patient context because it is nearer to the patient. This might be considered to be the process of review of QC and QA data, together with a review of the error log. Invariably, it is a more encompassing process in that it offers not only the opportunity to review the analytical performance but also the way in which POCT is used and its effectiveness in the wider healthcare setting. Thus in the management of diabetes, the opportunity to review the HbA1c at the time of the clinic visit embraces all aspects of self-monitoring of blood glucose, namely, both the quality of glucose testing and the way in which the results are used to guide therapy and life-style changes. A similar approach could be envisaged for anticoagulation therapy monitoring and it could be argued that these approaches are more relevant for the patient in helping to integrate testing into any chronic disease management regime.

Maintenance and Inventory Control

POCT by its very nature requires that stocks of devices be maintained at all times. It is also important to ensure that the reagents/devices are stored at the recommended conditions and released in time for any preanalytical preparation to be accommodated such as bringing up to room temperature. Operators should be aware of the stated shelf life of the consumables and to ensure that stocks are released for use well ahead of expiry dates. If there are multiple sites using the same materials, then a central purchasing, supply, and inventory control system should be put in place to ensure that individual systems are not supplied unknowingly with different batches of consumables. In addition, this enables the organization to gain the financial benefit from bulk purchasing.

The maintenance of reusable devices will vary from system to system and clear guidelines from the manufacturer should be adhered to rigorously. In larger institutions there may be a central register for POCT devices and other equipment used on the wards and in clinics. The central register holder is often the appropriate department to maintain the records for servicing and maintaining POCT systems. Features that usually require careful monitoring include:

- Expiry dates for components
- Effects of contamination with blood
- Electrical safety
- Maintenance of optics
- Inadvertent use of inappropriate consumables

Documentation

The adequacy of the patient record is crucial to good patient care and this includes keeping a record of all of laboratory investigations. This is particularly the case for POCT, where there are major challenges to the routine recording of accurate data. The minimal requirement is to keep an accurate record of the test request, the result, and the action taken. Some of the issues concerning documentation are now being resolved with the advent of the patient electronic record, electronic requesting, and better connectivity of POCT instrumentation to information systems and the patient record. This documentation should extend to the standard operating procedure (SOP) for each POCT system, to records of training and certification of operators, and to internal QC and QA together with error logs and any corrective action taken.

Accreditation and Regulation of POCT

The described organization and management of POCT are consistent with those for the accreditation of any diagnostic service (28). Accreditation of POCT can be part of the overall accreditation of laboratory medicine, as well as being an element of the accreditation of the full clinical service as is the case in countries such as the United States and the United Kingdom. Thus, the Clinical Laboratory Improvement Amendments of 1988 (CLIA) legislation in the United States demands that all POCT must meet certain minimum standards (35, 36). The Centers for Medicare and Medicaid Services, the Joint Commission on Accreditation of Healthcare Organizations, and the College of American Pathologists take on the responsibility for inspecting sites and ensuring compliance with testing regulations for POCT (37).

Accountability

An important feature of any service is the accountability for the provision of that service. Although accountability might ultimately be to the patient, there will be one person within the healthcare organization who takes on the role of being the patient's advocate such as the medical director for the institution. There will therefore need to be accountability that can be traced from the operator, through those who are responsible for directing and managing the service on a day-to-day basis, to the medical director. Lines of communication need to be developed such that this director is aware of the quality of the service and that any delivery or quality issues are highlighted and a means of resolution identified. Clearly, the responsibilities of each operator and each individual in the management team also need to be recognized.

Guidelines for POCT

Much of the material outlined in the preceding sections has been set out in a number of guideline documents published on behalf of a number of organizations concerned with the provision of laboratory medicine services. Some examples are given in the following references (3–6).

Connectivity and POCT

In recent times, the manufacturers of POCT devices have focused increasing attention on events that take place after the measurement process. These events include the management of processes which ensure that the raw patient result is converted into useful and timely clinical information. This process goes hand in hand with informatic processes that are designed to ensure the quality of all the transactions that take place and to provide evidence of this, e.g., audit trails and other quality statistics. All of these procedures are now an accepted part of laboratory practice, and processes such as real-time QC are demanded by organizations such as the Joint Commission on Accreditation of Healthcare Organizations in the United States.

The key to ensuring that both these informatic issues are dealt with appropriately is through linking measurement devices to information systems. This goal has proved difficult for POCT devices, of which there may be hundreds distributed over a wide area outside of the laboratory. For example, a major information management problem for many POCT devices is the lack of a database within the instrument. Thus, POCT data have often had to be entered manually into an information system, with the major risk of transcription error, or more likely, the data never reaching the patient record. Important clinical information may be lost with the additional possibility of costly duplicate testing. Newer devices have addressed this problem by incorporating a database, but linking this to information management systems remains a problem because each device has its own proprietary interface and the costs of interfacing every type of device is prohibitive. The extent of this problem was highlighted by a survey conducted by the Enterprise Corporation for the American Association for Clinical Chemistry in 1999 which showed that in more than 500 U.S. hospitals, only 17% of POCT data was sent to the LIS electronically while 67% never reached the LIS (38).

This lack of so-called **connectivity** has been addressed by the manufacturers of POCT devices who formed the Connectivity Industry Consortium (CIC), a group of more than 30 companies involved in the POCT industry, to develop a set of POCT communication standards. The latter ensure the fulfillment of critical user requirements such as bidirectionality, device connection commonality, commercial software intraoperability, security, and QC/regulatory compliance. The connectivity standard was approved by the Clinical and Laboratory Standards Institute (CLSI; formerly the National Committee for Clinical Laboratory Standards or NCCLS) in 2001 as the POCT1-A standard (11). Essentially if a POCT device incorporates this standard, it should easily communicate with laboratory and hospital information management systems, allowing exchange of data and information in a standardized format irrespective of vendor, location, or interface.

The availability of a POCT connectivity standard is a significant step forward for all those involved with this type of diagnostic testing, and it will help address the major issue of what happens to the patient data after the measurement process. The key questions in this area are:

- Do the data and related information become a permanent part of the patient's record?
- Are patient data accessible at the right time by those people who need the information?
- Are they combined with other data to provide useful clinical information?
- How can the laboratory enrich or add value to the data?

These questions are being driven by a number of broader informatic issues. First and foremost is the increasing attention being drawn to the incidence of medical error and ways to reduce its occurrence. The lack of POCT results or the incorrect transcription of manually reported POCT results can lead to errors in clinical management. Connectivity of POCT devices will ensure error-free, electronic transmission of POCT data. A second issue is the development of the electronic health, medical, or patient record (EHR/EMR/EPR). A distant goal in the past, it now seems to be a distinct possibility and with 60% of the EHR/EMR/EPR being diagnostic data, then connectivity of POCT devices is essential. Other developments include the availability of decision support systems to add value to diagnostic data and the need to integrate such information into clinical management systems. With a connectivity standard in place, it is likely that manufacturers will now develop applications around these informatic issues as a way of differentiating their products.

POCT AND HEALTH OUTCOMES

A health outcome can be considered in terms of the benefit to the patient (a clinical outcome), to the healthcare professional (an operational outcome), to the healthcare provider organization (an operational and/or economic outcome), to the purchasing organization/government (an economic outcome), and to society as a whole (an economic outcome). The outcome or benefit depends not only on the correct identification of the clinical question, on the choice of an appropriate test and satisfactory completion of the test, but also on completion of all of the other steps involved in the clinical process. As with clinical medicine in general, achieving a positive health outcome is dependent on compliance with all of the elements of the clinical process. In many respects, POCT helps to illustrate the role of laboratory medicine in improving patient care because it brings the testing closer to the patient. In particular it solves, at least in part, the problems that arise when the testing is performed away from the patient setting in which the test result is needed.

POCT can be used in a number of diagnostic scenarios. These include screening for the presence or absence of disease, ruling in or ruling out a diagnosis, and as an integral part of disease management where the test result is used to start, to stop, or to modify the use of a therapy, e.g., a drug. It has been recognized already in a systematic review of the literature on the use of POCT in the primary care setting that the majority of papers deal with the technical issues surrounding POCT, largely fail to explore the outcomes that derive from POCT, and generally contain a low level of quality evidence (39). The following discussion illustrates the application of POCT in a number of clinical settings using those examples from the peer-reviewed literature which contain evidence of POCT providing some benefit. In some instances, the review will highlight the potential benefits that can be achieved with POCT in the hope that the reader will be stimulated to embark on more robust outcome studies. The review will also point out some of the potential pitfalls that can arise from asking an inappropriate question or from a lack of compliance with the full process, leading to a failure to deliver outcomes.

POCT in the Home Setting

POCT in the home is increasing as a result of the trend to reduce the length of stay in hospital (40). While one pilot study of home care showed that only about 5% of visits were associated with laboratory-based testing, there were 10% return visits required to recollect specimens that were not suitable for analysis in the laboratory, thereby increasing the cost of care. Part of the trend to reducing hospital stay is to have more care undertaken in the community and implicitly for patients to become more involved in their own care. This is likely to become most common in the management of chronic diseases such as diabetes, anticoagulation therapy, and diuretic use. If testing is not done in the home, then the most convenient place for testing for many people is at the local pharmacy.

POCT in the Pharmacy Setting

POCT in the pharmacy setting has already shown some promise in the support of patients with diabetes. One study involved 260 patients who received three HbA1c tests from their local pharmacist, with those showing evidence of poor control targeted for healthcare intervention. Over the 6 months of the study, there was a slight improvement in the mean HbA1c of the group with 84.6% of the participants who were considered to have poor control showing an improvement. It was noticeable that there was a significant drop-out rate over the course of the study, which was mainly among those who had poorer control. This highlights the fact that successful use of test results depends on more than the test itself, and it is necessary to provide support for patients receiving results in order that the best use can be made of the service available. A number of such programs have been employed in rural communities for some time. In one report of an experimental project for a walk-in lipid screening program, it was found that 50% of the participants required intervention and 34% of the attendees were previously undiagnosed (41).

POCT in the Primary Care Setting

Primary care could include care in the home or at the local pharmacy, but at this point it will be defined as the environment in which the patient visits either a nurse or a doctor, usually located in a health center. As reported earlier, Hobbs et al. (39) undertook a systematic review of POCT in primary care and found little evidence to suggest that there were any benefits from the use of this testing. The authors pointed out that this was due to the fact that there were few studies designed to investigate the impact in terms of clinical outcomes. It is envisaged that this is likely to change with the increasing role of the primary care physician both in the initial diagnosis and triaging of patients to the hospital setting, as well as in chronic disease management. A systematic review of the devolved care of diabetics has illustrated some of the issues that need to be taken into account when seeking to devolve the management of chronic diseases. Griffin (42) found that there was some benefit seen with a fall in the HbA1c results, but the evidence from morbidity indicators did not favor the transfer of care to the primary sector. It was concluded that this dichotomy of findings might be due to the need for greater training in the earlier recognition of onset of secondary complications of the disease, with consequent referral to a diabetes specialist. If there is to be further movement of care to the primary care setting, then attention will have to be given to the use of POCT in the secondary care outpatient clinic setting, and to what steps are taken to deliver positive outcomes from a reliable service.

Rink et al. (43) in a study of a number of biochemical and microbiological tests in primary care found that there were few apparent benefits to the use of POCT, the main ones being the increased recording of risk factors in patients with cardiovascular disease, as well as a potential for reduction in the number of urines sent to the laboratory for testing when a urinary tract infection was suspected. They suggested that the tests available might not all be appropriate to the spectrum of clinical cases seen at the time and that the style of practice might have to change to be able to make the best use of POCT. The use of urinalysis strip tests at point-of-care has been the topic of many studies in a variety of clinical settings (44). Major differences in the predictive values of tests such as leukocyte esterase and nitrite have been attributed to the influence of interoperator variability in different studies, which illustrates the importance of reliable manufacture and storage of devices together with good operator training and continuing education.

The complaint of gastrointestinal discomfort is one of the most common presenting symptoms for the primary care physician and there have been a number of studies assessing the use of point-of-care type assays for *H. pylori* in patients presenting with dyspepsia. While one study using a simple device in the primary care setting found that almost all of the patients who tested positive could be treated with antibiotic therapy without any further intervention, a systematic review concluded that the sensitivity of a blood test varied between 77% and 92% with specificity varying between 56% and 69% (45). A more recent randomized controlled trial found that the point-of-care strategy did not lead to any improvement in clinical outcomes and was more expensive, although more patients with peptic ulcer were diagnosed (7.4% versus 2.1%). The urea breath test is considered to be the definitive test for the diagnosis of active *H. pylori* infection, and Opekun et al. (46) studied the use of this test in more than 300 ambulatory patients and found that 99.1% of results by POCT agreed with the reference laboratory result. These authors concluded that this was a practical alternative for use in primary care.

There is no doubt that POCT in primary care will increase but usage will be governed by the availability of the most appropriate tests and the ability of the physicians to integrate the testing procedure into the patient visit, which typically lasts for 8–10 minutes. There also needs to be a clearer understanding of the clinical challenges the primary care physician faces and the tests which will be of the greatest help with subsequent development of the POCT repertoire in order to meet these challenges.

POCT in Secondary Care and Chronic Disease Management

There are several clinical scenarios in which the test result provides a valuable means of both guiding the therapy dosage as well as providing some form of assessment of efficacy. There may be additional parameters that are then used to assess the long-term effectiveness of treatment. The test may then be used to assess the compliance with therapy, on the part of both the clinician and the patient. In this situation, POCT provides a means by which the clinician can assess the efficacy of treatment and alter the management or counsel the patient face to face at the time of the clinic visit.

Diabetes Mellitus

The findings of the Diabetes Control and Complications Trial (DCCT) and the United Kingdom Prospective Diabetes Study (UKPDS) have been responsible for the strategy that dictates the management of type 1 and type 2 diabetes. These studies showed that closer control of blood glucose levels reduces the rate of onset of complications. In the DCCT study, the blood glucose was monitored at least four times a day in order to guide treatment in the intensive therapy cohort while in the conventional therapy group the blood or urine glucose was measured daily. The UKPDS studied newly diagnosed type 2 diabetics, employing a number of clinical and biochemical endpoints to assess the potential benefit from tighter control of blood glucose. This study demonstrated that those patients allocated to the intensive therapy group experienced fewer diabetes related endpoints, e.g., cardiovascular events, blindness, and renal failure as well as a lower median HbA1c level. In addition, the study showed that for each 1% reduction in the mean updated HbA1c there was an associated reduction in risk of 21% for any diabetes-related endpoint. In both the DCCT and UKPDS studies, POCT was used for the routine disease management, while laboratory-based tests were used as surrogate markers for assessing the effectiveness of disease management and as outcome measures.

There are other observational studies which have shown that those diabetics who test their blood glucose level more frequently are more likely to have lower HbA1c levels. These studies take an holistic view to the management of diabetes and stress the complementary nature of several activities in which POCT play a part. Thus, improving communication (primarily to achieve greater accessibility to advice) through the use of interactive software support for the patient linked to a testing device and through telemedicine links with the diabetes specialists has also been shown to improve patient compliance with therapy protocols. There may be many reasons for poor compliance with the testing and therapy regime, which is then made worse by nonattendance at the regular clinic review. Thus, Piette et al. (47) investigated the efficacy of automated telephone disease management in a randomized controlled study and found more intensive care compared with a control group, together with better glycemic control and fewer adverse events.

The measurement of HbA1c is established as a surrogate marker for outcomes of glycemic control as demonstrated by its use in both the DCCT and UKPDS studies. It is effectively being used as a clinical QA tool in routine clinical practice. Guidelines for the management of diabetes suggest that HbA1c measurements should be made twice a year in diabetics who demonstrate good control, with greater frequency for patients with poor control. These figures are based primarily on the known half-life of the red cell and based on clinical experience with the test. In some countries, the levels are measured more frequently. There is now good evidence to show that access to the HbA1c result at the time of the diabetic's regular review leads to an improvement in compliance with disease management and a concomitant lowering of the HbA1c result. Grieve et al. (48) found the mean HbA1c level was 7.79% in a population of diabetics managed with the HbA1c result at the time of the clinic visit compared with 8.66% in a similar sized cohort managed by conventional means, i.e., data from the laboratory at a later date. A randomized trial of the provision of the HbA1c assay at the time of consultation reported a lowering of the results compared to the control group who were managed by conventional means (49). A further study found that rapid access to the HbA1c result at the time of the clinic visit led to more frequent intensification of therapy and a more rapid lowering of the HbA1c level during the course of the study (50).

Frequent blood glucose monitoring has also been shown to be very effective in reducing the incidence of complications associated with gestational diabetes. Langer et al. (51) found that blood glucose testing between four and seven times a day, supported by appropriate intervention with dietary changes and the use of insulin, led to a reduction in the incidence of complications for both mother and baby, while also reducing the length of hospital stay. An increase in urine albumin has been used as a surrogate marker for early diabetic nephropathy. With the availability of effective treatment for hypertension through angiotensin-converting enzyme inhibitors, there is now a good case for monitoring albumin excretion in the diabetes clinic. A recent review of the literature by the U.S. Agency for Health Research and Quality suggested that the measurement of urine albumin should be implemented on a regular basis 5 years after diagnosis in the type 1 diabetic and immediately after diagnosis in the type 2 diabetic (52).

Economic assessment of the impact of more intensive control of blood glucose has been undertaken in both the DCCT and UKPDS studies. These assessments have shown that there are longer term gains from using more intensive management as a consequence of the delay in onset of the complications, despite the increased cost associated with blood glucose testing and more intensive therapy. This is primarily due to a reduction in the hospital costs associated with more clinic visits and the treatment of the complications. A population-based study showed that when employing a more intensive disease management program there was a reduction in the referrals to specialist facilities and a concomitant reduction in hospital costs (53).

Anticoagulation Monitoring

Typically anticoagulation clinics have been located close to the laboratory to enable a rapid result to be provided with appropriate clinical advice for the routine management of patients. There have also been alternative approaches employed, in which either pharmacists, nurses, and/or primary care physicians have employed POCT technology to monitor anticoagulant status. Thus, it has been shown that a pharmacist-led service resulted in more patients being in control at a second visit compared with patients managed by physicians. This difference may have been due to frequent changes in clinic personnel which may have limited the opportunity to build a relationship between the adviser and the patient, again showing the importance of linking the result with advice and information on the meaning of the result. Another study using a mobile testing system which visited a number of doctors' office clinics found that the percentage of in-range international normalized ratios (INR) rose from 40.7% to 58.5% when using POCT. Fitzmaurice et al. (54) found that the assessment of coagulation status was as good in the nonhospital setting as the service provided by the laboratory, as judged by the INR and the incidence of adverse events. It has also been shown that the point-of-care approach led to a reduction in waiting times and improved patient satisfaction. As in the case of diabetes, a structured teaching and self-management program has been shown to improve outcomes with an improvement in the INR as well as quality of life measures (55). Monitoring of anticoagulation status has now extended to the home environment in many places.

Initial Treatment Optimization

Where a test is employed to monitor the efficacy of therapy, it is quite possible that such a test can also be of help in the optimization of therapy. However, there are few formal studies that have set out to demonstrate this outcome. As in the case of chronic disease management, the potential advantage with POCT is that having the result available at the time of the consultation can promote a more effective dialogue between the patient and the clinician, as well as enhancing the process of treatment optimization. A few years ago, a small study showed that the availability of anticonvulsant drug levels at the time of the consultation led to a significant reduction in the period required to achieve optimization of drug concentration, together with a reduction in the number of clinic visits (56). In another study, it was shown that it cost less to deliver a drug-monitoring service in the clinic compared with a laboratory service (57).

It has also been shown that treatment of patients with heart failure that is guided by the circulating brain natriuretic peptide (BNP) level can lead to a significant reduction (54%) in the cardiac events over the following 6 months compared to patients who were guided by clinical criteria (58). It is clear from several studies that if BNP levels can be provided at the point-of-care, then there will be both improved patient and clinician satisfaction from such a service. The advantages are that the drug-dosing regime is more effective and the healthcare costs are reduced as a consequence of fewer clinic visits.

POCT in the Hospital Setting

POCT provides a more rapid result service and consequently has always been associated with the measurement of critical parameters in seriously ill patients, when rapid decisions often with life-threatening consequences have to be made and interventions applied immediately. Thus, POCT is used in a number of settings within the hospital environment. There have also been several papers describing the use of blood gas and electrolyte measurement systems in paramedical transport support vehicles and space flight. Gruszecki et al. (59) reviewed experience over 6 years and found that POCT was reliable in this setting. Using questionnaires to assess the clinical impact of POCT, they found an improvement in the outcome was considered to have occurred in 14% of the patients (21 of 151), with a change in patient treatment being made in 30% of patients at the time testing was performed. POCT was performed in a total of 17% of the patients transported. In another very specific situation where the use of hand-bagging was compared with mechanical ventilation, it was shown that the latter was more effective at maintaining the pCO_2 level, and hence the likelihood of more effective cerebral blood flow. The authors concluded that monitoring in transit might help to further reduce the risk of complications associated with cerebral ischemia.

Emergency Room

It is likely that in emergency situations there will be more use of POCT for rule-out decision making than might be experienced in the intensive care environment. Furthermore, a larger repertoire of investigations might justifiably be called upon, some of which are given in Table 6. There have been several studies of POCT devices in the accident and emergency room, including two randomized controlled trials, both of which have made constructive observations. The first randomized controlled trial of a diagnostic test was reported by Kendall et al. (60) and investigated rapid access to blood gas and electrolyte results. In this study, the availability of rapid results had a very limited effect on clinical decisions and no significant change on clinical outcomes. Furthermore, there was no change in the length of stay and the authors concluded that the testing phase was not the rate-limiting step. However, it was not clear from this study whether the clinicians were available to make the decisions when the test results were produced or whether they had to wait for laboratory results before a decision could be made. A similar study found that the length of stay was reduced, but that this occurred in those patients with normal results and where the results were used to make an early discharge decision (61). Interestingly, the authors also found that the proportion of patients in whom only a POCT was required was

TABLE 6. Key tests that can be performed in the emergency room

Blood gases
Blood carbon monoxide
Blood D-dimer
Blood count
Blood activated prothrombin time
Plasma electrolytes
Urea and creatinine
Glucose
Acetaminophen
Salicylate
Alcohol
Troponin
Brain (b-type) natriuretic peptide
C-reactive protein
Urine human chorionic gonadotropin
Urine albumin
Urine drugs of abuse
Urine ketone bodies
Urine leukocyte esterase and nitrite
Fecal occult blood

quite low and consequently the full potential of POCT could not be explored because the clinicians had to wait for a laboratory result.

Other studies have found that electrolyte and urea measurements do not influence the initial management of major trauma patients but that occasionally the rapid availability of hemoglobin, glucose, blood gas, and lactate measurements can lead to improved clinical and economic outcomes in severe blunt-trauma-injured patients (62). In a study measuring the impact of POCT for blood glucose, cardiac markers, urinary chorionic gonadotropin, and routine urinalysis, it was found that the turnround time for test results decreased on average by 87%, and the length of stay decreased overall in those patients who received the pregnancy, urinalysis, and cardiac marker testing at the point of care. In addition, both clinician and patient satisfaction improved (63). Several of the general issues surrounding POCT in the emergency room are discussed in a systematic review of the literature by Fermann and Suyama (64). It is obvious that there will be no benefit if the data are not accessed immediately, and furthermore it is important to ensure that a full repertoire of tests is available or the clinician may have to wait for some results to come back from the laboratory.

It is clear that rapid access to the results does not impact on the length of stay or any other outcome measure unless the test has an influence on the clinical intervention required. The impact of rapid cardiac marker measurement in patients admitted with acute chest pain is therefore one of those situations where POCT may be of value. Thus, Ng et al. found that all patients with myocardial infarction were diagnosed within 90 minutes of admission (positive predictive value 47%, negative predictive value 100%) and coronary care unit admissions were reduced by 40% when using POCT. A total of 90% of patients with negative cardiac markers and ECG findings at 90 minutes were discharged home and only one returned with a infarction within the next 30 days (0.2%) (65). Similar results have been reported by others with sensitivity and negative predictive values of 96.9% and 99.6%, respectively, with a reduction in the length of stay in hospital (66). Zarich et al. (67) also showed that rapid testing for cardiac markers can lead to improved utilization of hospital resources and a reduction in costs.

While some of the outlined data concentrated on the earlier discharge of patients by effectively using a rule-out strategy, other studies have begun to look at the risk stratification of patients ruled-in by the use of biochemical tests. It has been shown that POCT for cardiac markers can be used effectively for risk stratification of patients admitted with acute chest pain, thus enabling more informed patient triage through a chest pain evaluation unit (68). It has also been shown that POCT for brain (b-type) natriuretic peptide together with other clinical observations can be helpful in establishing the presence or absence of congestive heart failure in patients admitted with dyspnea (69). Others have suggested that the use of BNP has a valuable role in the risk stratification of patients with congestive heart failure and can help to make better use of expensive diagnostic resources such as echocardiography.

A simple whole blood agglutination test for D-dimer, together with an assessment of alveolar dead space has been shown to help exclude pulmonary embolism in patients admitted to the emergency room. The authors concluded that a normal D-dimer test result was associated with a low prevalence of pulmonary embolism. A similar study concluded that a simple D-dimer test was useful for ruling out pulmonary embolism in patients with suspected venous thromboembolism (70). Thus, a POCT for D-dimer could usefully be added to a panel of tests for assessment of cardiovascular risk.

The measurement of toxic drugs and drugs of abuse has long been considered among the most important tests that should be available in the emergency room setting. Early recognition of the presence of the drug can help decision making, as well as prompting effective intervention. This would be particularly true for acetaminophen and salicylate intoxication. Rapid blood alcohol measurement can also help in the differential diagnosis of the unconscious patient.

Intensive Care

The assessment of blood gas and acid–base status, together with other parameters of gas exchange and electrolytes has long been established in the field of intensive care medicine. The maintenance of an adequate oxygen supply together with removal of carbon dioxide is vital to maintaining life as well as promoting the healing and recovery process. The maintenance of the correct extracellular potassium concentration is vital to cardiac and skeletal muscle function. Much of the evidence for use of POCT in intensive care is based on experience and observational data. Kilgore et al. (71) using modeling studies concluded that, in addition to the clinical benefits of a rapid delivery of results from POCT, annual savings in excess of $250,000 (at 1996 prices) could be made in a large hospital, despite the technology costs being greater. In the pediatric intensive care environment, the use of POCT devices ensures that less sample is required compared with a central laboratory procedure, a reduction of blood volume being a significant hazard in severely ill babies, with a concomitant reduction in the need for blood transfusions.

An increase in urine albumin excretion has been shown to be associated with poor morbidity and mortality in severely ill patients in both the intensive care and emergency room situations. It is claimed to be a good indicator of vascular permeability and that correction can improve the patient outcome (72). In particular, it can be used for the early recognition of those patients with imminent organ failure. The urine albumin-to-creatinine ratio has been used to predict acute respiratory distress syndrome with a positive predictive value of 64% at 8 hours and a negative predictive value of 73% being observed. The best performance was achieved 6 and 18 hours after admission to the intensive care unit and, based on a figure at 8 hours, 75% of the patients who developed acute respiratory distress syndrome would have received appropriate treatment.

Sepsis is a major issue in the intensive care unit, especially in neonates, and several markers have been proposed to aid its earlier recognition in order that early intervention with antibiotic therapy can be instigated. In a recent review, the diagnostic performance of C-reactive protein, interleukin-6, and procalcitonin were compared, and it is clear that these markers have some merit when used in combination to provide illness severity scores for the recognition of sepsis, particularly where the clinical signs are equivocal (73). However, the sensitivity of the tests has been shown to be only in the 70%–80% range at birth, rising over the next 48 hours, which is not sufficiently high enough for a rule-out test in this situation.

Intraoperative Testing

Blood gas and electrolyte status is a routine feature of intraoperative monitoring where complex and lengthy surgery is involved. There are other examples where monitoring of biochemical and hematological parameters is also invaluable. The measurement of ionized calcium during hepatic transplantation is used to assess the effect of the citrate burden from transfused blood, thereby reducing the risk of a cardiac arrest. There have also been papers describing the measurement of ionized magnesium; however, these show that the ionized fraction is not correlated with total magnesium in ICU patients, probably because of the changes in plasma protein concentration as well as changes in binding due to deranged acid–base status. In addition, there are no data at present to show that use of the ionized magnesium measurement to guide treatment for hypomagnesemia has led to improved outcomes. In an interesting observation, the provision of POCT for blood gas, electrolytes, urea, creatinine, glucose, and hematocrit measurements in an organ procurement program led to shorter turnround times than the laboratory service and enabled more effective oxygenation and fluid management of the donor (74).

The intraoperative monitoring of coagulation status, particularly during cardiopulmonary bypass procedures, has prompted considerable interest in POCT, primarily because it aids blood conservation and reduces the need for blood products. POCT supporting rapid decision making has led to a reduction in postoperative complications, reduced blood loss (therefore less utilization of transfused blood products), and reduced need for high dependency postoperative care (75). It has also been shown that the point-of-care assessment of platelet function can guide the use of desmopressin, with a resulting reduction in blood loss and less requirement for transfused blood products. The assessment of platelet status as an aid in guiding therapy with platelet aggregation inhibitors is still the subject of debate but is now attracting considerable attention, linked with the use of drugs to reduce platelet aggregation. It is thought to be important to find those patients who do not respond to certain platelet aggregation inhibitors, in order to consider an alternative therapy, e.g., to reduce the risk of developing thrombotic stent occlusion following elective coronary stent placement.

The intraoperative POCT for parathyroid hormone (PTH) has also been described during parathyroidectomy. Monitoring the circulating PTH level during the operation reduces the need for reoperation by ensuring all of the hyperplastic tissue is removed (76). Employing this strategy means that parathyroidectomy could be transferred to a day case procedure with improved patient satisfaction and significant reduction in hospital costs. A recent survey of intra-operative PTH testing services found that more than half were actually provided from a laboratory-based device, presumably with the logistic support to ensure rapid transport of the sample to the laboratory (77).

Screening

The term screening has been used to describe general rule-out testing although its correct use is in the testing of the asymptomatic population for early evidence of a disease, in a situation where there is a certain likelihood of the disease occurring and where a treatment exists, thereby leading to an improved outcome. Thus POCT has been used to rule-out myocardial infarction, *H. pylori* infection, chlamydia infection, influenza, preeclampsia, renal disease in diabetics, and a number of other disorders.

An exciting example of the use of POCT is in the screening for fetal anomalies in a one-stop clinic, where the patient can receive immediate counseling after the results of the tests have been produced. A high level of patient satisfaction has been found with this approach, which is thought to be responsible for the high level of compliance in the first trimester screening program and a concomitant high detection rate (78). This illustrates one of the key benefits from the use of POCT.

THE FUTURE OF POCT

The sophistication of the devices used in POCT means that the early concerns about reliability can now be dispelled and this form of testing can take its place alongside all of the other technology that is increasingly being used in the practice of medicine in all settings, home, community, or hospital. The challenge is for healthcare professionals, and patients, to use the technology effectively just as it was for the users of other new technologies such as cars, labor-saving devices in the home, computers, mobile phones, and other handheld devices. For POCT to be effective, it is essential to design processes that enable the caregiver to act quickly upon receipt of the test results.

The main stimulus to the use of POCT will come from changes in the way healthcare is delivered and patients needs and expectations. In many countries while there is consolidation of laboratories and an emphasis on more efficient and productive testing facilities, patient care is being moved away from the larger hospital unit. This will lead to an increase in either the logistics effort required to support the turnround times expected by clinicians and patients or a dramatic increase in the volume of POCT. If testing is truly going to be integrated into the patient consultation process, then POCT will be the only way forward. Also, patient expectations are increasing and will drive the trend toward more patient-focused style of care with fewer clinic visits, shorter waiting times, and an expectation of better care. The challenge will lie in ensuring greater investment in POCT which can be achieved by reducing the expenditure in other areas, e.g., associated with hospital stay. However, this also requires a considerable change in practice style, and this may prove to be the greatest challenge.

Technological innovation will continue to be a driver as it will continue to identify the opportunities to provide a more efficient and acceptable service. Thus, the trend toward miniaturization of devices will produce smaller, more portable instruments as well as helping to achieve the goal of an implantable device. In parallel there is the whole field of noninvasive devices which will certainly be popular in the case of patients with chronic diseases requiring regular testing.

REFERENCES

1. Price CP. Point-of-care testing. BMJ 2001;322:1285–8.
2. Price CP. Medical and economic outcomes of point-of-care testing. Clin Chem Lab Med 2002;40:246–51.
3. Briedigkeit L, Muller-Plathe O, Schlebusch H, Ziems J. Recommendations of the German Working Group on medical laboratory testing (AML) on the introduction and quality assurance of procedures for point-of-care testing (POCT) in hospitals. Clin Chem Lab Med. 1999;37:919–25.
4. England JM, Hyde K, Lewis SM, Mackie IJ, Rowan RM. Guidelines for near patient testing:haematology. Clin Lab Haem 1995;17:300–9.
5. Kost GJ. Guidelines for point-of-care testing. Improving patient outcomes. Am J Clin Pathol 1995;104(4 Suppl 1):S111–27.
6. National Committee for Clinical Laboratory Standards. Point-of-care in vitro diagnostic (IVD) testing; approved guideline. NCCLS Document AST2-A, Wayne, PA: NCCLS, 1999.
7. Turner APF. In: Karube I, Wilson GS, eds. Biosensors: fundamentals and applications. New York: Oxford University Press, 1987:1–770.
8. Kricka LJ. Microchips: the hitchhiker's guide to analytical microchips. Washington, DC: AACC Press, 2002:1–94.
9. Khandurina J, Guttman A. Bioanalysis in microfluidic devices. J Chromatogr A 2002;943: 159–83.
10. Jones R. Informatics and point-of-care testing. In: Price CP, Hicks JM, eds. Point-of-care testing. Washington, DC: AACC Press, 1999:175–95.
11. National Committe for Clinical Laboratory Standards. Point-of-care connectivity; approved standard. NCCLS Document POCT1-A, Wayne, PA: NCCLS, 2001.
12. Kost GJ, ed. Principles and practice of point-of-care testing. Philadelphia: Lippincott Williams & Wilkins, 2002:1–654.

13. Price CP, Hicks JM, eds. Point-of-care testing. Washington, DC: AACC Press, 1999:1–580.
14. Zipp A, Hornby WE. Solid phase chemistry: its principles and application in clinical analyses. Talanta 1984;31:863–77.
15. Spitznagel TM, Clark DS. Surface density and orientation effects on immobilized antibodies and fragments. Biotechnology 1993;11:825–9.
16. Antman EM, Grudzien C, Sacks DB. Evaluation of a rapid bedside assay for detection of serum cardiac troponin T. JAMA 1995;273:1279–82.
17. Harbeck RJ. Evaluation of two rapid antigen assays, BioStar Strep A OIA and Pacific Biotech CARDS O.S., and culture for detection of group A streptococci in throat swabs. J Clin Microbiol 1995;33:3365–7.
18. Henning TP, Cunningham TP. Biosensors for personal diabetes management. In: Ramsay G, ed. Commercial biosensors. New York: Wiley, 1998:3–46.
19. Steinhausen RL, Price CP. Principles and practices of dry chemistry systems. In: Price CP, Alberti KGMM, eds. Recent advances in clinical biochemistry. Edinburgh: Churchill Livingstone, 1985:273–96.
20. Davis G. Microfabricated sensors and the commercial development of the i-Stat® point-of-care system. In: Ramsay G, ed. Commercial biosensors. New York: Wiley, 1998:47–76.
21. Lubbers DW. Optical sensors for clinical monitoring. Acta Anaesthesiol Scand (Suppl) 1995;104:37–54.
22. Jacobs E, Nowakowski M, Colman N. Performance of Gem Premier blood gas/electrolyte analyzer evaluated. Clin Chem 1993;39:189–93.
23. Hirst D, St John A. Keeping the spotlight on quality from a distance. Accred Qual Assur 2000;5:9–13.
24. Hyltoft Petersen P, Fraser CG, Kallner A, Kenny D, eds. Strategies to set global analytical quality specifications in laboratory medicine. Scand J Clin Lab Invest 1999;59:475–585.
25. Fraser CG. Optimal analytical performance for point of care testing. Clin Chim Acta 2001;307:37–43.
26. Jacobs E, Hinson KA, Tolnai J, Simson E. Implementation, management and continuous quality improvement of point-of-care testing in an academic health care setting. Clin Chim Acta 2001;307:49–59.
27. Freedman DB. Clinical governance: implications for point-of-care testing. Ann Clin Biochem 2002;39:421–3.
28. Burnett D. Accreditation and point-of-care testing. Ann Clin Biochem 2000;37:241–3.
29. National Committes for Clinical Laboratory Standards. Evaluation of precision performance of clinical chemistry devices; approved guideline. NCCLS Document EP5-A, Wayne, PA: NCCLS, 1999.
30. Westgard JO. Electronic quality control, the total testing process, and the total quality system. Clin Chim Acta 2001;307:45–8.
31. National Committee for Clinical Laboratory Standards. Quality management for unit-use testing; approved guideline. NCCLS Document EP18-A, Wayne, PA: NCCLS, 2002.
32. College of American Pathologists:www.cap.org/lap/fudt.html (e.g., drugs of abuse testing program).
33. United Kingdom National External Quality Assessment Scheme. Available at http://www.ukneqas.org.uk/Directory/CC/lipids.htm. Accessed March 23, 2005.
34. Wales External Quality Assessment Scheme: www.weqas.co.uk (e.g., urinalysis program).
35. U.S. Department of Health and Human Services. Medicare, Medicaid, and CLIA programs: regulations implementing the Clinical Laboratory Improvement Amendments of 1988 (CLIA). Final rule. Federal Register 1992;57:7002–186.
36. U.S. Department of Health and Human Services. Medicare, Medicaid and CLIA programs: regulations implementing the Clinical Laboratory Improvement Amendments of 1988 (CLIA) and Clinical Laboratory Act program fee collection. Federal Register 1993;58:5215–37.
37. Ehrmeyer SS, Laessig RH. Regulation, accreditation and education for point-of-care testing. In: Kost G, ed. Principles and practice of point-of-care testing. Philadelphia: Lippincott Williams and Wilkins, 2002:434–43.

38. Stephens EJ. Developing open standards for point-of-care connectivity. IVD Technology 1999;10:22–5.
39. Hobbs FD, Delaney BC, Fitzmaurice DA, Wilson S, Hyde CJ, Thorpe GH, et al. A review of near patient testing in primary care. Health Technol Assess 1997;1(5):1–230.
40. Lehmann CA. The future of home testing—implications for traditional laboratories. Clin Chim Acta 2002;323:31–6.
41. Mahtabjafari M, Masih M, Emerson AE. The value of pharmacist involvement in a point-of-care service, walk-in lipid screening program. Pharmacotherapy 2001;21:1403–6.
42. Griffin S. Diabetes care in general practice: meta-analysis of randomised control trials. BMJ 1998;317:390–6.
43. Rink E, Hilton S, Szczepura A, Fletcher J, Sibbald B, Davies C, et al. Impact of introducing near patient testing for standard investigations in general practice. BMJ 1993;307:775–8.
44. Hurlbut TA, Littenberg B, and the Diagnostic Technology Assessment Consortium. The diagnostic accuracy of rapid dipstick tests to predict urinary tract infection. Am J Clin Pathol 1991;96:582–8.
45. Roberts AP, Childs SM, Rubin G, de Wit NJ. Tests for *Helicobacter pylori*: a critical appraisal from primary care. Fam Pract 2000;17:S12–20.
46. Opekun AR, Abdalla N, Sutton FM, Hammoud F, Kuo GM, Torres E, et al. Urea breath testing and analysis in the primary care office. J Fam Pract. 2002;51:1030–2.
47. Piette JD, Weinberger M, McPhee SJ, Mah CA, Kraemer FB, Crapo LM. Do automated calls with nurse follow-up improve self-care and glycemic control among vulnerable patients with diabetes? A randomized controlled trial. Am J Med 2000;108:20–7.
48. Grieve R, Beech R, Vincent J, Mazurkiewicz J. Near patient testing in diabetes clinics: appraising the costs and outcomes. Health Technol Assess 1999;3(15):1–74.
49. Cagliero E, Levina E, Nathan D. Immediate feedback of HbA1c levels improves glycemic control in type 1 and insulin-treated type 2 diabetic patients. Diabetes Care 1999;22:1785–9.
50. Miller CD, Barnes CS, Phillips LS, Ziemer DC, Gallina DL, Cook CB, et al. Rapid alc availability improves clinical decision-making in an urban primary care clinic. Diabetes Care 2003;26:1158–63.
51. Langer O, Rodriguez DA, Xenakis EM, McFarland MB, Berkus MD, Arrendondo F. Intensified versus conventional management of gestational diabetes. Am J Obstet Gynecol 1994;170: 1036–47.
52. Agency for Healthcare Research and Quality. Use of glycated hemoglobin and microalbuminuria in the monitoring of diabetes mellitus. Available at http://www.ahrq.gov/clinic/epcsums/glycasum.htm. Accessed March 23, 2005.
53. Stratton IM, Adler AI, Neil HA, Matthews DR, Manley SE, Cull CA, et al. Association of glycaemia with macrovascular and microvascular complications of type 2 diabetes (UKPDS 35): prospective observational study. BMJ 2000;321:405–12.
54. Fitzmaurice DA, Hobbs FD, Murray ET, Holder RL, Allan TF, Rose PE. Oral anticoagulation management in primary care with the use of computerized decision support and near-patient testing. Arch Intern Med 2000;160:2343–8.
55. Sawicki PT. A structured teaching and self-management program for patients receiving oral anticoagulation. JAMA 1999;281:145–50.
56. Patsalos PN, Sander JW, Oxley J. Immediate anticonvulsive drug monitoring in management of epilepsy. Lancet 1987;2:39.
57. Price CP. Point of care testing. Potential for tracking disease management outcomes. Dis Manage Health Outcomes 2002;10:749–61.
58. Troughton RW, Frampton CM, Yandle TG, Espiner EA, Nicholls MG, Richards AM. Treatment of heart failure guided by plasma aminoterminal brain natriuretic peptide (N-BNP) concentrations. Lancet 2000;355:1126–30.
59. Gruszecki AC, Hortin G, Lam J, Kahler D, Smith D, Vines J, et al. Utilization, reliability, and clinical impact of point-of-care testing during critical care transport: six years of experience. Clin Chem. 2003;49:1017–9.

60. Kendall J, Reeves B, Clancy M. Point of care testing: randomised, controlled trial of clinical outcome. BMJ 1998;316:1052–7.
61. Murray RP, Leroux M, Sabga E, Palatnick W, Ludwig L. Effect of point of care testing on length of stay in an adult emergency department. J Emer Med 1999;17:811–4.
62. Asimos AW, Gibbs MA, Marx JA, Jacobs DG, Erwin RJ, Norton HJ, Thomason M. Value of point-of-care testing in emergent trauma management. J Trauma 2000;48:1101–8.
63. Lee-Lewandrowski E, Corboy D, Lewandrowski K, Sinclair J, McDermot S, Benzer TJ. Implementation of a point-of-care satellite laboratory in the emergency department of an academic medical center. Impact on test turnaround time and patient emergency department length of stay. Arch Pathol Lab Med 2003;127:456–60.
64. Fermann GJ, Suyama J. Point of care testing in the emergency department. J Emerg Med 2002;22:393–404.
65. Ng SM, Krishnaswamy P, Morissey R, Clopton P, Fitzgerald R, Maisel AS. Ninety-minute accelerated critical pathway for chest pain evaluation. Am J Cardiol 2001;88:611–7.
66. McCord J, Nowak RM, McCullough PA, Foreback C, Borzak S, Tokarski G, et al. Ninety-minute exclusion of acute mycardial infarction by use of quantitative point-of-care testing of myoglobin and troponin I. Circulation 2001;104:1483–7.
67. Zarich S, Bradley K, Seymour J, Ghali W, Traboulsi A, Mayall ID, Bernstein L. Impact of troponin T determinations of hospital resource utilization and costs in the evaluation of patients with suspected myocardial ischemia. Am J Cardiol 2001;88:732–6.
68. Ohman EM, Armstrong PW, White HD, Granger CB, Wilcox RG, Weaver WD, et al. Risk stratification with a point-of-care cardiac troponin T test in acute myocardial infarction. Am J Cardiol 1999;84:1281–6.
69. Maisel AS, Krishnaswamy P, Nowak RM, McCord J, Hollander JE, Duc P, et al. Rapid measurement of B-type natriuretic peptide in the emergency diagnosis of heart failure. N Engl J Med 2002;347:161–7.
70. Bates SM, Grand'Maison A, Johnston M, Naguit I, Kovacs MJ, Ginsberg JS. A latex D-dimer reliably excludes venous thromboembolism. Arch Intern Med 2001;161:447–53.
71. Kilgore ML, Steindel SJ, Smith JA. Cost analysis for decision support: the case of comparing centralized versus distributed methods for blood gas testing. J Health Manag 1999;44:207–15.
72. Gosling P, Brudney S, McGrath L, Riseboro S, Manji M. Mortality prediction at admission to intensive care: a comparison of microalbuminuria with acute physiology scores after 24 hours. Crit Care Med 2003;31:98–103.
73. Chiesa C, Pellegrini G, Panero A, Osborn JF, Signore F, Assumma M, Pacifico L. C-reactive protein, interleukin-6, and procalcitonin in the immediate postnatal period: influence of illness severity, risk status, antenatal and perinatal complications, and infection. Clin Chem 2003;49: 60–8.
74. Baier KA, Markham LE, Flaigle SP, Nelson PW, Shield CF, Muruve NA, et al. Point-of-care testing in an organ procurement organization donor management setting. Clin Transplant 2003;17(Suppl 9):48–51.
75. Despotis GJ, Joist JH, Goodnough LT. Monitoring of hemostasis in cardiac surgical patients: impact of point-of-care testing on blood loss and transfusion outcomes. Clin Chem 1997;43: 1684–96.
76. Irvin GL, Molinari AS, Figueroa C, Carneiro DM. Improved success rate in reoperative parathyroidectomy with intraoperative PTH assay. Ann Surg 1999;229:874–9.
77. Hortin GL, Carter AB. College of American Pathologists Point-of-Care Testing Resource Committee. Intraoperative parathyroid hormone testing: survey of testing program characteristics. Arch Pathol Lab Med 2002;12:1045–9.
78. Spencer K, Spencer CE, Power M, Dawson C, Nicolaides KH. Screening for chromosomal abnormalities in the first trimester using ultrasound and maternal serum biochemistry in a one-stop clinic: a review of three years prospective experience. BJOG. 2003;110:281–6.

Index